Medical Imaging: Fundamentals, Tools and Techniques

Medical Imaging: Fundamentals, Tools and Techniques

Edited by **Aaron Jackson**

FOSTER ACADEMICS

New Jersey

Published by Foster Academics,
61 Van Reypen Street,
Jersey City, NJ 07306, USA
www.fosteracademics.com

Medical Imaging: Fundamentals, Tools and Techniques
Edited by Aaron Jackson

International Standard Book Number: 978-1-63242-440-2 (Hardback)

Printed in China.

Contents

Preface

The main aim of this book is to educate learners and enhance their research focus by presenting diverse topics covering this vast field. This is an advanced book which compiles significant studies by distinguished experts. This book addresses successive solutions to the challenges arising in the area of application, along with it; the book provides scope for future developments.

This book contains some path-breaking studies in the field of medical imaging. It sheds light on some new techniques and latest advances in this field. Medical Imaging refers to the process of visually presenting the interior of a human body for examination and analysis and also to the techniques of monitoring the functioning of the internal organs. It uses the technologies like x-rays, ultrasounds, radiography, endoscopy, etc. This book presents researches and studies performed by experts across the globe. It also includes a detailed explanation of the various fundamentals and tools of medical imaging. It will prove to be a beneficial text for students and researchers in this field.

It was a great honour to edit this book, though there were challenges, as it involved a lot of communication and networking between me and the editorial team. However, the end result was this all-inclusive book covering diverse themes in the field.

Finally, it is important to acknowledge the efforts of the contributors for their excellent chapters, through which a wide variety of issues have been addressed. I would also like to thank my colleagues for their valuable feedback during the making of this book.

Editor

1

T1 mapping: characterisation of myocardial interstitial space

Rosario J. Perea · Jose T. Ortiz-Perez · Manel Sole · M. Teresa Cibeira · Teresa M. de Caralt · Susanna Prat-Gonzalez · Xavier Bosch · Antonio Berruezo · Marcelo Sanchez · Joan Blade

Abstract

Myocardial fibrosis is always present in end-stage heart failure and is a major independent predictor of adverse cardiac outcome. Cardiac magnetic resonance (CMR) is an imaging method that permits a non-invasive assessment of the heart and has been established as the "gold standard" for the evaluation of cardiac anatomy and function, as well as for quantifying focal myocardial fibrosis in both ischaemic and non-ischaemic heart disease. However, cardiac pathologies characterised by diffuse myocardial fibrosis cannot be evaluated by late gadolinium enhancement (LGE) imaging, as there are no reference regions of normal myocardium. Recent improvements in CMR imaging techniques have enabled parametric mapping of relaxation properties (T1, T2 and T2*) clinically feasible within a single breath-hold. T1 mapping techniques performed both with and without contrast enable the quantification of diffuse myocardial fibrosis and myocardial infiltration. This article reviews current imaging techniques, emerging applications and the future potential and limitations of CMR for T1 mapping.

R. J. Perea (✉) · T. M. de Caralt · M. Sanchez
Radiology Department. Hospital Clinic, University of Barcelona, Barcelona, Spain
e-mail: rjperea@clinic.ub.es

J. T. Ortiz-Perez · S. Prat-Gonzalez · X. Bosch · A. Berruezo
Cardiology Department. Hospital Clinic, University of Barcelona, Barcelona, Spain

M. Sole
Pathology Department. Hospital Clinic, University of Barcelona, Barcelona, Spain

M. T. Cibeira · J. Blade
Haematology Department. Hospital Clinic, University of Barcelona, Barcelona, Spain

Teaching points

- *Myocardial fibrosis is a common endpoint in a variety of cardiac diseases.*
- *Myocardial fibrosis results in myocardial stiffness, heart failure, arrhythmia and sudden death.*
- *T1-mapping CMR techniques enable the quantification of diffuse myocardial fibrosis.*
- *Native T1 reflects myocardial disease involving the myocyte and interstitium.*
- *The use of gadolinium allows measurement of the extracellular volume fraction, reflecting interstitial space.*

Keywords Magnetic resonance imaging · T1 mapping · Extracellular volume fraction · Diffuse myocardial fibrosis · Interstitial space

Abbreviations

CMR	cardiac magnetic resonance
LGE	late gadolinium enhancement
ECM	extracellular matrix
CVF	collagen volume fraction
GBCA	gadolinium based contrast agents
ECV	extracellular volume fraction
MOLLI	modified Look-Locker inversion recovery
ShMOLLI	shortened modified Look-Locker inversion recovery
SASHA	saturation recovery single-shot acquisition
SAPPHIRE	saturation pulse prepared heart rate independent inversion recovery
LL	Look-Locker
IR	inversion recovery
SSFP	steady-state free-precession
SENSE	sensitivity encoding
TI	inversion times
ROI	region of interest
EQ-CMR	equilibrium contrast-CMR

Introduction

The normal myocardium is composed of cardiac cells, blood vessels and nerves embedded within a complex three-dimensional space, the interstitium or extracellular space. The interstitium is a complex and dynamic environment, vital for normal cardiac structure and function. In the normal human heart, the extracellular matrix (ECM) is predominantly made up of collagen scaffolding [1, 2] and contains a ground substance of proteoglycans and glycosaminoglycans, as well as fibroblasts and immune cells [3]. One of the distinctive factors of its pathology is interstitial space expansion, normally through the development of fibrosis. Myocardial fibrosis is associated with worsening ventricular function, abnormal cardiac remodelling and increased ventricular stiffness [4]. Moreover, fibrosis plays an important role in the development of arrhythmia and sudden death [5], having been shown that it is an independent predictor of major adverse cardiac events (heart failure, arrhythmia and death) [6].

Currently, the only method to quantify diffuse fibrosis is invasive biopsy, which carries significant morbidity, is prone to sampling error and fibrotic involvement of the whole left ventricle cannot be determined [7]. Blood biomarkers for fibrosis assessment are also known to have complex confounding factors. Late gadolinium enhancement (LGE) imaging with cardiac magnetic resonance (CMR) has been the "gold standard" for detecting focal myocardial fibrosis in clinical practice. While LGE is clinically useful [8], reliance on relative signal intensity changes and nulling of "normal appearing" myocardium make it difficult to identify subtle abnormalities such as diffuse interstitial fibrosis [9]. A unique feature of CMR is its ability to use proton relaxation times, such as T1 to characterise myocardial tissue [9]. These relaxation times can be quantified using recently created mapping sequences [10, 11].

This article describes the emerging techniques of myocardial T1 mapping and extracellular volume quantification, evaluates its capacity to characterise myocardial tissue and demonstrates its clinical relevance.

Etiophysiopathology of myocardial fibrosis

The healthy myocardium contains an ECM that is a major determinant of its structural integrity and mechanical functions [3]. Normally, the ECM and fibrillar collagen network form only 6 % and 2-4 %, respectively, of the structural space within the heart [12]. However, the interstitium is actively maintained by the relationships between itself, myocytes, the neurohormonal system, mechanical forces and cardiac fibroblasts [13]. Within these coexisting matrices, a constant flux of tissue and collagen turnover takes place, coordinated by regulatory cytokines, growth factors, enzymes, hormones and direct cell-to-cell communication [14].

Diffuse myocardial fibrosis is a covert process that occurs as a part of normal ageing [8] but is accelerated in disease [15, 16, 17, 18]. Although fibrotic remodelling is not completely understood, after a specific cardiovascular stress (e.g. an ischaemic or mechanical injury), a cascade of chemokines, cytokines, neurohormonal factors and matrix metalloproteinases lead to local cell activation and collagen synthesis [19]. Myocardial fibrosis, defined as a significant increase in the collagen volume fraction (CVF) of myocardial tissue, is a common endpoint in a variety of cardiac diseases [20]. The distribution of myocardial fibrosis, however, varies according to the underlying pathology [20]. The progressive accumulation of collagen develops a range of ventricular dysfunctional processes that generally affect diastolic and subsequently systolic function [4]. Usually, myocardial fibrosis is classified as interstitial or replacement fibrosis.

Replacement or scarring fibrosis corresponds to the replacement of myocytes after cell damage or necrosis by plexiform fibrosis [21]. It may have localised (Fig. 1) (ischaemic cardiomyopathy, myocarditis, hypertrophic cardiomyopathy and sarcoidosis) or diffuse distribution (chronic renal insufficiency, toxic cardiomyopathies and inflammatory diseases) depending on the underlying aetiology. The most common cause of replacement fibrosis is scarring from myocardial infarction. LGE is a validated way to identify focal replacement fibrosis [8].

Interstitial fibrosis has a diffuse distribution within the interstitium and its subtypes include reactive and infiltrative fibrosis. Reactive fibrosis has a progressive onset and follows the increase in collagen synthesis by myofibroblasts under the influence of different stimuli. It has mostly been described in hypertension [15] and diabetes [16], but it is also present in the ageing heart [22], in idiopathic dilated cardiomyopathy [23], and in left ventricular pressure-overload and volume-overload states induced

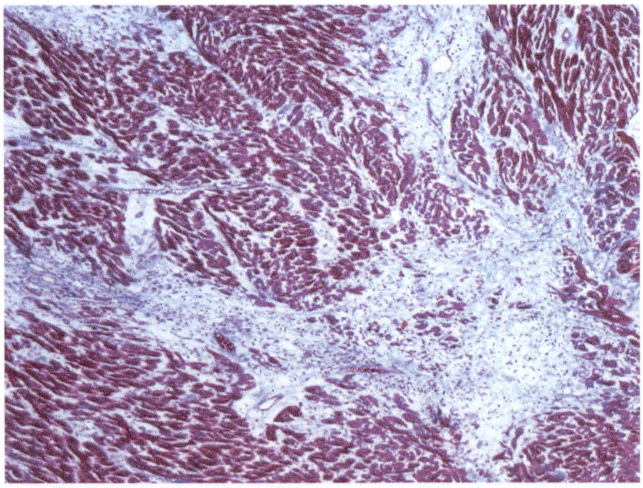

Fig. 1 Scarring or replacement fibrosis after myocardial infarction: a stellate fibrous scar (*blue areas*) replaces myocardial parenchyma (Masson trichrome staining ×40)

by chronic aortic valve regurgitation and stenosis [24]. It has also been reported in the remote non-infarcted myocardium after infarction [18]. Infiltrative fibrosis is more unusual and is induced by the progressive deposit of insoluble proteins (amyloidosis) [25] (Fig. 2) or glycosphingolipids (Anderson-Fabry disease) [26] in the cardiac tissue. Their pathophysiology follows similar patterns as reactive fibrosis. Interstitial fibrosis precedes irreversible replacement fibrosis [27]. Reactive and infiltrative fibrosis may be reversible under specific therapy [28]. Therefore, the early detection of cardiac involvement is of critical importance to therapeutic management.

Detection of myocardial fibrosis

Until now, the only approach to assess myocardial fibrosis has been endomyocardial biopsy. This methodology allows qualitative macroscopic assessment with Masson Trichrome staining [29] and quantitative morphometry (quantification of CVF) with picrosirius red [30] (Fig. 3). However, this technique is invasive and prone to sampling errors. CMR T1 mapping of the myocardium has the potential to quantify myocardial fibrosis in a non-invasive way. Preliminary studies suggest that these techniques are reproducible and may be more reliable than the current biopsy gold standard, because the biopsy sample represents less than a thousandth of the total myocardial volume. Furthermore, these techniques can potentially quantify the fibrosis of the whole heart, which truly reflects the global myocardial fibrosis burden. These new biological parameters have the ability to detect early disease, guide therapy and predict outcomes [31].

Myocardial T1 mapping

Quantitative myocardial T1 mapping is a CMR technique that provides in vivo tissue characterisation [10]

In CMR images, the pixel signal intensity is based on the relaxation of hydrogen nuclei protons in a static magnetic field. T1 relaxation time depends on the molecular environment of the water molecules in the tissue and therefore characterises each tissue very specifically. T1 relaxation time varies from one type of tissue to another, but also within the same tissue depending on its physiopathological status (inflammation, oedema, fat, fibrosis, etc.).

Gadolinium-based contrast agents (GBCAs) shorten T1. These low-molecular-weight extracellular agents are small enough to pass across the vascular wall into the extracellular space, yet are large enough that they do not penetrate cells with intact membranes. They accumulate passively in the gaps between cells and the increased volume of distribution of interstitial expansion in "scar" tissue [32]. This forms the basis of the LGE for detection of focal fibrosis and recent developments have built upon this, further allowing scrutiny of diffuse interstitial expansion (Fig. 4).

A T1 map of the myocardium is a parametric reconstructed image, where each pixel's intensity directly corresponds to the T1 relaxation time of the corresponding myocardial voxel. Therefore, it allows signal quantification (in milliseconds) on a standardised scale of each myocardial voxel with high spatial resolution [10]. Compared with LGE images, T1 mapping CMR techniques eliminate the influences of windowing and variations in signal enhancement by directly measuring the underlying T1 relaxation times. Pre-contrast or native T1 times in normal myocardium are longer than post-contrast T1, due to the small amount of residual gadolinium in the myocardial interstitium (Fig. 5). Native and post-contrast T1 mapping can be performed to measure the extracellular volume fraction (ECV) [32], which has important prognostic value [31] and shows promise for the detection of diffuse myocardial fibrosis [33, 34]. These techniques will solve the problem of detecting the processes that diffusely affect the myocardium.

T1 mapping methodology

T1 mapping sequences

T1 maps originate from a series of co-registered images acquired at different times of T1 recovery, typically following a magnetisation preparation by inversion or saturation [35]. Raw images used for T1 mapping have to be acquired at

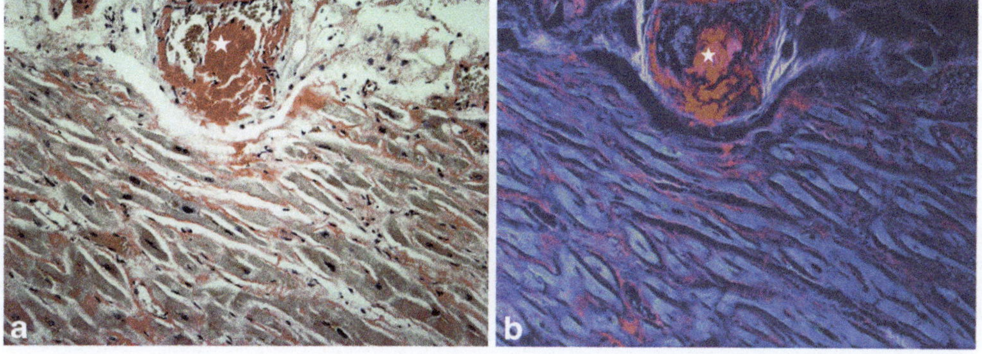

Fig. 2 Cardiac AL amyloidosis with interstitial (perimyocytic) and vascular involvement (*star*). (Congo red stain with **a** normal light and **b** ultraviolet light microscopy×100). *Red areas* represent amyloid deposition

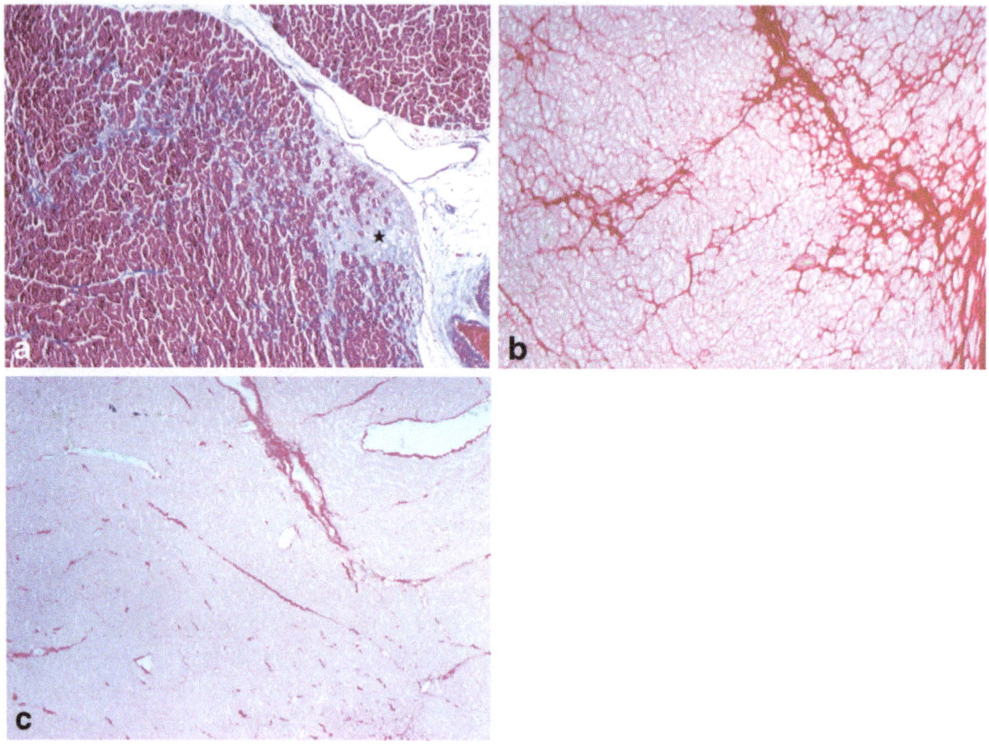

Fig. 3 Dilated cardiomyopathy of toxic origin with myocardial focal replacement containing fibrous tissue (*star*) and interstitial widening for fibrosis (Masson trichrome staining). *Blue areas* depict fibrosis, *red areas* are cardiomyocytes. (**b**) Picrosirius red stain enhances the perimyocytic pattern of fibrosis (*red areas* represent fibrosis). (**c**) Picrosirius red stain of normal myocardium for comparison. (Original magnification ×40)

identical times in the cardiac cycle. Different CMR acquisition sequences have been used to obtain myocardial T1 maps, including the modified Look-Locker inversion recovery (MOLLI) [10], shortened MOLLI (ShMOLLI) [36], saturation recovery single-shot acquisition (SASHA) [37] and saturation pulse prepared heart rate independent inversion recovery (SAPPHIRE) [38].

T1 measurements can be altered by several factors, such as the acquisition scheme, magnetisation transfer, flow, T2 effect and motion [35, 36, 37, 39, 40]. This is an essential point to consider before performing myocardial T1 maps, because it directly influences the accuracy and reproducibility of the final T1 measurements. This will also be considered when comparing results between different studies. Different T1 mapping strategies will have varying sensitivities to motion artefacts, heart rate, and intrinsic T1 values ranges [41]; Table 1 shows normal values of myocardial T1 mapping at different studies.

The most assessed T1-mapping sequence has been described by Messroghli et al. [10, 41] and is the MOLLI sequence that provides high-resolution T1 maps of human myocardium. Although it is sensitive to extreme heart rate values and tends to slightly underestimate the true T1 value, the method allows a rapid and highly reproducible T1 map of heart with high levels of intra- and inter-observer agreement

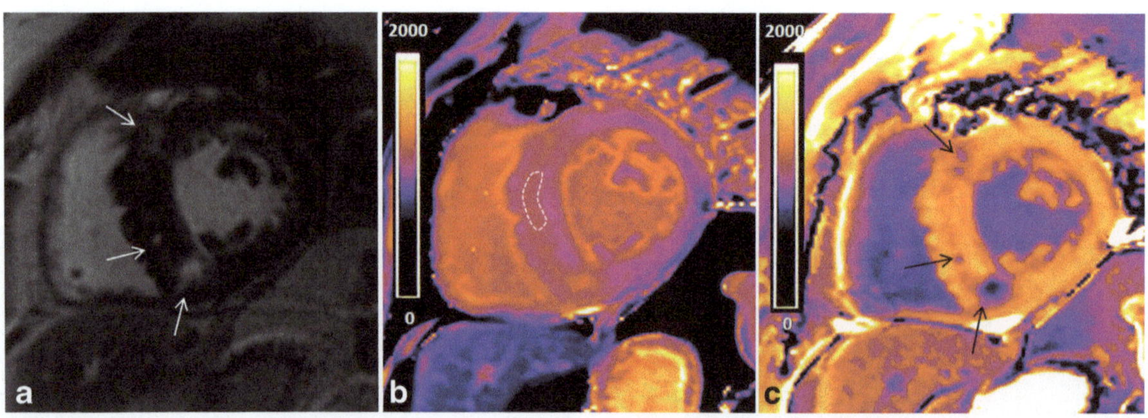

Fig. 4 T1 mapping in hypertrophic cardiomyopathy. **a** LGE imaging demonstrating patchy mid-wall enhancement in the septum (*white arrows*). **b** MOLLI T1 map at 3 T (Magneton Trio-Tim; Siemens, Erlangen, Germany) demonstrating increased T1 value (1,161 ms) in an area without LGE (ROI) because of diffuse fibrosis. The T1 value in the area with LGE (focal fibrosis) is 1,281 ms. **c** Post-contrast T1 map illustrating excellent agreement between LGE (*black arrows*). Post-contrast T1 values are shortened in the area with late enhancement (301 ms) as well as in the rest of the septum (465 ms)

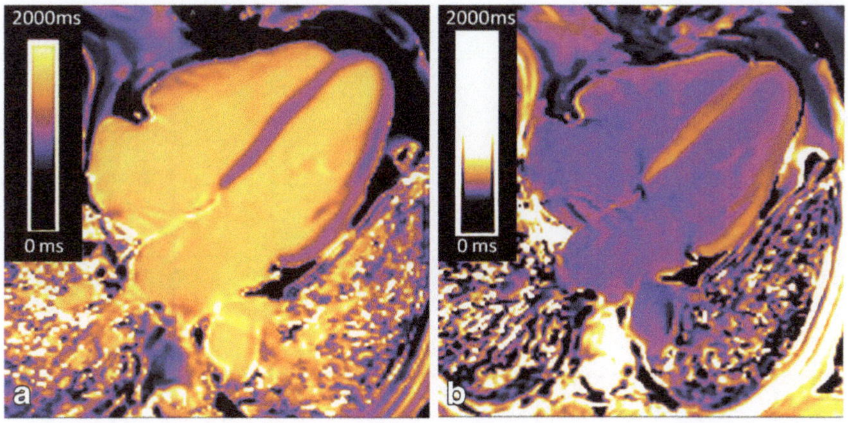

Fig. 5 Quantification of native T1 values of a healthy volunteer in a four-chamber view obtained at 3 T. The resulting pixel by pixel colour native T1 map is displayed using a customised table where normal myocardium is *purple* and increasing T1 ranges from *orange* to *yellow*. Normal values of native T1 at 3 T (Magneton Trio-Tim; Siemens) with MOLLI sequence are 1,031±24 ms. Post-contrast T1 values at 15 min are much shorter (557 ms, in the range of *orange* in the colour scale), due to the relaxing effect of the residual gadolinium in the myocardial interstitium

[42]. The MOLLI method [10, 41] overcame the limitations of motion and prolonged acquisition time of Look-Locker (LL) sequences [43], incorporating an efficient sampling of the T1 relaxation curve. The MOLLI sequence employs selective data acquisition at a given time of the cardiac cycle over successive heartbeats and merges data from multiple LL experiments into one data set. Each MOLLI study consists of three successive LL inversion recovery (IR) experiments with different inversion times (TI) which are performed consecutively within one breath-hold, for a total of 11 images over 17 heartbeats. Images are acquired in late diastole using a single-shot steady-state free-precession (SSFP) technique combined with sensitivity encoding (SENSE) [44]. By combining the three inversions, the relaxation curve is sampled in an interleaved manner, resulting in a sufficient number of points for accurate T1 quantification (Fig. 6) [10]. With some vendors, these data are automatically entered into three-parameter curve fitting at the scanner and T1 times are calculated on a per-pixel basis. To generate the inline T1 map, the acquired IR images are first registered using a motion correction algorithm which is based on estimating synthetic images presenting contrast changes similar to the acquired images solving a variational energy minimisation problem [45] (Fig. 7).

The ShMOLLI sequence requires a short breath-hold [36] and can generate rapid and high-resolution myocardial T1 maps. The imaging time with ShMOLLI is 9.0±1.1 s, compared with the 17.6±2.9 s required with MOLLI. In order to shorten the breath-hold, ShMOLLI does not achieve a full recovery of the longitudinal magnetisation between sequential inversion pulses. ShMOLLI uses a similar effective TI principle to MOLLI but over only nine heartbeats. ShMOLLI has less heart rate dependency, which may improve accuracy. The

Table 1 Reference values of native myocardial T1 mapping at different studies

	Field strength	Scanner	Reception coil	T1 mapping sequence	T1 values (ms)
Messroghli et al. [42] 2006	1.5 T	Gyroscan Intera CV, Philips	–	MOLLI	980±53
Piechnik et al. [36] 2010	1.5 T	Avanto, Siemens	32-channel	ShMOLLI	966±48
	1.5 T	Avanto, Siemens	32-channel	MOLLI	976±46
	3 T	Trio, Siemens	16-channel	ShMOLLI	1,166±60
	3 T	Trio, Siemens	16-channel	MOLLI	1,169±45
Lee et al. [58] 2011	3 T	Verio, Siemens	32-channel	MOLLI	1,315±39
Rogers et al. [59] 2013	1.5 T	Philips, Best	32-channel	MOLLI	976±37
	3 T	Philips, Best	32-channel	MOLLI	1,108±67
Von Knobelsdorff et al. [49] 2013	3 T	Verio, Siemens	32-channel	MOLLI	1,158 (range, 1,005–1,295)
Kellman et al. [82] 2013	1.5 T	Avanto, Siemens	32-channel	MOLLI	1,012±25
Piechnik et al. [83] 2013	1.5 T	Avanto, Siemens	16-channel	ShMOLLI	962±25
	1.5 T	Avanto, Siemens	32-channel	ShMOLLI	962±25
Puntmann et al. [74] 2013	3 T	Achieva TX, Philips	32-channel	MOLLI	1,070±55
Fontana et al. [76] 2014	1.5 T	Avanto, Siemens	16-channel	ShMOLLI	967±34
Liu et al. [84] 2014	3 T	Trio, Siemens	12-channel	MOLLI	1,232±51

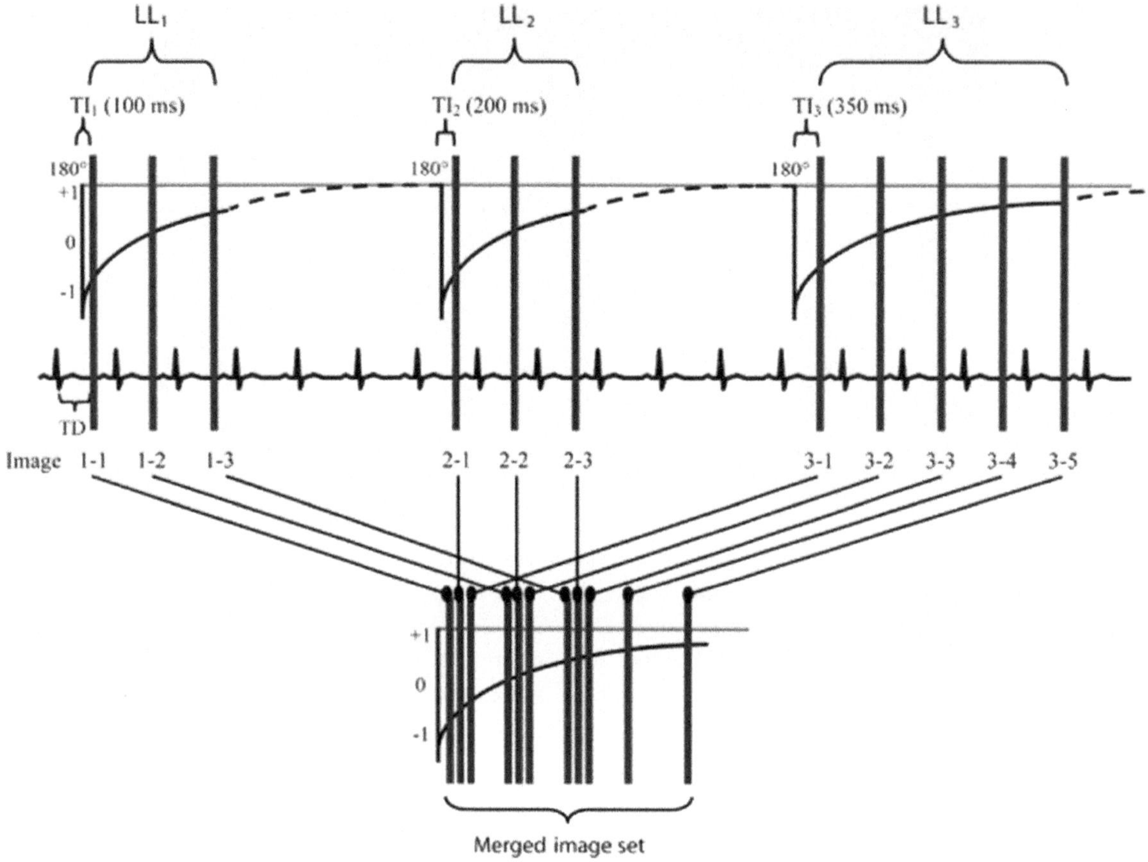

Fig. 6 MOLLI pulse sequence scheme. *Vertical bars* represent image acquisition. *Dashed lines* represent undisturbed signal recovery. Three sets of LL experiments are performed successively with increasing TI within one breath-hold's time. Images are acquired with a specific trigger delay (TD) to select end-diastole. For post-processing (calculation of T1 values), the images are regrouped into one data set according to their effective TI. (Reprinted, with permission, from Messroghli et al. [10])

measurements of myocardial T1 by ShMOLLI are in good agreement with previous measurements using MOLLI [36].

The recently described SASHA sequence [37] uses a single-shot balanced SSFP readout to provide good signal-to-noise ratio and blood–tissue contrast. This approach will overcome the limitations of MOLLI that underestimate T1 values [10, 41, 36] and which are known to have greater underestimation in short T2 tissues such as the myocardium [46]. This sequence consists of ten electrocardiogram-triggered single-shot balanced SSFP images in a breath-hold. The first image is acquired without magnetisation preparation and the remaining nine images follow saturation pulses with variable saturation recovery times [37]. The accuracy of SASHA T1 values is independent of absolute T1, T2, heart rate, flip angle and off-resonant frequencies up to 696 Hs.

In the presence of arrhythmias, a common co-morbidity in patients with heart failure, T1 mapping image quality is usually sub-optimal. Arrhythmia-insensitive inversion recovery sequences have been developed with the purpose of generating a technique insensitive to heart rate variability [38]. The novel preparation pre-pulse, called SAPPHIRE, which consists of a combination of saturation and inversion pulses, is introduced to remove the magnetisation history in each heartbeat and eliminate the need for rest periods in T1 mapping.

T1 mapping: acquisition protocol and post-processing

The most widely used and most extensively validated sequences for T1 mapping are MOLLI-based sequences [10, 42, 47]. Data may be acquired in basal, mid-ventricular and apical short-axis and in four-chamber views. To quantify T1 values, a region of interest (ROI) can be drawn in the septum in a four-chamber plane (excluding areas of focal fibrosis), assuming this to be representative of the whole myocardium. The ROI can be placed, as well, in the short-axis if it is more convenient for avoiding scar areas. The ROI has to be within the myocardium and does not include blood or epicardial fat (Fig. 8) [48] Another strategy to quantify T1 values is segmental analysis, but it is time-consuming and can also be problematic due to ventricular motion artefacts, which occur most frequently in the inferolateral region [49].

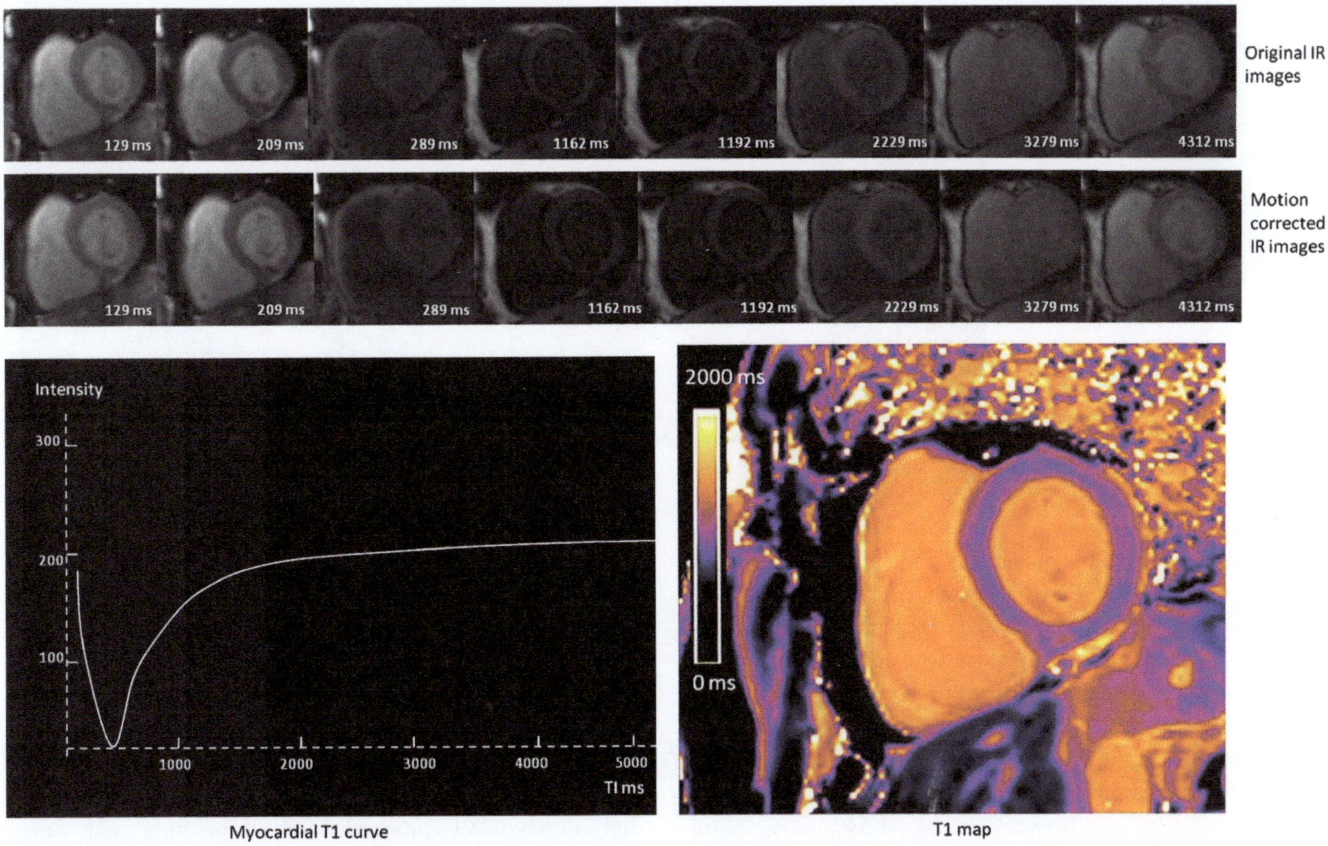

Fig. 7 MOLLI T1 mapping in a healthy subject acquired at 3 T (Magneton Trio-Tim; Siemens). The *top row* shows the original images acquired at different TI times. The *bottom row* shows the motion corrected images using a non-rigid registration algorithm. By merging these source images into one data set, T1 values can be computed for every pixel with three-parameter curve fitting; a map of T1 in the imaging section can then be generated from these pixel values

Post-contrast T1 mapping and ECV

The use of an extrinsic contrast agent adds another dimension to CMR tissue characterisation. The interstitial space can be directly assessed using standard gadolinium chelates. The post-contrast T1 maps are evaluated at different time points after contrast administration and may be used to obtain a curve of myocardial T1 recovery reflecting the contrast agent washout [42] (Fig. 9).

At a fixed time after contrast administration, T1 may be reduced in cardiac disease, suggesting increased interstitial space [34]. However, in addition to heart rate and acquisition-related confounders, isolated post-contrast T1 values are influenced by a number of factors, including body fat percentage, reduced renal function, altered haematocrit, native T1, delay time in measurement after contrast administration and gadolinium characteristics (dose, concentration and water exchange rate). Consequently, native T1 mapping and ECV are currently preferred for T1 quantification [35]. If, instead, the ratio of signal change in blood and myocardium after contrast administration is calculated, corrected by the haematocrit, the ECV, which reflects the interstitial space, can be calculated, avoiding confounding factors.

The ECV technique introduces a potentially important new method to examine the myocardium because it is sensitive to the distribution of the left ventricular myocardium into its cellular and ECM compartments. Alterations in these compartments occur from different pathophysiological processes [50]. The ECV reflects the volume fraction of heart tissue that is not taken by cells. ECV may be measured using manual regions of interest (ROIs) drawn on T1 maps (Fig. 10), by performing a manual or semi-automatic image registration of T1 maps [51] or by a fully automated method calculating pixel-wise ECV parametric maps [52], if native and post-contrast T1 images are co-registered, quantified and adjusted for the haematocrit.

Expansion of the ECV represents a non-specific increase in free water in the myocardium and occurs in a variety of pathologies, including focal and diffuse fibrosis, oedema, and amyloidosis. In the absence of amyloid or oedema [53], expansion of the myocardial CVF is responsible for most ECM expansion, which culminates in mechanical, electrical and vasomotor dysfunction.

The myocardial ECV may be estimated from the concentration of extracellular contrast agent in the myocardium relative to the blood in a steady state. The contrast agent

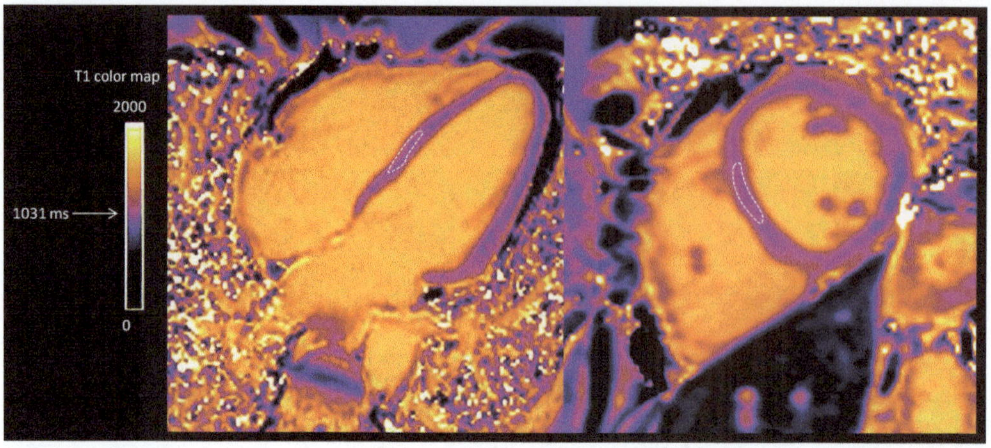

Fig. 8 Quantification of native T1 values from a healthy volunteer in a four-chamber plane (**a**) and in a short-axis (**b**) view. A ROI is drawn in the septum. Care is particularly taken to avoid "contamination" with signal from the blood pool and the epicardial fat. Normal values of native T1 at 3 T with MOLLI sequence are 1,031±24 ms. (Reprinted and modified, with permission, from Perea et al. [48])

distributes between extracellular space and blood plasma such that the relative pre- and post-contrast signal changes measure the myocardial ECV [32, 54]. The measurements are only valid for tissues where contrast agent concentration is in equilibrium (steady state) or dynamic equilibrium (dynamic steady state) with the contrast agent concentration in the blood pool. Following an intravenous injection, contrast agents are continuously cleared from the blood via renal clearance. If the contrast exchange rate between the blood and the tissue of interest is faster than the renal clearance, then the ratio of contrast agent concentration in the tissue and the blood will, after the short initial period, achieve a dynamic equilibrium and remain unchanged over time [32]. By then substituting in the blood contrast volume of distribution (equal to one minus the haematocrit) the myocardial contrast volume of distribution is obtained, reflecting the fraction of the tissue which is interstitial space, also referred to as myocardial ECV. The ECV in the myocardium is then calculated as follows:

$$ECV_{myo} = [1-\text{haematocrit}] \times \Delta R1_{myo}/\Delta R1_{blood}$$

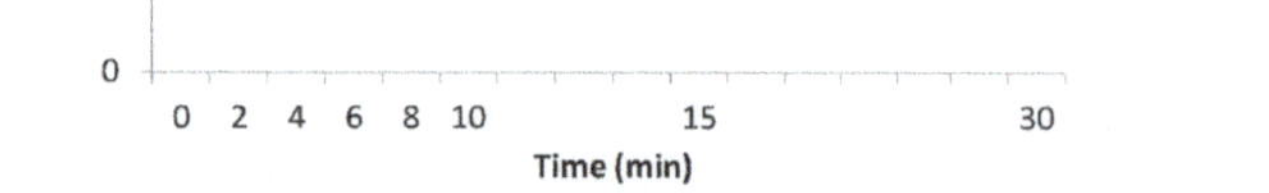

Fig. 9 Myocardial T1 values obtained in a healthy volunteer from minute 0 to minute 30 after administration of 0.15 mmol/kg of gadopentetate dimeglumine. T1 values are expressed as means. The exponential recovery of myocardial T1 reflects the washout of the contrast agent from the myocardium

Where $\Delta R1$ is (1/T1 pre-contrast – 1/T1 post-contrast)

Equilibrium distribution can be achieved with a primed contrast infusion (equilibrium contrast-CMR [EQ-CMR]) [55] or might be approximated by the dynamic equilibration achieved by delayed post-bolus measurement [56, 57].

EQ-CMR is a robust, non-invasive method to quantify diffuse myocardial fibrosis, which has been validated against the current gold standard of surgical myocardial biopsy CVF quantification in patients with aortic stenosis and hypertrophic cardiomyopathy [55]. EQ-CMR is achieved by primed infusion (a loading bolus of 0.1 mmol/kg followed by a slow continuous infusion of 0.001 mmol/kg/min [equivalent to 0.1 mmol/kg over 90 min]) [55]. Standard LGE imaging is possible after the bolus, although the sensitivity of LGE may decline since doses as low as 0.1 mmol/kg have reduced sensitivity for myocardial infarction. This technique is time-consuming, but continuous infusion removes contrast kinetic effects, measuring diffuse fibrosis in vivo.

The bolus only technique assumes that at a sufficient time after a single-contrast bolus, a dynamic equilibrium exists [56] allowing the equivalent ECV measurement. Post-gadolinium ECV is stable from approximately 8.5 min after administration of a bolus and remains at a steady state up to 50 min after gadolinium injection [56, 58] The contrast dose varies across groups (0.15 [51] or 0.2 [56] mmol/kg), enabling a quality LGE imaging 10–15 min after bolus. ECV can be measured with simple gadolinium contrast bolus as accurately as with an infusion, but with slightly less precision [56]. The bolus strategy to measure myocardial ECV is preferred against the primed infusion because it simplifies the data acquisition protocol and facilitates its integration into routine CMR practice. This technique has been validated histologically in distinct disease groups and the correlation with CVF is similar to that with the infusion technique and does not differ statistically [57]. Bolus only is sufficient for ECV measurement across a range of cardiac diseases. However, when ECV is >40 %

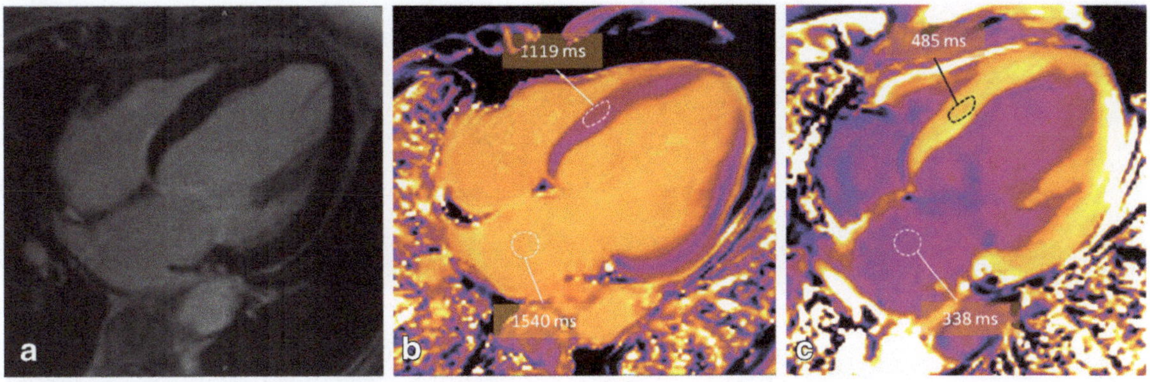

Fig. 10 ECV measured using manual ROIs drawn on T1 maps in a patient with idiopathic dilated cardiomyopathy. **a** Four-chamber myocardial delayed enhancement CMR image shows absence of late contrast enhancement. **b**, **c** T1 maps using MOLLI; pre-contrast (**b**) and post-contrast (**c**) showing marked T1 shortening. The two T1 maps are combined with 1-haematocrit blood correction to calculate ECV. Haematocrit in this patient was 38 % and ECV 31 % (slightly elevated, reflecting diffuse fibrosis)

(amyloid, LGE areas of hypertrophic cardiomyopathy and myocardial infarction), the bolus only technique consistently measures ECV higher compared with infusion, therefore, in selected cases (especially amyloidosis) the infusion method is preferred.

T1 values are affected by confounding variables mentioned before. Due to these factors, T1 times cannot be readily compared to T1 data from other centres. There are different normal T1 values in the literature depending on the field strength, the scanner manufacturer, the kind of sequence and other parameters related with the acquisition protocol and the post-processing [36, 58, 59, 49]. In order to use native myocardial T1 mapping to accurately identify disease states, it is advisable to obtain the reference values in each scenario by performing a study with healthy volunteers. In contrast, ECV is an inherent physiological property that should not be affected by these variables. The ECV data of normal volunteers do not significantly differ between the different studies, being in the range of 24–28 % [56, 58, 59, 60, 61, 62]; *see* Table 2.

Clinical applications of interstitial imaging

Native T1 distinguishes normal from abnormal myocardium, indicating myocardial disease involving both the myocyte and interstitium. Measurement requires no exogenous contrast administration, making it feasible in patients with severe renal dysfunction or pregnancy. Cardiac T1-mapping without the use of a GBCA has been shown to be sensitive to a variety of pathologies where increased water is present, such as oedema [63,

Table 2 Normal values of myocardial ECV at different studies

	Field strength	Scanner	Contrast	Technique	Dose (mmol/kg)	T1 mapping sequence	ECV (%)
Broberg et al. [60] 2010	1.5 T/*3 T*	Achieva/Intera, Philips	Gadodiamida	Only bolus	0.15	Look-Locker	24.8
Schelbert et al. [56] 2011	1.5 T	Espree, Siemens	Gadoteridol	Only bolus	0.2	MOLLI	24.1
Lee et al. [58] 2011	3 T	Verio, Siemens	Gadopentetate Dimeglumine	Only bolus	0.15	MOLLI	26.7
Kellman et al. [61] 2012	1.5 T	Avanto/Espree, Siemens	Gd-DTPA	Only bolus	0.15	MOLLI	25.4
Sado et al. [85] 2012	1.5 T	Avanto, Siemens	Gadoterate Meglumine	Bolus+infusion	0.1+0.002/min[a]	FLASH IR	25.3
Salerno et al. [62] 2013	1.5 T	Avanto, Siemens	Gd-DTPA	Bolus+infusion	0.1+0.001/min[b]	MOLLI	28.5
Liu et al. [86] 2013	1.5 T	Avanto/Espree, Siemens	Gadopentetate Dimeglumine	Only bolus	0.15	MOLLI	26.9

[a] Bolus of 0.1 mmol/kg followed by infusion of 0.002 mmol/kg/min

[b] Bolus of 0.1 mmol/kg followed by infusion of 0.001 mmol/kg/min

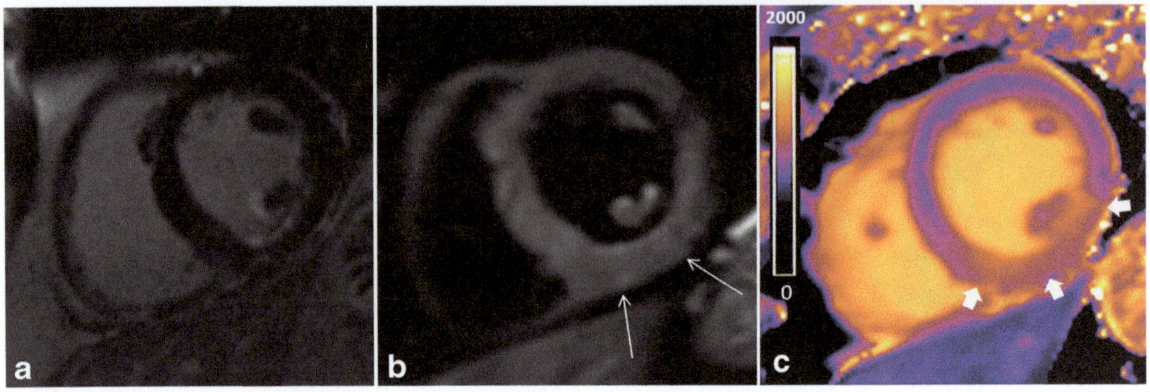

Fig. 11 T1 mapping in acute myocardial infarction. Subendocardial enhancement (**a**) in the inferolateral, midventricular segment of the left ventricle. Although the T2-weighted images (**b**) show only a mild increase in brightness (*long arrows*), there is an area of increased T1 values (1,208 ms, into the *orange* range of the colour scale) (*short arrows*) (**c**) exceeding the area of LGE enhancement

64], focal or diffuse fibrosis [65] and amyloidosis [66]. Acute myocardial injury is accompanied by intracellular and interstitial oedema and is traditionally detected by increased T2 signal, although pre-contrast T1 mapping may prove to be equally effective and robust [64]. The oedema in myocardial ischaemia and infarction can be recognised by increases in T1 with high sensitivity and specificity [67, 68, 69] (Fig. 11). In chronic myocardial infarction, there is replacement of myocardial cells by fibrosis with an increase in extracellular collagen. Consequently, T1 values are higher than in normal myocardium, but not as high as in acute myocardial infarction [67]. For determining the area at risk, native T1 and T2 mapping provide similar results and closely match the area at risk as defined by microspheres in animal models [64]. Native T1 mapping is superior compared with T2-weighted and LGE techniques in detecting acute myocarditis [70, 71], which is helpful in subtle focal disease [72] and may detect pathology missed by LGE technique, such as pan-myocarditis [72]. Native T1 values provide diagnostic accuracy to discriminate between normal and diffuse fibrosis in patients with non-ischaemic dilated cardiomyopathies [73, 74] and hypertrophic cardiomyopathy [73, 74], having the potential to become a test in patients with suspected diffuse fibrosis, which may be missed by classic LGE imaging. Furthermore, native T1 is significantly elevated in patients with aortic stenosis and correlates with the CVF quantified at biopsy [65]. Diffuse fibrosis is an important clinical parameter in aortic stenosis and is also reflected in the degree of postoperative recovery. However, fibrosis is a potentially reversible phenomenon under several therapies [75]. Cardiac amyloidosis shows markedly increased non-contrast T1 relaxation times in the myocardium [66, 76], even more pronounced that in aortic stenosis [66] (Fig. 12). Myocardial T1 mapping is an accurate technique for the detection of cardiac involvement in amyloidosis, avoiding the administration of GBCA that frequently is problematic in this group of patients [66]. Other pathologies may result in a decrease

Fig. 12 T1 mapping in amyloidosis. MOLLI non-contrast T1 map in a normal volunteer (**a**), and cardiac amyloid patient (**b**). Note the markedly elevated myocardial T1 time in the cardiac amyloid patient (1,195 ms, into the *orange* range of the colour scale) compared with the normal control (1,048 ms, in *purple* range of the scale)

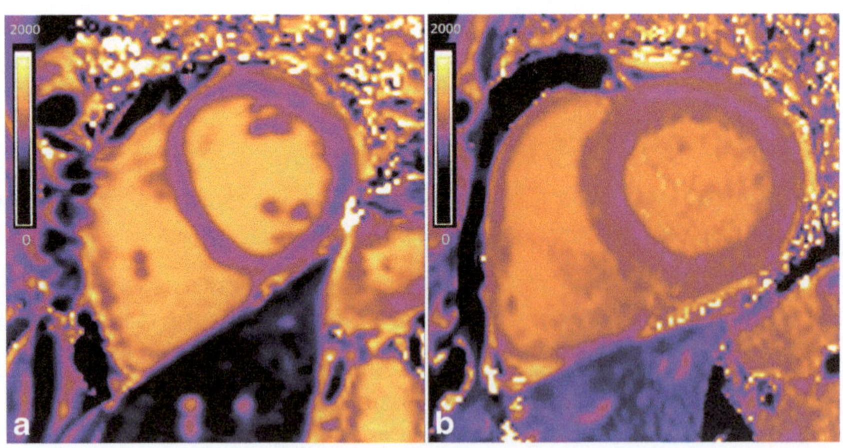

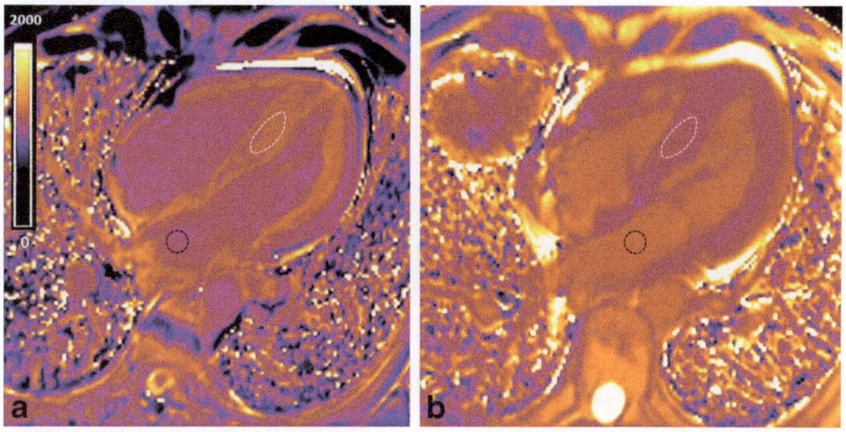

Fig. 13 Native (**a**) and post-contrast with the EQ-CMR technique (**b**) T1 maps in a patient with AL amyloidosis. A ROI is placed in the septum (*white ROI*) and in the blood (*black ROI*) in the native and post-contrast T1 maps. Native T1 value is increased (1,219 ms; *N*, 1,031±24) and post-contrast T1 time is shortened (481 ms). The two T1 maps values combined with 1-haematocrit blood correction enable the calculation of the ECV that is increased (68 %) in this patient. (Native blood T1, 1,121 ms; post-contrast blood T1, 541 ms; haematocrit, 48 %)

of native T1 values, like Anderson-Fabry disease, because of the intracellular lipid accumulation [77], and iron overload where T1 mapping is superior to the classic T2* sequence for the detection of early iron overload [78].

The use of GBCA allows a direct measurement of the size of the extracellular space, reflecting interstitial disease. The values of myocardial ECV are increased in cardiac diseases (hypertrophic [55] and dilated [79] cardiomyopathy, aortic stenosis [55], infarction [51], diabetes [80] and congenital heart diseases with myocardial dysfunction [60]) reflecting diffuse myocardial fibrosis. In myocarditis, where expansion of ECV is due to oedema/inflammation/necrosis, the ECV quantification with LGE imaging improve the diagnostic accuracy of CMR compared with standard "Lake Louise" criteria [81]. Expansion of the myocardial ECV in amyloidosis is higher than in any other disease generating diagnostic specificity above a certain threshold [53] (Fig. 13). Myocardial ECV measurement has the potential to become the first non-invasive test to quantify cardiac amyloid burden.

These new techniques might help us to detect subclinical myocardial changes in cardiovascular risk populations that otherwise could be missed by traditional imaging techniques, enabling an improvement in therapeutic strategies, monitoring the treatment effect and improving clinical outcome.

Conclusions

The T1 mapping techniques and ECV imaging by CMR appear to be sufficiently robust methods for diagnosis of many cardiac diseases. Just as native T1 mapping may be considered an intrinsic myocardial contrast, the ECV after GBCA is a direct measurement of the size of the extracellular space, reflecting interstitial disease. This technique separates the myocardium into its cellular and interstitial components. These techniques promise early detection of the disease and have the potential to provide a more individualised therapy. Consequently, native T1 mapping and ECV might supply a CMR biomarker for myocardial fibrosis, justifying their use in clinical practice. However, more research is required before a large-scale application for clinical decision-making can be recommended.

Acknowledgments The authors have no conflict of interest in relation to the subject matter of this article. This review has been supported in part by grant FIS PI12/01290 from the Ministerio de Economía y Competitividad, Instituto de Salud Carlos III, Spain.

References

1. Bashey RI, Martinez-Hernandez A, Jimenez SA (1992) Isolation, characterization, and localization of cardiac collagen type VI. Associations with other extracellular matrix components. Circ Res 70:1006–1017
2. Rossi MA (1998) Pathologic fibrosis and connective tissue matrix in left ventricular hypertrophy due to chronic arterial hypertension in humans. J Hypertens 16:1031–1041
3. Weber KT (1989) Cardiac interstitium in health and disease: the fibrillar collagen network. J Am Coll Cardiol 13:1637–1652
4. Conrad C, Brooks W, Hayes J et al (1995) Myocardial fibrosis and stiffness with hypertrophy and heart failure in the spontaneously hypertensive rat. Circulation 91:161–170
5. Wu KC, Weiss RG, Thiemann DR et al (2008) Late gadolinium enhancement by cardiovascular magnetic resonance heralds an adverse prognosis in nonischemic cardiomyopathy. J Am Coll Cardiol 51:2414–2421
6. Kwong RY, Sattar H, Wu H et al (2008) Incidence and prognostic implication of unrecognized myocardial scar characterized by cardiac

magnetic resonance in diabetic patients without clinical evidence of myocardial infarction. Circulation 118:1011–1020
7. Schalla S, Bekkers SC, Dennert R, van Suylen RJ, Waltenberger J, Leiner T, Wildberger J, Crijns HJ HS (2010) Replacement and reactive myocardial fibrosis in idiopathic dilated cardiomyopathy: comparison of magnetic resonance imaging with right ventricular biopsy. Eur J Hear Fail 12:227–31
8. Kim RJ, Wu E, Rafael A et al (2000) The use of contrast-enhanced magnetic resonance imaging to identify reversible myocardial dysfunction. N Engl J Med 343:1445–1453
9. Mongeon FP, Jerosch-Herold M, Coelho-Filho OR et al (2012) Quantification of extracellular matrix expansion by CMR in infiltrative heart disease. JACC Cardiovasc Imaging 5:897–907
10. Messroghli DR, Radjenovic A, Kozerke S et al (2004) Modified look-locker inversion recovery (MOLLI) for high-resolution T 1 mapping of the heart. Magn Reson Med 52:141–146
11. Kellman P, Aletras AH, Mancini C et al (2007) T2-prepared SSFP improves diagnostic confidence in edema imaging in acute myocardial infarction compared to turbo spin echo. Magn Reson Med 57: 891–897
12. Rossi M (2001) Connective tissue skeleton in the normal left ventricle and in hypertensive left ventricular hypertrophy and chronic chagasic myocarditis. Med Sci Monit 7:820–32
13. Souders CA, Bowers SLK, Baudino TA (2009) Cardiac fibroblast: The renaissance cell. Circ Res 105:1164–1176
14. Baudino TA, Carver W, Giles WBT (2006) Cardiac fibroblasts: friend or foe? Am J Physiol Hear Circ Physiol 291:H1015–26
15. Schwartzkopff B, Frenzel H, Dieckerhoff J et al (1992) Morphometric investigation of human myocardium in arterial hypertension and valvular aortic stenosis. Eur Heart J 13 Suppl D:17–23
16. Konduracka E, Gackowski A, Rostoff P et al (2007) Diabetes-specific cardiomyopathy in type 1 diabetes mellitus: No evidence for its occurrence in the era of intensive insulin therapy. Eur Heart J 28:2465–2471
17. St John Sutton MG, Lie JT, Anderson KR et al (1980) Histopathological specificity of hypertrophic obstructive cardiomyopathy. Myocardial fibre disarray and myocardial fibrosis. Br Heart J 44:433–443
18. Marijianowski MMH, Teeling P, Becker AE (1997) Remodeling after myocardial infarction in humans is not associated with interstitial fibrosis of noninfarcted myocardium. J Am Coll Cardiol 30: 76–82
19. Spinale FG (2007) Myocardial matrix remodeling and the matrix metalloproteinases: influence on cardiac form and function. Physiol Rev 87:1285–1342
20. Schaper J, Speiser B (1992) The extracellular matrix in the failing human heart. Basic Res Cardiol 303–309
21. Sutton MG, Sharpe N (2000) Left ventricular remodeling after myocardial infarction: pathophysiology and therapy. Circulation 101: 2981–2988
22. Song Y, Yao Q, Zhu J, Luo BLS (1999) Age-related variation in the interstitial tissues of the cardiac conduction system; and autopsy study of 230 Han Chinese. Forensic Sci Int 104:133–42
23. Brooks A, Schinde V, Bateman ACGP (2003) Interstitial fibrosis in the dilated non-ischaemic myocardium. Heart 89:1255–6
24. Schwarz F, Flameng W, Schaper J, Langebartels F, Sesto M, Hehrlein FSM (1978) Myocardial structure and function in patients with aortic valve disease and their relation to postoperative results. Am J Cardiol 41:661–9
25. Shah KB, Inoue Y, Mehra MR (2006) Amyloidosis and the heart: a comprehensive review. Arch Intern Med 166:1805–1813
26. Zarate YA, Hopkin RJ (2008) Fabry's disease. Lancet 372:1427–1435
27. Martos R, Baugh J, Ledwidge M et al (2007) Diastolic heart failure: Evidence of increased myocardial collagen turnover linked to diastolic dysfunction. Circulation 115:888–895
28. Diez J, Querejeta R, Lopez B et al (2002) Losartan-dependent regression of myocardial fibrosis is associated with reduction of left ventricular chamber stiffness in hypertensive patients. Circulation 105:2512–2517
29. Roberts WC, Siegel RJ, McManus BM (1987) Idiopathic dilated cardiomyopathy: analysis of 152 necropsy patients. Am J Cardiol 60:1340–1355
30. De Leeuw N, Ruiter DJ, Balk AH et al (2001) Histopathologic findings in explanted heart tissue from patients with end-stage idiopathic dilated cardiomyopathy. Transpl Int 14:299–306
31. Wong TC, Piehler K, Meier CG et al (2012) Association between extracellular matrix expansion quantified by cardiovascular magnetic resonance and short-term mortality. Circulation 126: 1206–1216
32. Arheden H, Saeed M, Higgins CB et al (1999) Measurement of the distribution volume of gadopentetate dimeglumine at echo-planar MR imaging to quantify myocardial infarction: comparison with 99mTc-DTPA autoradiography in rats. Radiology 211:698–708
33. Mewton N, Liu CY, Croisille P et al (2011) Assessment of myocardial fibrosis with cardiovascular magnetic resonance. J Am Coll Cardiol 57:891–903
34. Iles L, Pfluger H, Phrommintikul A et al (2008) Evaluation of diffuse myocardial fibrosis in heart failure with cardiac magnetic resonance contrast-enhanced T1 mapping. J Am Coll Cardiol 52: 1574–1580
35. Moon JC, Messroghli DR, Kellman P et al (2013) Myocardial T1 mapping and extracellular volume quantification: a Society for Cardiovascular Magnetic Resonance (SCMR) and CMR Working Group of the European Society of Cardiology consensus statement. J Cardiovasc Magn Reson 15:92
36. Piechnik SK, Ferreira VM, Dall'Armellina E et al (2010) Shortened Modified Look-Locker Inversion recovery (ShMOLLI) for clinical myocardial T1-mapping at 1.5 and 3 T within a 9 heartbeat breathhold. J Cardiovasc Magn Reson 12:69
37. Chow K, Flewitt JA, Green JD et al (2013) Saturation recovery single-shot acquisition (SASHA) for myocardial T1 mapping. Magn Reson Med. doi:10.1002/mrm.24878
38. Weingärtner S, Akçakaya M, Basha T et al (2014) Combined saturation/inversion recovery sequences for improved evaluation of scar and diffuse fibrosis in patients with arrhythmia or heart rate variability. Magn Reson Med 71:1024–1034
39. Robson MD, Piechnik SK, Tunnicliffe EM, Neubauer S (2013) T1 measurements in the human myocardium: The effects of magnetization transfer on the SASHA and MOLLI sequences. Magn Reson Med 70:664–670
40. Kellman P, Hansen MS (2014) T1-mapping in the heart: accuracy and precision. J Cardiovasc Magn Reson 16:2
41. Messroghli DR, Greiser A, Fröhlich M et al (2007) Optimization and validation of a fully-integrated pulse sequence for modified look-locker inversion-recovery (MOLLI) T1 mapping of the heart. J Magn Reson Imaging 26:1081–1086
42. Messroghli DR, Plein S, Higgins DM et al (2006) Human myocardium: single-breath-hold MR T1 mapping with high spatial resolution-reproducibility study. Radiology 238:1004–1012
43. Look DC, Locker DR (1970) Time saving in measurement of NMR and EPR relaxation times. Rev Sci Instrum 41:250–251
44. Pruessmann KP, Weiger M, Scheidegger MB, Boesiger P (1999) SENSE: Sensitivity encoding for fast MRI. Magn Reson Med 42: 952–962
45. Xue H, Shah S, Greiser A et al (2012) Motion correction for myocardial T1 mapping using image registration with synthetic image estimation. Magn Reson Med 67:1644–1655
46. Gai ND, Stehning C, Nacif M, Bluemke DA (2013) Modified Look-Locker T1 evaluation using Bloch simulations: human and phantom validation. Magn Reson Med 69:329–336

47. Nacif MS, Turkbey EB, Gai N et al (2011) Myocardial T1 mapping with MRI: Comparison of look-locker and MOLLI sequences. J Magn Reson Imaging 34:1367–1373
48. RJ, Perea, Ortiz JT, Cibeira MT, Caralt TM, Prat S, Bosch X, Arguis P, Sanchez M, Sole M (2014) Characterising the myocardial interstitial space: clinical relevance of T1 and extracellular volume mapping. Eur Congr Radiol C–0416. doi: 10.1594/ecr2014/C-0416
49. Von Knobelsdorff-Brenkenhoff F, Prothmann M, Dieringer MA et al (2013) Myocardial T1 and T2 mapping at 3 T: reference values, influencing factors and implications. J Cardiovasc Magn Reson 15: 53
50. Weber KT, Brilla CG (1991) Pathological hypertrophy and cardiac interstitium. Fibrosis and renin-angiotensin-aldosterone system Circulation 83:1849–1865
51. Ugander M, Oki AJ, Hsu LY et al (2012) Extracellular volume imaging by magnetic resonance imaging provides insights into overt and sub-clinical myocardial pathology. Eur Heart J 33:1268–1278
52. Kellman P, Wilson JR, Xue H et al (2012) Extracellular volume fraction mapping in the myocardium, part 1: evaluation of an automated method. J Cardiovasc Magn Reson 14:64
53. Banypersad SM, Sado DM, Flett AS et al (2013) Quantification of myocardial extracellular volume fraction in systemic AL amyloidosis: An equilibrium contrast cardiovascular magnetic resonance study. Circ Cardiovasc Imaging 6:34–39
54. Flacke SJ, Fischer SE, Lorenz CH (2001) Measurement of the gadopentetate dimeglumine partition coefficient in human myocardium in vivo: normal distribution and elevation in acute and chronic infarction. Radiology 218:703–710
55. Flett AS, Hayward MP, Ashworth MT et al (2010) Equilibrium contrast cardiovascular magnetic resonance for the measurement of diffuse myocardial fibrosis: Preliminary validation in humans. Circulation 122:138–144
56. Schelbert EB, Testa SM, Meier CG et al (2011) Myocardial extravascular extracellular volume fraction measurement by gadolinium cardiovascular magnetic resonance in humans: slow infusion versus bolus. J Cardiovasc Magn Reson 13:16
57. White SK, Sado DM, Fontana M et al (2013) T1 mapping for myocardial extracellular volume measurement by CMR: Bolus only versus primed infusion technique. JACC Cardiovasc Imaging 6:955–962
58. Lee JJ, Liu S, Nacif MS et al (2011) Myocardial T1 and extracellular volume fraction mapping at 3 tesla. J Cardiovasc Magn Reson 13:75
59. Rogers T, Dabir D, Mahmoud I et al (2013) Standardization of T1 measurements with MOLLI in differentiation between health and diseas-the ConSept study. J Cardiovasc Magn Reson 15:78
60. Broberg CS, Chugh SS, Conklin C et al (2010) Quantification of diffuse myocardial fibrosis and its association with myocardial dysfunction in congenital heart disease. Circ Cardiovasc Imaging 3:727–734
61. Kellman P, Wilson JR, Xue H et al (2012) Extracellular volume fraction mapping in the myocardium, part 2: initial clinical experience. J Cardiovasc Magn Reson 14:64
62. Salerno M, Janardhanan R, Jiji RS et al (2013) Comparison of methods for determining the partition coefficient of gadolinium in the myocardium using T1 mapping. J Magn Reson Imaging 38:217–224
63. Ferreira V, Piechnik S, Dall'Armellina E et al (2012) Non-contrast T1-mapping detects acute myocardial edema with high diagnostic accuracy: a comparison to T2-weighted cardiovascular magnetic resonance. J Cardiovasc Magn Reson 14:42
64. Ugander M, Bagi PS, Oki AJ et al (2012) Myocardial edema as detected by pre-contrast T1 and T2 CMR delineates area at risk associated with acute myocardial infarction. JACC Cardiovasc Imaging 5:596–603
65. Bull S, White SK, Piechnik SK et al (2013) Human non-contrast T1 values and correlation with histology in diffuse fibrosis. Heart 99: 932–7
66. Karamitsos TD, Piechnik SK, Banypersad SM et al (2013) Noncontrast T1 mapping for the diagnosis of cardiac amyloidosis. JACC Cardiovasc Imaging 6:488–497
67. Messroghli DR, Walters K, Plein S et al (2007) Myocardial T1 mapping: application to patients with acute and chronic myocardial infarction. Magn Reson Med 58:34–40
68. Dall'armellina E, Piechnik SK, Ferreira VM et al (2012) Cardiovascular magnetic resonance by non contrast T1 mapping allows assessment of severity of injury in acute myocardial infarction. J Cardiovasc Magn Reson 14:15
69. Goldfarb JW, Arnold S, Han J (2007) Recent myocardial infarction: assessment with unenhanced T1-weighted MR imaging. Radiology 245:245–250
70. Ferreira VM, Piechnik SK, Dall'Armellina E, Karamitsos TD, Francis JM, Ntusi N, Holloway C, Choudhury RP, Kardos A, Robson MD, Friedrich MG NS (2014) Native T1-mapping detects the location, extent and patterns of acute myocarditis without the need for gadolinium contrast agents. J Cardiovasc Magn Reson 16:36
71. Luetkens JA, Doerner J, Thomas DK et al (2014) Acute myocarditis: multiparametric cardiac MR imaging. Radiology 273:383–392
72. Ferreira VM, Piechnik SK, Dall'Armellina E et al (2013) T1 mapping for the diagnosis of acute myocarditis using CMR: comparison to T2-weighted and late gadolinium enhanced imaging. JACC Cardiovasc Imaging 6:1048–1058
73. Dass S, Suttie JJ, Piechnik SK et al (2012) Myocardial tissue characterization using magnetic resonance noncontrast T1 mapping in hypertrophic and dilated cardiomyopathy. Circ Cardiovasc Imaging 5:726–733
74. Puntmann VO, Voigt T, Chen Z et al (2013) Native T1 mapping in differentiation of normal myocardium from diffuse disease in hypertrophic and dilated cardiomyopathy. JACC Cardiovasc Imaging 6: 475–484
75. Hein S, Arnon E, Kostin S et al (2003) Progression from compensated hypertrophy to failure in the pressure-overloaded human: Heart structural deterioration and compensatory mechanisms. Circulation 107:984–991
76. Fontana M, Banypersad SM, Treibel TA et al (2014) Native T1 mapping in transthyretin amyloidosis. JACC Cardiovasc Imaging 7: 157–165
77. Sado DM, White SK, Piechnik SK et al (2013) Identification and assessment of Anderson-Fabry disease by cardiovascular magnetic resonance noncontrast myocardial T1 mapping. Circ Cardiovasc Imaging 6:392–8
78. Sado DM, Maestrini V, Piechnik SK et al (2014) Noncontrast myocardial T1 mapping using cardiovascular magnetic resonance for iron overload. J Magn Reson Imaging. doi:10.1002/jmri.24727
79. Aus dem Siepen F, Buss SJ, Messroghli D, Andre F, Lossnitzer D, Seitz S, Keller M, Schnabel PA, Giannitsis E, Korosoglou G, Katus HASH (2014) T1 mapping in dilated cardiomyopathy with cardiac magnetic resonance: quantification of diffuse myocardial fibrosis and comparison with endomyocardial biopsy. Hear. J Cardiovasc Imaging, Eur
80. Wong TC, Piehler KM, Kang IA et al (2014) Myocardial extracellular volume fraction quantified by cardiovascular magnetic resonance is increased in diabetes and associated with mortality and incident heart failure admission. Eur Heart J 35:657–664
81. Radunski UK, Lund GK, Stehning C et al (2014) CMR in patients with severe myocarditis: Diagnostic value of quantitative tissue markers including extracellular volume imaging. JACC Cardiovasc Imaging 7:667–675

82. Kellman P, Arai AE, Xue H (2013) T1 and extracellular volume mapping in the heart: estimation of error maps and the influence of noise on precision. J Cardiovasc Magn Reson 15:56
83. Piechnik SK, Ferreira VM, Lewandowski AJ et al (2013) Normal variation of magnetic resonance T1 relaxation times in the human population at 1.5 T using ShMOLLI. J Cardiovasc Magn Reson 15:13
84. Liu CY, Bluemke DA, Gerstenblith G, Zimmerman SL, Li J, Zhu H, Lai SLH (2014) Reference values of myocardial structure, function, and tissue composition by cardiac magnetic resonance in healthy African-Americans at 3 T and their relations to serologic and cardiovascular risk factors. Am J Cardiol 114:789–95
85. Sado DM, Flett AS, Banypersad SM et al (2012) Cardiovascular magnetic resonance measurement of myocardial extracellular volume in health and disease. Heart 98:1436–41
86. Liu CY, Liu YC, Wu C et al (2013) Evaluation of age-related interstitial myocardial fibrosis with cardiac magnetic resonance contrast-enhanced T1 mapping: MESA (Multi-Ethnic Study of Atherosclerosis). J Am Coll Cardiol 62:1280–1287. This review article is based on a electronic poster publised in EPOS 2014. Characterising the myocardial interstitial space: clinical relevance of T1 and extracellular volume mapping. *Eur Congr Radiol.* 2014:C-0416. doi:10.1594/ecr2014/C-0416.

2

Visual grading characteristics and ordinal regression analysis during optimisation of CT head examinations

Francis Zarb · Mark F. McEntee · Louise Rainford

Abstract

Objectives To evaluate visual grading characteristics (VGC) and ordinal regression analysis during head CT optimisation as a potential alternative to visual grading assessment (VGA), traditionally employed to score anatomical visualisation.

Methods Patient images (n=66) were obtained using current and optimised imaging protocols from two CT suites: a 16-slice scanner at the national Maltese centre for trauma and a 64-slice scanner in a private centre. Local resident radiologists (n=6) performed VGA followed by VGC and ordinal regression analysis.

Results VGC alone indicated that optimised protocols had similar image quality as current protocols. Ordinal logistic regression analysis provided an in-depth evaluation, criterion by criterion allowing the selective implementation of the protocols. The local radiology review panel supported the implementation of optimised protocols for brain CT examinations (including trauma) in one centre, achieving radiation dose reductions ranging from 24 % to 36 %. In the second centre a 29 % reduction in radiation dose was achieved for follow-up cases.

Conclusions The combined use of VGC and ordinal logistic regression analysis led to clinical decisions being taken on the implementation of the optimised protocols. This improved method of image quality analysis provided the evidence to support imaging protocol optimisation, resulting in significant radiation dose savings.

Main Messages

- *There is need for scientifically based image quality evaluation during CT optimisation.*
- *VGC and ordinal regression analysis in combination led to better informed clinical decisions.*
- *VGC and ordinal regression analysis led to dose reductions without compromising diagnostic efficacy.*

Keywords CT · Optimisation · Image quality · Visual grading characteristics · Ordinal regression

F. Zarb (✉)
Department of Radiography, Faculty of Health Sciences, University of Malta, Msida, Malta
e-mail: francis.zarb@um.edu.mt

M. F. McEntee
Discipline of Medical Radiation Sciences and Brain and Mind Research Institute, Faculty of Health Sciences, The University of Sydney, Sydney, Australia
e-mail: mark.mcentee@sydney.edu.au

L. Rainford
School of Medicine & Medical Science, Health Science Centre, University College Dublin, Belfield, Dublin 4, Ireland
e-mail: louise.rainford@ucd.ie

Introduction

Producing high-quality images in computerised tomography (CT) is important for image interpretation to ensure that the maximum diagnostic information is available to facilitate the visualisation of discrete changes in anatomy indicating early pathological processes [1–3]. Higher quality CT images, however, normally imply a higher radiation dose to the patient since changes in scan parameters are required to facilitate high resolution [4]. The standard of image quality mainly depends on the preferences of radiologists and their willingness to balance low-noise, high-quality CT images with the impact upon radiation levels administered. Noise is a major factor in determining acceptable image quality and often dictates the radiation dose for a particular CT protocol. Increases in noise degrade both low-contrast resolution and spatial resolution and therefore influence the radiologists' perception of the image [5–8]. However, an increase in noise up to certain levels may not necessarily impair the image diagnosis [9, 10].

The aim of image quality optimisation is to provide an image that is suitable for the clinical task with the lowest radiation dose given to the patient. '*It is whether the clinical information required is contained in the image and can be interpreted by the observer that is important rather than whether the appearance of the image is pleasing to the eye*' [11]. The threshold of image quality should be one able to deliver enough information to the radiologist to permit a medical decision to be taken with an acceptable amount of assurance [11].

Hence, there is a need to have a keen understanding of image quality evaluation tools and methods of data analysis to identify the required level of image quality required for diagnosis in the development of optimised scan protocols using the lowest possible radiation dose. Effective and scientifically accepted methods of assessing image quality are needed for the implementation of such optimised imaging protocols across all imaging modalities including CT [1–3, 12–15].

To limit any uncertainties in interpretation, observer performance tests on images obtained using CT scanning protocols should be carried out testing visualisation of anatomical structures or known pathologies. The usefulness of observer performance studies where observers visually grade image quality is attributed to the following characteristics [16]:

- The validity of such studies is assumed to be high since the observer's ratings take into account all technical factors in reproducing anatomical structures on the image together with the experience and confidence of the observer in identifying and interpreting the image.
- Image assessment is based on the visualisation of clinically relevant anatomical structures using established standards such as the European guidelines on quality criteria.
- The studies are easy to conduct following a clear and reproducible methodology and take practical consideration of radiology availability increasing the chances for participation.

Observer performance methods such as image criteria (IC) studies, visual grading analysis (VGA) and receiver-operating characteristic (ROC) analysis are now established methods for the analysis of image quality. IC and VGA are useful in the majority of cases where the patient examinations present as normal anatomy [17]. ROC is of value for the identification and location of pathologies [18].

CT examinations producing anatomical structures obtained from either anthropomorphic phantoms or animal models make it easier to produce large numbers of images with no concern about the ethical issues associated with the irradiation of patients. Results of such studies facilitate the comparison of optimised protocols with current ones prior to their implementation on patients in the clinical setting [13, 19–21].

Established methods in performing observer and diagnostic performance tests make it possible to measure image quality by the evaluation of anatomical structures seen on the CT images against a set of criteria that have to be fulfilled [21–24]. Visual grading analysis (VGA) facilitates the quantification of subjective opinions and involves grading of the visibility of anatomical structures on the images. In relative VGA, the visibility of anatomical structures is compared and graded against the visibility of the same structures within a reference image. The observers grade the visibility of the structure with an arbitrary ordinal scale where '0' implies a visibility equal to the structure within the reference image, while negative or positive values imply inferior or superior visibility respectively. In absolute VGA, the visibilities of anatomical structures within the images are graded against each other. The scales are ordinary and are usually given a description facilitating interpretation and improving the agreement between observers. A VGA score calculated from the results of such analysis allows statistical analysis of the differences [13, 21].

In 2007 Bath and Mansson indicated the inappropriate analysis of visual grading data using parametric tests and recommended a novel method of analysing such data called Visual Grading of Characteristics: VGC analysis. VGC treats the scale steps as ordinal with no assumptions on the distribution of the data [25]. The resemblance between VGC and receiver-operator characteristic (ROC) analysis leads to the possibility of using the well-established ROC evaluation methods in analysing VGC data. The variation in the visual grading of the reviewers of two imaging techniques can be used to describe the variation between the two techniques in the same way as in an ROC study. VGC can be considered as a repeated image criteria scoring, where reviewers change their threshold for the necessity of fulfilling each criterion in a similar way to the scale steps in an ROC study. The reviewers therefore state their confidence concerning the fulfilment of a criterion obtaining an ordinal scale. As in ROC analysis, the different ratings do not necessarily correspond to the same numerical intervals on the decision scale nor do all reviewers use the ratings with the same meaning since the ordinal scale is just used to test the probability distribution for each imaging technique [25].

In 2010, Smedby and Fredrikson proposed a method for analysing ranked visual grading data using ordinal logistic regression analysis [26]. Ordinal logistic regression is a statistical technique able to process data on an ordinal scale that handles situations involving several factors that could potentially influence the outcome [27, 28]. Scott (1997) states that a lack of a full review of ordinal data increases the potential for lost information and that ordinal regression facilitates the analysis whilst taking account of a number of explanatory variables, accounting for the effects of each in the form of an odds ratio, so excluding unverifiable assumptions [27]. In

2011, Smedby presented a study quantifying potential radiation dose reduction with visual grading regression at the Medical Imaging Perception Society's (MIPS) 14th Conference held in August 2011 in Dublin, Ireland [26]. This study was published in the British Journal of Radiology (BJR) in 2012 [29]. Although ordinal logistic regression analysis is an established statistical method for analysing ordinal data, only recently have publications specifically recommended its use in the investigation of diagnostic efficacy [26].

Effective and scientifically accepted methods of assessing image quality are needed for the clinical implementation of optimised CT protocols [1–3, 12–15]. This study investigated image quality evaluation using VGC during optimisation of CT examinations of the head. Image quality scores obtained from this visual grading assessment were analysed using VGC and ordinal regression analysis and the impact of their findings upon the achieved radiation dose savings during the review of the optimised scanning protocols. Detail of the optimisation process for the Maltese data set was previously published [30, 31].

Materials and methods

Ethical approval was obtained from the clinical centres and from the governing ethics institution (UREC Ref No: 001/2009).

Image data set: collation and review

This research group had previously identified CT examinations of the head (43 %) as the most commonly requested and performed CT examination in Malta [21]. Head CT examinations using the locally optimised protocols were performed in each participating CT suite (n=2): a GE BrightSpeed Elite16-slice CT scanner at a public hospital with an annual CT referral rate of 6,460 head CT examinations and a Philips Brilliance 64-slice CT scanner in a private centre with an annual CT referral rate of 300 head CT examinations. The resulting 66 CT data sets for image quality evaluation included the current protocol (n=30), optimised protocol (n=30) and duplicate examinations (n=6) to facilitate inter- and intra- reviewer reliability.

The coded CT data sets were reviewed by six local resident radiologists including: two consultant radiologists, one with more than 20 years' experience in CT reporting and the second having more than 5 years, two senior radiology registrars, both with more than two years' experience and two radiology trainees. These images were presented using ViewDex, a Java-based software for presentation and evaluation of medical images in reviewer performance studies developed at Sahlgrenska University Hospital, Goteborg University and Sodra Alvsborg Hospital [32].

The images were displayed on primary monitors using a General Electric (GE) Advantage Workstation (AW) v.4.3_07, previously tested and satisfying the recommendations by the American Association of Physicists in Medicine (AAPM) as outlined in task group 18 [33], having 3-megapixel monitors (1,536 * 2,048 pixels) driven by a BarcoMed Coronis graphics card, with a maximum luminance of 725.22 cd/m^2 [34]. Ambient lighting levels adhered to AAPM recommendations for diagnostic reading workstations (15–60 lux) [33, 35] and were measured with a calibrated Unfors Light-O-Meter photometer (Billdal, Sweden).

The radiologists declared their confidence for each of the EU CT anatomical criteria [36] using a five-point scale [16] as follows:

- 1: confident that the criterion is not fulfilled;
- 2: somewhat confident that the criterion is not fulfilled;
- 3: indecisive whether the criterion is fulfilled of not;
- 4: somewhat confident that the criterion is fulfilled;
- 5: confident that the criterion is fulfilled.

The image data sets predominantly consisted of normal cases. Clinical indications included head trauma, cerebrovascular accident (CVA) or stroke and headaches. Eight cases presented abnormal findings: four subdural haematomas and four infarcts, all classified as obvious pathologies by a consultant radiologist. The pathologies were deemed not to distort the anatomy indicated in the evaluation criteria. VGC curves and ordinal regression analysis were employed to analyse the data.

Quantification of dose reduction recorded between systems

The overall reductions in radiation dose measured in terms of radiation dose quantities: volume CT dose index (CTDIvol) and dose length product (DLP) following optimisation are summarised in Table 1. CTDIvol is the main radiation dose indicator in spiral CT, integrating the radiation dose for a single slice delivered both within and beyond the scanned volume, representing the average radiation dose for a single slice in the scanned volume for contiguous scans. CTDIvol given in milligrays (mGy) is an accurate indicator of the radiation dose per slice within the scanned volume [1, 36–39]. The CTDIvol multiplied by the total scan length in centimetres is given as the dose length product (DLP) given in milligray cm (mGy cm) [2, 36–38, 40]. DLP correlates better with the patient radiation dose than CTDIvol and can easily be used as an indicator of the given radiation dose. There is a linear relationship between DLP and radiation dose and a linear relationship between radiation dose and the stochastic risk. Hence, DLP can be used to compare the stochastic risk between different CT examinations [41]. DLP is a more realistic indicator of the radiation dose and, in calculating the DLP, the measure of CTDIvol is still required. While

Table 1 Comparison of mean CT doses between current and optimised protocols (confidence interval p<0.05)

CT head Independent samples t-test	GE BrightSpeed Current n =24	Optimised n =20	p	Philips Brilliance Current n =24	Optimised n =20	p
CTDIvol (mGy)	35.8	33.1	0.00	39.6	28.3	0.00
(Range)	(30.0-37.6)	(29.8-36.1)		(39.6-39.6)	(28.3-28.3)	
DLP (mGy-cm)	489.4	461.5	0.03	694.8	637.3	0.03
(Range)	(420.0-564.0)	(389.2-575.1)		(491.0-820.0)	(541.1-823.1)	

CTDIvol is estimated based on the selected scan parameters prior to imaging, DLP is calculated after the examination has taken place.

Data analysis

Image quality scores obtained from the evaluation of the image data sets by local radiologists were analysed using VGC. VGC analysis is performed in three steps:

1. A frequency table ($2 \times n$ frequency table, where n=number of categories) summarises the results for the two scan protocols separately.
2. The VGC data points in the frequency table represent the coordinates of the VGC curve. As in an ROC curve the origin of a VGC curve per definition is "0". The data points are arranged according to the cumulative (relative) frequencies of the corresponding categories. The last point includes all decisions and therefore is "1" [16].
3. The VGC points are plotted to produce a VGC curve indicating the sensitivity or true positive fraction (TPF). The curves are produced using the same software for obtaining ROC curves [13]. The VGC curves for this study were created using the ROC analysis web-based calculator for ROC curves developed by John Eng, M.D., and Russell H. Morgan at the Department of Radiology and Radiological Science, Johns Hopkins University, Baltimore, MD, USA (available online at: http://www.rad.jhmi.edu/jeng/javarad/roc/JROCFITi.html).

The area under the curve (AUC_{VGC}) can be considered as a measure or accuracy index of the difference in image quality between the two techniques. A VGC curve situated on or near the diagonal (AUC_{VGC} =0.5) indicates that the two scan protocols produce identical image quality. The greater the AUC_{VGC} (>0.5) indicates better image quality for the scan protocol on the vertical axis of the plot [16, 25].

Image quality scores together with radiation dose measurements and protocol type were also analysed using ordinal regression analysis. Ordinal logistic regression analysis takes into account potential confounders of the association between two cohorts: the independent variables and the end result (dependent variable), with the measure of association being the odds ratio [42]. In this study, random effects include the patients and the radiologists participating in the study while the independent variables are the scan protocols and the radiation dose administered as the DLP. The dependent variable is the rating scores as an indication of image quality. The ordinal logistic regression model (proportional odds model) is the appropriate model for analysing rating scores since these are ordinal categorical responses.

Ordinal regression analysis was performed using the IBM Statistical Package for Social Sciences (SPSS version 19), where differences were considered significant outside the 95 % confidence interval ($p \leq 0.05$).

Results

Image quality evaluation: VGC

VGC curves (Figs. 1 and 2) indicate that the optimised protocols do not differ significantly from the current protocols in terms of image quality. A one-sample t-test on the values of the area under the curve (AUC_{VGC}) (Table 2) demonstrated no significant difference from the 0.5 value ($p \geq 0.05$) despite radiation dose reductions.

Image quality evaluation: ordinal regression analysis

Ordinal regression analysis was applied to further identify differences between the protocols and their effect on the quality of the images produced and therefore as predictors of image quality.

Overall results presented in Table 3 show that DLP and criteria have no significant impact on the rating scores ($p \leq 0.05$). The protocol used however does have a significant impact on the quality of the images in terms of rating scores ($p \leq 0.05$). The difference in the protocols is based on the imaging parameters selected with the optimised protocol administering a significantly lower radiation dose (Table 1).

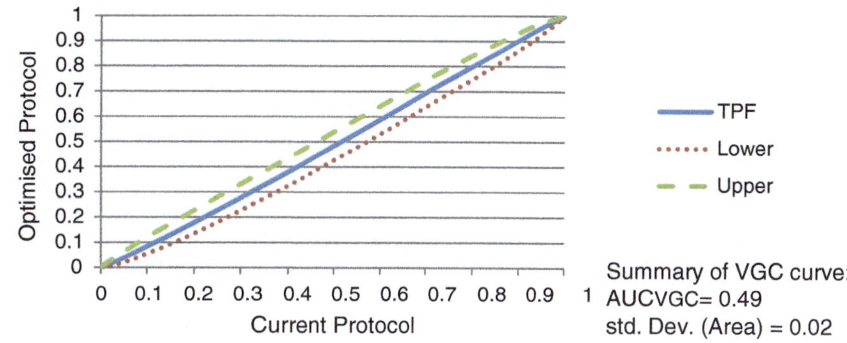

Fig. 1 VGC curve—GE BrightSpeed

Results presented in Table 4 indicate that only criteria 2 (*visually sharp reproduction of the basal ganglia*) had a negative odd for the GE BrightSpeed, while criteria 1 (*visually sharp reproduction of the border between white and grey matter*) and again criteria 2 had a negative odd for the Philips Brilliance. For every one-unit increase, the odds that the selected protocol is the current protocol rather than the optimised protocol increase by: *(Odds Ratio (B) – 1)* × *100* [42].

The kappa (k) values for resident radiologists (n=6) ranged between 0.33 and 0.59 showing fair to moderate agreement in their interpretation of the repeated scans, while the p-value was ≤0.05, implying significant agreement between the two interpretations of the repeated scans. Cronbach's alpha (α) measured 0.76, indicating an acceptable level of internal consistency within the local resident radiologist, with inter-reviewer correlations ranging between 0.26 and 0.45.

Discussion

The advantages of using visual grading studies in the evaluation of clinical images are that these can be carried out with clinically available images and there is no need for a gold standard during the evaluation. However the use of appropriate data analysis methods should be emphasised. The terminology in this field is somewhat confusing as some authors use VGA to denote standard statistical tests with assumptions that may not be appropriate since the data in a VGA str ordinal. Analysing visual grading analysis methods with parametrical statistical tests such as t-tests and analysis of variance (ANOVA) incorrectly assumes the grading data are an interval variable; VGC and ordinal regression analysis correctly treat visual grading data as ordinal and categorical [29].

An added advantage of the logistic regression model is that it can simultaneously consider multiple factors influencing the quality of the image. The inclusion of multiple factors in the logistic statistical model means that more complete detailed information can be obtained [27, 28]. Based on this information a specific clinical decision can be taken.

The findings of the VGC and ordinal regression analysis also led to consultation with participating resident radiologists highlighting the importance of image quality criteria for CT head imaging, which could be weighted differently depending on the pathology being investigated. Asked to rate the five criteria in order of importance, they concluded that criterion 1 (*visually sharp reproduction of the border between white and grey matter*) and criterion 5 (*visually sharp reproduction of the cerebro-spinal fluid space over the brain*) are the two most important. The majority of brain pathologies such as infarcts and brain tumours require image quality levels that allow differentiation between these structures. In the

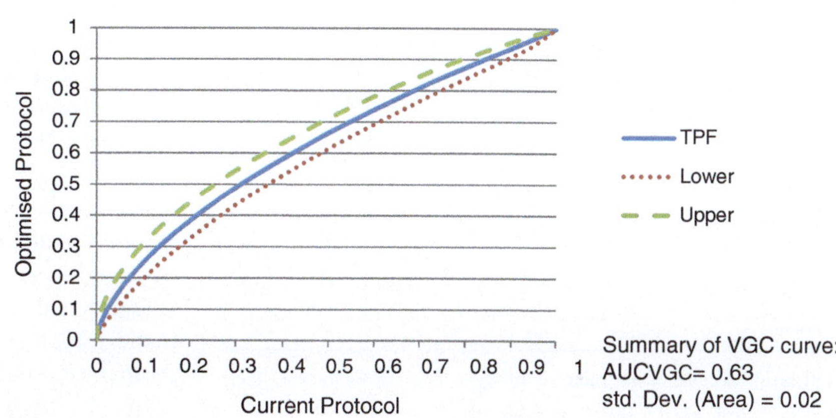

Fig. 2 VGC curve—Philips Brilliance

Table 2 AUC_{VGC} results of one-paired sample t-test

Head	Test value =0.5								
	N	Mean	SD	SE mean	t	df	p-value	Mean difference	95 % confidence interval of the difference	
Malta AUC_{VGC}	4	0.56	0.06	0.03	1.89	3	0.16	0.06	−0.04	0.15

case of suspected fresh haemorrhage, since it is hyperdense in relation to the surrounding brain tissue, a lower image quality may be sufficient for diagnosis. No specific criteria were indicated for white matter disease as this is normally determined by MRI.

Based on the results of both VGC and ordinal regression analysis performed in this study, the optimised protocols were implemented for all patient presentations (inclusive of trauma) for general brain on the GE BrightSpeed scanner as the negative odds did not affect any of the two most important criteria. However, the optimised protocol was limited to follow-up cases on the Philips Brilliance as criteria 1 findings were affected by the optimisation process and this was considered important for initial diagnosis by the radiology experts.

While low-dose CT has been shown to be viable in high contrast imaging [6], it is still unclear whether the same radiation dose reductions are possible in areas of low contrast differences such as intracranial brain structures. Initial CT examinations are mainly targeted for the diagnosis of subtle changes in intracranial structures such as lacunar infarcts requiring optimal contrast resolution and therefore it may not be appropriate to use low-dose, high-noise scan protocols [43]. Follow-up CT examinations on the other hand are performed with the purpose of identifying gross morphological changes involving structures with high contrast or large structures and can therefore benefit from the use of radiation dose reduced protocols especially if performed for repeat patient imaging. The indications of follow-up brain scans are frequently gross imaging findings that may change or affect the clinical management of the patient. Examples include follow-up for traumatic or non-traumatic haemorrhage, raptured aneurysms, stroke or evaluation of ventricular size in cases of hydrocephalus [6, 43, 44].

Table 3 Overall results: ordinal regression analysis

Omnibus test			
	Likelihood ratio Chi-square	df	p-value
Philips Brilliance	170.19	6	0.00
GE BrightSpeed	310.00	6	0.00
Tests of model effects			
Type III			
Source	Wald chi-square	df	p-value
Philips Brilliance			
DLP	1.25	1	0.26
Criteria	1.25	1	0.26
Protocol	44.53	1	0.00
GE BrightSpeed			
DLP	0.02	1	0.90
Criteria	11.81	1	0.00
Protocol	278.47	4	0.00

Dependent variable: rating score

Model: (Threshold), DLP, criteria, protocol

A limitation of this study is that image quality evaluation was based primarily on morphologically normal anatomical structures. Radiologists were not asked to evaluate or comment on any pathology present in the image data sets. So the question still remains as to whether this low radiation dose is applicable for specific brain pathologies, which frequently present as low contrast differences in comparison to normal brain tissue [6, 43–45]. The inclusion of pathologies together with an ROC analysis to investigate the applicability of the optimised protocols in the diagnosis of subtle to obvious pathologies is recommended. Consideration of different weighting levels for anatomical criteria is suggested by the authors to be incorporated in future image quality research.

The absence of a significant finding may be related to an insufficient number of observations rather than as a result of the statistical approaches applied; however the number of observations involving six expert readers and 66 CT data sets pre and post optimisation aligns with similar observer studies and exceeds several [46–49]. Additionally, as the CT images were of the brain, the variability in subject matter was minimal with respect to anatomical criteria due to patient size differences compared to studies that have looked at other anatomical regions such as the chest or abdomen. It is therefore suggested that the findings are representative of the statistical tool employed. Currently research incorporating both VGC and ordinal regression analysis in review of clinical images and anatomical criteria is limited and

Table 4 Criteria results: ordinal regression analysis

Parameter	Parameter estimates		95 % Wald confidence interval		Hypothesis test		
	Odds (B)	S E	Lower	Upper	Wald chi-square	Df	p-value
GE BrightSpeed							
Threshold [rating score=1]	−1.87	0.57	−2.98	−0.75	10.73	1	0.00
[Rating score=2]	−0.60	0.57	−1.71	0.51	1.12	1	0.29
[Rating score=3]	0.44	0.57	−0.67	1.55	0.61	1	0.44
[Rating score=4]	1.46	0.57	0.35	2.58	6.62	1	0.01
DLP	0.00	0.00	−0.00	0.00	0.02	1	0.90
[Criteria=1]	0.61	0.20	0.23	1.02	9.42	1	0.00
[Criteria=2]	−1.17	0.15	−1.46	−0.87	60.80	1	0.00
[Criteria=3]	0.95	0.15	0.65	1.24	39.22	1	0.00
[Criteria=4]	0.38	0.15	0.09	0.67	6.622	1	0.01
[Criteria=5]	0.00	.	.	.	.	.	.
[Protocol=1]	0.35	0.1005	0.15	0.54	11.81	1	0.00
[Protocol=2]	0	.	.	.	.	.	.
(Scale)	1						
Philips Brilliance							
Threshold [rating Score=1]	−4.46	0.56	−5.56	−3.36	63.45	1	0.00
[Rating score=2]	−2.47	0.53	−3.50	−1.44	22.01	1	0.00
[Rating score=3]	−1.16	0.52	−2.18	−0.14	4.97	1	0.03
[Rating score=4]	1.28	0.52	0.26	2.29	6.01	1	0.01
DLP	−0.00	0.00	−0.00	0.00	1.25	1	0.26
[Criteria=1]	−1.02	0.20	−1.42	−0.62	24.86	1	0.00
[Criteria=2]	−1.37	0.20	−1.77	−0.10	45.34	1	0.00
[Criteria=3]	0.62	0.20	0.23	1.02	9.42	1	0.00
[Criteria=4]	0.03	0.20	−0.37	0.43	0.02	1	0.90
[Criteria=5]	0.00	.	.	.	.	.	.
[Protocol=1]	0.86	0.129	0.61	1.12	44.53	1	0.00
[Protocol=2]	0	.	.	.	.	.	.
(Scale)	1						

Dependent variable: rating score model: (Threshold), DLP, criteria, protocol

therefore further research involving these statistical test tools is recommended.

The use of image quality criteria facilitates the use of visual grading studies. European guidelines on quality criteria for computed tomography (EUR 16262) list anatomical structures for the visualisation for specific CT examinations such as the cranium (general brain and skull base); face and neck (face, sinuses, petrous bone, orbits, sella, salivary glands, pharynx and larynx); spine (vertebral and paravertebral structures, lumbar spine, disc herniation and spinal cord); chest (general chest, mediastinal vessels and high resolution CT); abdomen and pelvis (general abdomen, liver, spleen, kidneys, pancreas, adrenal glands and general pelvis); bones and joints (pelvis and shoulder) [36]. Additional research is recommended to encompass the range of CT examinations indicated in the European guidelines with increased focus upon anatomical structural criterion definition and the weighting of criteria with respect to the diversity of patient presentation.

Conclusion

This work has confirmed the utility of VGC and ordinal regression during optimisation of radiation dose and image quality in CT. These are valid statistical methods for the data generated during VGA experiments. The use of this method should be encouraged over statistical tests for VGA that assume normality or continuous data.

References

1. Mayo J, Aldrich J, Muller N (2003) Radiation exposure at chest CT: a statement of the Fleischner Society. Radiology 228:15–21
2. Kalra M, Maher M, Toth T, Hamberg L, Blake M, Shepard J et al (2004) Strategies for CT radiation dose optimization. Radiology 230: 619–628
3. Mattson S, Soderberg M (2011) Radiation dose management in CT, SPECT/CT and PET/CT techniques. Radiat Prot Dosim 147(1–2): 13–21
4. Watson S, Jones A, Oatway W, Hughes J. Ionising radiation exposure of the UK population: 2005 review. Health Protection Agency/ Radiation Protection Division. HPA-RPD-001, May, 2005. p 1–104
5. Manning D (1998) Evaluation of diagnostic performance in radiography. Radiography 4:40–60
6. Cohnen M, Fischer H, Hamacher J, Lins E, Kotter R, Modder U (2000) CT of the head by use of reduced current and kilovoltage: relationship between image quality and dose reduction. AJNR 215: 1654–1660
7. Primak A, McCollough C, Bruesewitz M, Zhang J, Fletcher J (2006) Relationship between noise, dose, and pitch in cardiac multidetector row CT. RadioGraphics 26:1785–1794
8. McNitt-Gray M (2006) Tradeoffs in CT image quality and dose. Med Phys 33(6):2154–2162
9. Wessling J, Fischbach R, Meier N, Allkemper T, Klusmeier J, Ludwig K et al (2003) CT Colonography: protocol optimization with multi-detector row CT—Study in an anthropomorphic colon phantom. Radiology 228:753–759
10. Kalender W (2005) Computed tomography: fundamentals, system technology, image quality, applications. Publicis Corporate Publishing, Erlangen
11. Martin C, Sutton D, Sharp P (1999) Balancing patient dose and image quality. Appl Radiat Isot 50:1–19
12. Marmolya G, Wiesen E, Yagan R, Harija C, Shah A (1991) Paranasal sinuses: low dose CT. Radiology 181:689–691
13. Mansson L (2000) Methods for the evaluation of image quality: a review. Radiat Prot Dosim 90(1–2):89–99
14. Haaga J (2001) Radiation dose management: weighing risk versus benefit. AJR 177:289–291
15. Kalra M, Prasad S, Saini S, Blake M, Varghese J, Halpern E et al (2002) Clinical comparison of standard dose and 50 % reduced dose abdominal CT: effect on image quality. AJR 179:1101–1106
16. Ludewig E, Richter A, Frame M (2010) Diagnostic Imaging—evaluating image quality using visual grading characteristic (VGC) analysis. Vet Res Commun 34:473–479
17. Jurik A, Petersen J, Jessen K, Bongartz G, Geleijns J, Golding S et al (2000) Clinical use of image quality criteria in computed tomography: a pilot study. Radiat Prot Dosim 90(1–2):47–52
18. Chakraborty D (2006) A search model and figure of merit for observer data acquired according to the free-response paradigm. Phys Med Biol 51:3449–3462
19. Pachoud M, Verdun F, Moeckli R, Hessler C, Lepori D, Valley J (2000) New screen-film characterisation by means of objective and subjective methods. Radiat Prot Dosim 90(1–2):177–180
20. Ciantar D, Fitzgerald M, Cotterill D, Pettett A, Cook V, Beluffi G et al (2000) Correlation between quantitative and subjective assessment of image quality in pediatric radiology. Radiat Prot Dosim 90(1–2):185–188
21. Zarb F, Rainford L, McEntee M (2010) AP diameter shows the strongest correlation with CTDI and DLP in abdominal and chest CTRadiat Prot Dosimetry 140(3):266–273. doi:10.1093/rpd/ncq115
22. Jurik A, Jessen K, Hansen J (1997) Image quality and dose in computed tomography. Eur Radiol 7:77–81
23. Crawley M, Booth A, Wainwright A (2001) A practical approach to the first iteration in the optimizatiion of radiation dose and image quality in CT: estimates of the collective dose savings achieved. BJR 74:607–614
24. Gerber T, Kuzo R, Morin R (2005) Techniques and parameters for estimating radiation exposure and dose in cardiac computed tomography. Int J Cardiovasc Imaging 21:165–176
25. Bath M, Mansson L (2007) Visual grading characteristics (VGC) analysis: a non-parametric rank-invariant statistical method for image quality evaluation. BJR 80:169–176
26. Smedby O, Fredrikson M, De Geer J, Borgen L, Sandborg M. Quantifying the potential for dose reduction with visual grading regression. [Conference proceedings.]. MIPS XIV conference, Dublin, Ireland., August, 2011, 2011
27. Scott S, Goldberg M, Mayo N (1997) Statistical assessment of ordinal outcomes in comparative studies. J Clin Epidemiol 50(1): 45–55
28. Smedby O, Fredrikson M (2010) Visual grading regression: analysing data from visual grading experiments with regression models. BJR 83:767–775
29. Smedby O, Fredrikson M, De Geer J, Borgen L, Sandborg M (2012) Quantifying the potential for dose reduction with visual grading regression. BJR. doi:10.1259/bjr/31197714, Published ahead of print June 20, 2012
30. Zarb F, Rainford L, McEntee M (2011) Developing optimized CT scan protocols: Phantom measurements of image quality. Radiogr 17 (1):109–114
31. Zarb F, McEntee M, Rainford L (2013). CT radiation dose and image quality optimization using a porcine model. Radiol Technol (85): 127–36
32. Borjesson S, Hakansson M, Bath M, Kheddache S, Svensson S, Tingberg A et al (2005) A software tool for increased efficiency in observer performance studies in radiology. Radiat Prot Dosim 114(1–3):45–52
33. Samei E, Badano A, Chakraborty D, Compton K, Cornelius C, Corrigan K et al (2005) Assessment of display performance for medical imaging systems: executive summary of AAPM TG18 report. Med Phys 32(4):1205–1225
34. GE Health Care, 2010, *GE Health Care Advantage Work Station* <http://www.gehealthcare.com/usen/aw/index.html>. Accessed 10 Aug 2010
35. Brennan P, McEntee M, Evanoff M, Philips P, O'Connor W et al (2007) Ambient lighting: effect of illumination on soft-copy viewing of radiographs of the wrist. AJR 188:W177–W180
36. European Commission (1999) Guidance on diagnostic reference levels (DRLs) for medical exposures. Radiation Protection 109
37. McNitt-Gray M (2002) Radiation dose in CT. RadioGraphics 22: 1541–1553
38. ICRU (2005) Patient dosimetry for x-rays used in medical imaging. J ICRU 5(2):1–19
39. Flohr T, Ohnesorge B (2006) Developmens in CT. Imaging 18:45–61
40. Hatziioannou K, Papanastassiou E, Delichas M, Bousbouras P (2003) A contribution to the establishment of diagnostic reference levels in CT. BJR 76:541–545

41. Hidajat N, Maurer J, Schroder R, Nunnemann AWM, Pauli K, Felix R (1999) Relations between physical dose quantities and patient dose in CT. BJR 72:556–561
42. Daly L, Bourke G, McGilvray J (2000) Interpretation and uses of medical statistics, 5th edn. Blackwell Science, Oxford
43. Mullins M, Lev M, Bove P, O'Reilly C, Saini S, Rhea J et al (2004) Comparison of image quality between conventional and low dose enhanced head CT. AJNR 25:533–538
44. Britten A, Crotty M, Kiremidjian H, Grundy A (2004) The addition of computer simulated noise to investigate radiation dose and image quality in images with spatial correlation of statistical noise: an example application to X-ray CT of the brain. BJR 77:323–328
45. Gundogdu S, Mahmutyazicioglu K, Ozdemir H, Savranlar A, Asil K (2005) Assessment of image quality of a standard and three dose reducing protocols in adult cranial CT. Eur Radiol 15(9):1959–1968
46. Foley S, McEntee M, Achenbach S, Brennan P, Rainford L, Dodd J (2011) Breast surface radiation dose during coronary CT angiography: reduction by breast displacement and lead shielding. AJR 197:367–373
47. McNulty J, Ryan J, Evanoff M, Rainford L (2012) Flexible image evaluation: IPad versus secondary-class monitors for review of MR spinal emergency cases, a comparative study. Acad Radiol 19(8): 1023–1028
48. Robinson J, Ryan J, McEntee M, Lewis S, Evanoff M, Rainford L et al (2013) Grey-scale inversion improves detection of lung nodules. Br J Radiol 86, 20110812
49. Leong D, Rainford L, Haygood T, Whitman G, Tchou P, Geiser W et al (2013) Verification of DICOM GSDF in complex backgrounds. J Digit Imaging 25:662–669

3

Cross-sectional imaging of common and unusual complications after endoscopic retrograde cholangiopancreatography

Massimo Tonolini · Alessandra Pagani · Roberto Bianco

Abstract Endoscopic retrograde cholangiopancreatography (ERCP) is currently a primarily therapeutic procedure that is extensively employed to treat several biliopancreatic disorders. Although widely considered a safe procedure, ERCP is associated with a non-negligible morbidity and occasional mortality. Due to the number and complexity of operative ERCPs performed, radiologists are increasingly faced with urgent requests for investigation of suspected post-procedural complications, which often have similar clinical and laboratory manifestations. This pictorial essay reviews the usual post-procedural CT findings, the clinical features and imaging appearances of common and unusual post-ERCP occurrences including interstitial oedematous and necrotising acute pancreatitis, haemorrhages, retroperitoneal and intraperitoneal duodenal perforations, infections and stent-related complications. Emphasis is placed on the pivotal role of multidetector CT, which is warranted after complex or prolonged ERCP procedures as it represents the most effective modality to detect and grade ERCP-related complications and to monitor nonsurgically treated patients. Timely diagnosis and optimal management require a combination of clinical and laboratory data with imaging appearances; therefore, this article aims to provide an increased familiarity with interpretation of early post-ERCP studies, particularly to triage those occurrences that require interventional or surgical treatment. In selected patients MRI allows imaging pancreatitis and abnormal collections without the use of ionising radiation.

Teaching Points

- *Endoscopic retrograde cholangiopancreatography (ERCP) allows treating many biliopancreatic disorders.*
- *Due to the number and complexity of procedures, post-ERCP complications are increasingly encountered.*
- *Main complications include acute pancreatitis, haemorrhages, duodenal perforation and infections.*
- *Diagnosis and management of complications rely on combined clinical, laboratory and imaging data.*
- *Multidetector CT is most effective to diagnose, categorise and monitor post-ERCP complications.*

Keywords Endoscopic retrograde cholangiopancreatography (ERCP) · Complications · Computed tomography (CT) · Acute pancreatitis · Duodenal perforation

Introduction

Background

Due to the widespread availability of non-invasive imaging techniques such as magnetic resonance cholangiopancreatography (MRCP) and multidetector computed tomography (CT), during the last decade endoscopic retrograde cholangiopancreatography (ERCP) has evolved from a diagnostic tool towards a primarily therapeutic procedure. Currently indispensable in surgical practice, ERCP is extensively used to treat several disorders of the biliopancreatic system so that over 500,000 procedures are performed yearly in the USA [1].

M. Tonolini (✉) · A. Pagani · R. Bianco
Department of Radiology, "Luigi Sacco" University Hospital, Via G.B. Grassi 74, 20157 Milan, Italy
e-mail: mtonolini@sirm.org

The growing number of indications for ERCP encompass retained or recurrent choledocholithiasis, benign and malignant biliary strictures, ampullary stenosis, sphincter of Oddi dysfunction (SOD), postoperative and traumatic ductal injuries, acute gallstone and chronic pancreatitis. Widely considered a safe procedure that often obviates the need for surgery (particularly in frail patients with poor performance status), ERCP has limited contraindications such as upper aerodigestive obstruction, severe coagulopathy, oesophageal and/or gastric varices, anaphylactic reaction to iodinated contrast medium (CM), acute nonbiliary pancreatitis, severe cardiopulmonary impairment and recent myocardial infarction. ERCP is technically challenging in patients with pancreatico-duodenectomy or Billroth type II surgical reconstruction, unfeasible with the previous Roux-en-Y anastomosis. Following identification and cannulation of the ampullary orifice and CM injection under fluoroscopy, current endoscopic equipment allows performing sphincterotomy, extraction of common bile duct (CBD) stones, lithotripsy, biliary drainage, stricture dilatation, brush cytology and biopsy [1–3].

Furthermore, endoscopic positioning of biliary prostheses allows minimally invasive management of obstructive jaundice from benign and neoplastic causes with high technical (over 90 %) and clinical (approximately 80 %) success rates. Plastic stents are commonly used to treat benign strictures, postoperative bile leaks and pancreatic diseases. Conversely, self-expanding metal stents (SEMS) may provide effective palliation of malignant biliary obstruction [4, 5].

However, ERCP is associated with a non-negligible post-procedural morbidity (estimated in the range 4–10 % overall). The most common short-term (occurring within 3 days) complications include more or less severe cardiopulmonary problems (hypoxia, arrhythmia and aspiration) commonly associated with medications used for sedation and analgesia. The reported incidence of ERCP-specific complications ranges from 5 to 40 %, depending on the underlying diagnosis, patient age and comorbidities, complexity of the procedure, and operator experience. The most common occurrences include post-ERCP acute pancreatitis (PEAP, 2–9 %), haemorrhage (1.3–3.7 %), infection (1.9–3.6 %) and duodenal perforation (DP) in descending order of frequency. Additionally, a variety of rare complications have been occasionally reported, including pneumothorax, portal venous air embolism, splenic injury and perforation of colonic diverticula [2, 6–9].

The risk of complications is increased by operative techniques such as use of balloons and dilating catheters, tissue sampling, mechanical lithotripsy and wire baskets for stone extraction, and plastic and metallic biliary stents. Mostly related to operative procedures, ERCP-related mortality (0.5–1.4 %) may result from any of the above-mentioned complications and is particularly high in elderly patients with comorbidities and in centres with limited caseloads [2, 6–8, 10].

Aim

According to the guidelines issued by the American Society for Gastrointestinal Endoscopy (ASGE) and the World Society of Emergency Surgery (WSES), diagnosis and management of ERCP-related complications should rely upon a combination of clinical, laboratory and imaging data. Since iatrogenic complications represent a non-negligible cause of litigation and lawsuits, early recognition and prompt appropriate intervention are essential in optimising patient management and outcome [6, 11, 12].

Based upon 8 years of personal experience at a university-based general hospital where approximately 230 ERCPs are performed each year, this pictorial essay reviews and illustrates the normal post-procedural appearances observed shortly after ERCP, and the imaging findings associated with common and unusual complications, aiming to provide radiologists with an increased familiarity with interpretation of early post-procedural studies for an optimal triage of complications. Most of the emphasis is placed on the pivotal role of multidetector CT, which represents, according to the WSES guidelines for management of intra-abdominal infections, the preferred and most effective modality to comprehensively investigate the abdomen and pelvis to search for possible iatrogenic complications [6, 12–15].

Early post-ERCP imaging: indications, techniques, usual findings and reactive changes

Clinical features and indications for imaging

In the vast majority of cases, the clinical suspicion of early iatrogenic complications is based on a combination of intraprocedural findings (difficult or repeated cannulation, suspected or confirmed DP), symptoms and physical signs (sudden or worsening abdominal pain, distension, fever, haemodynamic impairment) and laboratory data (decreasing haemoglobin, elevated leukocyte count, acute phase reactants, serum lipase or amylase). The key role of CT imaging to investigate patients who become acutely ill hours or days after ERCP results from the limited value of physical examination (due to the retroperitoneal location of most iatrogenic changes) and the similar clinical and laboratory manifestations observed in most complications, particularly AP and DP [2, 6, 12].

Furthermore, ERCP duration may represent a surrogated marker for challenging cannulation and/or operative manoeuvres that can lead to papillary oedema and compromise ductal outflow, thus resulting in an increased risk and severity of complications, particularly PEAP. According to both the literature and personal experience, planned CT may be warranted in patients after prolonged ERCP procedures, particularly with sphincterotomy or multiple cannulations [16].

CT technique, usual post-procedural findings and reactive changes

A preliminary unenhanced CT acquisition without intravenous and peroral CM is helpful to visualise extraluminal air (particularly using image review at lung or bone window settings) and hyperattenuating (35–70 Hounsfield units, HU) fresh blood. Afterwards, following standard-dose intravenous CM injection we recommend a biphasic (arterial-dominant and venous) acquisition, particularly to identify pancreatic necrosis and CM extravasation indicating active bleeding. Additionally, in selected cases gastroduodenal opacification by means of peroral ingestion of diluted enteral CM may be beneficial to confirm or exclude leakage indicating DP (Fig. 1) [6, 13–15].

After ERCP the presence of air in the biliary tree is an expected, common finding. Intra- and extrahepatic pneumobilia is visible in the majority of patients studied with CT within a few weeks from the procedure and may persist for months or years in patients who underwent sphincterotomy (Fig. 2). Shortly after ERCP retained CM is commonly seen in the biliary tree and gallbladder, often with a characteristic stratified appearance (Fig. 2) [13, 15].

Multiplanar CT reformations (Figs. 2 and 3) provide high-resolution visualisation of biliary endoprostheses, whether of plastic or metallic reticular "mesh" material, and of their anatomical relationships. When interpreting post-procedural studies, the stent type should be reported along with the integrity, patency and position including proximal and distal extremities [13, 17].

In up to 29 % of asymptomatic patients, limited retroperitoneal air observed within 24 h from ERCP may result from excessive insufflation during and after endoscope withdrawal. Although this occurrence is categorised as type IV perforation according to the Stapfer classification (Table 1), we suggest not to emphasise the term "perforation" in the radiological report, since its does not require treatment [8, 18, 19].

Finally, reversible oedematous-type mural thickening consistent with acute duodenitis (Fig. 3) may be observed following therapeutic ERCP [20].

Role and limitations of ultrasound and magnetic resonance imaging (MRI)

Compared to CT, sonographic investigation of patients with suspected post-ERCP complications is strongly limited by the usual abdominal distension due to ileus, pneumoperitoneum or pneumoretroperitoneum and by its inability to assess pancreatic necrosis and bleeding. Practically, ultrasound may be useful for rapid assessment of the gallbladder and biliary tree (with or without stents) and for follow-up of known collections, and its use is not recommended by current practice guidelines [6, 12, 14, 21].

An increasingly attractive alternative modality, MRI can image PEAP and abnormal collections without use of ionising radiation, and it is particularly beneficial in young patients. Unenhanced T1- and T2-weighted sequences with and without fat suppression may be

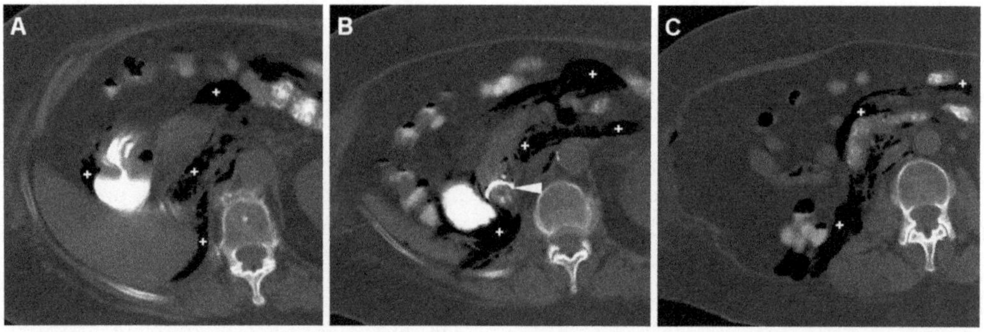

Fig. 1 During endoscopic retrograde cholangiopancreatography (*ERCP*), a 65-year-old female with sphincter of Oddi dysfunction experienced duodenal perforation (*DP*), which was recognised intraprocedurally and treated with endoluminal clipping. Twenty-four hours later, unenhanced multidetector CT obtained after peroral ingestion of enteral contrast medium (*CM*) and viewed at the bone window setting showed a well-opacified gastroduodenal lumen without extraluminal CM leak, consistent with sealed DP. Note the persistent extensive retroperitoneal air (+) and metallic clips (*arrowhead in B*)

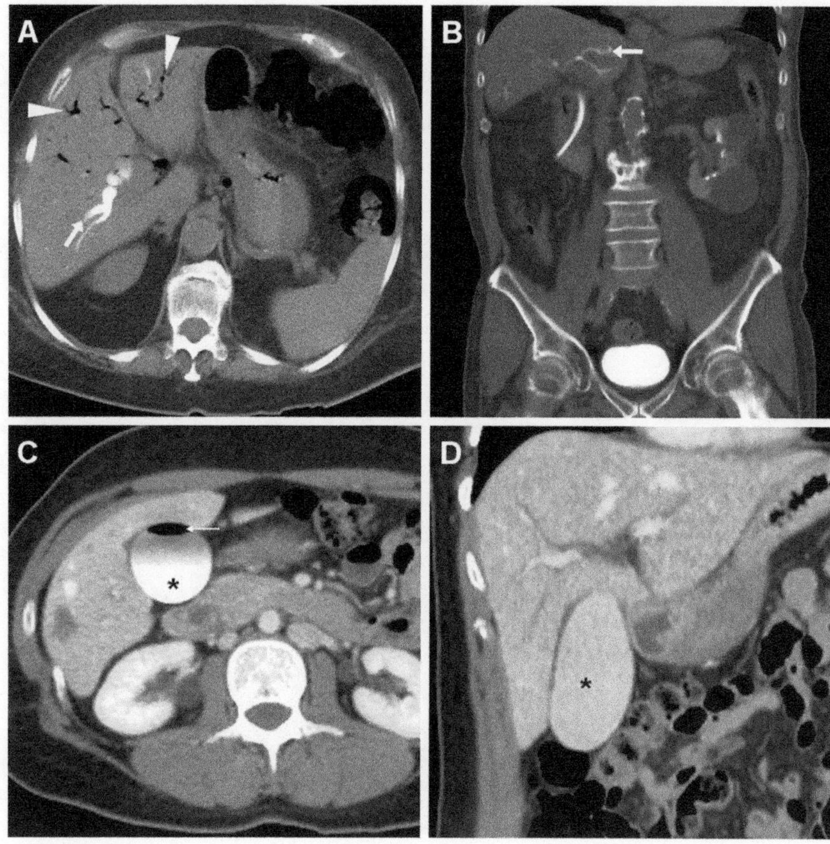

Fig. 2 Normal findings observed hours after operative ERCP in a 75-year-old male investigated with unenhanced CT (**c**, **d**) to verify correct placement of a plastic biliary stent, including dependent contrast medium (*arrows*) and air (*arrowheads*) in the intrahepatic bile ducts. In a different patient, a 44-year-old female patient suffering from acute post-procedural pain, contrast-enhanced CT (**a**, **b**) 2 days after ERCP excluded signs of acute complications and showed stratified iodinated contrast medium (*), bile and air (*thin arrow*) in the gallbladder

complemented with MRCP sequences to assess the biliary and pancreatic ducts and with additional dynamic fat-suppressed T1-weighted gradient echo sequences during intravenous gadolinium contrast when pancreatic necrosis is suspected. Furthermore, diffusion-weighted MRI may be more sensitive in detecting cases of mild pancreatic inflammation. However, despite recent technical advancements MRI remains limited in acutely ill or uncooperative patients, and the presence or pneumobilia often renders MRCP sequences uninformative or confusing [13, 22, 23].

Acute pancreatitis

Arguably the most common serious adverse event, PEAP has been reported with variable incidence (2–9 % overall, approximately 3.5 % in a meta-analysis of several prospective studies, and up to 30 % of high risk cases) according to patient selection. A transient asymptomatic increase in serum pancreatic enzymes occurs in the majority (70–75 %) of patients within 4 h after ERCP and resolves within 4 days. According to the widely used consensus definition adopted by the ASGE guidelines, diagnosis of PEAP requires at least two of the three following criteria: (1) consistent new-onset or worsening abdominal pain (persistent, severe, epigastric pain often radiating to the back); (2) new or prolongation of hospitalisation for at least 2 days; (3) abnormally elevated (at least three times above the upper normal limit) serum lipase or amylase 24 h after the procedure [2, 6, 21].

The multifactorial pathogenesis of PEAP involves mechanical factors (such as direct trauma from endoscopy, difficult bile duct cannulation and multiple pancreatic duct injections) along with enzymatic, microbiological and patient-related factors including history of allergy [24–26]. The role of iodinated CM as one of the cofactors in causing PEAP has been extensively studied. In experimental models of acute pancreatitis, digestive enzyme activation occurs rapidly within acinar cells following an initiating event: secretion blockage leads to accumulation of zymogen granules within cells, their fusion into large vacuoles, enzyme activation and finally cellular injury [24]. Besides the reduced pancreatic blood flow due to CM hyperviscosity, controversy exists on the role of the chemical effect of CM osmolality. Earlier studies reported reduced rates of pancreatic damage and decreased with newer low- or iso-osmolar compared to high-osmolar contrast medium, but other

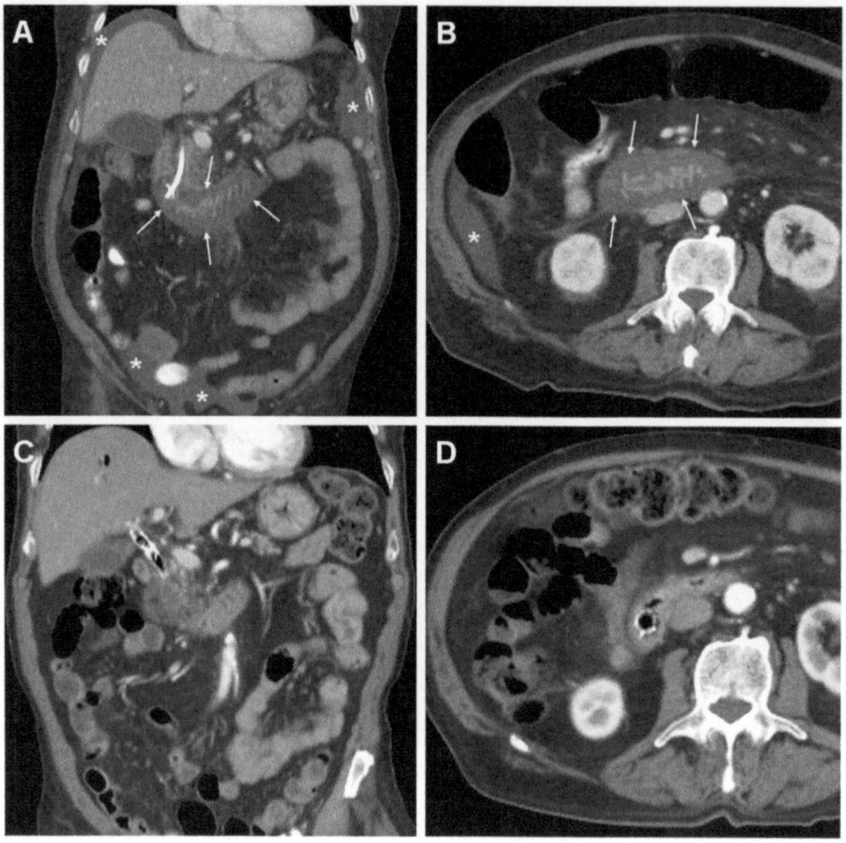

Fig. 3 Acute reversible duodenitis following ERCP. A 78-year-old male with common bile duct (*CBD*) carcinoma causing concentric stenosis of the proximal choledochus suffered from acute diffuse abdominal pain without peritonitis 24 h after ERCP including cytological brushing and positioning of a 10-French plastic biliary stent. Urgent contrast-enhanced CT (**a**, **b**) showed a correctly placed biliary stent, appearance of moderate ascites (*) and of marked circumferential thickening of the duodenum from the Vaterian papilla to the Treitz angle, with enhancing mucosa and hypoattenuating oedematous submucosa ("*target sign*", *thin arrows*), and minimal associated inflammatory changes in the periduodenal fat. Imaging findings, laboratory data and the subsequent course excluded iatrogenic pancreatitis, haemorrhage and DP. Three weeks later, the plastic biliary stent was removed and replaced with a self-expanding metal stent (*SEMS*). Follow-up CT (**d**) showed imaging resolution of both biliary obstruction and acute duodenal inflammatory changes [partly reprinted from Ref. 20]

reports including a meta-analysis did not confirm a significantly different risk and outcome of PEAP [25–28].

Probably unavoidable even in the hands of experienced endoscopists, PEAP is associated with established risk conditions including patient-specific (age below 55 years, female gender, SOD, history of AP) and procedure-related factors (difficult cannulation, standard or pre-cut sphincterotomy). Whereas the risk of bleeding and perforation is similar to that of younger patients, the elderly are less likely to experience PEAP. Clinical guidelines increasingly suggest pharmacologic prophylaxis with nonsteroidal anti-inflammatory drugs, glyceryl trinitrate or somatostatin; furthermore, in patients with SOD, the use of temporary pancreatic duct stenting has been proposed to limit the risk and severity of PEAP.

Table 1 Classification of duodenal perforations according to Stapfer et al. (Ref. 8)

Type	Description	Comment
I	Endoscope-related lateral or medial duodenal wall perforations	Often large and distant from the ampulla, requires surgical intervention in most cases
II	Retroperitoneal peri-Vaterian perforations resulting from (pre-cut) sphincterotomy	Of variable severity but most often discrete and amenable to conservative management
III	Distal common bile duct injuries secondary to guidewire insertion or instrumentation for stone extraction	Amenable to conservative management
IV	Isolated retroperitoneal air from excessive insufflation	Does not require specific treatment

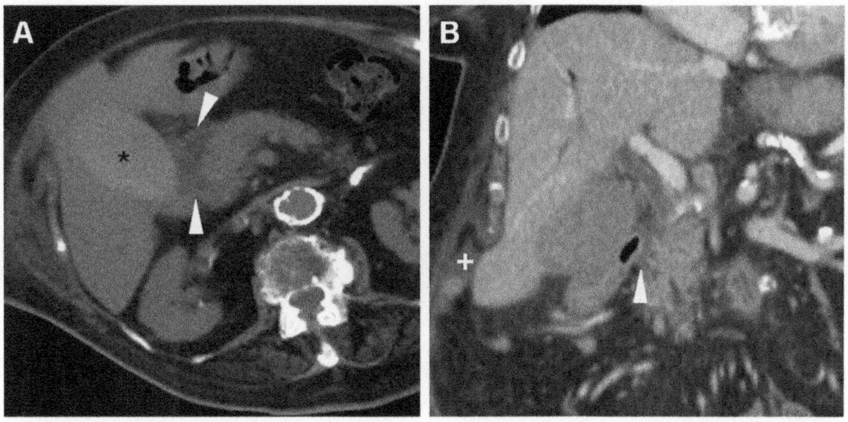

Fig. 4 Oedematous acute pancreatitis (*AP*) in a 77-year-old female 3 days after endoscopic treatment of choledocholithiasis including sphincterotomy. Unenhanced (**a**) and post-contrast (**b**) CT images showed persistent moderately hyperattenuating contrast medium (*) in the gallbladder, oedema and fluid in the pancreatico-duodenal groove (*arrows*), minimal ascites (+) consistent with clinical and laboratory features of mild AP, and excluded abnormal collections and non-enhancing parenchyma indicating pancreatic necrosis. The patient had an uneventful course with conservative treatment

Treatment is analogous to that of non-iatrogenic AP, and mortality reaches 3 % of cases [2, 6, 21].

In patients with consistent above-mentioned clinical and laboratory criteria following ERCP, early imaging is generally unnecessary to diagnose PEAP, and during the first week organ failure and systemic inflammatory response syndrome (SIRS) may be present with few local complications. Although not specifically developed for iatrogenic occurrences, the revised Atlanta classification differentiates morphologically interstitial oedematous (IEP) from necrotising acute pancreatitis (NAP), the latter associated with a high probability of infection, subsequent organ failure and increased mortality (12–30 % versus below 3 %). CT diagnosis of IEP relies on diffuse or localised enlargement of the pancreatic parenchyma with preserved homogeneous enhancement (to 80–150 HU) after intravenous CM, accompanied by peripancreatic fat stranding or by hypoattenuating (0–30 HU) acute peripancreatic fluid collections (APFCs). Containing a mixture of exudates, necrosis and blood, APFCs are adjacent to the pancreas and confined by normal fascial planes, and they display homogeneous low (0–30 HU) attenuation without a discernible wall and enhancement [22, 23].

Nevertheless, in our experience CT is requested within 24–72 h in most patients with clinical and laboratory features indicating PEAP to exclude other complications (particularly DP) with similar manifestations. Therefore, a majority of patients with IEP are imaged with near-normal or subtle CT findings, including a homogeneously enhancing pancreas, fat stranding and minimal fluid around the head and neck of the pancreas (Figs. 4 and 5). Borrowing from experience with gallstone AP, early contrast-enhanced CT obtained within 2–3 days from the onset of symptoms may underestimate the severity of PEAP including confident exclusion of necrosis so that repeated scanning may be required during post-ERCP hospitalisation [13, 15, 16, 22, 23].

Fig. 5 Oedematous AP with markedly increased serum lipase 48 h after ERCP treatment of choledocholithiasis in a 55-year-old male with previous history of biliary AP and laparoscopic cholecystectomy. Unenhanced CT (**a**) and T2-weighted MRI (**b**) images show mild peripancreatic and retroperitoneal fascial fluid (*thin arrows*) without abnormal collections. Clinical symptoms and laboratory changes regressed within 72 h

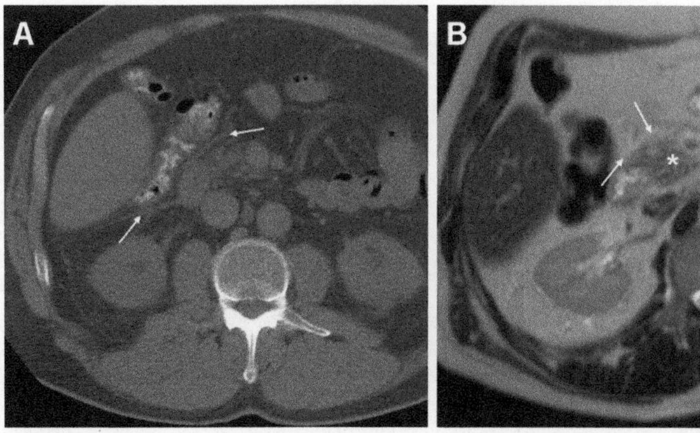

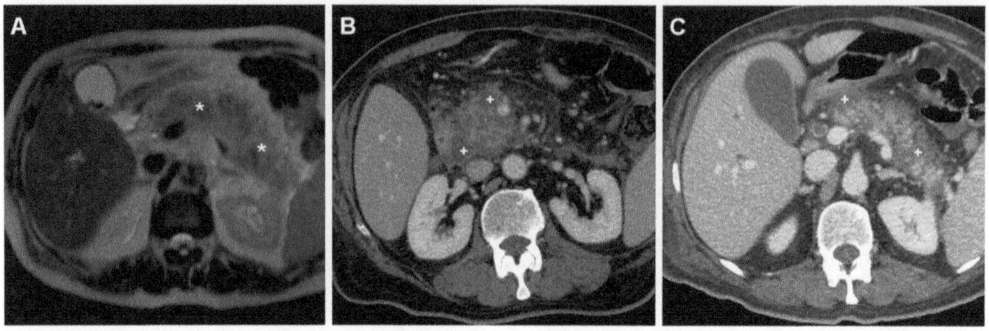

Fig. 6 Necrotising AP in a 73-year-old male after ERCP including endoscopic treatment of mild bleeding after papillotomy. Urgent MRI (T2-weighted image in **a**) requested because of increased C-reactive protein (*CRP*), leukocyte count and serum lipase showed a markedly enlarged pancreatic gland (*) with peripancreatic oedema. Contrast-enhanced CT (**b**, **c**) confirmed severe AP with inhomogeneous enhancement of the enlarged pancreas due to diffuse peripancreatic necrosis (+). The patient finally recovered after 2 weeks of in-hospital conservative treatment

Conversely, NAP includes fatty tissue necrosis in either the pancreatic parenchyma or peripancreatic tissue and corresponds at imaging to pancreatic enlargement, heterogeneous because of single or multiple areas of diminished or absent enhancement consistent with necrosis (Figs. 6 and 7). In NAP, post-necrotic peripancreatic fluid collections (PNPFCs) are commonly observed in the pancreas, peripancreatic tissue or both. PNPFCs contain fluid, necrosis and/or loculation in varying degrees. Differentiation from APFCs is very difficult in the early phase and is generally based on the presence or absence of glandular necrosis. PNPFCs may become progressively more organised and encapsulated later and are termed walled-off pancreatic necrosis after 4 weeks of symptom onset (Fig. 7) [13, 15, 16, 22, 23].

Therefore, the radiologist's role mostly relies in the identification of the presence and extent of necrosis. Severity of AP may be graded according to the modified CT severity index (M-CTSI), which takes into account the presence of pancreatic and/or peripancreatic inflammatory changes, APFCs, necrosis (<30 %, 30–50 % and over 50 %) and extrapancreatic complications such as pleural effusion, ascites, vascular or gastrointestinal involvement. The only large specific series graded PEAP severity according to M-CTSI scores as mild (≤2 points), moderate (4–6) and severe (≥8) in 53.6, 42.8 and 3.6 % of cases respectively [13, 15, 16, 22, 23].

Furthermore, peripancreatic and glandular changes consistent with PEAP are well demonstrated by MRI (Figs. 5 and 6). Typical MRI findings of AP include variable degrees of glandular enlargement with mildly increased T2-weighted signal intensity corresponding to oedema, normal signal on fat-saturated T1-weighted acquisitions, peripancreatic inflammatory fat stranding, fluid or collections. Similarly to CT, pancreatic enhancement may appear homogeneous (in IEP), diminished or heterogeneous (in NAP) after intravenous gadolinium CM. In the setting of gallstones, it has been proposed that a limited noncontrast MRI protocol has high correlation with

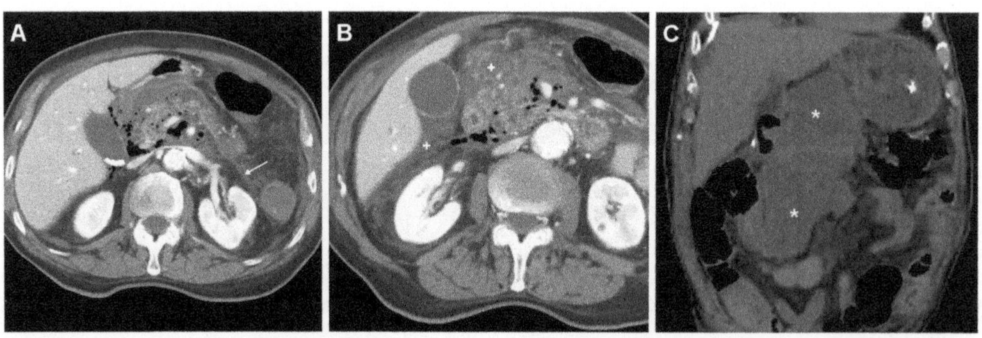

Fig. 7 Necrotising AP plus retroperitoneal air in a 79-year-old male occurring 48 h after ERCP treatment of choledocholithiasis, including sphincterotomy. Contrast-enhanced CT (**a**, **b**) showed an enlarged, markedly inhomogeneous, poorly enhancing pancreas with fascial (*thin arrow* in **a**), peripancreatic and infrahepatic (+ in **b**) fluid, gas bubbles along the superior mesenteric vessels and in the periduodenal region. Pleural effusion was present bilaterally. Urgent laparotomic surgery confirmed severe necrotic-haemorrhagic pancreatitis. During his prolonged stay in the intensive care unit, follow-up unenhanced CT (**c**) showed the appearance of a vast walled-off postnecrotic collection (*)

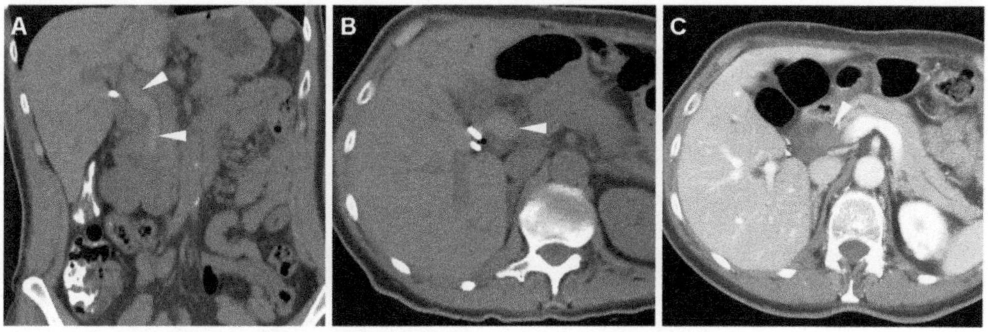

Fig. 8 Haemobilia following ERCP in a 57-year-old female with benign papillary stenosis and previous cholecystectomy, manifesting with abdominal pain and mild haemoglobin drop. Unenhanced (**a**, **b**) and post-contrast (**c**) CT images showed moderate dilatation and hyperattenuating (45 HU) content of the CBD (*arrowheads*) corresponding to endoluminal haemorrhage but initially misinterpreted as retained CM injected during the procedure, without signs of active bleeding. This complication was self-limiting and resolved on conservative treatment

contrast-enhanced CT in the assessment of mild AP. Furthermore, the use of diffusion-weighted MRI including measurement of apparent diffusion coefficients (ADCs) may allow differentiation among normal, inflamed and necrotic pancreas before or without CM administration [22, 23, 29, 30].

Haemorrhage

Primarily a complication related to sphincterotomy rather than to diagnostic ERCP, bleeding may be immediate or delayed up to 2 weeks (in up to 50 % of cases) and is clinically suggested by haematemesis, melaena or haemoglobin drop. Whereas variable degrees of bleeding occur in approximately 1–2 % of treated patients, haemorrhage is graded as mild (according to blood loss and transfusion need) in approximately 70 % of cases, with occasional mortality (0.3 %). Specific risk factors include coagulopathy, therapeutic anticoagulation, haemodialysis, acute cholangitis or papillary stenosis, pre-cut or extended sphincterotomy [2, 6].

Although clinically significant haemorrhage requiring angiographic, endoscopic or surgical intervention is rare (less than 1/1,000 sphincterotomies), CT imaging may help in the diagnosis by showing hyperattenuating fluid consistent with blood in the choledochus (Fig. 8) or duodenal lumen. Residual diluted CM in the duodenal or jejunal lumen may sometimes be confused with fresh haemorrhage. Alternatively, intramural bleeding may appear as high-attenuation duodenal wall thickening. Arterial-phase acquisition completed with maximum-intensity projection (MIP) reconstructions at vascular window settings may effectively show active contrast extravasation in the duodenum, indicating ongoing bleeding (Fig. 9). Furthermore, following operative ERCP bleeding may occasionally form intrahepatic or subcapsular hepatic haematomas with associated haemoperitoneum (Fig. 10) [13, 31, 32].

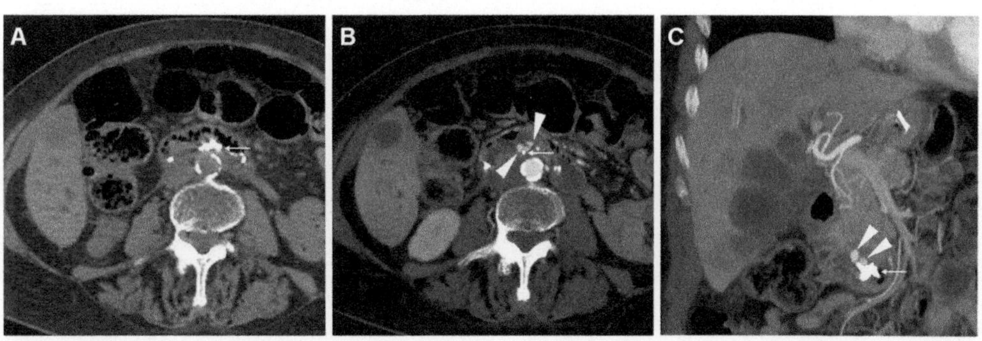

Fig. 9 Acute intraluminal bleeding in the duodenum manifesting with acute abdominal pain and impending haemodynamic shock, hours after an unsuccessful endoscopic attempt to relieve the intrahepatic biliary obstruction in 77-year-old female with recently diagnosed infiltrating gallbladder carcinoma. Operative ERCP was interrupted after sphincterotomy because of duodenal haemorrhage, which was treated with epinephrine injection and endoluminal clipping. Comparison of unenhanced (**a**) and arterial-phase (**b**, **c**) CT images detected active contrast extravasation in the duodenal lumen (*arrowheads*) abutting the metallic clips (*thin arrows*), consistent with persistently ongoing arterial haemorrhage. Endovascular therapeutic embolisation of the gastroduodenal artery was necessary to control bleeding

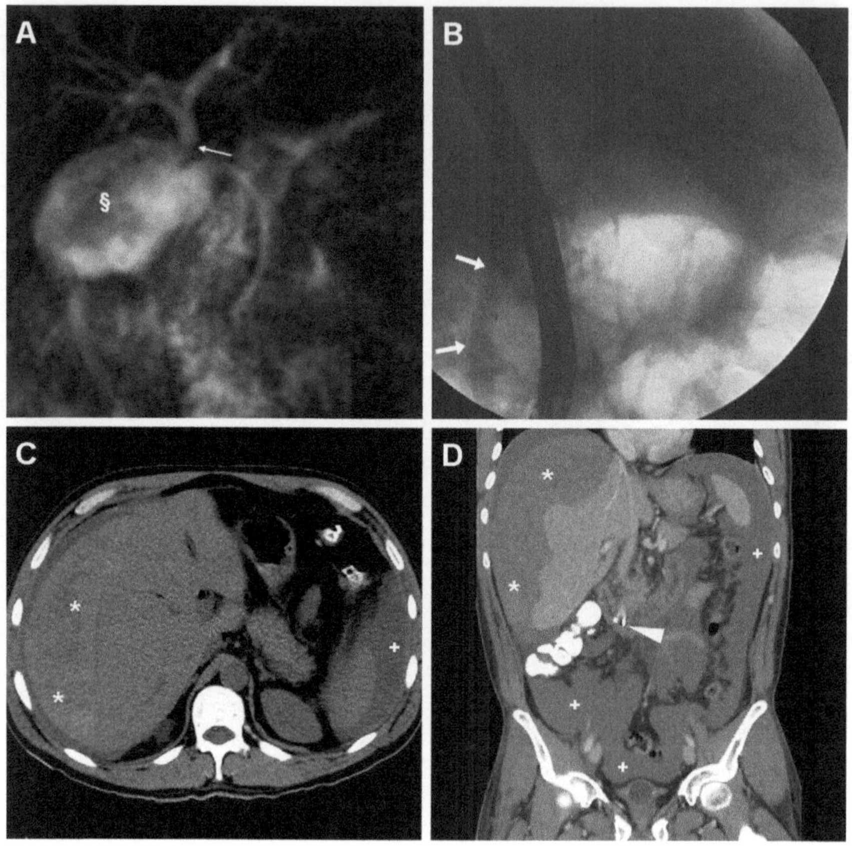

Fig. 10 A 39-year-old male with previous Bismuth type II iatrogenic bile duct injury during laparoscopic cholecystectomy 10 months earlier, shown in a coronal thick-slab MR cholangiography (*MRCP*) image (*thin arrows in* **a**), which required immediate reintervention to remove the surgical clips plus temporary plastic biliary stenting. Note haematoma in the gallbladder fossa (§). Twenty-four hours after endoscopic positioning of the covered metallic biliary stent (**b**), he suffered from sudden abdominal pain, vomiting and hypotension, and unenhanced (**c**) CT images detected a large hyperattenuating subcapsular liver haematoma (*) and haemoperitoneum (+) attributed to guidewire manoeuvres, which progressed at repeated contrast-enhancement CT on the next day (**d**), thus dictating immediate surgical evacuation

The CT detection of active bleeding represents an indication for endoscopic, interventional or surgical treatment. The generally accepted first-line treatment to control bleeding is repeated endoscopy with several haemostatic methods such as flushing with epinephrine solution, balloon tamponade, haemostatic (fibrin glue) injection, hemoclip placement, electrocoagulation or temporary stent placement. When endoscopic procedures fail, bleeding control requires interventional radiological embolisation or surgery [33–36].

Duodenal perforation

Representing the rarest yet most feared occurrence, DP complicates 0.1–1 % of ERCP procedures and is associated with a non-negligible mortality rate (9–18 %). DP is mostly associated with standard (using an electrical papillotome catheter) or pre-cut (with a needle knife) sphincterotomy extending beyond the intramural CBD portion and with guidewire manipulation. Other risk factors for ERCP-related perforation include dilated CBD, stricture dilatation, SOD, presence of peripapillar diverticula and previous Billroth II surgery [2, 6–8, 14, 19, 37, 38].

In a variable proportion (26–48 %) of patients DP is suspected or verified during ERCP by means of CM injection through the endoscope showing extraluminal CM leakage (Fig. 11). Alternatively, clinical presentation occurs hours or days later, may be closely similar to those associated with PEAP and is not unusually mild compared to the imaging findings [2, 6–8, 14, 37, 38].

The classification system proposed by Stapfer et al. (Table 1) categorises DP into four classes in descending order of severity, on the basis of the mechanism and anatomical location, in order to predict the need for surgery [8].

Although controversy exists about the optimal approach, the management of ERCP-related DP should be individualised according to its type, clinical picture and imaging findings. Whereas type I (endoscope-related) duodenal wall perforations invariably require early surgery, the majority (approximately 70 %) of patients with peri-Vaterian (type II) DP tend to seal spontaneously and thus are amenable to endoclipping (Fig. 1) or conservative management (nasogastric drainage, nil-by-mouth and parenteral nutrition, intravenous hydration and antibiotics). Currently, the therapeutic approach to management of stable patients is increasingly

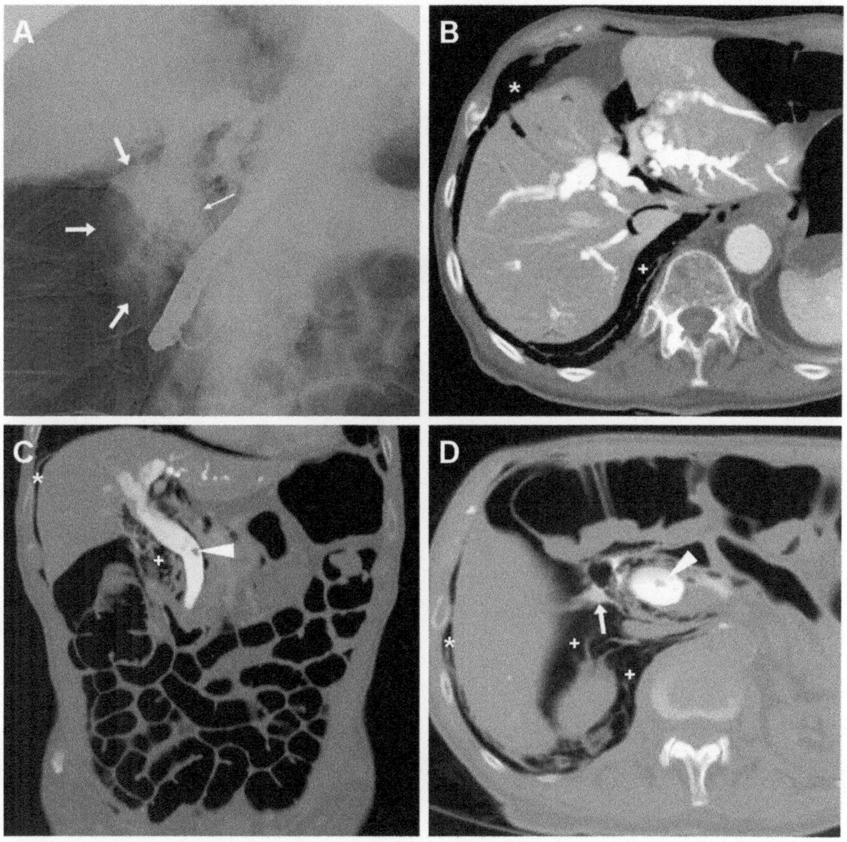

Fig. 11 An elderly 80-year-old male with multiple comorbidities underwent endoscopic treatment of choledocholithiasis, including precut sphincterotomy of the Vaterian papilla and stone retrieval using a basket device. During ERCP, fluoroscopy (**a**) showed opacification of dilated intrahepatic and common bile ducts and of a sizeable extraluminal CM collection (*thin arrows*) from lateral duodenal wall perforation (type I according to the Stapfer classification system). A few hours later CT (**b**–**d**) showed diffuse gaseous bowel distension from insufflation during endoscopy, presence of posterior pneumomediastinum, perihepatic and right parietocolic pneumoperitoneum (*), and extensive retroperitoneal emphysema in the right perirenal, posterior and anterior pararenal spaces (+). Note persistently opacified intrahepatic and common bile ducts with residual lithiasis fragments (*arrowheads*), persistently extravasated CM (*arrow* in **d**). Imaging findings and worsening clinical conditions with peritonitis dictated urgent laparotomy, which confirmed intra-abdominal free air, and included opening and toilette of common bile duct and positioning of a Kehr T-tube. The patient finally recovered after a prolonged hospital stay

nonsurgical and proves successful in approximately two-thirds of cases: unfortunately, delayed recognition of type I perforations and failure of conservative treatment are associated with a high death rate (50 %) from sepsis. As from the WSES guidelines, accepted indications for surgical treatment include clinical features such as sepsis and peritonitis, imaging features (free intraperitoneal air, periduodenal or retroperitoneal fluid collections, contrast extravasation at ERCP, CT or upper gastrointestinal study with water-soluble CM, retained stones or basket/wire endoscopic instruments) and failure of conservative management. Surgery may include perforation closure or duodenal exclusion, retroperitoneal drainage, CBD exploration and T-tube insertion [2, 6, 8, 12, 14, 38–42].

The CT imaging hallmark of DP is represented by extraluminal air, which may sometimes be located in the duodenal wall, but most commonly dissects through the retroperitoneal compartments. Due to the anatomic location of the CBD, the typical appearance of a type II DP includes air collecting posteriorly to the duodenum and pancreatic head, in the anterior pararenal and right perirenal space, surrounding the inferior vena cava, portal vein and splanchnic vessels, and sometimes crossing the midline (Figs. 11, 12, 13 and 14). Occasionally, air may track cranially in the posterior mediastinum [2, 8, 9, 13, 38].

However, the presence and amount of retroperitoneal air at imaging do not linearly correlate with the severity of the injury or with the need for invasive treatment since it rather reflects the degree of continuous endoscopic air insufflation and manipulation after an undetected injury occurred. Therefore, successful nonoperative management of type II DP with extensive retroperitoneal air is possible, provided that the patient does not

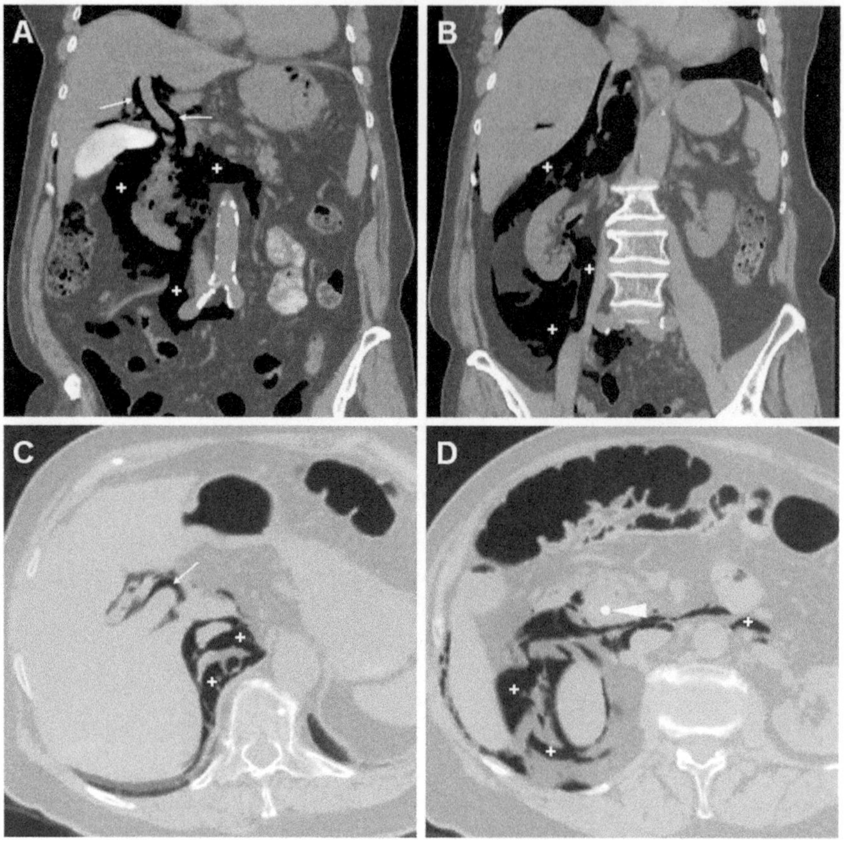

Fig. 12 Severe retroperitoneal (type II) DP in an 80-year-old female following ERCP with sphincterotomy, incomplete removal of choledocholithiasis and positioning of a plastic CBD prosthesis (*arrowhead*). Post-procedural unenhanced CT viewed at both soft-tissue (**a**, **b**) and bone (**c**, **d**) window settings showed extensive retroperitoneal air (+) predominantly located in the right peri- and pararenal spaces, around the descending duodenum and tracking along the inferior vena cava and portal vein (*thin arrows*). Surgical exploration dictated by sepsis failed to detect a perforation site, and the patient recovered fully

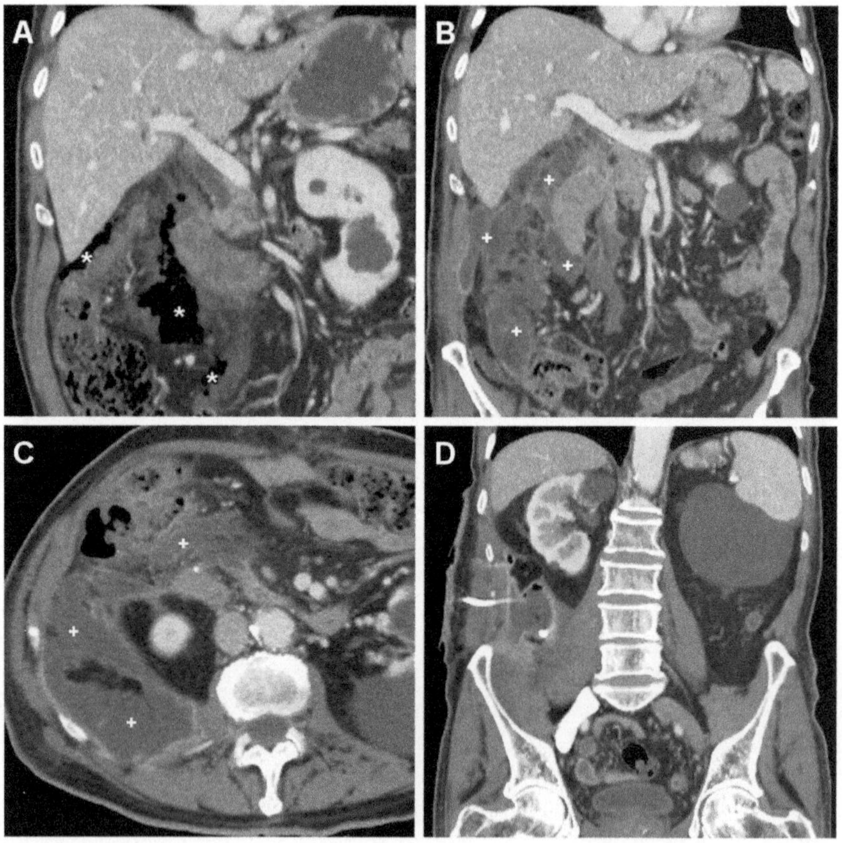

Fig. 13 Failed conservative treatment of DP in an 83-year-old male with chronic duodenal stricture who underwent ERCP to prevent further episodes of infectious cholangitis. The next day, contrast-enhanced CT (**a**) showed moderate right-sided retroperitoneal gas (*). Follow-up CT (**b**, **c**) 4 days later showed formation of multiple confluent periduodenal and right parietocolic fluid-like infected collections (+), with extensive occupation of the ipsilateral posterior pararenal space, which required percutaneous drainage (**d**) to relieve sepsis

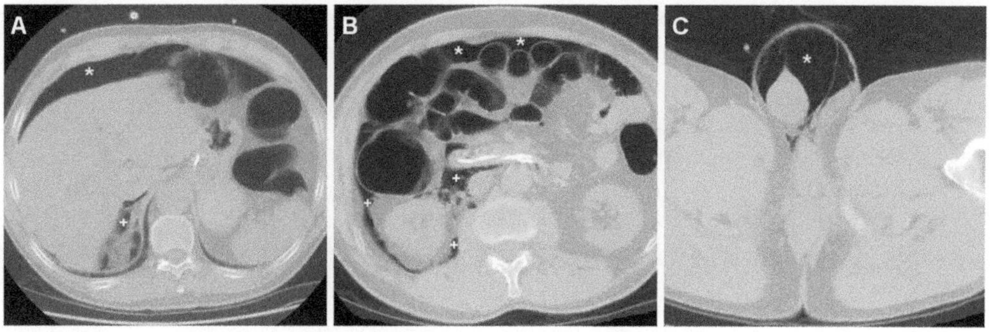

Fig. 14 Stapfer type I DP with moderate retroperitoneal air (+) plus pneumoperitoneum extending to the scrotum (*) shown by emergency unenhanced CT in a 62-year-old male undergoing ERCP treatment of choledocholithiasis. Laparotomic surgery included duodenotomy and suture of a posterior duodenal wall discontinuity, toilette and drainage of the peritoneal cavity. The subsequent course was uneventful and repeated CT with oral CM at discharge (*not shown*) excluded extraluminal contrast leak

develop peritonitis, fever or impending shock. However, negative physical findings do not reliably exclude surgery since severe DP may be masked clinically by the retroperitoneal site especially in elderly or chronically ill patients. Extraluminal CM leak (Fig. 11), pneumoperitoneum (Fig. 14) and fluid collections represent the key imaging findings, which usually shift the therapeutic approach towards surgery. During conservative treatment, repeat CT may be warranted after a 48–72-h interval to confirm sealed leaks and absent fluid collections as well as to monitor the patient until recovery [2, 6, 12, 13, 15].

Post-procedural infections

Although the current guidelines recommend antibiotic prophylaxis in known or suspected biliary obstruction, bacteraemia is a common event (15–27 %) after diagnostic or therapeutic ERCP. The reported incidence of

Fig. 15 Acute cholecystitis in a 66-year-old female manifesting with fever and transverse upper abdominal pain 3 days after ERCP with sphincterotomy and biopsy of ampullary adenoma including antibiotic prophylaxis. Multiplanar contrast-enhanced CT images show a thickened gallbladder wall (*arrows*) with focal perforation (*arrowhead* in **c**) and localised collection (*), which required emergency laparotomic cholecystectomy.

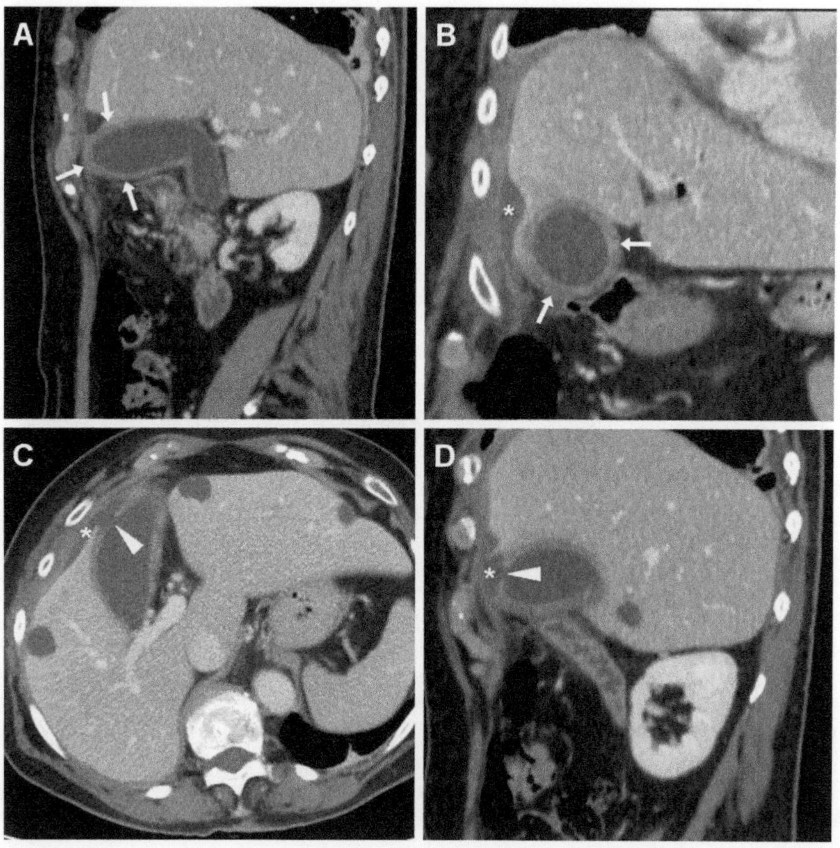

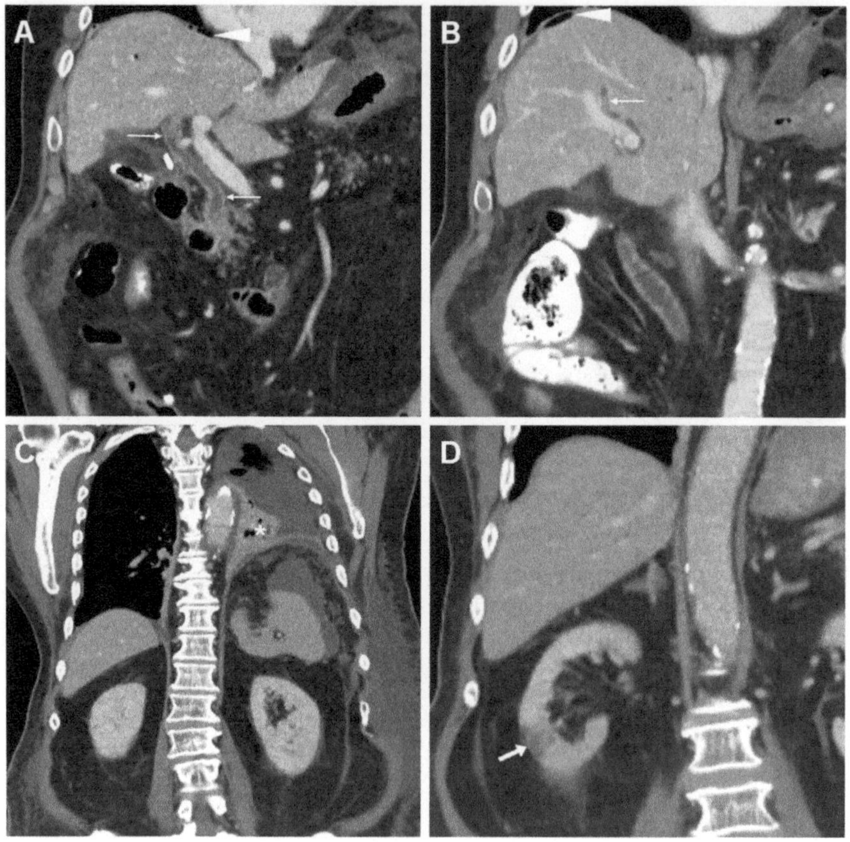

Fig. 16 Cholangitis and sepsis in an 81-year-old female following endoscopic stone removal using a Fogarty catheter. Multiplanar contrast-enhanced CT images showed minimal pneumoperitoneum (*arrowheads*) and peritoneal effusion, thickened enhancing walls of CBD and main intrahepatic ducts (*thin arrows*). Additionally, left-sided pneumonia (* in **c**) and a limited renal infarct (*arrow* in **d**) were seen. Worsening clinical conditions dictated surgery, which revealed biliary peritonitis from contained cystic duct injury. The patient recovered after a long intensive care unit stay

clinically significant iatrogenic infections is limited (1–3 %), but sepsis represents a common cause of death. Specific risk factors for infection include stenting across tumours, obstructed ducts and jaundice, combined percutaneous-endoscopic procedures, primary sclerosing cholangitis, incomplete or failed biliary drainage [2, 6].

The spectrum of post-ERCP infectious complications encompasses cholecystitis, septic cholangitis, liver abscess and systemic sepsis. Occurring in approximately 0.2–0.5 % of patients, cholecystitis has been correlated to cholelithiasis and intraprocedural filling of the gallbladder with CM, and it is heralded by the appearance

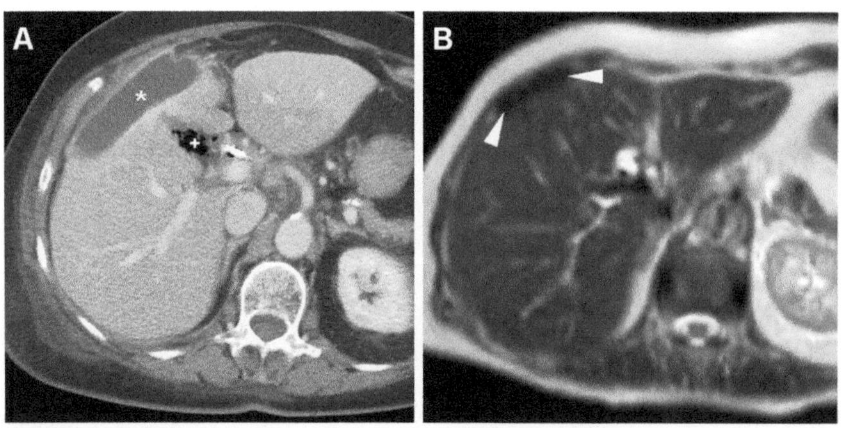

Fig. 17 Perihepatic abscess diagnosed 10 days after endoscopic stent positioning through a cytologically benign distal CBD stricture in a 78-year-old female. Contrast-enhanced CT (**a**) requested because of fever and right hypochondrium pain revealed a fluid-like collection (*) with an enhancing peripheral rim and minimal extraluminal air (+) predominantly in the right-sided retroperitoneum. Urgent surgery included cholecystectomy and abscess drainage. Postoperatively, unenhanced T2-weighted MRI (**b**) depicted resolution of the abscess (*arrowheads*)

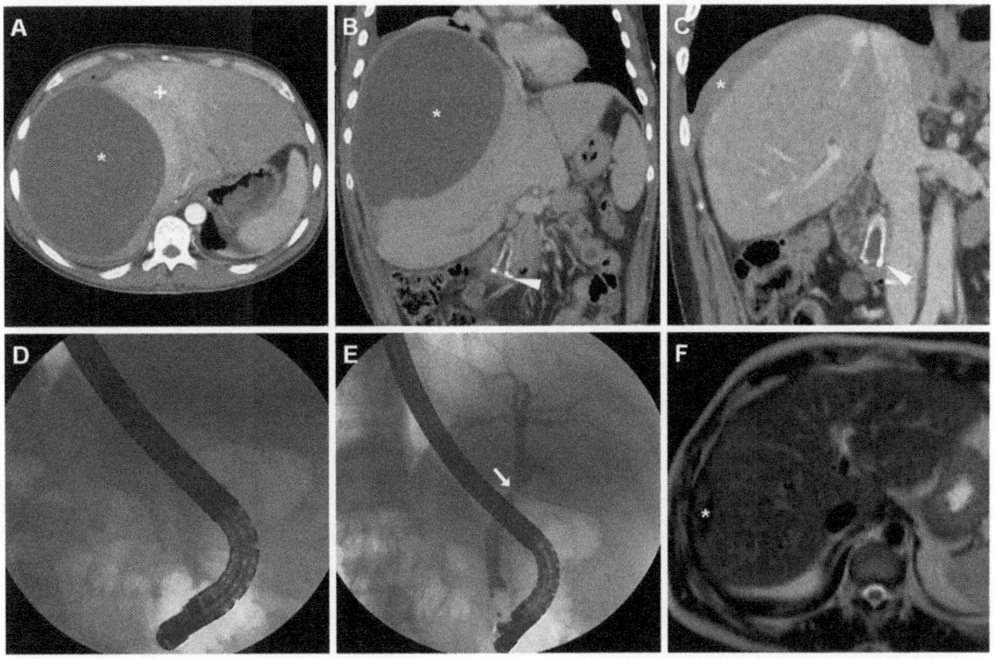

Fig. 18 One month after evacuation of the haemoperitoneum and subcapsular hepatic haematoma, the same patient in Fig. 10 suffered form right-sided thoraco-abdominal pain and fever. Arterial- (**a**) and venous-phase (**b**) CT showed a huge, fluid-attenuating (15 HU) subphrenic collection (*) with inflammatory enhancement of the surrounding, compressed liver parenchyma (+) and thin peripheral enhancement, consistent with an abscess. Ipsilateral pleural effusion and basal lung atelectasis were associated. Percutaneous drainage yielded 3 l of stinking pus. Note the correctly positioned metallic CBD stent (*arrowheads*), and clinical, laboratory and imaging (* in **c**) resolution was obtained. During endoscopic replacement, the biliary stent was not found anymore (**d**), displaced and probably lost with stools. Endoscopic cholangiogram (**e**) confirmed persistent iatrogenic biliary stricture (*arrow*). Follow-up MRI (T2-weighted image in **f**) showed resolved subphrenic abscess with low signal intensity consistent with fibrosis (*)

of luminal overdistension and circumferential mural thickening (Fig. 15). Septic cholangitis is suggested by thickened enhancing CBD and intrahepatic duct walls (Fig. 16). Accessory signs of sepsis such as atelectasis/pneumonia, splenic or renal infarcts may be observed (Fig. 16). Alternatively, sepsis may result from superinfection of PNPFCs or abnormal collections from DP (Fig. 13). Abscess collections usually display enhancing mural thickening, similar attenuation to that of non-infected fluid collections and sometimes internal gas bubbles (Figs. 17 and 18) [6, 13, 15].

Stent-related complications

Relatively rare, early complications after biliary stenting include haemorrhage (Fig. 10), PEAP, stent misplacement, perforation (Fig. 19) and injury to the CBD or main pancreatic duct [13, 17].

Chronic stent-related complications are more common and include stent obstruction (25–35 % of patients), migration, fracture or collapse, infections such cholangitis, liver abscess (Fig. 18) or sepsis. Biliary stent dislodgement (Fig. 18) occurs after a variable time interval in up to 6 % of patients

Fig. 19 In a 60-year-old male with severe chronic calcific pancreatitis, after ERCP positioning of the metallic pancreatic stent (*arrowhead* in **a**) contrast-enhanced CT showed minimal intraperitoneal air (*), which was treated conservatively with success. Note pneumobilia (*arrows*) and retained CM in the gallbladder

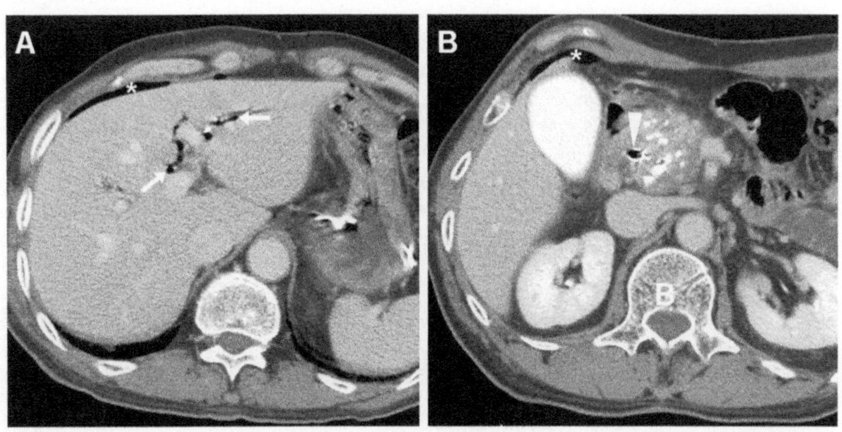

and is more frequent with plastic stents compared to SEMS. Displacement may be proximal, particularly in patients with malignant obstruction, or alternatively distal to the intestine, the latter not unusually asymptomatic [4, 5, 17, 43, 44].

Conclusion

Diagnosis and management of post-ERCP complications should combine clinical and laboratory data with imaging appearances. Urgent CT imaging is crucial to promptly identify and categorise the most common and unusual complications after ERCP, particularly to triage those occurrences that require prolonged in-hospital treatment or surgical reoperation. Knowledge of ERCP procedural details, the appropriate CT acquisition technique and familiarity with normal appearances are needed to diagnose and grade oedematous or necrotic PEAP, bleeding, DP and infections, which may have similar, nonspecific clinical and laboratory manifestations [2, 6, 12].

References

1. Adler DG, Baron TH, Davila RE et al (2005) ASGE guideline: the role of ERCP in diseases of the biliary tract and the pancreas. Gastrointest Endosc 62:1–8
2. Silviera ML, Seamon MJ, Porshinsky B et al (2009) Complications related to endoscopic retrograde cholangiopancreatography: a comprehensive clinical review. J Gastrointestin Liver Dis 18:73–82
3. Glomsaker TB, Hoff G, Kvaloy JT et al (2013) Patient-reported outcome measures after endoscopic retrograde cholangiopancreatography: a prospective, multicentre study. Scand J Gastroenterol 48:868–876
4. Siriwardana HP, Siriwardena AK (2005) Systematic appraisal of the role of metallic endobiliary stents in the treatment of benign bile duct stricture. Ann Surg 242:10–19
5. van Boeckel PG, Vleggaar FP, Siersema PD (2009) Plastic or metal stents for benign extrahepatic biliary strictures: a systematic review. BMC Gastroenterol 9:96
6. Anderson MA, Fisher L, Jain R et al (2012) Complications of ERCP. Gastrointest Endosc 75:467–473
7. Kapral C, Duller C, Wewalka F et al (2008) Case volume and outcome of endoscopic retrograde cholangiopancreatography: results of a nationwide Austrian benchmarking project. Endoscopy 40:625–630
8. Stapfer M, Selby RR, Stain SC et al (2000) Management of duodenal perforation after endoscopic retrograde cholangiopancreatography and sphincterotomy. Ann Surg 232:191–198
9. Kwon CI, Song SH, Hahm KB et al (2013) Unusual complications related to endoscopic retrograde cholangiopancreatography and its endoscopic treatment. Clin Endosc 46:251–259
10. Glomsaker T, Hoff G, Kvaloy JT et al (2013) Patterns and predictive factors of complications after endoscopic retrograde cholangiopancreatography. Br J Surg 100:373–380
11. Cotton PB (2006) Analysis of 59 ERCP lawsuits; mainly about indications. Gastrointest Endosc 63:378–382, quiz 464
12. Sartelli M, Viale P, Catena F et al (2013) 2013 WSES guidelines for management of intra-abdominal infections. World J Emerg Surg 8:3
13. Pannu HK, Fishman EK (2001) Complications of endoscopic retrograde cholangiopancreatography: spectrum of abnormalities demonstrated with CT. Radiographics 21:1441–1453
14. Paspatis GA, Dumonceau JM, Barthet M et al (2014) Diagnosis and management of iatrogenic endoscopic perforations: European Society of Gastrointestinal Endoscopy (ESGE) position statement. Endoscopy 46:693–711
15. Wax BN, Katz DS, Badler RL et al (2006) Complications of abdominal and pelvic procedures: computed tomographic diagnosis. Curr Probl Diagn Radiol 35:171–187
16. Woods RW, Akshintala VS, Singh VK et al (2014) CT severity of post-ERCP pancreatitis: results from a single teriary medical center. Abdom Imaging 39:1162–1168
17. Catalano O, De Bellis M, Sandomenico F et al (2012) Complications of biliary and gastrointestinal stents: MDCT of the cancer patient. AJR Am J Roentgenol 199:W187–W196
18. Dubecz A, Ottmann J, Schweigert M et al (2012) Management of ERCP-related small bowel perforations: the pivotal role of physical investigation. Can J Surg 55:99–104
19. Zissin R, Shapiro-Feinberg M, Oscadchy A et al (2000) Retroperitoneal perforation during endoscopic sphincterotomy: imaging findings. Abdom Imaging 25:279–282
20. Tonolini M (2014) Reversible acute duodenitis as a complication of endoscopic biliary stenting. J Gastrointestin Liver Dis 23:8
21. Dumonceau JM, Andriulli A, Elmunzer BJ et al (2014) Prophylaxis of post-ERCP pancreatitis: European Society of Gastrointestinal Endoscopy (ESGE) Guideline-updated June 2014. Endoscopy 46: 799–815
22. Zaheer A, Singh VK, Qureshi RO et al (2013) The revised Atlanta classification for acute pancreatitis: updates in imaging terminology and guidelines. Abdom Imaging 38:125–136
23. Sheu Y, Furlan A, Almusa O et al (2012) The revised Atlanta classification for acute pancreatitis: a CT imaging guide for radiologists. Emerg Radiol 19:237–243
24. Pezzilli R, Romboli E, Campana D et al (2002) Mechanisms involved in the onset of post-ERCP pancreatitis. JOP 3:162–168
25. Pfau PR, Mosley RG, Said A et al (2006) Comparison of the effect of non-ionic and ionic contrast agents on pancreatic histology in a canine model. JOP 7:27–33
26. Johnson GK, Geenen JE, Johanson JF et al (1997) Evaluation of post-ERCP pancreatitis: potential causes noted during controlled study of differing contrast media. Midwest Pancreaticobiliary Study Group. Gastrointest Endosc 46:217–222
27. Goebel C, Hardt P, Doppl W et al (2000) Frequency of pancreatitis after endoscopic retrograde cholangiopancreatography with iopromid or iotrolan: a randomized trial. Eur Radiol 10:677–680
28. George S, Kulkarni AA, Stevens G et al (2004) Role of osmolality of contrast media in the development of post-ERCP pancreatitis: a metanalysis. Dig Dis Sci 49:503–508
29. Miller FH, Keppke AL, Dalal K et al (2004) MRI of pancreatitis and its complications: part 1, acute pancreatitis. AJR Am J Roentgenol 183:1637–1644
30. de Freitas Tertulino F, Schraibman V, Ardengh JC et al (2014) Diffusion-weighted magnetic resonance imaging indicates the severity of acute pancreatitis. Abdom Imaging
31. Horton KM, Jeffrey RB Jr, Federle MP et al (2009) Acute gastrointestinal bleeding: the potential role of 64 MDCT and 3D imaging in the diagnosis. Emerg Radiol 16:349–356

32. Jaeckle T, Stuber G, Hoffmann MH et al (2008) Acute gastrointestinal bleeding: value of MDCT. Abdom Imaging 33: 285–293
33. So YH, Choi YH, Chung JW (2012) Selective embolization for post-endoscopic sphincterotomy bleeding: technical aspects and clinical efficacy. Korean J Radiol 13:73–81
34. Katsinelos P, Kountouras J, Chatzimavroudis G (2010) Endoscopic hemostasis using monopolar coagulation for postendoscopic sphincterotomy bleeding refractory to injection treatment. Surg Laparosc Endosc Percutan Tech 20:84–88
35. Tsou YK, Lin CH, Liu NJ (2009) Treating delayed endoscopic sphincterotomy-induced bleeding: epinephrine injection with or without thermotherapy. World J Gastroenterol 15:4823–4828
36. Maleux G, Bieden J, Laenen A et al (2014) Embolization of post-biliary sphincterotomy bleeding refractory to medical and endoscopic therapy: technical results, clinical efficacy and predictors of outcome. Eur Radiol 24:2779–2786
37. Kim J, Lee SH, Paik WH et al (2012) Clinical outcomes of patients who experienced perforation associated with endoscopic retrograde cholangiopancreatography. Surg Endosc 26: 3293–3300
38. Miller R, Zbar A, Klein Y et al (2013) Perforations following endoscopic retrograde cholangiopancreatography: a single institution experience and surgical recommendations. Am J Surg 206:180–186
39. Avgerinos DV, Llaguna OH, Lo AY et al (2009) Management of endoscopic retrograde cholangiopancreatography: related duodenal perforations. Surg Endosc 23:833–838
40. Machado NO (2012) Management of duodenal perforation post-endoscopic retrograde cholangiopancreatography. When and whom to operate and what factors determine the outcome? A review article. JOP 13:18–25
41. Polydorou A, Vezakis A, Fragulidis G et al (2011) A tailored approach to the management of perforations following endoscopic retrograde cholangiopancreatography and sphincterotomy. J Gastrointest Surg 15:2211–2217
42. Rabie ME, Mir NH, Al Skaini MS et al (2013) Operative and non-operative management of endoscopic retrograde cholangiopancreatography-associated duodenal injuries. Ann R Coll Surg Engl 95:285–290
43. Matlock J, Freeman ML (2005) Endoscopic therapy of benign biliary strictures. Rev Gastroenterol Disord 5:206–214
44. Judah JR, Draganov PV (2007) Endoscopic therapy of benign biliary strictures. World J Gastroenterol 13:3531–3539

4

Role of interventional radiology in the management of complications after pancreatic surgery: a pictorial review

Giovanni Mauri · Chiara Mattiuz · Luca Maria Sconfienza · Vittorio Pedicini · Dario Poretti · Fabio Melchiorre · Umberto Rossi · Fabio Romano Lutman · Marco Montorsi

Abstract Pancreatic resections are surgical procedures associated with high incidence of complications, with relevant morbidity and mortality even at high volume centres. A multidisciplinary approach is essential in the management of these events and interventional radiology plays a crucial role in the treatment of patients developing post-surgical complications. This paper offers an overview on the interventional radiological procedures that can be performed to treat different type of complications after pancreatic resection. Procedures such as percutaneous drainage of fluid collections, percutaneous transhepatic biliary procedures, arterial embolisation, venous interventions and fistula embolisation are viable treatment options, with fewer complications compared with re-look surgery, shorter hospital stay and faster recovery. A selection

G. Mauri · L. M. Sconfienza
Servizio di Radiologia, IRCCS Policlinico San Donato,
San Donato Milanese, Milano, Italy

L. M. Sconfienza
e-mail: io@lucasconfienza.it

G. Mauri
Dipartimento Aziendale di Oncologia, Struttura Complessa di Radiologia Oncologica Interventistica, Azienda Ospedaliera Ospedale di Circolo di Busto Arsizio, Varese, Italy

C. Mattiuz
Facoltà di Medicina e Chirurgia, Scuola di Specializzazione in Radiodiagnostica, Università degli Studi di Milano, Milano, Italy
e-mail: chiara.mattiuz@gmail.com

L. M. Sconfienza
Dipartimento di Scienze Biomediche per la Salute, Università degli Studi di Milano, San Donato Milanese, Milano, Italy

V. Pedicini · D. Poretti · F. R. Lutman
Dipartimento di Diagnostica per Immagini,
IRCCS Istituto Clinico Humanitas, Rozzano, Italy

V. Pedicini
e-mail: vittorio.pedicini@humanitas.it

D. Poretti
e-mail: dario.poretti@humanitas.it

F. R. Lutman
e-mail: Romano.lutman@humanitas.it

F. Melchiorre
Dipartimento di Diagnostica per Immagini,
Azienda Ospedaliera San Paolo, Milano, Italy
e-mail: fabio.melchiorre@ao-sanpaolo.it

U. Rossi
Dipartimento di Scienze Diagnostiche,
Azienda Ospedaliera San Carlo Borromeo, Milano, Italy
e-mail: urossi76@hotmail.com

M. Montorsi
Dipartimento di Chirurgia, Azienda Ospedaliera Humanitas (Humanitas Research Hospital), Rozzano, Italy
e-mail: marco.montorsi@humanitas.it

G. Mauri (✉)
Servizio di Radiologia, IRCCS Policlinico San Donato,
Piazza Malan 2, 20097 San Donato Milanese, Milano, Italy
e-mail: vanni.mauri@gmail.com

of cases of complications following pancreatic surgery managed with interventional radiological procedure are presented and discussed.

Teaching Points

- *Interventional radiology is crucial to treat complications after pancreatic surgery*
- *Percutaneous drainage of collections can be performed under ultrasound or computed tomography guidance*
- *Percutaneous biliary procedures can be used to treat biliary complications*
- *Venous procedures can be performed effectively through transhepatic or transjugular access*
- *Fistulas can be treated effectively by percutaneous embolisation*

Keywords Interventional radiology · Duodenopancreasectomy · Complication · Embolisation · Biliary drainage

Introduction

Pancreatic resection is a surgical procedure associated with significant morbidity and mortality even at specialised high-volume centres [1–3]. Although in recent years refinements in surgical technique and perioperative management have led to a reduction in perioperative mortality, the incidence of post-operative complications (including intra-abdominal abscesses and leakages [4–9], biliary complications [10–14] and vascular complications [15–18]) still remains high. Moreover, in case of complications, surgical re-operation is associated with a high mortality rate [1–3]. In a large series of 650 patients, Yeo et al. [2] reported an overall mortality of 1.4 % and a morbidity of 41 %, with a mean length of hospital stay of 13 days. They reported re-operation in 26/650 patients (4 %) and identified the absence of reoperation as an independent predictor of prolonged survival [2].

Interventional radiology (IR) provides a minimally invasive alternative for managing post-surgical complications [19, 20]. Several different IR procedures, such as percutaneous drainage, aspiration of abscesses or fluid collections [4, 5], percutaneous transhepatic biliary drainage [6], and arterial embolisation [21–23] have been introduced in clinical practice to treat post-surgical complications. IR procedures are an alternative approach to manage post-surgical complications less invasive than surgical re-intervention, and may lead to a reduction in hospital stay and re-operation rate [10, 11].

In the present pictorial review, we offer an overview on the IR procedures that can be performed to treat different types of complications after pancreatic resection.

Percutaneous drainage

Intra-abdominal collections and abscesses represent the most common complication following pancreatic surgery [1–3]. Once an intra-abdominal collection is identified, in most cases it is possible to place a percutaneous drainage under image guidance. When the collection is well visible using ultrasound (US), US-guided percutaneous drainage placement is generally the preferred choice, as US is widely available, easy to handle and allows for real-time monitoring of the drainage placement, being also free from ionising radiation [24]. When the collection is located deep in the abdomen and is not well seen at US, computed tomography (CT) generally offers good anatomical definition to guide the safe placement of a percutaneous drainage. Drainage placement can be performed using the trocar or Seldinger technique. In the trocar technique, the drainage catheter containing a trocar needle is inserted directly into the collection. The trocar technique provides a fast deployment of the drainage that can be extremely helpful in critically ill or agitated patients. The Seldinger technique implies multiple steps: the collection is punctured with a small calibre needle, different calibre guidewires are inserted and the drainage is then advanced up to the collection over the guidewire. The Seldinger technique is particularly helpful when there is a small window to reach the collection, as typically happens when a retroperitoneal collection has to be drained through an anterior approach. The main disadvantage of this technique is that it may require considerably longer time than the trocar technique. The correct location of the needle or drainage can be confirmed by aspiration of a small amount of material. Furthermore, a small amount of iodinated contrast may be injected through the catheter to identify the presence of an underlying fistula.

In a series of 373 subjects who underwent pancreaticoduodenectomy reported by Zink et al. [5], percutaneous drainage was required in 22.2 % of patients after surgery. They report an immediate technical and overall success rate of 97.6 and 79.6 %, respectively.

A case of a patient with fluid collection after pancreaticoduodenectomy successfully managed with percutaneous CT guided drainage is shown in Fig. 1.

Percutaneous transhepatic biliary procedures

In patients treated by pancreaticoduodenectomy with Roux-en-Y bilio-enteric reconstruction, endoscopical access to the biliary tree is not feasible. Thus, in this kind of patient, a percutaneous transhepatic route is the only approach to the biliary system in case of biliary complications. The access to the biliary system is obtained by puncturing a peripheral bile duct under US and/or fluoroscopic guidance.

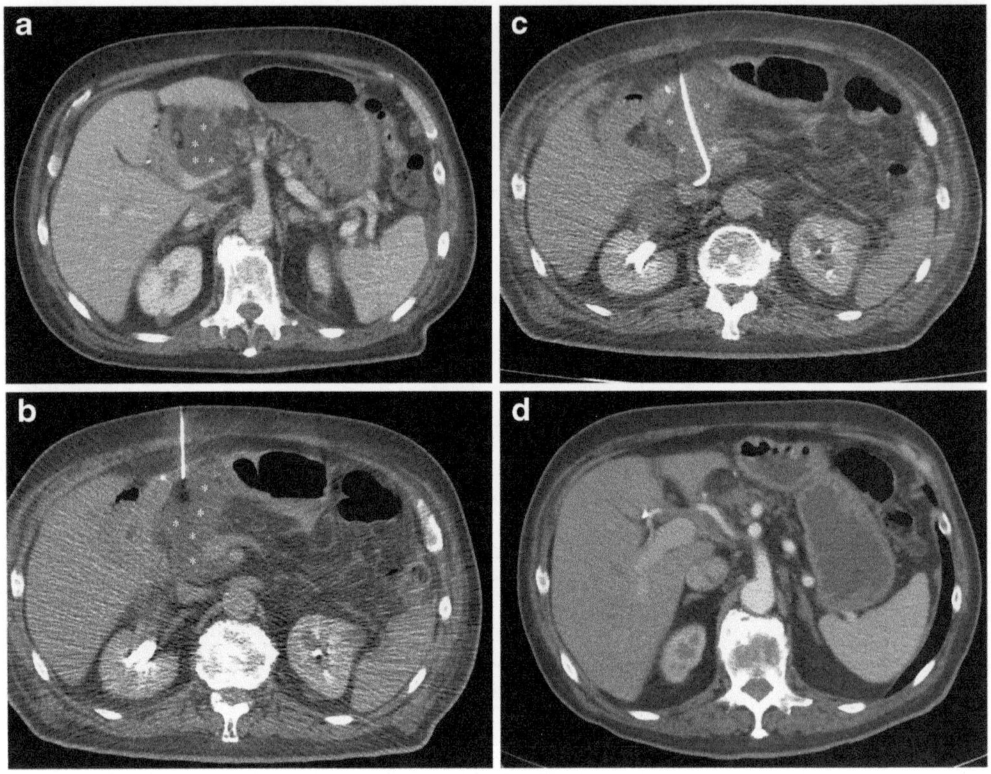

Fig. 1 Use of a percutaneous drainage to treat a post-pancreaticoduodenectomy fluid collection. **a** CT scan shows post-pancreaticoduodenectomy retroperitoneal fluid collection (*asterisks*). **b** The fluid collection (*asterisks*) is punctured with a small needle under CT guidance. **c** A percutaneous drainage (*arrow*) is inserted into the collection (*asterisks*) using the Seldinger technique. **d** At the end of the treatment complete resolution of the collection is obtained

Percutaneous biliary procedures can be particularly helpful in postoperative biliary leaks. They have been reported in about 3–4 % of cases after pancreatic surgery [1–3]. These complications are often associated with others, in particular with pancreatic fistula and fluid collections. In patients who develop such complication after surgery, percutaneous transhepatic biliary drainage—by allowing for a bile diversion from the site of the fistula—has been proven to be feasible and effective in the majority of cases [6, 20, 21]. The positioning of an occlusion balloon to obstruct the biliary duct above the site of the fistula, by allowing for complete external drainage of the bile, may represent a valuable option to treat post-surgical biliary leaks [7, 10]. A different and more recent technique is to use a covered stent that can close the bile leak and subsequently be retrieved percutaneously. Gwon et al. [25] used this approach successfully in 11 patients with post-operative bile leak, with no recurrence in the 1-year follow-up. A case of a patient with post-surgical biliary leak successfully treated with percutaneous transhepatic biliary drainage is shown in Fig. 2.

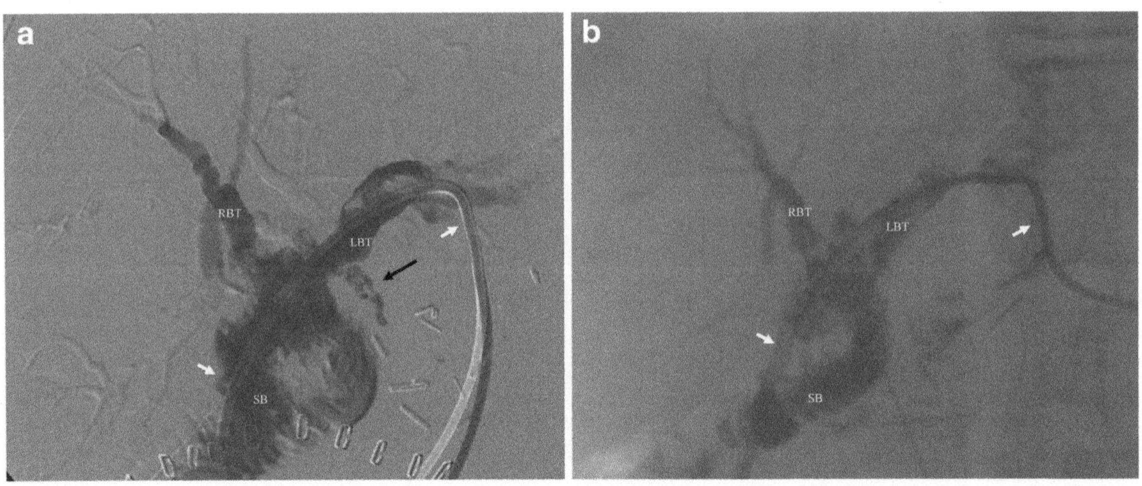

Fig. 2 Use of a percutaneous transhepatic biliary drainage to treat a post-surgical biliary leak. **a** Percutaneous colangiography demonstrates a biliary leak (*arrow*) and a biliary drainage (*white arrows*) is inserted via segment III left lobe approach; *RBT* right biliary tree, *LBT* left biliary tree, *SB* small bowel. **b** Final result with complete healing of the leak and absence of contrast leakage; *RBT* right biliary tree, *LBT* left biliary tree, *SB* bowel

After bilio-pancreatic surgery, stricture of a biliary duct may represent a serious complication, [26]. Surgical re-intervention is associated with morbidity and mortality rates as high as 28 and 2.6 % respectively [26]. Percutaneous treatments represent an effective alternative to surgery in the treatment of such complication [27–29]. To achieve resolution of the stenosis, subsequent larger biliary drainage catheter may be inserted and left in place and balloon dilation can be performed. However, recurrence of stenosis may occur in up to 29–58 % of cases [27–29], and multiple treatment sessions may be required. Stents are rarely used in the treatment of benign strictures, as they have to be removed after a period because the tube itself may stimulate inflammatory reaction, fibrosis and stone formation. A novel option may be represented by the use of biodegradable biliary stents, which may improve the long-term patency rate, without requiring a subsequent procedure for removal [13].

A case of a patient with a post-surgical biliary stricture successfully treated with balloon dilation and placement of a biodegradable biliary stent is shown in Fig. 3.

Arterial embolisation

Postoperative intra-abdominal arterial haemorrhage is still one of the most serious complications, with a reported incidence between 1.5 and 15 %, and a reported mortality rate of 20–50 % [15–17]. Haemorrhage is defined as 'early' when occurring within 24 h after surgery, while 'late' haemorrhages occur after 24 h [30]. Early haemorrhage requires immediate

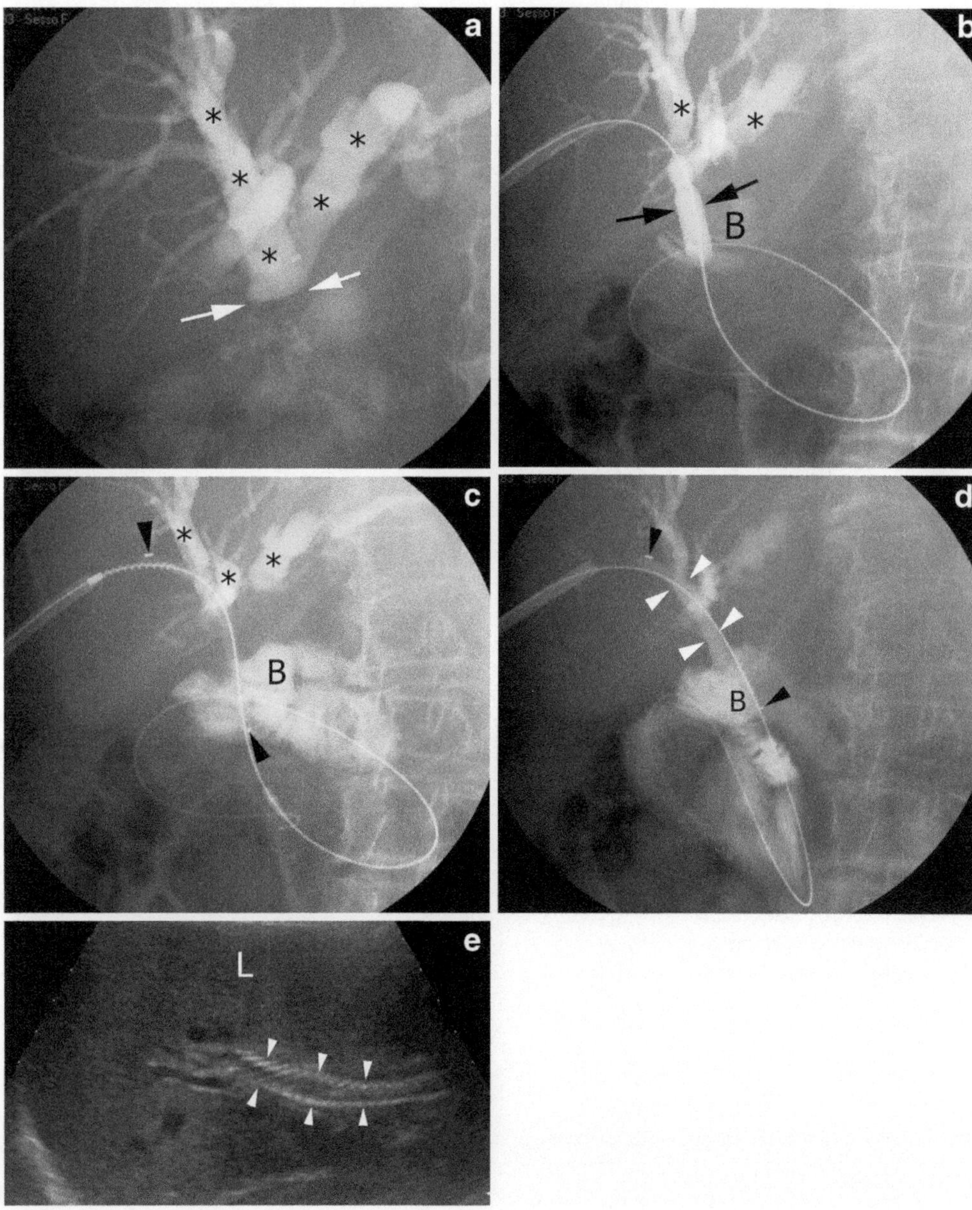

Fig. 3 Percutaneous treatment of a benign stricture of the common bile duct by a bioabsorbable biliary stent. **a** Percutaneous transhepatic cholangiography demonstrates remarkably dilated bile ducts (*asterisks*). The obstruction can be clearly spotted (*white arrows*). **b** Bilioplasty procedure. The balloon (*black arrows*) is fully inflated to dilate the stricture. Radiopaque contrast agent can be detected in the bowel (*B*); *asterisks* dilated bile ducts. **c** A bioabsorbable stent is positioned to keep the stricture open. The stent is radiolucent, but two platinum, radiopaque markers can be seen (*black arrowheads*); *asterisks* dilated bile ducts, *B* bowel. **d** The stent is fully expanded and radiopaque bile can be seen flowing through the patent common bile duct (*white arrowheads*); *black arrows* radiopaque stent markers; *B* bowel. **e** US follow-up at 3 months demonstrating good visibility of the stent (*arrowheads*) that was correctly expanded, and no dilation of the intrahepatic biliary ducts; *L* liver

laparotomy, as it is generally caused by a technical failure or underlying coagulopathy, while the most appropriate management of delayed haemorrhage still remains controversial. In haemodynamically stable patients, CT is crucial to address the suspicion of a delayed haemorrhage and is extremely useful prior to angiography as it may avoid it or guide it. In unstable patients, direct visceral angiography has been suggested as the best method to elucidate the site of bleeding, with the advantage of sparing time for a subsequent immediate intra-arterial treatment.

Transcatheter arterial embolisation has been reported to be safe and effective, with a reported success rate of 50–100 %, gaining acceptance for the treatment of intra-abdominal bleeding [15–17]. Once the site of bleeding has been identified, several different techniques may be used to stop bleeding and achieve haemostasis. In case of terminal vascularisation, a proximal embolisation of the bleeding vessel may be enough to achieve the haemostasis, while in the presence of collaterals, it is crucial to embolise both the inflow and outflow vessels in order to avoid re-bleeding ("isolation technique") [22]. Different materials are nowadays available to obtain vascular occlusion, and have to be chosen according to the desired type of vascular occlusion (transient or permanent). Transient embolisation, generally required due to a traumatic haemorrhage, is reached by resorbable materials, which allows for restoring the blood flow in a variable window of time (inter alia: autologous blood clot, gelatine or fibrin sponge). The main advantage of such materials is to avoid definitive occlusion of the treated vessel. However, a non-negligible risk of re-bleeding has to be considered once the material has been absorbed. Permanent embolisation is reached using non-resorbable materials (polyvynilic alcohol, bucrilate, metallic coils or detachable balloons) that induce a permanent vessel occlusion. At the present, an ideal material does not exist, thus the choice of the most appropriate embolic material and technique for embolisation, crucial to minimise failure and complications, requires the presence of a IR team with high experience and the availability of several different materials.

Stent grafting of the artery at the site of bleeding has been proposed as an alternative or in addition to embolisation, with the advantage of maintaining the patency of the end organ, thus minimising the risk of ischaemia deriving from embolisation [21]. A recent meta-analyisis comparing laparotomy and transarterial embolisation for the management of delayed

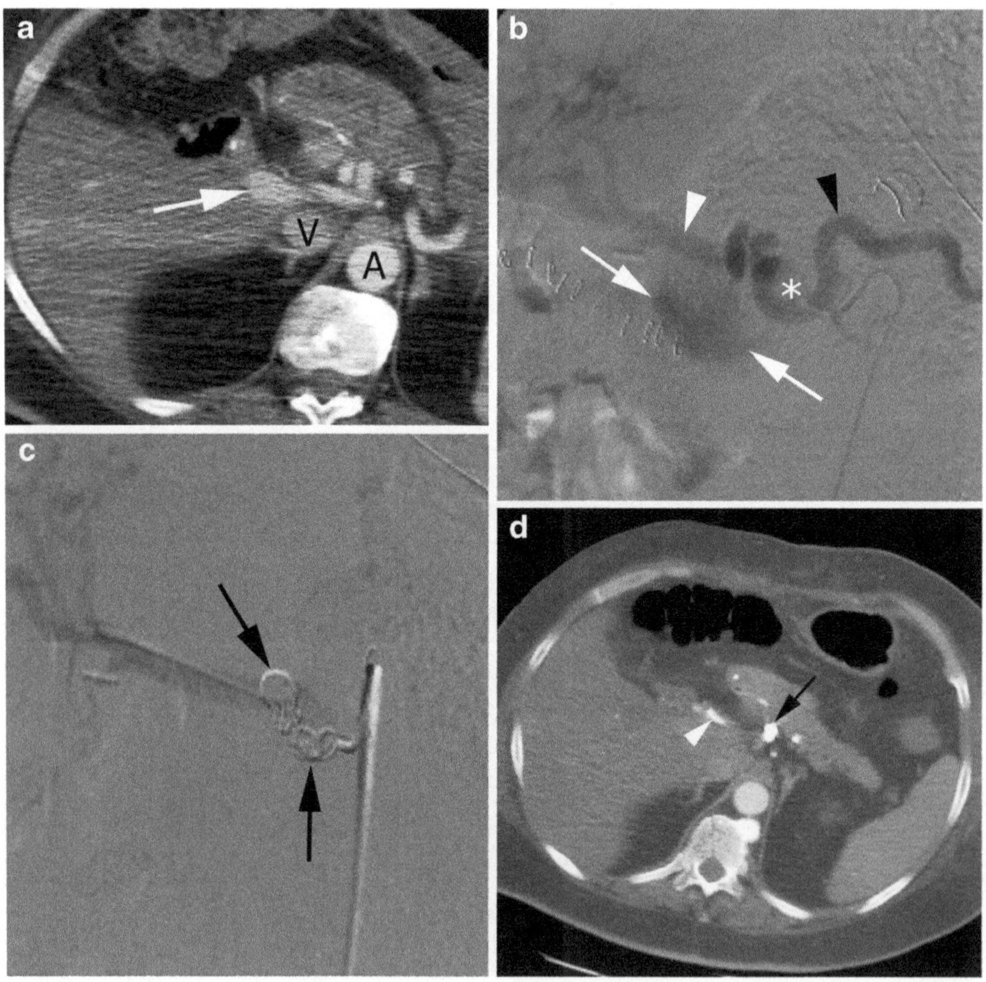

Fig. 4 Arterial embolisation of a post-surgical haemorrhage. **a** CT scan showing contrast extravasation (*arrow*) from the celiac trunk at the level of the bifurcation between hepatic and splenic artery; *V* inferior vena cava, *A* abdominal aorta. **b** Angiographic appearance of the active bleeding with contrast extravasation (*arrows*); *asterisk* celiac trunk, *black arrowhead* splenic artery, *white arrowhead* hepatic artery. **c** Angiography after embolisation with coils (*arrows*) demonstrating absence of contrast extravasation at the level of previous bleeding. **d** CT scan at 2 years, demonstrating absence of contrast extravasation at the level of previous bleeding and preserved patency of proper hepatic artery (*white arrow*), even in the presence of part of a coil in its lumen (*arrowhead*); *black arrow* clustered metallic coils in the focus of arterial lesion properly embolised

postoperative haemorrhage found a reduction in mortality (43 % vs 20 %) and morbidity (77 % vs 35 %) in the IR group, even if not reaching the statistical significance. Authors conclude that the appropriate treatment pathway for late haemorrhage ultimately will be decided by the clinical status of the patient and the institution preference [16].

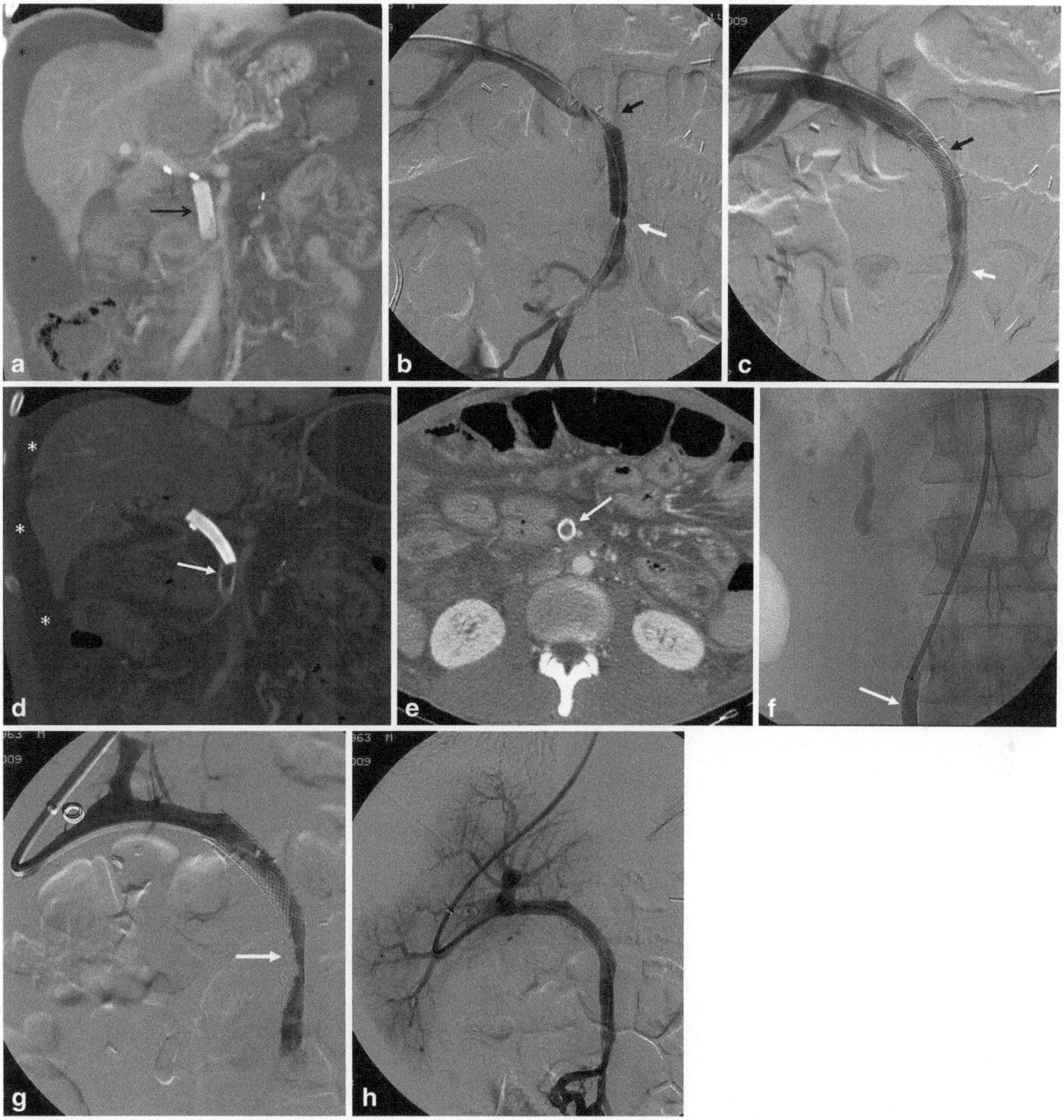

Fig. 5 Treatment of a patient with postoperative mesenteric vein stenosis and thrombosis by percutaneous transhepatic stenting, thromboaspiration, and thrombolysis through a transjugular approach (the case has been partially previously reported [18]). **a** Maximum intensity projection reconstruction of abdominal MDCT shows surgical vascular graft (*black arrow*) at the level of the superior mesenteric vein and ascitic fluid (*asterisks*) **b** Percutaneous transhepatic angiography demonstrates stenosis at the level of proximal (*black arrow*) and distal (*white arrow*) anastomoses of the PTFE graft. **c** Angiography after stent placement (*black arrow* proximal stent, *white arrow* distal stent) demonstrating resolution of the stenosis. **d** MDCT MIP reconstruction and **e** axial image showing intra-stent thrombosis (*white arrow*) and ascitic fluid (*asterisks*). **f** Contrast injection in SMV (*arrow*) demonstrates complete vessel occlusion. **g** Angiography after aspiration thrombectomy and angioplasty shows residual thrombus (*arrow*). **h** Complete resolution and calibre restoration after direct thrombolysis with rt-PA

A case of transcatheter arterial embolisation for a post-surgical haemorrhage is shown in Fig. 4.

Venous interventions

In some cases, post-surgical complications may involve the portal and mesenteric veins, which may develop stenosis or thrombosis after surgical treatment. Moreover, with the recent advancement of vascular reconstruction with polytetrafluoroethylene graft, this occurrence may happen more frequently in the future. Percutaneous endovascular treatment, such as transjugular portosystemic shunt, direct and indirect thrombolysis, stenting and mechanical thrombectomy, described mainly in liver-transplant patients, may represent a valuable option in the management of these conditions after pancreatic surgery [2, 5, 18]. The access to the portal system may be achieved through a transhepatic route, with the direct image guided puncture of a peripheral portal branch, or through a transjugular approach, by puncturing the portal system from the hepatic veins. Transhepatic access is generally easier than transjugular access and represents the first choice strategy in patients with normal coagulation parameters. In patients with thrombosis of the portal or mesenteric vein, in which anticoagulation treatment has been undertaken, the best choice is represented by the transjugular approach, in order to minimise the risk of peritoneal haemorrhage correlated with direct liver puncture [18]. Once the access to the portal system has been achieved, it is possible to perform balloon dilation and stenting of post-surgical strictures using the several different commercially available devices. In case of thrombosis, direct trombo-aspiration through a catheter or infusion of trombolitic agents has been reported as a feasible and effective treatment [18].

A case of post-surgical mesenteric vein stenosis and thrombosis treated percutaneously is shown in Fig. 5.

Fistula embolisation

Fistulas are the most common complication following pancreatic surgery after presence of fluid collections [1–3]. The most frequent type is pancreatic fistula, followed by enteric and biliary fistulas [1–3]. This kind of complication is frequently associated with others, in particular the presence of an intra-abdominal fluid collection. Recent reports highlighted how this kind of complication can be successfully managed

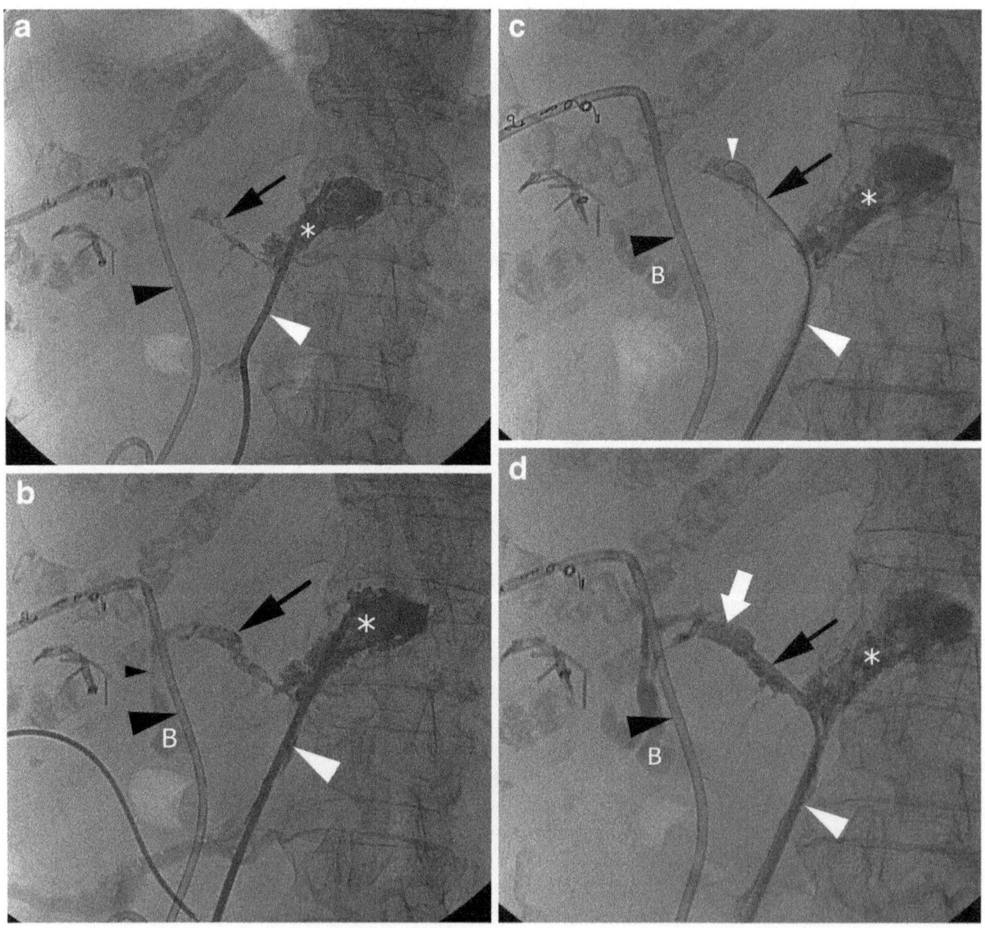

Fig. 6 Successful percutaneous embolisation with cyanoacrilic glue of a postoperative fistula. **a**, **b** Contrast injection through a previously placed percutaneous drainage (*white arrowhead*) at the level of a fluid collection (*asterisk*) demonstrating a fistula (*black arrow*) with a communication (*small black arrowhead*) with the biliary system and bowel (*B*); *large black arrowhead* percutaneous transhepatic biliary drainage. **c** A guidewire (*small white arrowhead*) is advanced through the percutaneous drainage (*large white arrowhead*) into the fistula (*black arrow*); *asterisk* fluid collection, *black arrowhead* percutaneous transhepatic biliary drainage, *B* bowel. **d** A microcatheter (*white arrowhead*) is advanced over the wire at the level of the fistula (*black arrow*), and glue is injected (*white arrow*); *asterisk* fluid collection, *black arrowhead* percutaneous transhepatic biliary drainage, *B* bowel

without surgery in over 90 % of patients [9]. In the non-operative management of such complications, IR plays a crucial role.

In presence of a fluid collection, a percutaneously placed drainage may be enough to treat the collection, and in several cases to allow for the spontaneous closure of the fistula [4, 5]. If the main component of a fistula is biliary material, the transhepatic insertion of a biliary drainage, by diverting the bile from the site of the fistula, may be enough to determine the fistula closure. In cases with persisting biliary leak, the placement of an occlusion balloon above the fistula, by interrupting completely the bile flow towards the site of the fistula, has been reported as an effective tool [7–10].

Some authors reported the direct embolisation of the site of the fistula as a feasible and effective procedure. Reaching perfectly the site of the fistula is crucial to perform a correct procedure. This can be done through a previously placed surgical drainage, through an image-guided percutaneously placed drainage, or even through a transhepatic approach. Once the site of the fistula has been reached, several different materials can be used to perform embolisation, including ethanol, particles or different kind of glues [31–33]. Inter alia, cyanoacrilic glues seem to represent optimal materials for fistula percutaneous treatment, due to their high adhesive and haemostatic properties and fast polymerisation [31].

A case of embolisation of a fistula with cyanoacrilic glue is shown in Fig. 6.

Conclusions

IR plays an increasing, crucial role in the multidisciplinary management of complications after pancreatic surgery, providing a minimally invasive therapy also in critical patients, reducing recovery times and avoiding re-operation morbidity. IR procedures such as percutaneous drainage of fluid collections, percutaneous transhepatic biliary procedures, arterial embolisation, venous interventions and fistula embolisation are viable treatment options and have been reported as feasible, safe and effective techniques with fewer complications compared with re-look surgery, with a shorter hospital stay and faster recovery in the management of complications after pancreatic surgery.

Conflict of interest Giovanni Mauri declares sponsored research and consulting from Esaote S.p.A, Italy. All other authors declare no conflicts of interest.

References

1. Buchler MW, Wagner M, Schmied BM, Uhl W, Friess H, Z'Graggen K (2003) Changes in morbidity after pancreatic resection: toward the end of completion pancreatectomy. Arch Surg 138(12):1310–1314
2. Yeo CJ, Cameron JL, Sohn TA et al (1997) Six hundred fifty consecutive pancreaticoduodenectomies in the 1990s: pathology, complications, and outcomes. Ann Surg 226(3):248–257
3. Sohn TA, Yeo CJ, Cameron JL et al (2000) Resected adenocarcinoma of the pancreas-616 patients: results, outcomes, and prognostic indicators. J Gastrointest Surg 4(6):567–579
4. Gervais DA, Fernandez-del Castillo C, O'Neill MJ, Hahn PF, Mueller PR (2001) Complications after pancreatoduodenectomy: imaging and imaging-guided interventional procedures. Radiographics 21(3):673–690
5. Zink SI, Soloff EV, White RR et al (2009) Pancreaticoduodenectomy: frequency and outcome of post-operative imaging-guided percutaneous drainage. Abdom Imaging 34(6):767–771
6. Cozzi G, Severini A, Civelli E et al (2006) Percutaneous transhepatic biliary drainage in the management of postsurgical biliary leaks in patients with nondilated intrahepatic bile ducts. Cardiovasc Intervent Radiol 29(3):380–388
7. Pedicini V, Poretti D, Mauri G et al (2010) Management of post-surgical biliary leakage with percutaneous transhepatic biliary drainage (PTBD) and occlusion balloon (OB) in patients without dilatation of the biliary tree: preliminary results. Eur Radiol 20(5):1061–1068
8. Winter JM, Cameron JL, Yeo CJ, Lillemoe KD, Campbell KA, Schulick RD (2008) Duodenojejunostomy leaks after pancreaticoduodenectomy. J Gastrointest Surg 12(2):263–269
9. Shrikhande SV, D'Souza MA (2008) Pancreatic fistula after pancreatectomy: evolving definitions, preventive strategies and modern management. World J Gastroenterol 14(38):5789–5796
10. Cozzaglio L, Cimino M, Mauri G et al (2011) Percutaneous transhepatic biliary drainage and occlusion balloon in the management of duodenal stump fistula. J Gastrointest Surg 15:1977–1981
11. Kim JH, Ko GY, Sung KB et al (2008) Bile leak following living donor liver transplantation: clinical efficacy of percutaneous transhepatic treatment. Liver Transpl 14:1142–1149
12. Mauri G, Sconfienza LM (2014) Few comments on "Defining treatment and outcomes of hepaticojejunostomy failure following pancreaticoduodenectomy". J Gastrointest Surg 18(4):880–881
13. Mauri G, Michelozzi C, Poretti D et al (2013) Bioabsorbable biliary stent implantation in the treatment of benign bilioplastic-refractory biliary strictures: preliminary experience. Eur Radiol 23(12):3304–3310
14. Mauri G, Sconfienza LM (2013) A few thoughts on "Interventional radiology in the management of benign biliary stenoses, biliary leaks and fistulas: a pictorial review" Insights. Imaging 4(2):253
15. Blanc T, Cortes A, Goere D et al (2007) Hemorrhage after pancreaticoduodenectomy: when is surgery still indicated? Am J Surg 194(1):3–9
16. Limongelli P, Khorsandi SE, Pai M et al (2008) Management of delayed postoperative hemorrhage after pancreaticoduodenectomy: a meta-analysis. Arch Surg 143(10):1001–1007
17. Yekebas EF, Wolfram L, Cataldegirmen G et al (2007) Postpancreatectomy hemorrhage: diagnosis and treatment: an analysis in 1669 consecutive pancreatic resections. Ann Surg 246(2):269–280
18. Mauri G, Monti L, Pedicini V (2011) Interventional management of in-stent thrombosis after superior mesenteric vein stenting. EJVES Extra 22(3):27–29
19. Baker TA, Aaron JM, Borge M, Pierce K, Shoup M, Aranha GV (2008) Role of interventional radiology in the management of complications after pancreaticoduodenectomy. Am J Surg 195(3):386–390

20. Sohn TA, Yeo CJ, Cameron JL et al (2003) Pancreaticoduodenectomy: role of interventional radiologists in managing patients and complications. J Gastrointest Surg 7(2):209–219
21. Lee HG, Heo JS, Choi SH, Choi DW (2010) Management of bleeding from pseudoaneurysms following pancreaticoduodenectomy. World J Gastroenterol 16(10):1239–1244
22. Rossi UG, Seitun S, Ferro C (2013) Endovascular embolization of a third jejunal artery aneurysm: isolation techinique using the Amplatzer vascular plug 4. Catheter Cardiovasc Interv 81(6):1049–1052
23. Miura F, Asano T, Amano H et al (2009) Management of postoperative arterial haemorrhage after pancreato-biliary surgery according to the site of bleeding: re-laparotomy or interventional radiology. J Hepatobiliary Pancreat Surg 16(1):56–63
24. Sconfienza LM, Mauri G, Grossi F et al (2013) Pleural and peripheral lung lesions: comparison of US- and CT-guided biopsy. Radiol 266(3):930–935
25. Gwon DI, Ko GY, Sung KB, Kim JH, Yoon HK (2011) Percutaneous transhepatic treatment of postoperative bile leaks: prospective evaluation of retrievable covered stent. J Vasc Interv Radiol 22(1):75–83
26. Shimada H, Endo I, Shimada K, Matsuyama R, Kobayashi N, Kubota K (2012) The current diagnosis and treatment of benign biliary stricture. Surg Today 42:1143–1153
27. Mueller PR, vanSonnenberg E, Ferrucci JT Jr, Weyman PJ, Butch RJ, Malt RA et al (1986) Biliary stricture dilatation: multicenter review of clinical management in 73 patients. Radiol 160(1):17–22
28. Born P, Rosch T, Bruhl K et al (1999) Long-term results of endoscopic and percutaneous transhepatic treatment of benign biliary strictures. Endosc 31(9):725–731
29. Krokidis M, Orgera G, Rossi M, Matteoli M, Hatzidakis A (2013) Interventional radiology in the management of benign biliary stenoses, biliary leaks and fistulas: a pictorial review. Insights Imaging 4:77–84
30. Wente MN, Veit JA, Bassi C et al (2007) Postpancreatectomy haemorrhage (PPH): an International Study Group of Pancretic Surgery (ISGPS) definition. Surg 142(1):20–25
31. Mauri G, Sconfienza LM, Fiore B et al (2013) Post-surgical enteric fistula treatment with image-guided percutaneous injection of cyanoacrylic glue. Clin Rad 68(1):59–63
32. Sconfienza LM, Mauri G (2014) Interventional options to treat post-operative duodenal stump leaks. Cardiovasc Intervent Radiol. doi:10.1007/s00270-014-0937-7
33. Mtsumoto T, Iwaki K, Hagino Y et al (2002) Ethanol injection therapy of an isolated bile duct associated with a biliary-cutaneous fistula. J Gastroenterol Hepatol 17(7):807–810

5

Morphological MR imaging of the articular cartilage of the knee at 3 T—comparison of standard and novel 3D sequences

Pieter Van Dyck [1] · Floris Vanhevel [1] · Filip M. Vanhoenacker [1,2,3] · Kristien Wouters [4] · David M. Grodzki [5] · Jan L. Gielen [1] · Paul M. Parizel [1]

Abstract

Objectives This study sought to compare various 3D cartilage sequences and to evaluate the usefulness of ultrashort TE (UTE) imaging, a new technique to isolate signal from the osteochondral junction.

Methods Twenty knees were examined at 3 T with 3D spoiled GRE (FLASH), double-echo steady-state (DESS), balanced SSFP, 3D turbo spin-echo (TSE), and a prototype UTE sequence. Two radiologists independently evaluated all images. Consensus readings of all sequences were the reference standard. Statistical analysis included Friedman and pairwise Wilcoxon tests. Retrospective analysis of UTE morphology of osteochondral tissue in normal and abnormal cartilage seen at conventional MR was also performed.

Results Three-dimensional TSE was superior to other sequences for detecting cartilage lesions. FLASH and DESS performed best in the subjective quality analysis. On UTE images, normal cartilage exhibited a high-intensity linear signal near the osteochondral junction. Retrospective analysis revealed abnormal UTE morphology of the osteochondral junction in 50 % of cartilage lesions diagnosed at conventional MR.

Conclusions Cartilage imaging of the knee at 3 T can be reliably performed using 3D TSE, showing high accuracy when compared to standard sequences. Although UTE depicts signal from the deep cartilage layer, further studies are needed to establish its role for assessment of cartilage.

Main Messages

- *MRI is the best available imaging method for assessment of knee cartilage.*
- *Cartilage imaging can be reliably performed using 3D TSE.*
- *UTE cannot be used as a single sequence to assess cartilage.*

Keywords Knee · Magnetic resonance imaging · Cartilage · 3 T-isotropic

✉ Pieter Van Dyck
pieter.van.dyck@uza.be

1 Department of Radiology, Antwerp University Hospital and University of Antwerp, Wilrijkstraat 10, 2650 Antwerp (Edegem), Belgium

2 Department of Radiology, Ghent University Hospital and University of Ghent, De Pintelaan 185, 9000 Ghent, Belgium

3 Department of Radiology, AZ St-Maarten, Rooienberg 25, 2570 Antwerp (Duffel), Belgium

4 Department of Biostatistics, Antwerp University Hospital and University of Antwerp, Wilrijkstraat 10, 2650 Antwerp (Edegem), Belgium

5 Siemens Healthcare, Allee am Röthelheimpark 2, 91052 Erlangen, Germany

Introduction

Magnetic resonance (MR) imaging is generally regarded as the best available noninvasive method for evaluating injury and repair of the articular cartilage of the knee [1–3]. Currently, most evaluation of knee cartilage is done with two-dimensional (2D) acquisition techniques, such as turbo spin-echo (TSE) sequences, as they provide excellent tissue contrast and high in-plane spatial resolution [4]. However, 2D sequences have relatively thick slices (≥2 mm) and small gaps (0.2 mm) between slices, which can obscure pathology because of partial volume averaging [4, 5].

Three-dimensional (3D) imaging has the great potential of acquiring volumetric data sets with isotropic resolution, providing thin (0.5–0.6 mm) contiguous slices through the knee joint, thereby reducing partial volume artefacts. Multiplanar reformats along any user-defined imaging plane can be generated from the source data without loss of resolution [4–6].

Techniques for morphological 3D MR imaging of cartilage have changed rapidly in the past 2 decades. Gradient-echo (GRE) sequences were the first 3D sequences used for cartilage imaging [4, 7, 8]. They are classically divided into dark fluid sequences (e.g. spoiled gradient echo or FLASH) and bright fluid sequences (e.g. double echo steady-state or DESS) based upon the signal intensity of synovial fluid [4, 8]. These traditional GRE methods have been shown to be highly accurate for cartilage lesions in various studies and are still considered the standard of reference for high-resolution 3D isotropic imaging of cartilage [5–8]. A water-excited DESS sequence has been used in various knee osteoarthritis trials and is currently being used in the Osteoarthritis Initiative to assess the articular cartilage of the knee joint [9]. Many different methods of steady-state free-precession-based imaging (SSFP), a new variant of the GRE method, are also available for imaging cartilage, and all have higher cartilage signal compared with conventional GRE methods [10]. However, major disadvantages of 3D GRE imaging include their sensitivity to susceptibility artefacts and their suboptimal tissue contrast [4–8].

The increased availability of high-field 3-T imaging systems combined with improved coil technology facilitate the use of novel isotropic 3D sequences in clinical practice. Recently, 3D TSE sequences (e.g. SPACE) were developed for 3-T scanners. The important advantage of the 3D TSE acquisitions is their capability of mimicking the contrast properties of conventional 2D TSE intermediate-weighted acquisitions, allowing for better tissue contrast and higher conspicuity of cartilage lesions [5, 11].

In the knee, the superficial and middle layers of articular cartilage have T2 values of~50 ms, while the deep cartilage layer has much shorter T2 values, in the range of 1 to 2 ms or less [12]. Therefore, with a practical minimum echo time (TE) of about 10 ms for a spin-echo (SE) sequence and of about 2 ms for a GRE sequence, conventional MR imaging lacks the ability to display signal near the osteochondral junction. Through the use of ultrashort TE (UTE) sequences, now becoming available on clinical 3-T scanners, the minimum TE can be considerably reduced and the signal detected before it has totally decayed. As a result, signal can now be acquired from these previously 'invisible' tissues at the bone-cartilage interface, allowing for direct visual assessment [12, 13].

Controversy remains as to which is the single best 3D sequence for clinical cartilage imaging of the knee at 3 T [14, 15]. Also, clinical UTE imaging of the knee has been performed in healthy volunteers [16, 17], but studies investigating the role of morphological UTE imaging in patients with cartilage lesions are lacking. Thus, the main purpose of the present study was to compare standard and novel 3D cartilage MR sequences at 3 T. It was hypothesised that 3D TSE acquisitions compare favourably to the standard of reference GRE sequences for clinical cartilage imaging. In addition, we sought to explore how the normal UTE signal patterns change in normal and abnormal cartilage seen at conventional MR.

Materials and methods

Patient selection

This prospective study was approved by the Institutional Review Board of the Antwerp University Hospital according to the ICH Good Clinical Practice rules (registration no. B300201421002). Written informed consent was obtained from all of the participants after the nature of the examinations had been fully explained. From 1 March to 31 May 2014, a total of 20 subjects were prospectively enrolled in this study, including 10 healthy volunteers (8 males and 2 females; mean age 25 years; range 23–32 years; mean body mass index 22.6 kg/m^2) and 10 patients (2 males and 8 females; mean age 49 years; range 27–61 years; mean body mass index 26.4 kg/m^2). All volunteers were medical or paramedical personnel (e.g. medical students, residents, and nurses), and none of them had known musculoskeletal disease or prior knee symptoms. A patient was enrolled in the study if they (1) had a clinical suspicion of a cartilage abnormality at the knee (pain and stiffness for more than 6 months, n=5; anterior knee pain aggravating when climbing stairs, n=3; recent episodes of pain and functional limitation in nonprofessional marathon runners, n=2), (2) had no history of prior knee surgery, and (3) consented to undergo a 3-T MRI of the knee with dedicated cartilage imaging sequences. Subjects with contra-indications to the use of MRI (e.g. aneurysm clip, cardiac pacemaker, claustrophobia) were not included in the study. The right knee was imaged in all study participants.

MR imaging protocol

All images were acquired with a 3-T MR imaging system (Magnetom SKYRA, Siemens, Erlangen, Germany) by using a transmit/receive 15-channel knee coil (Quality Electrodynamics, Mayfield, OH, USA). The MR protocol consisted of five different isotropic 3D sequences: water-excited (we) 3D Fast-Low Angle Shot (FLASH), we Double-Echo Steady-State (DESS), we True Fast Imaging with Steady-State Free Precession (TrueFISP), fat-saturated (fs) intermediate-weighted 3D Turbo Spin-Echo Sampling Perfection with Application optimised Contrasts using variable flip angle Evolutions (SPACE), and a prototype 3D Ultrashort Echo-Time (UTE) sequence. All sequences had a sagittal plane of acquisition and used a 0.6 mm^3 voxel volume, except for the 3D UTE sequence, which employed a 0.8 mm^3 voxel size. Detailed parameters for all imaging sequences are provided in Table 1. In our study, a dual echo 3D UTE sequence was used consisting of a 60-μs nonselective RF pulse followed by 3D radial ramp sampling from the centre to the surface of a sphere. In order to achieve the shortest possible TE, data acquisition started already during ramp-up time of the readout gradient. Frequency-based fat suppression was available as an additional option. Difference images were formed to suppress signals from long T2 components by subtracting the later echo time (TE=3.92 ms) images from the first image (TE=60 μs) (Fig. 1). The scan time of the 3D UTE sequence was 6 min 48 s, which is feasible for routine clinical use.

MR imaging analysis

All images were independently reviewed during separate sessions by two readers [with 25 years (reader A) and 10 years (reader B) of experience in musculoskeletal radiology at the time of the study]. Images were obtained without any annotation. At the time of review, the readers were blinded to the patient's clinical history and clinical findings. A total of 100 MRI data sets (5 data sets per subject for a total of 20 study subjects) were reviewed in 5 separate sessions at least 96 h apart to prevent recall bias. Each session consisted of 20 data sets that were presented randomly except that different data sets of the same patient were never reviewed in the same session. The readers used sagittal source data to create multiplanar reformatted (MPR) images in the axial and coronal plane. Subjective image quality was assessed by using the following criteria: edge sharpness, artefacts, amount of noise, tissue contrast, and reformat quality. The quality score consisted of an ordinal 5-point Likert-scale and was defined as (1) poor, unacceptable for diagnostic purposes; (2) adequate but poorer than average quality; (3) average quality of a diagnostic acceptable image; (4) above average quality; (5) best quality. The readers graded each of the six articular surfaces of the knee as follows: (1) normal; (2) low-grade cartilage defect (<50 % of total cartilage thickness); (3) high-grade cartilage defect (>50 % of total cartilage thickness). Each reader was asked to assign a confidence level to the diagnosis as follows: (1) definitely normal; (2) probably normal; (3) probably abnormal; (4) definitely abnormal. Presence of bone marrow oedema was also recorded using the same 4-point Likert scale. On UTE images, the readers prospectively evaluated the morphology of the deep osteochondral tissues to predict the status of the overlying cartilage: a distinct, continuous high linear signal at the cartilage/bone interface was considered normal (indicating normal cartilage) and thinning, interruption, or complete absence of that signal was considered abnormal (indicating cartilage lesion), according to previously described criteria by Bae et al [12, 18]. Finally, the UTE morphology of the osteochondral tissue was retrospectively assessed in consensus and with knowledge of the findings on conventional MR sequences.

Standard of reference

The standard of reference for the MR abnormalities was based on image analysis by two senior radiologists in consensus with all available MR sequences as well as clinical findings. Both radiologists had more than 25 years of experience in musculoskeletal radiology at the time of the study and were not involved in the blinded study readings.

Table 1 MRI parameters for 3D sequences

	3D cartilage imaging sequence				
Imaging parameter*	FLASH	DESS	TruFISP	SPACE	UTE
TR (ms)	10.1	14.8	7.18	1200	10
TE (ms)	4.92	5.0	3.18	30	0.06/3.92
Acquistion matrix	256×233	256×240	256×240	256×256	256×256
FOV (mm)	150×150	150×140	150×140	160×160	200×200
Flip angle	10	25	28	120	15
Averages	1	1	3	1	1
PAT	2	2	2	2	no
No. of slices	160	160	192	192	256
Imaging time (min:s)	3:02	3:42	9:09	10:04	6:48

* TR = repitition time; TE = echo time; FOV = field of view; PAT = parallel acquisition technique

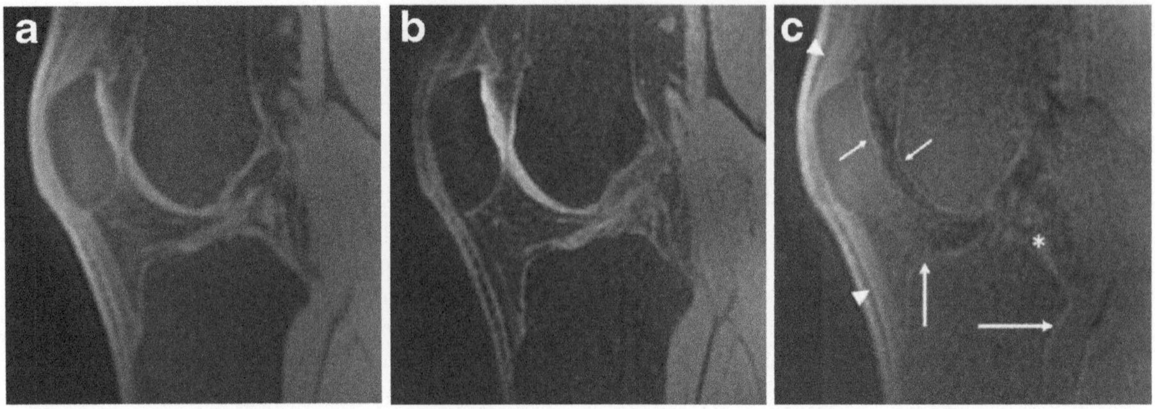

Fig. 1 UTE imaging of the articular cartilage of the knee in a 24-year-old healthy volunteer. Two echos with varying TE were acquired. **a** First echo, obtained at a minimum TE (=60 μs), and **b** second echo, obtained at longer TE (=3.92 ms). The second echo image was then digitally subtracted (**c**) from the first one to suppress signal from the long T2 tissue components, improving visualisation of the deep layer of cartilage. UTE subtraction image shows distinct high-intensity linear signal near the osteochondral junction at the patella and trochlea (small arrows). Also note bright signal at the cortical margins (large arrows), extensor apparatus (arrowheads), and posterior cruciate ligament (*)

Statistical analysis

Statistical analysis was performed by a statistician with use of R software (version 3.1.1.; R Foundation for Statistical Computing, Vienna, Austria). Differences between the MR sequences were considered to be statistically significant if $p<0.05$. The Friedman test and pairwise Wilcoxon tests with Bonferroni-Holm correction for multiple testing were used to compare the performance and subjective image quality gradings of all sequences [19]. Interreader agreement was determined using the weighted kappa (κ) statistic with κ value≥0.8 indicating excellent agreement. To increase statistical power for the performance analysis, calculations were made for all articular surfaces, all grades of severity, and both readers combined. Therefore, a bootstrapping procedure with 1000 samples at the level of the patients was used to calculate standard errors. Finally, the proportion of definite MR diagnoses (i.e. definitely normal or definitely abnormal) was calculated for each sequence.

Results

Diagnostic performance and confidence analysis

Consensus readings of all available MR sequences revealed 20 cartilage defects (low grade <50 %, n=7; high grade >50 %, n=13) in 10 patients (medial tibia, n=2; lateral tibia, n=1; medial femoral condyle, n=5; lateral femoral condyle, n=1; patella, n=9; trochlea, n=2). Since 120 articular cartilage surfaces were each evaluated by 2 readers, we had a total of 240 individual surface interpretations. A summary of the performance of all sequences in detecting cartilage defects is given in Table 2. For the detection of cartilage lesions, the highest sensitivity was achieved with SPACE (98 %), being significantly higher than TruFISP (sensitivity=55 %, p=0.014) and UTE (sensitivity=20 %, p=0.010) (Figs. 2 and 3). There were no significant differences in specificity and accuracy for diagnosing cartilaginous lesions among FLASH, DESS, TruFISP, and SPACE (all values≥90 %). Accuracy of UTE was 86 %, being significantly lower than FLASH (accuracy=95 %, p=0.010) and DESS (accuracy=94 %, p=0.036).

A review of the radiologists' confidence scores in diagnosing cartilage lesions revealed that readers were most confident with DESS sequence (88 % definite diagnoses for both readers). For the detection of subchondral bone marrow oedema, the readers were most confident with SPACE (95 % definite diagnoses for both readers).

Image quality analysis

There were no significant differences in overall image quality among FLASH, DESS, and SPACE, but all three performed significantly better than TruFISP and UTE (p<0.0001) (Table 3). Mild blurring artefacts were seen with the SPACE sequence; TruFISP image quality was degraded by susceptibility artefacts. Although UTE images exhibited high signal intensity at the osteochondral junction in all subjects, the UTE sequence was ranked lowest for contrast at the cartilage/bone interface because of poor image quality and blurring artefacts. DESS, TruFISP, and SPACE performed significantly better than FLASH (p≤0.0001) for separating between the surface layer of the articular cartilage and joint fluid. There were no significant differences in reformat quality among FLASH, DESS, and SPACE. Agreement between readers for the subjective assessment of overall image quality was excellent (κ=0.90).

Table 2 Performance of 3D sequences in detecting cartilage defects

Sequence	Sensitivity	SE*	Specificity	SE*	Accuracy	SE*
FLASH	0.80 (32/40)	0.09	0.98 (195/200)	0.01	0.95 (227/240)	0.02
DESS	0.68 (27/40)	0.13	0.99 (198/200)	0.01	0.94 (225/240)	0.03
TruFISP	0.55 (22/40)	0.13	0.97 (194/200)	0.02	0.90 (216/240)	0.03
SPACE	0.98 (39/40)	0.03	0.96 (192/200)	0.02	0.96 (231/240)	0.01
UTE	0.20 (8/40)	0.08	0.99 (198/200)	0.01	0.86 (206/240)	0.04

*SE = standard error

Note: Data are given for all articular surfaces, all grades of cartilage lesion severity, and both readers combined

Analysis of UTE morphology of the osteochondral junction

On UTE images, normal cartilage exhibited a high-intensity linear signal near the osteochondral junction. Retrospective analysis of UTE morphology of the osteochondral junction in subjects diagnosed with cartilage lesions (n=20) on conventional MRI revealed ten abnormalities (irregular, n=5; disruption, n=4; absence, n=1). Of these, six were diagnosed with high-grade cartilage lesions and four with low-grade cartilage lesions on conventional MRI (Fig. 4). Ten cartilage lesions showed a normal appearance of the osteochondral junction on UTE images. Of these, seven were diagnosed with high-grade cartilage lesions and three with low-grade cartilage lesions on conventional MRI (Fig. 2).

Discussion

The most important findings of the present study are that, first, morphological cartilage imaging of the knee can be reliably performed using 3D TSE MRI, showing good image quality

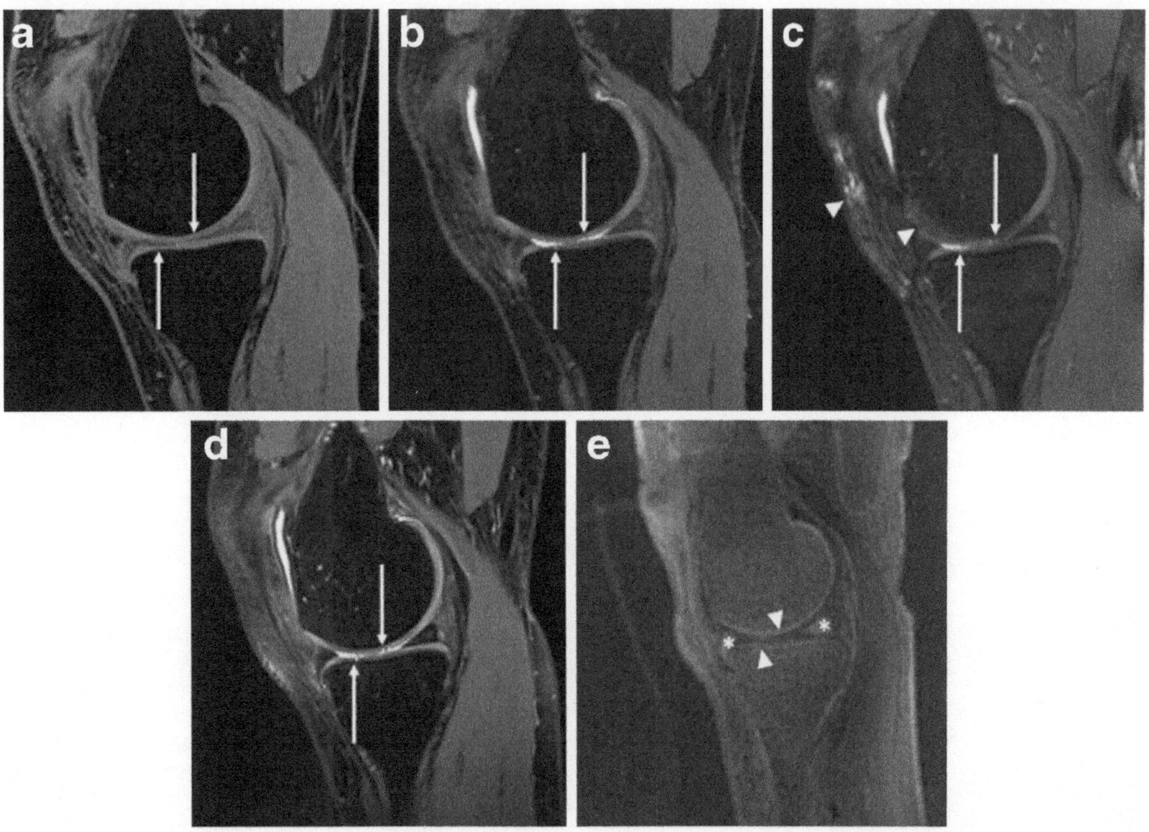

Fig. 2 A 32-year-old female marathon runner with episodes of medial knee pain. Comparison of sagittal FLASH (**a**), DESS (**b**), TruFISP (**c**), and SPACE (**d**) showing cartilage defects (arrows) at the medial knee compartment. Lesion conspicuity is highest on SPACE sequence. Susceptibility artefacts are seen on TruFISP (arrowheads). UTE subtraction image (**e**) shows normal appearance of deep osteochondral tissue at the medial knee compartment (arrowheads). Also note that, whereas the meniscus appears dark on conventional sequences, bright meniscal signal is seen on the UTE image (*)

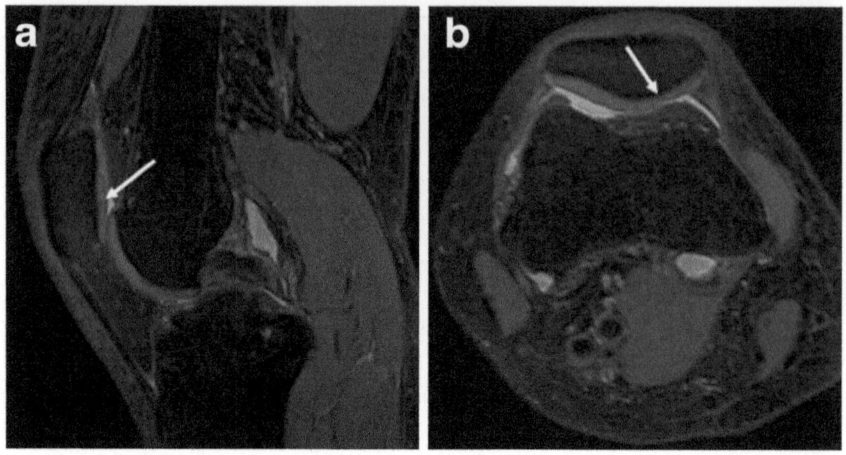

Fig. 3 A 46-year-old female patient with episodes of anterior knee pain. **a** Sagittal SPACE image shows signal heterogeneity (arrow) at the patellar cartilage. **b** Axial reformatted SPACE image shows superficial cartilage loss on the medial patellar facet (arrow)

Table 3 Qualitative image analysis

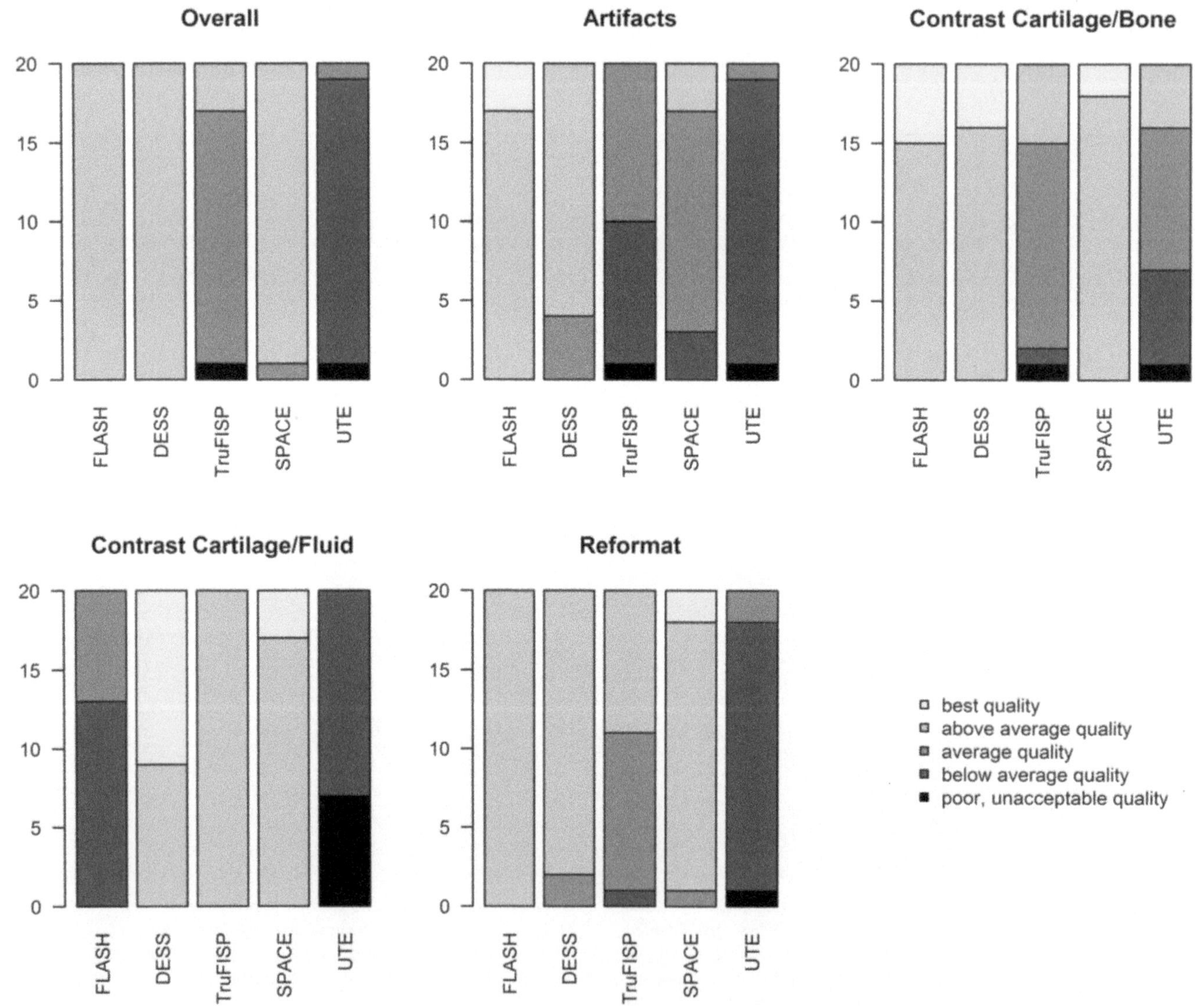

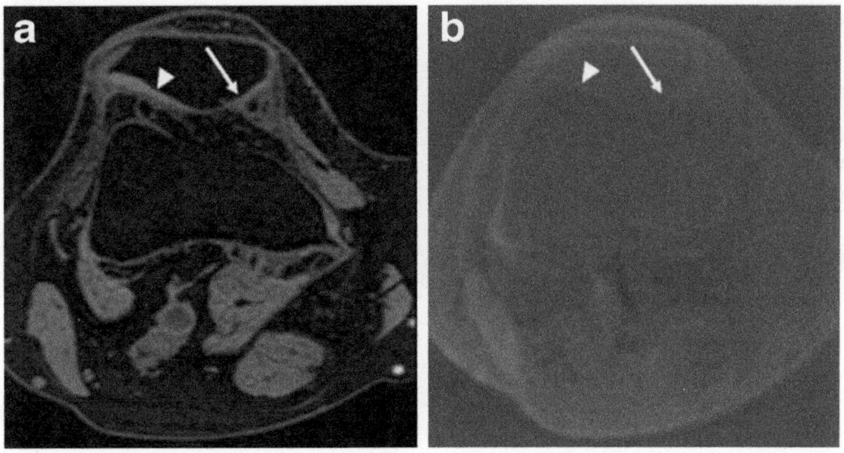

Fig. 4 A 59-year-old female with chronic knee pain. **a** Axial reformatted FLASH image shows extensive cartilage loss at the medial patella (arrow). Normal cartilage is seen on the lateral patellar facet (arrowhead). **b** Axial reformatted UTE subtraction image shows absence of high-intensity linear signal near the osteochondral junction at the medial patella (arrow). Normal UTE appearance of the osteochondral junction on the lateral patellar facet is demonstrated (arrowhead)

and high accuracy when compared to the standard of reference sequences. Second, although the newly available UTE sequence can distinguish between superficial and deep cartilage layers, it cannot be used as a single sequence to assess the articular cartilage at present.

The most common 3D sequences used in clinical practice to evaluate the articular cartilage of the knee are GRE-based methods, e.g. FLASH or DESS sequences. These sequences are available on most MR imaging systems and have been successfully used to evaluate cartilage. In addition, these sequences can be used to perform cartilage volume measurements in osteoarthritis research studies [4–8]. Although dark-fluid sequences have lower contrast between cartilage and fluid than bright-fluid sequences [4, 7], there was no significant difference in the performance of both sequences to evaluate cartilage in our study.

The development of balanced SSFP imaging, a variant of the GRE technique, was promising to improve 3D MRI of the musculoskeletal system. Several studies have shown excellent synovial fluid-cartilage contrast with these sequences. They are also useful in the imaging of other internal structures of the knee, such as the ligaments and menisci, a capability that makes it an attractive option for use in clinical practice [10, 20]. Although our study results confirm good contrast properties between cartilage and synovial fluid, the TruFISP sequence yielded more severe susceptibility artefacts and poorer overall image quality than did the conventional GRE methods.

Despite these developments, GRE imaging displays image contrast characteristics different from those of the TSE pulse sequences commonly used in assessment of joints. Recently, 3D TSE sequences (e.g. SPACE) have been used to assess the knee joint with high spin-echo contrast resolution and isotropic spatial resolution, improving conspicuity of cartilage lesions [5, 21]. Therefore, 3D TSE retains the advantages of 2D TSE while also addressing its limitations. The 3D TSE sequence typically uses variable flip angle modulation to constrain T2 decay over an extended echo train. This allows for intermediate-weighted images of the knee with bright fluid to be acquired with minimal blurring [11]. Our study results are in concordance with prior studies demonstrating superior performance of 3D SPACE in assessing cartilage lesions [14, 21]. A disadvantage of the SPACE sequence is its long acquisition time (10 min 4 s). This limitation, however, is counterbalanced by the fact that SPACE, due to its favourable tissue contrast, allows for comprehensive knee joint assessment. A single acquisition of 3D SPACE may therefore replace multiple 2D FSE acquisitions, which increases the time efficiency when used in a clinical knee MR protocol [21].

The osteochondral junction has been implicated in the pathogenesis of OA [22] and cartilage repair [23]. Thus, direct visualisation of these tissue components is clinically relevant. To date, MR imaging has, however, not been capable of assessing the deep radial and calcified layers of cartilage. These deep layers of cartilage have short T2 characteristics (<1 ms), and conventional pulse sequences are unable to acquire data in this range. UTE sequences are designed to target tissue components with very short T2 and allow signal to be detected in the deep layer of cartilage [24]. In a recent study, Bae et al. [18] compared UTE MRI and histology of experimental preparations and determined that the presence of the deepest layer of uncalcified cartilage and the calcified cartilage, but not the subschondral bone, results in this linear signal intensity in UTE MRI.

The term UTE imaging has generally been applied to techniques using shorter RF excitation pulses and faster readout methods than conventional methods to produce images with very short TEs, typically in the range of 8–250 μs [24]. A number of UTE techniques focussing on the method of image acquisition have been developed [25, 26]. These include both

2D and 3D sequences. They are typically combined with some form of long T2 component reduction in order to isolate the signal from the short T2 components and thus demonstrate change in disease [24].

Although a characteristic pattern of high linear signal near the osteochondral junction and low signal in the superficial cartilage layer could be observed in all subjects, sensitivity of our 3D UTE sequence in the detection of cartilage lesions was significantly lower compared to conventional sequences. Poor performance was probably related to blurring artefacts in the radial UTE acquisition together with field heterogeneity or potential gradient delays. Even at retrospective analysis, focal or diffuse abnormalities in the linear signal were found in only 10 of the 20 cartilage lesions. Most of these had high-grade cartilage lesions diagnosed on conventional MR sequences. In ten cartilage lesions, no abnormality in the UTE morphology of the osteochondral junction could be found. Of note, seven of these ten were apparent high-grade cartilage lesions on conventional MR sequences. This finding may suggest that these lesions were rather low-grade defects and overestimated on conventional MR images. Larger studies with arthroscopic correlation are needed to explore how the normal UTE signal pattern changes with disease and injury.

As with conventional MR techniques, UTE can also be used for quantitative mapping of tissues. A recent in vitro study [25] has evaluated UTE T2* and T1rho values of the patellar osteochondral junction in cadaveric samples and found that these measurements were useful for non-invasive assessment of the deep calcified layer of cartilage, including understanding the involvement of this tissue component in osteoarthritis.

There were several limitations to this study. First, and most important, the small number of patients limited the statistical analysis. However, in this era of limited resources and cost savings in health care, a larger study including more patients would not be possible in our busy clinical practice. Second, there was no arthroscopic correlation available. Great care was taken to obtain the best possible standard of reference using all available MR sequences and consensus readings. High accuracy of these sequences for detecting cartilage lesions is well documented in the literature [4–6]. Furthermore, arthroscopy also has limitations and should be considered an imperfect reference standard for grading of cartilage defects [27]. Third, all readers were employed in centres equipped with the sequences tested in our study; this may have introduced an interpretation bias, since the readers were very probably able to identify the sequence from the overall appearance of the blinded MR images. Fourth, in our study, we evaluated only subjective image quality, without quantitative analysis of the signal-to-noise (SNR) or contrast-to-noise (CNR) ratio. However, quantitative analysis of images acquired with parallel imaging requires that the "difference method" be used [28]. This would have been at the cost of doubling the total imaging time leading to motion artefacts again disturbing the methodological improvement.

Conclusion

Our study, comparing various isotropic 3D sequences at 3 T, confirmed that 3D TSE MRI can be reliably performed for morphological cartilage imaging of the knee. In addition, further studies with arthroscopic correlation are needed to explore the role of clinical UTE sequences in the MR imaging assessment of cartilage lesions.

Acknowledgments The UTE sequence was made available through a clinical research agreement with Siemens Healthcare.

Conflict of interest David M. Grodzki, PhD, is employed by Siemens Healthcare, Erlangen, Germany.

References

1. Brittberg M, Winalski CS (2003) Evaluation of cartilage injuries and repair. J Bone Joint Surg Am 85-A(Suppl 2):58–69
2. Guermazi A, Hayashi D, Eckstein F, Hunter DJ, Duryea J, Roemer FW (2013) Imaging of osteoarthritis. Rheum Dis Clin N Am 39: 67–105
3. Mosher TJ, Walker EA, Petscavage-Thomas J, Guermazi A (2013) Osteoarthritis year 2013 in review: imaging. Osteoarthr Cartil 21: 1425–1435
4. Kijowski R, Gold GE (2011) Routine three-dimensional magnetic resonance imaging of joints. J Magn Reson Imaging 33: 758–771
5. Crema MD, Roemer FW, Marra MD, Burstein D, Gold GE, Eckstein F et al (2011) Articular cartilage in the knee: current MR imaging techniques and applications in clinical practice and research. Radiographics 31:37–61
6. Gold GE, Hargreaves BA, Stevens KJ, Beaulieu CF (2006) Advanced magnetic resonance imaging of articular cartilage. Orthop Clin N Am 37:331–347
7. Hargreaves BA (2012) Rapid gradient-echo imaging. J Magn Reson Imaging 36:1300–1313
8. Recht MP, Goodwin DW, Winalski CS, White LM (2005) MRI of articular cartilage: revisiting current status and future directions. AJR Am J Roentgenol 185:899–914
9. Peterfy CG, Schneider E, Nevitt M (2008) The osteoarthritis initiative: report on the design rationale for the magnetic resonance imaging protocol for the knee. Osteoarthr Cartil 16:1433–1441
10. Duc SR, Pfirrmann CWA, Koch PP, Zanetti M, Hodler J (2008) Internal knee derangement assessed with 3-minute three-dimensional isovoxel True FISP MR sequence: preliminary study. Radiology 246:526–535
11. Roemer FW, Crema MD, Trattnig S, Guermazi A (2011) Advances in imaging of osteoarthritis and cartilage. Radiology 260:332–354
12. Bae WC, Biswas R, Chen K, Chang EY, Chung CB (2014) UTE MRI of the osteochondral junction. Curr Radiol Rep 2:35
13. Gatehouse PD, Bydder GM (2003) Magnetic resonance imaging of short T2 components in tissue. Clin Radiol 58:1–19
14. Chen CA, Kijowski R, Shapiro LM, Tuite MJ, Davis KW, Klaers JL et al (2010) Cartilage morphology at 3.0 T: assessment of three-

dimensional MR imaging techniques. J Magn Reson Imaging 32: 173–183

15. Friedrich KM, Reiter G, Kaiser B, Mayerhöfer M, Deimling M, Jellus V et al (2011) High-resolution cartilage imaging of the knee at 3 T: basic evaluation of modern isotropic 3D MR-sequences. Eur J Radiol 78:398–405
16. Goto H, Fujii M, Iwama Y, Aoyama N, Ohno Y, Sugimura K (2012) Magnetic resonance imaging (MRI) of articular cartilage of the knee using ultrashort echo time (UTE) sequences with spiral acquisition. J Med Imaging Radiat Oncol 56:318–323
17. Lee YH, Kim S, Song HT, Kim I, Suh JS (2014) Weighted subtraction in 3D ultrashort echo time (UTE) imaging for visualization of short T2 tissues of the knee. Acta Radiol 55:454–461
18. Bae WC, Dwek JR, Znamirowski R, Statum SM, Hermida JC, D'Lima DD et al (2010) Ultrashort echo time MR imaging of osteochondral junction of the knee at 3 T: identification of anatomic structures contributing to signal intensity. Radiology 254:837–845
19. Holm S (1979) A simple sequentially rejective multiple test procedure. Scand J Stat 6:65–70
20. Jung JY, Yoon YC, Kim HR, Choe B-K, Wang JH, Jung JY (2013) Knee derangements: comparison of isotropic 3D fast spin-echo, isotropic 3D balanced fast field-echo, and conventional 2D fast spin-echo MR imaging. Radiology 268:802–813
21. Crema MD, Nogueira-Barbosa MH, Roemer FW, Marra MD, Niu J, Chagas-Neto FA et al (2013) Three-dimensional turbo spin-echo magnetic resonance imaging (MRI) and semiquantitative assessment of knee osteoarthritis: comparison with two-dimensional routine MRI. Osteoarthr Cartil 21:428–433
22. Muir P, McCarthy J, Radtke CL, Markel MD, Santschi EM, Scollay MC et al (2006) Role of endochondral ossification of articular cartilage and functional adaptation of the subchondral plate in the development of fatigue microcracking of joints. Bone 38:342–349
23. Frisbie DD, Morisset S, Ho CP, Rodkey WG, Steadman JR, McIlwraith CW (2006) Effects of calcified cartilage on healing of chondral defects treated with microfracture in horses. Am J Sports Med 34:1824–1831
24. Gatehouse PD, Thomas RW, Robson MD, Hamilton G, Herlihy AH, Bydder GM (2004) Magnetic resonance imaging of the knee with ultrashort TE pulse sequences. Magn Reson Imaging 22: 1061–1067
25. Du J, Carl M, Bae WC, Statum S, Chang E, Bydder GM et al (2013) Dual inversion recovery ultrashort echo time (DIR-UTE) imaging and quantification of the zone of calcified cartilage (ZCC). Osteoarthr Cartil 21:77–85
26. Grodzki DM, Jakob PM, Heismann B (2012) Ultrashort echo time imaging using pointwise encoding time reduction with radial acquisition (PETRA). Magn Reson Med 67:510–518
27. Cameron ML, Briggs KK, Steadman JR (2003) Reproducibility and reliability of the outerbridge classification for grading chondral lesions of the knee arthroscopically. Am J Sports Med 31:83–86
28. Dietrich O, Raya JG, Reeder SB, Reiser MF, Schoenberg SO (2007) Measurement of signal-to-noise ratios in MR images: influence of multichannel coils, parallel imaging, and reconstruction filters. J Magn Reson Imaging 26:375–385

6

Magnetic resonance imaging of sellar and juxtasellar abnormalities in the paediatric population: an imaging review

Rachel Shields · Rajiv Mangla · Jeevak Almast · Steven Meyers

Abstract The sellar and juxtasellar regions in the paediatric population are complex both anatomically and pathologically, with magnetic resonance imaging (MRI) being the "gold standard" imaging modality due to the high contrast of detail. Assessment requires a detailed understanding of the anatomy, embryology, pathophysiology and normal signal characteristics of the pituitary gland and surrounding structures in order to appropriately characterise abnormalities. This article aims to provide an overview of the imaging characteristics of developmental/congenital and acquired disease processes which affect the sellar and juxtasellar region in the paediatric population.

Main Messages

- *The sellar region is anatomically complex and covers a wide pathology spectrum.*
- *MRI is the key imaging modality to assess sellar and juxtasellar pathology.*
- *Numerous developmental anomalies may not be discovered until adulthood.*
- *Knowledge of pathology alerts and guides the clinician towards appropriate management.*

Keywords Magnetic resonance imaging · Paediatrics · Pituitary gland · Pituitary diseases · Sella turcica

R. Shields (✉) · R. Mangla · J. Almast · S. Meyers
Department of Imaging Sciences, University of Rochester Medical Center, 601 Elmwood Ave., Rochester, NY 14642-0001, USA
e-mail: rachel_shields@urmc.rochester.edu

Pituitary function and anatomy

The pituitary gland is comprised of two dominant lobes, the neurohypophysis and the adenohypophysis. It is situated within the sella turcica, a depression in the sphenoid bone which is covered by the diaphragm sella with a defect for the passage of the infundibulum. The pituitary stalk extends inferiorly as a continuation of the hypothalamic infundibulum (Fig. 1).

The neurohypophysis receives its hormonal supply through direct contiguity with the hypothalamus, with axons extending from the hypothalamic supraoptic and paraventricular nuclei into the neurohypophysis. The hormonal supply includes oxytocin and vasopressin-containing vesicles. The adenohypophysis does not have axonal contiguity between the hypothalamus and the anterior gland and relies on the hypothalamic-hypophyseal portal system. Parvocellular messengers are transported from the hypothalamic median eminence into the capillaries surrounding the anterior gland. Hormones from the adenohypophysis include: follicle stimulating hormone, luteinising hormone, corticotropin (ACTH), thyroid-stimulating hormone, prolactin and growth hormone.

Embryology

The pituitary gland develops through a complex mechanism involving the developing diencephalon and the primitive oral stomodeum [1]. The adenohypophysis derives from Rathke's pouch, which originates rostral to the oropharyngeal membrane. This begins at approximately 24 days of gestation, in which Rathke's pouch forms as an ectodermal outpouching of stomodeum and the infundibulum which forms in the floor of the diencephalon. The infundibulum grows ventrally, while simultaneously Rathke's pouch grows dorsally. Rathke's pouch eventually loses its connection with the stomodeum

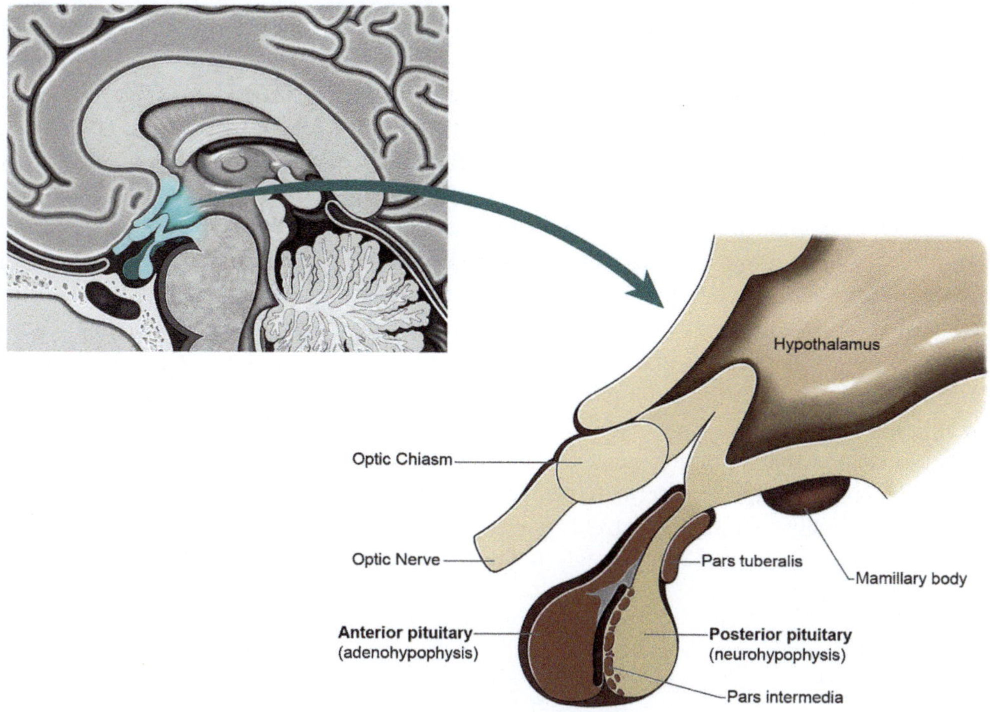

Fig. 1 Normal pituitary anatomy

and forms a sac which adheres to the infundibular process. This sac continues to differentiate into the adenophyophysis and the distal aspect of the infundibulum differentiates to form the neurohypophysis (Fig. 2).

Imaging characteristics in the paediatric population

The pituitary gland exhibits a wide range of appearances during the first 2 years of life, with considerable variability in

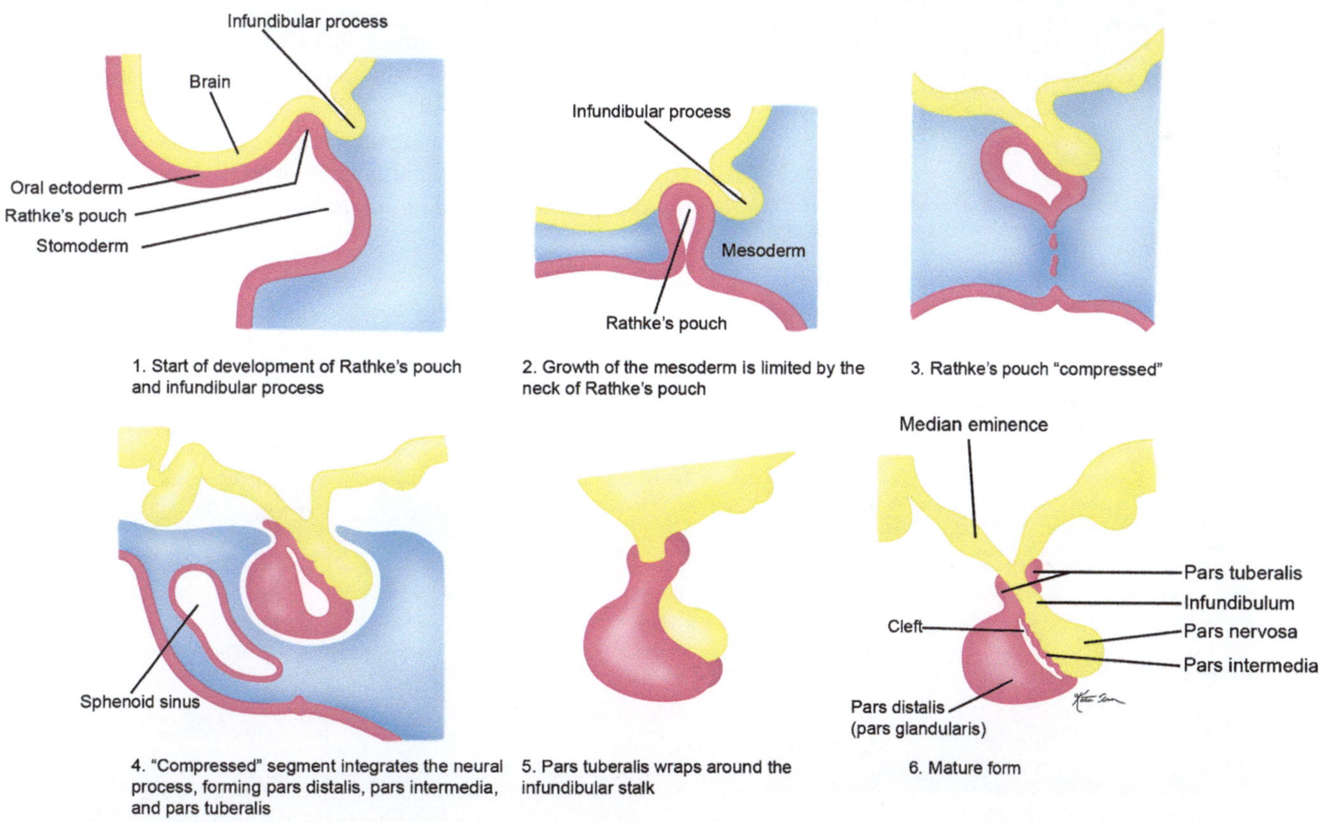

Fig. 2 Normal development of the pituitary gland

size, shape, and signal. At birth, both the anterior and posterior pituitary gland have high signal intensity on T1-weighted images (Fig. 3). The anterior pituitary progressively decreases in signal intensity on T1-weighted images with signal drop to near isointensity with the posterior pons by 6 weeks of age [1, 2]. The posterior pituitary gland retains its high signal intensity on T1-weighted images throughout adulthood, with several papers supporting that this high signal results from neurosecretory granules or the protein neurophysin [3–5]. The normal gland enhances symmetrically after intravenous gadolinium with the anterior gland enhancement appearing more noticeable given the posterior gland is already high signal at baseline.

At birth, the gland is physiologically enlarged with a corresponding concave superior margin, flattening with age. The gland is traditionally symmetric in size; however there can be asymmetry in normally functioning glands. In preterm infants, the gland is taller than in normal-term infants, even when correcting for gestational age. This is thought to be the result of reduced insulin-like growth factor 1 and higher levels of growth hormone in premature infants [6]. The pituitary height is fairly stable for the first 2 years of life in normal-term children. Gender-associated differences in the rate of gland growth tend to occur after 5 years of age, with linear growth of the gland up to that point in both boys and girls [7]. Typically, the normal pituitary measures between 2 to 6 mm in height during childhood and up to 10 mm or slightly higher at puberty. In adults, the female glands are slightly larger than their male counter parts [1]. Standards for assessing the pituitary stalk size are not well established, and are based on experience rather than age-appropriate measurements. The stalk is best visualised on post-contrast T1-weighted images because of the strong enhancement.

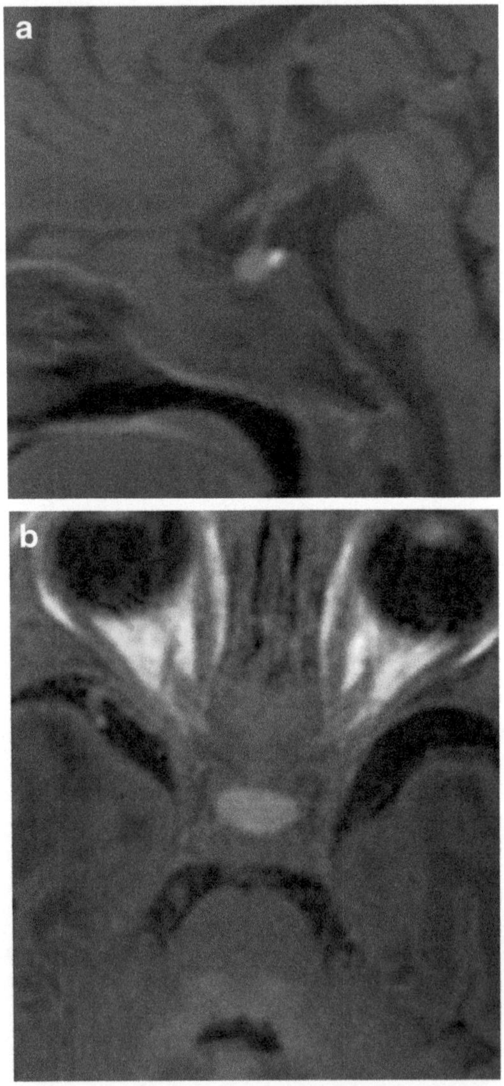

Fig. 3 Normal physiological T1 sagittal (**a**) and axial (**b**) hyperintensity of the anterior pituitary in a 1-month-old baby

Developmental anomalies of the pituitary gland

Agenesis of the adenohypophysis (Fig. 4) This is a rare congenital anomaly with a neonatal presentation. The neonates can present with metabolic acidosis, thyroid and adrenal insufficiency, hypoglycaemia, and/or seizures. Associated anomalies of the forebrain and midline craniofacial bones can be present. Newborns are normal in size at birth, which has been explained by the presence of maternal growth hormone. Standard treatment includes replacement of growth hormone, thyroid hormone and glucocorticoids. Magnetic resonance imaging (MRI) findings include the absence of the anterior pituitary gland with an associated shallow sella, and variable length of the infundibulum and position of the posterior pituitary, ranging from the hypothalamus to the sella [8].

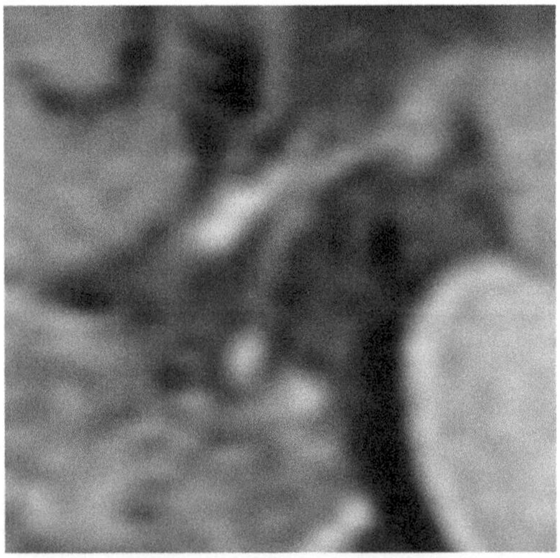

Fig. 4 Agenesis of the anterior pituitary gland (adenohypophysis) in an infant with hypopituitarism. Sagittal T1-weighted imaging (T1WI) shows absence of the adenohypophisis. The stalk terminates into a bulbous neurohypophysis with high signal in the dorsal portion of the sella

The infundibulum may be thinned and terminate into a partially formed bulbous posterior pituitary gland.

Hypoplasia of the adenohypophysis (Fig. 5) This rare anomaly consists of hypoplasia of the anterior pituitary gland, and also potentially the infundibulum and posterior pituitary gland. It can be associated with varying degrees of endocrine dysfunction, including panhypopituitarism and other congenital anomalies. Some research suggests that traumatic transection of the pituitary stalk during birth or hypoxic injury to the hypothalamus could result in hypoplasia, whereas others suggest an error during embryogenesis [9–12]. MRI findings include varying degrees of hypoplasia of the anterior pituitary gland with variable size and length of the infundibulum. As with agenesis of the adenohypophysis, the posterior pituitary position can range from the hypothalamus to the sella.

Ectopic posterior pituitary (Fig. 6) This congenital anomaly results in an aberrant position of the neurohypophysis, often located at the undersurface of the hypothalamus. It is associated with pituitary dwarfism, delayed skeletal maturation, Kallman syndrome, septo-optic dysplasia, dysgenesis of the corpus callosum, lobar holoprosencephaly, Chiari 1 malformation or a persistent/enlarged craniopharyngeal canal. It affects males more than females. MRI may show a small

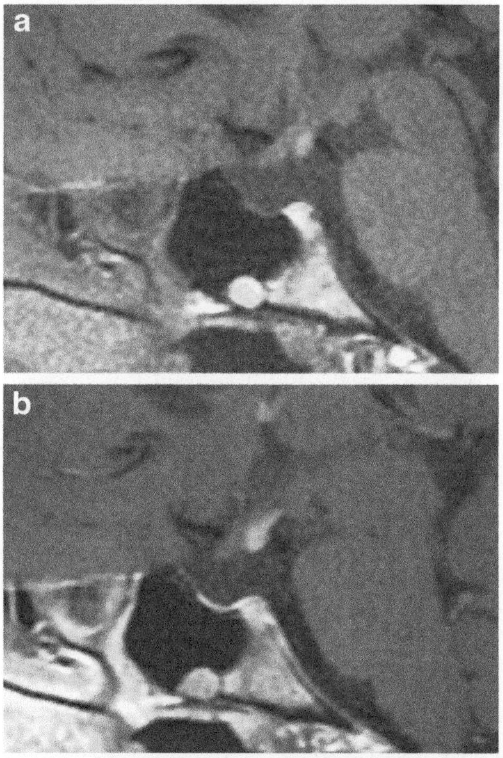

Fig. 5 Severe hypoplasia of the anterior pituitary gland. Pre-contrast (**a**) and post-contrast (**b**) MR images show severe hypoplasia of the anterior pituitary gland which shows only minimal contrast enhancement along the floor of the sella. The ectopic posterior pituitary is located adjacent to the optic chiasm

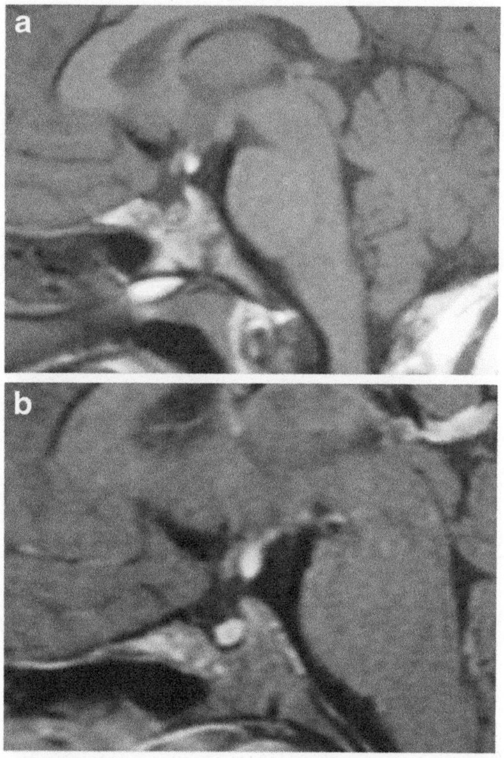

Fig. 6 Ectopic posterior pituitary gland. Pre-contrast (**a**) and post-contrast (**b**) MR images show a normal anterior pituitary gland with contrast enhancement and an ectopic posterior pituitary located adjacent to the optic chiasm

anterior pituitary gland with the posterior "bright spot" on T1-weighted imaging (T1WI) located within the upper portion of the infundibulum or the undersurface of the hypothalamus instead of the dorsal portion of the sella [1, 13–15].

Pituitary duplication (Fig. 7) This congenital anomaly is related to abnormal separation of the anterior portion of the notochord and prechordal plate during embryogenesis, likely due to teratogenic factors occurring during early embryogenesis [16, 17]. Clinical findings include precocious puberty, facial dysmorphism, hypothyroidism and/or increased prolactin levels. Pituitary duplication may be associated with other anomalies such as dysgenesis of the corpus callosum, absent olfactory bulbs, cerebellar hypoplasia, midline defects, and teratomas. MRI findings include duplicated pituitary stalks and glands within separate pituitary fossa in the sphenoid bone. Abnormal thickening, "pseudohamartoma", of the hypothalamus with duplication of the infundibular recess of the third ventricle is often seen [16, 18]. Pituitary duplication can also be associated with duplication of the basilar artery [19].

Hypothalamic hamartoma (Figs. 8 and 9) Congenital developmental non-neoplastic grey matter heterotopia involving the tuber cinereum, inferior hypothalamus and/or mammillary bodies which are composed of small neuronal cells within a neutrophil-like stroma and scattered fibrillary astrocytes.

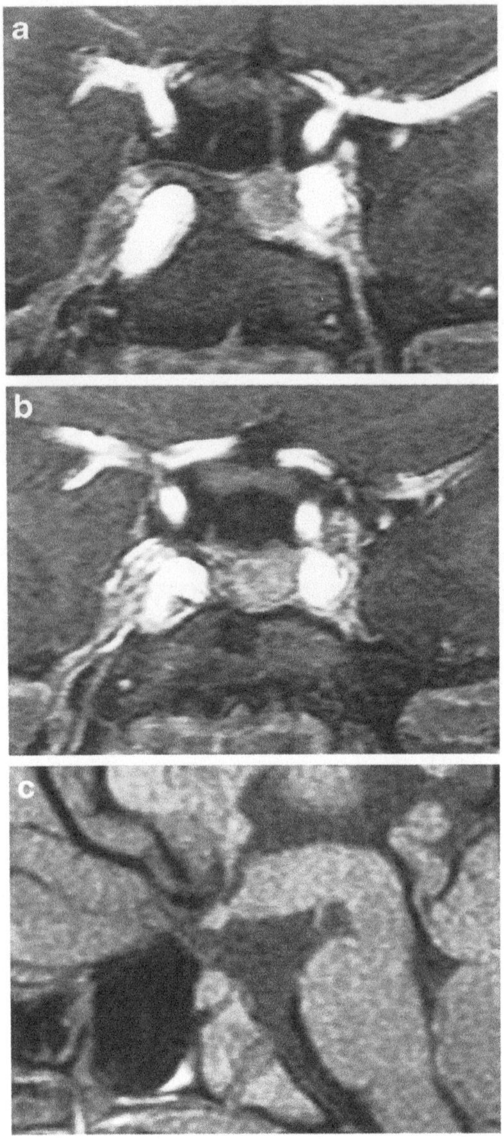

Fig. 7 Pituitary duplication. Coronal post-contrast images (**a** and **b**) show two pituitary stalks which extend inferiorly into separate duplicated pituitary glands. Sagittal T1WI (**c**) shows marked thickening of the hypothalamus, referred to as a pseudohamartoma, which has intermediate signal. The pseudohamartoma showed no contrast enhancement (not shown)

These lesions typically occur in children with isosexual precocious puberty (0-8 years) or seizures, both gelastic or partial complex, in the second decade [20, 21]. They can be associated with holoprosencephaly, midline facial, cardiac and renal anomalies. MRI demonstrates sessile or pedunculated lesions at the tuber cinereum of the hypothalamus, often intermediate signal on T1WI and T2WI similar to grey matter. Lesions occasionally have slightly high signal on T2WI, with no contrast enhancement or restricted diffusion. Rarely contain cystic and/or fatty portions may be seen in a small minority of cases. The absence of long-term change in size or signal intensity supports the diagnosis [22]. Ictal FDG-PET and SPECT show hyperperfusion during seizures. On MR spectroscopy, there may be an elevated myoinositol peak.

Persistent craniopharyngeal canal (Fig. 10) Lack of involution of the craniopharyngeal canal, which can contain pituitary tissue. The adenohypophysis develops from evagination of ectodermal cells at the upper posterior portion of the primitive oropharynx, Rathke's pouch, at 4-5 weeks of gestation. Rathke's pouch passes between the developing presphenoid and basisphenoid chondrification centres at the upper clivus and sella, where it associates with the descending neuroectoderm of the infundibulum and will go on to form the neurohypophysis. The pathway of Rathke's pouch is the craniopharyngeal canal, which progressively involutes by 6-7 weeks of gestation. The persistent craniopharyngeal canal on MRI can be associated with trans-sphenoidal meningoencephaloceles, ectopic pituitary tissue, sphenoid teratoma and infrasellar craniopharyngiomas [23, 24]. On MRI, the persistent canal has low T1 signal intensity compared with the high T1 signal of the clivus [13].

Rathke's cleft cyst (Fig. 11) Benign cystic lesion containing fluid and variable amounts of protein, mucopolysaccharides and/or cholesterol [25, 26]. The cysts arise from epithelial rests of the craniopharyngeal canal. They are 2-3 times more common in women than men, and occasionally become symptomatically related to compression of adjacent structures. The frequency of these cysts on MRI in one study was 1.2 % in childhood [27]. MRI will show a well-circumscribed lesion with variable low, intermediate or high signal on T1WI and T2WI. On T2WI, a small low-signal nodule may be seen within the predominant high signal of the lesion, which does not enhance after contrast administration. The incidence of these intracystic nodules varies from 17 to 78 % [28, 29]. There is no contrast enhancement centrally; however, occasionally there may be a thin peripheral rim of enhancement from associated inflammation. The majority are located in the intrasellar region or combined intrasellar and suprasellar region with reports that only 8.3 % are exclusively suprasellar [30, 31]. Most are stable in size, and some may disappear spontaneously. Pars intermedia cysts (Fig. 12) can also form along the posterior margin of Rathke's pouch, are typically less than 3 mm, with many considered Rathke's cleft cysts on imaging as they are difficult to distinguish from one another and Rathke's cleft cysts are more common [1].

Cephaloceles (meningoceles or meningoencephaloceles) (Fig. 13) Congenital malformation involving the lack of separation of neuroectoderm from surface ectoderm with resultant localised failure of bone formation. There is a wide range of abnormalities which affect the skull base within the sella turcica, ranging from a persistent craniopharyngeal canal to trans-sphenoidal and sphenoethmoidal cephaloceles, many

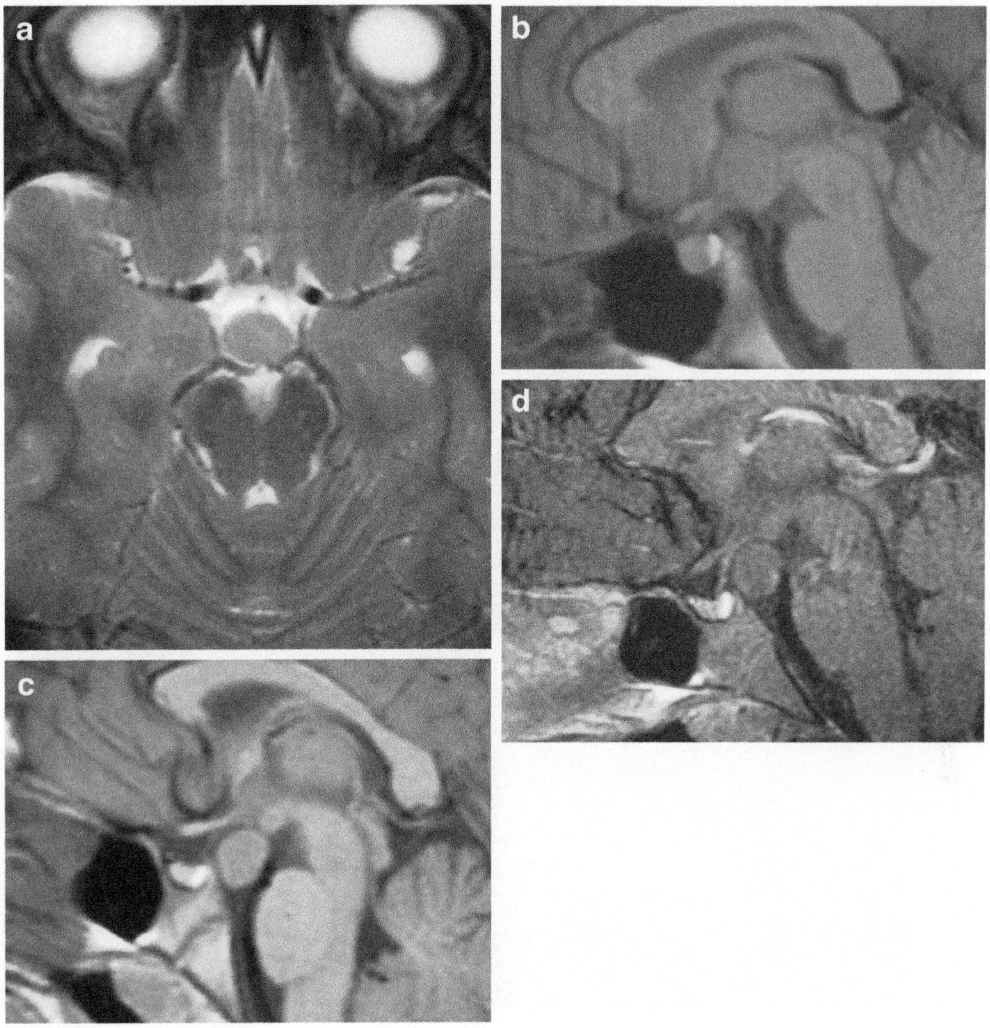

Fig. 8 Hypothalamic hamartoma. Axial T2WI (**a**) and sagittal T1WI (**b**) shows a sessile type of hypothalamic hamartoma which has intermediate signal similar to grey matter. Pre-contrast (**c**) and post-contrast (**d**) sagittal T1WI in another patient shows a pedunculated hypothalamic hamartoma with intermediate signal and lacks contrast enhancement

presentations of which are extremely rare. For example, the reported incidence of trans-sphenoidal meningoencephaloceles is 1 per 700,000 live births [13, 32]. Clinical findings include difficulty in feeding and nasal obstruction in the first year, and potential for cerebrospinal fluid (CSF) leaks and meningitis. MRI will show a defect in the skull, through which there is either herniation of meninges and CSF (meningocele), or meninges, CSF and brain tissue (meningoencephaloceles).

Epidermoid (congenital cholesteatoma) (Fig. 14) Non-neoplastic congenital or acquired extra-axial off-midline lesion filled with desquamated cells and keratinaceous debris, usually with mild mass effect on the adjacent brain. Epidermoids grow by accumulation of desquamated epithelial cells into the centre of the cyst [33–35]. MRI will show a well circumscribed spheroid or multilobulated extra-axial ectodermal inclusion cystic lesion with low-intermediate signal on T1WI, high signal on T2WI and no contrast enhancement. They can be distinguished from arachnoid cysts, as they are typically high signal on FLAIR and DWI sequences, with corresponding low signal on ADC [36].

Dermoid (Fig. 15) Non-neoplastic congenital or acquired ectodermal inclusion cystic lesion, which like an epidermoid, is lined by squamous epithelium, and are filled with lipid material, cholesterol, desquamated cells and keratinaceous debris. They are distinguished from epidermoids by containing deeper dermal elements and commonly arise from the midline. They typically present in the 20- to 30-year age range, but can also be seen in adolescence, with males slightly more affected than females [36]. MRI will show a well-circumscribed spheroid or multilobulated extra-axial lesion, usually with high signal on T1WI, variable signal on T2WI and no contrast enhancement. Fluid/fluid or fluid/debris levels may be present. They can cause a chemical meningitis if the dermoid cyst ruptures into the subarachnoid space [37, 38].

Arachnoid cyst (Fig. 16) Congenital arachnoid cysts are found in 0.16 % of all newborns with approximately 9-15 % occurring in the sellar region, with suprasellar cysts more commonly seen than intrasellar cysts. Most cases are asymptomatic; however, they may cause headache, optic nerve compression, psychomotor retardation, endocrine dysfunction or

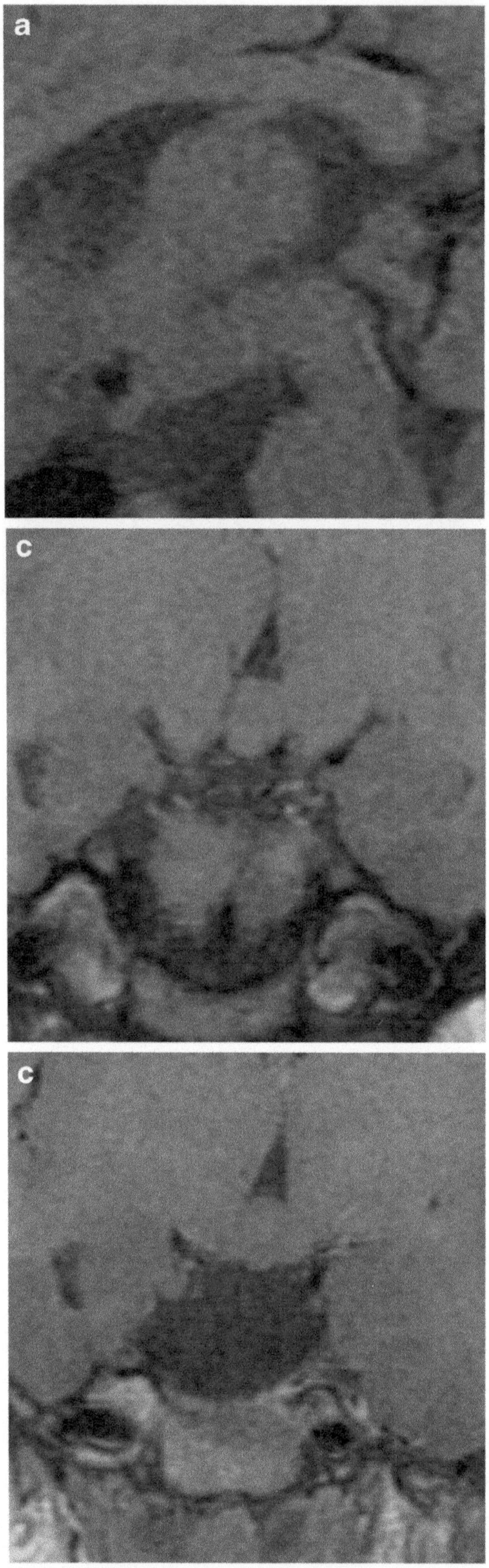

Fig. 9 Tuber cinerum hamartoma. Sagittal (**a**) and coronal (**b**) T1WI, and coronal post-contrast T1WI (**c**) show a non-enhancing bulky soft tissue mass in the region of the of the tuber cinerum

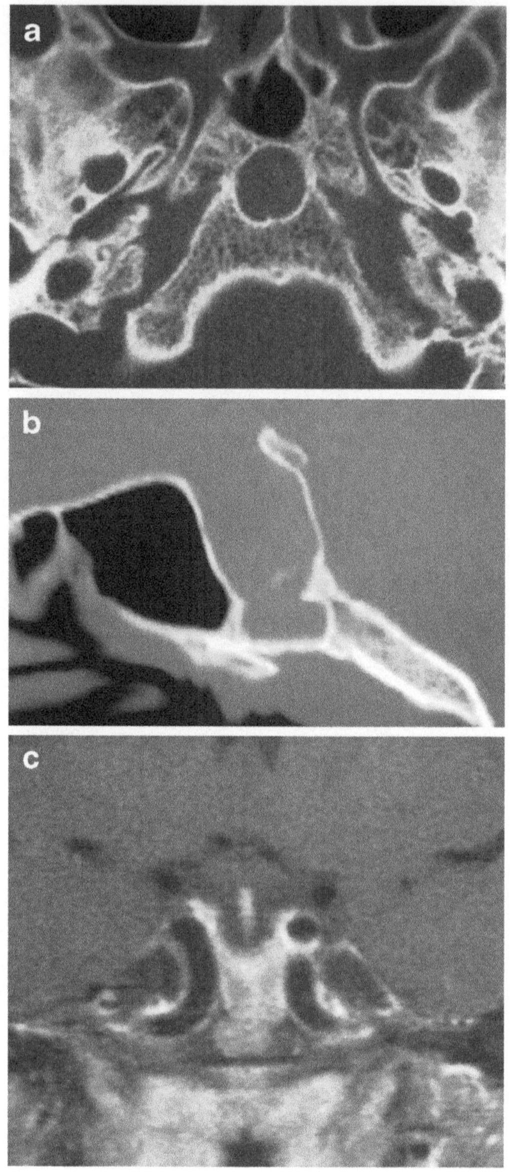

Fig. 10 Persistent craniopharyngeal canal. Axial (**a**) and sagittal (**b**) CT shows a markedly enlarged persistent craniopharyngeal canal. Coronal fat-suppressed T1WI shows inferior extension of enhancing pituitary tissue within the abnormally enlarged craniopharyngeal canal (**c**)

hydrocephalus [39, 40]. Secondary arachnoid cysts may result from trauma, haemorrhage or infection [41]. On imaging, the cysts have low signal intensity on T1WI, FLAIR and DWI, high signal intensity on T2WI, no contrast enhancement, and may cause mild mass effect on adjacent brain.

Lipoma (Fig. 17) Benign fatty lesions resulting from a congenital malformation, often located at or near the midline. In the sellar region, they occur along the surface of the infundibulum, floor of the third ventricle, or adjacent to cranial nerves, and are usually discovered incidentally, unless they cause a mass effect [42, 43]. They may contain calcifications and/or traverse blood vessels. MRI signal is

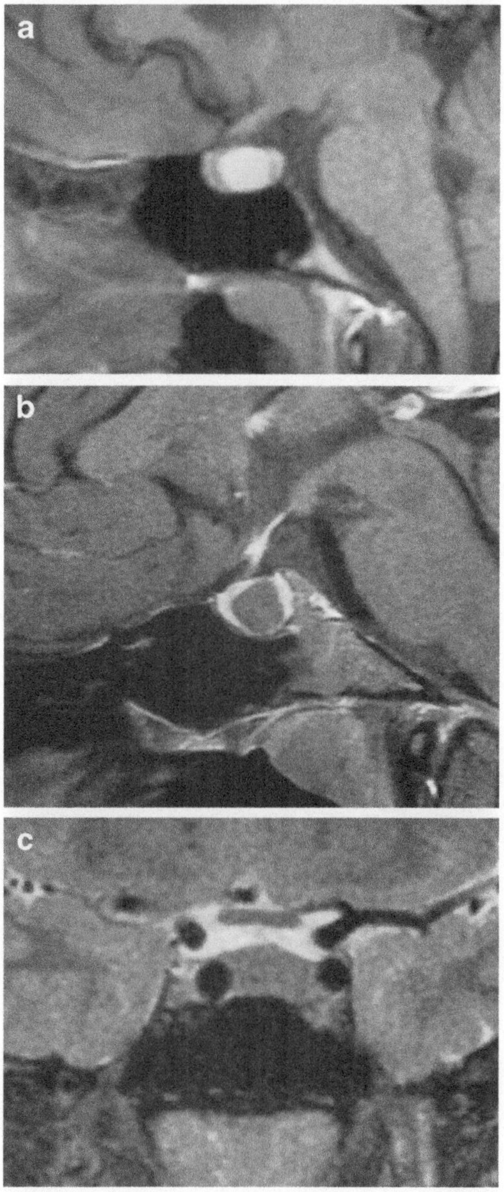

Fig. 11 Rathke's cleft cyst. Sagittal T1WI (**a**) shows a lesion in the central portion of the pituitary gland which has high signal. Post-contrast sagittal fat-suppressed T1WI (**b**) shows lack of enhancement of the Rathke cleft cyst. The cyst has intermediate signal on T2WI (**c**) secondary to slightly elevated protein content

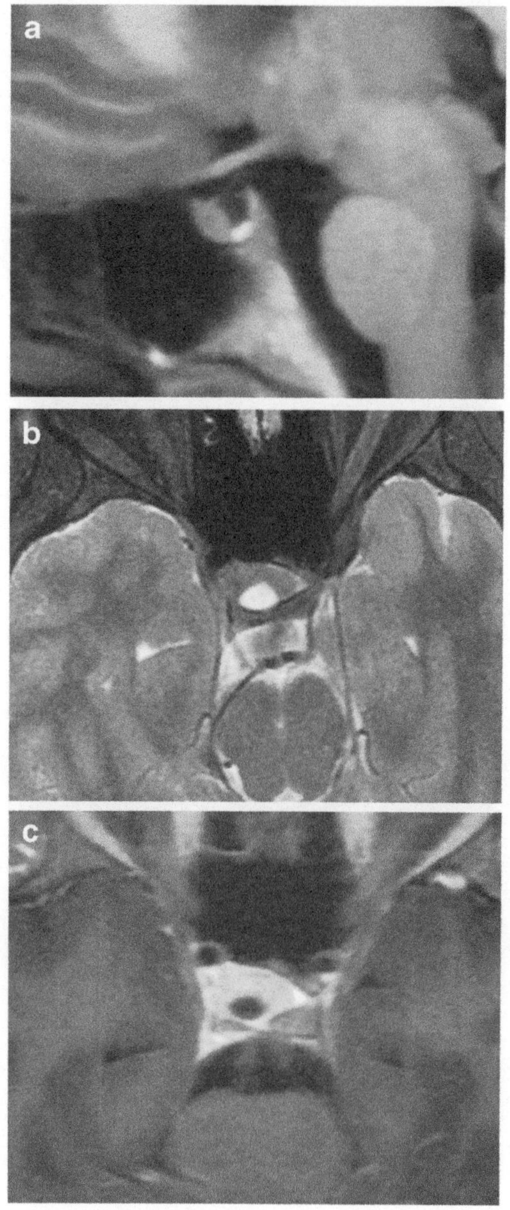

Fig. 12 Pars intermedia cyst. Sagittal T1WI (**a**) and axial T2WI (**b**) shows a small cyst between the anterior and posterior pituitary which lacks contrast enhancement on axial fat-suppressed T1WI (**c**)

isointense to subcutaneous fat on all sequences, with fat suppressed images useful in distinguishing from haemorrhagic or proteinaceous lesions.

Empty sella (Fig. 18) Common incidental finding involving the pituitary gland and sella, which can result from a weakened or fenestrated diaphragma sella allowing CSF pulsations to flatten the pituitary gland. They are associated with elevated intracranial pressure, a posteriorly placed optic chiasm, and are considered a normal variant or termed "primary empty sella turcica" in the absence of surgery, radiation therapy or medically treated intrasellar tumour [44]. In children, the incidence of an empty sella is seen more often in boys and is more likely to be associated with clinical symptoms and endocrinopathies, particularly growth hormone or multiple pituitary hormone deficiencies [45]. MRI findings include a thinned/flattened pituitary gland along the floor of the sella, with the infundibulum in its normal midline position. The flattened pituitary gland has normal MRI signal characteristics and contrast enhancement.

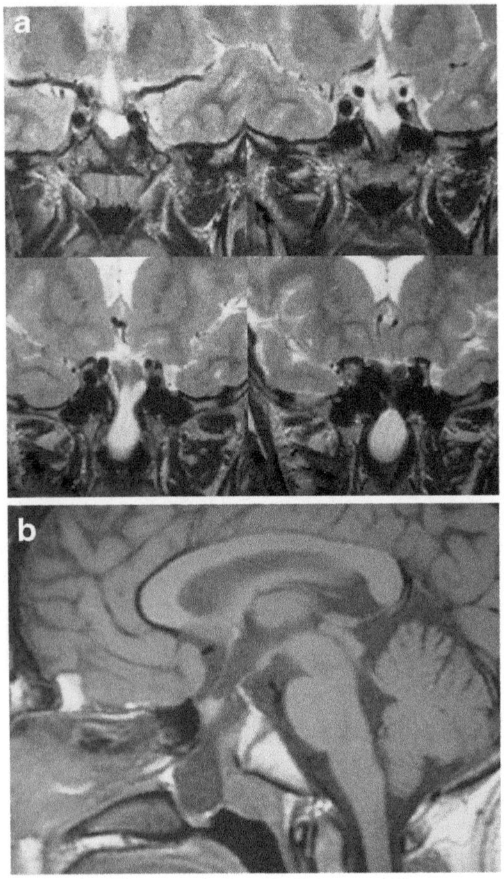

Fig. 13 Cephalocele in a 17-year-old girl. Coronal T2WI (**a**) and sagittal T1WI (**b**) shows a meningocele extending inferiorly into the nasopharynx through an osseous defect in the sphenoid bone posterior to the pituitary gland

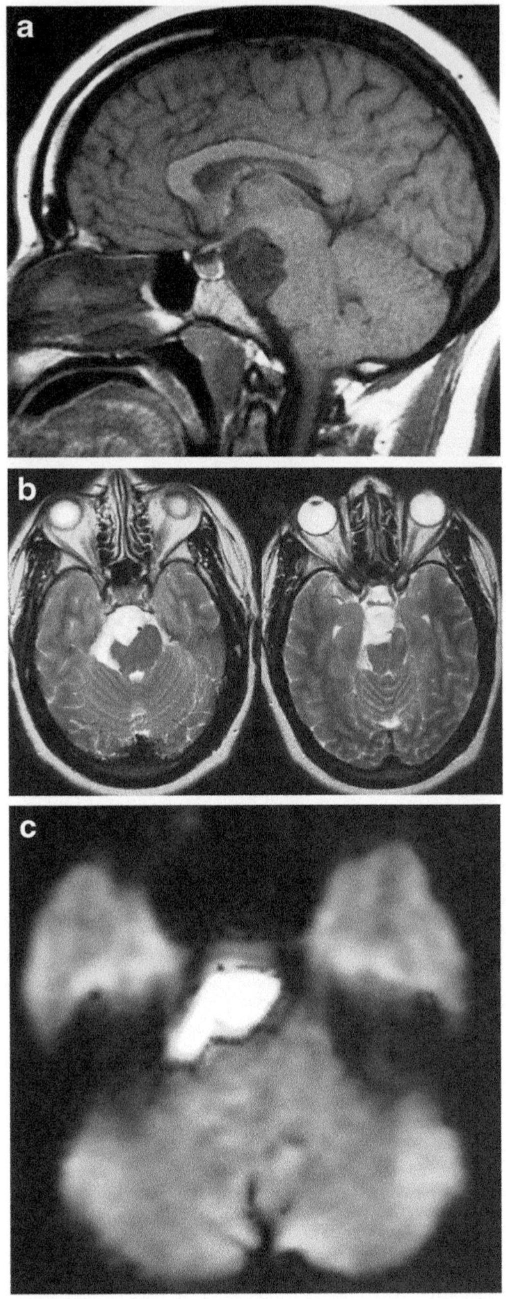

Fig. 14 Epidermoid. Sagittal T1WI (**a**) shows an extra-axial lesion along the endocranial surface which has heterogeneous mostly low-intermdiate signal, and on T2WI has high signal (**b**). Diffusion-weighted imaging (DWI) (**c**) shows restricted diffusion

Pituitary lesions

Pituitary adenoma (Fig. 19) In comparison to adults, pituitary adenomas are rare in the paediatric population, accounting for approximately 2.7 % of all supratentorial tumours. Most paediatric adenomas are functioning, with only 3-6 % non-functioning, compared to one-third of non-functioning adenomas in adults [46–48]. Microadenomas may be associated with endocrine abnormalities related to over-secretion of hormones, with prolactinomas being the most common. Rarely, extensive haemorrhage can occur involving the adenoma, resulting in pituitary apoplexy (Sheehan syndrome). Macroadenomas with suprasellar extension can cause compression and displacement of the optic chiasm with associated visual disturbances (bitemporal hemianiopsia). Most pituitary adenomas arise from sporadic mutations; however, 5 % can be associated with inherited disorders such as McCune Albright syndrome, Carney complex and multiple endocrine neoplasia type 1 (MEN 1).

MRI findings of a microadenoma (<10 mm) commonly have intermediate signal on T1WI and T2WI, and may show characteristics of cysts, haemorrhage or necrosis. They typically show less contrast enhancement than normal pituitary tissue, often best visualised with dynamic early-phase imaging. In macroadenomas (>10 mm), they commonly have intermediate signal on T1WI and T2WI similar to grey matter, and may

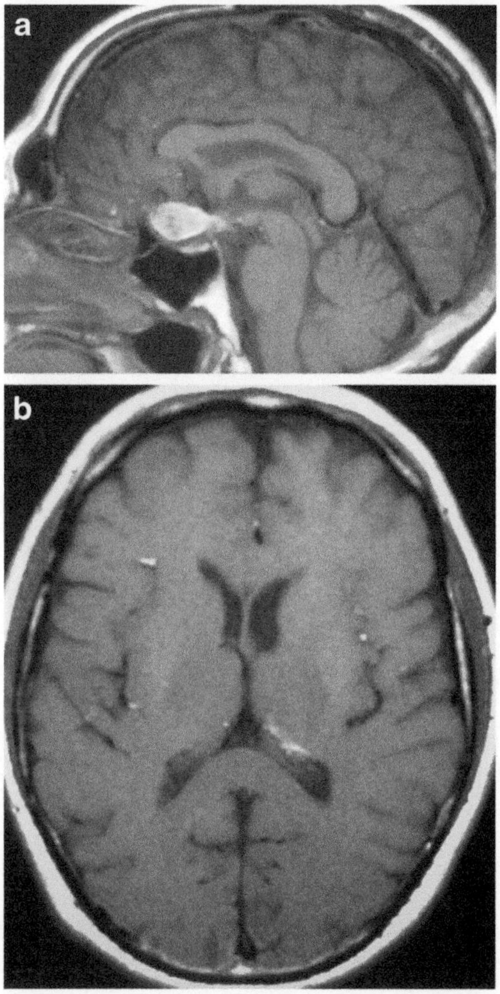

Fig. 15 Dermoid. Sagittal (**a**) and axial (**b**) T1WI shows an extra-axial lesion in the suprasellar cistern which has high signal. Multiple small foci with high signal are seen in the sulci and within the left lateral ventricle representing ruptured dermoid contents in the leptomeninges

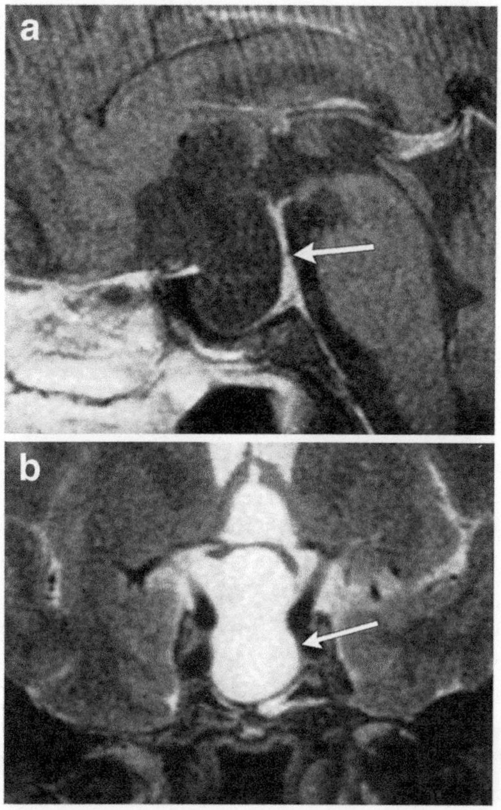

Fig. 16 Arachnoid cyst. Sagittal T1WI (**a**) and coronal T2WI (**b**) show a well defined cystic mass with low T1 and high T2 signal intensity with sellar and suprasellar components

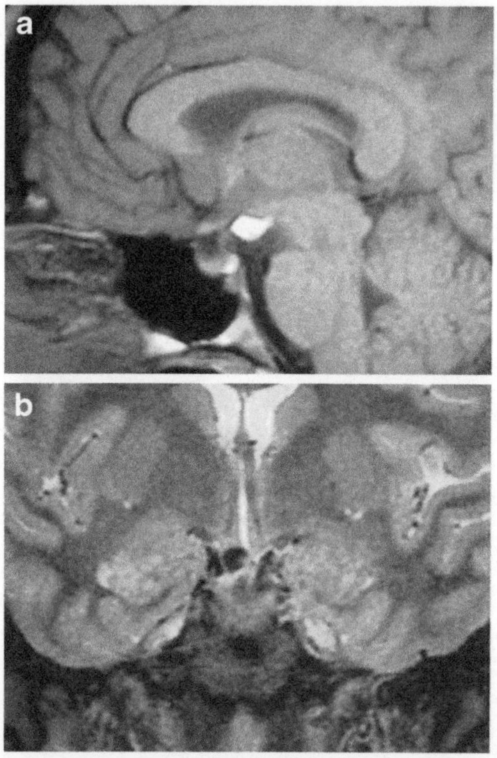

Fig. 17 Lipoma. Sagittal T1WI (**a**) shows a lipoma with high signal along the inferior surface of the hypothalamus. The signal on the lipoma is nulled on coronal fat-suppressed T2WI (**b**)

also have cystic, haemorrhagic or necrotic components. They can extend into the suprasellar cistern with a waist at the diaphragm sella or into the cavernous sinus, with occasional invasion into the skull base.

Juxtasellar lesions

Craniopharyngioma (Fig. 20) Usually histologically benign locally aggressive lesions which arise from squamous epithelial rests along Rathke's cleft, occurring in a bimodal age distribution, in children (<10 years) and adults (>40 years). Craniopharyngioma's account for 3 % of all intracranial tumours. They are categorised into adamantinomatous and squamous-papillary types. The adamantinomatous type is more common and has a bimodal age distribution occurring in children and adults, whereas the squamous-papillary type usually occurs in adults. Although histologically benign, their

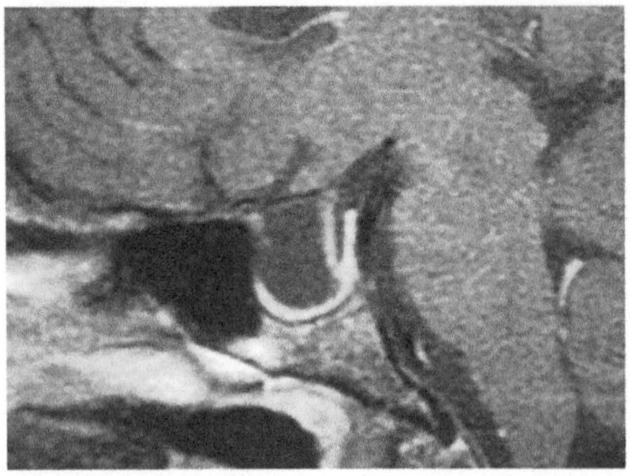

Fig. 18 Empty sella. Sagittal post-contrast T1WI with fat-suppression show an enlarged sella mostly filled with CSF. The enhancing flattened pituitary tissue is located along the floor of the sella

insinuating pattern of growth makes complete surgical excision very difficult and not often possible.

The adamantinomatous type usually demonstrates circumscribed lobulated margins on MRI, with the suprasellar location seen at a greater frequency than intrasellar. They show variable low, intermediate and/or high signal on T1WI and T2WI, with or without a nodular or rim of contrast enhancement. They may contain cysts, lipid components and calcifications. In children, the cystic parts tend to predominate, and frequently contain highly proteinaceous fluid, which may be bright on T1WI [49].

Glioma (Fig. 21) Lesions which may occur anywhere along the optic pathway and account for 4-6 % of brain tumours in children, with a median age of diagnosis from 5-9 years. Approximately half of patients with optic pathway gliomas have neurofibromatosis type 1 (NF1), with symptomatic lesions only occurring in 1-5 % of patients [50]. Most tumours are slow growing WHO grade I-II astrocytomas, often the pilocytic type, however tumours may show a wide spectrum of progression. On MRI, there is fusiform and/or nodular enlargement of the optic chiasm and/or optic nerves with thickening of the third ventricular floor and hypothalamus. They usually have low-intermediate signal on T1WI, intermediate-high signal on T2WI and variable contrast enhancement. Larger lesions may have cystic components and grow directly into the pituitary stalk [1].

Pilomyxoid astrocytoma (Fig. 22) Rare neoplasms (WHO grade II) which contain prominent mucoid matrix and angiocentric pattern of bipolar neoplastic astrocytes. Typically, they occur in children in the first and second decades, with a mean age of 7 years [51]. They tend to occur at a younger age and are more aggressive with a higher rate of local recurrence than pilocytic astromcytomas. They have a strong predilection for the hypothalamus and suprasellar cistern [52]; however, they can also occur in the thalamus, cerebellum,

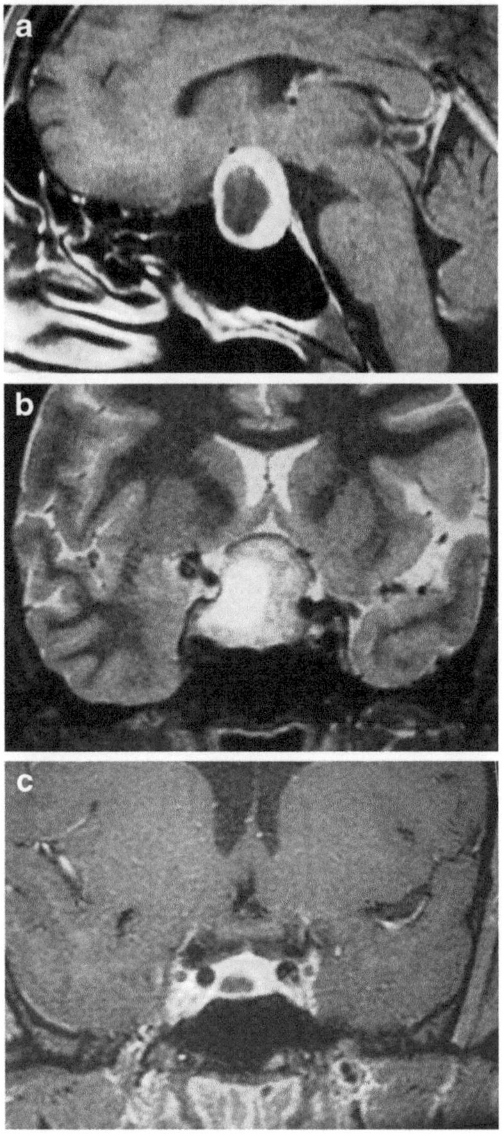

Fig. 19 Pituitary adenomas. Sagittal post-contrast fat-suppressed T1WI (**a**) shows an heterogenously enhancing pituitary macroadenoma which contains a non-enhancing portion with high signal on T2WI (**b**). secondary to cystic degeneration. Coronal post-contrast fat-suppressed T1WI (**c**) shows a pituitary microadenoma which shows less early contrast enhancement than the normal pituitary tissue

brainstem, temporal lobe and spinal cord. The presence of intra-tumoural haemorrhage is the most prominent imaging characteristic to suggest a pilomyxoid astrocytoma over a pilocytic astrocytoma, 25 % versus 8 %, respectively [51]. MRI demonstrates a solid/cystic focal lesion with low-intermediate signal on T1WI, high signal on T2WI and FLAIR, variable contrast enhancement and may show increased ADC values.

Germ cell tumours—germinoma (Fig. 23) Extra-gonadal germ cell tumours include: germinoma (most common), mature teratoma, malignant teratoma, yolk sac tumour, embryonal carcinoma and choriocarcinoma. They account for 0.6 %

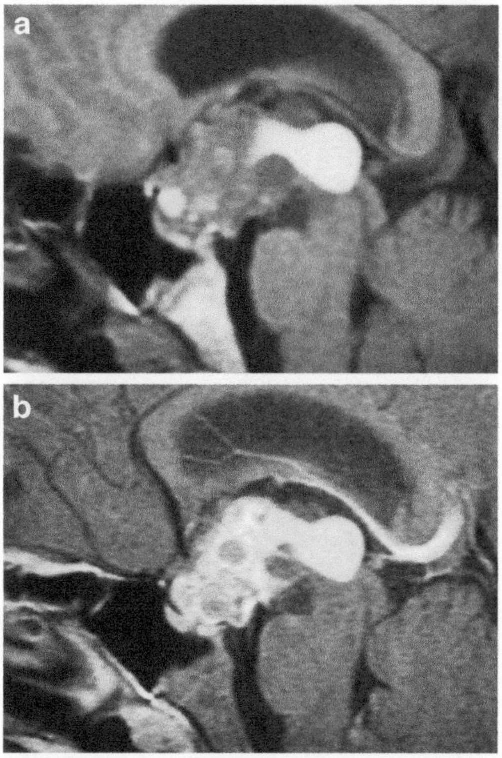

Fig. 20 Craniopharyngioma. Sagittal T1WI (**a**) shows a lobulated lesion filling the suprasellar cistern which contains zones of low, intermediate and high signal. Sagittal post-contrast T1WI (**b**) shows the lesion to have heterogeneous contrast enhancement

of primary intracranial tumours, with an incidence of 0.09 per 100,000. Peak incidence occurs between 10 and 14 years, with 90 % occurring in patients less than 25 years. They occur more frequently in males. Prognosis depends on the histological subtype, with a 10 year survival rate for germinomas of over 85 %. Other germ cell tumours have a lower survival rate, particularly those containing non-germinomatous malignant cells. Tumours often have intermediate signal on T1WI, slightly high signal on T2WI, and show contrast enhancement. They are typically centred on the pituitary stalk with the posterior pituitary bright spot often absent. They may look similar to Langerhans' cell histiocytosis (LCH) or lymphocytic hypophysitis [53]. Contrast-enhancing disseminated subarachnoid and/or intraventricular tumour may occur through CSF seeding.

Germ cell tumours—teratoma (Fig. 24) The second most common type of germ cell tumour behind a germinoma. They occur in children, with a greater frequency in boys, accounting for 0.5-1.5 % of all childhood brain tumours, and >50 % of intracranial tumours in infants less than 2 months [54, 55]. Histologically, they demonstrate benign or malignant types, composed of derivatives of ectoderm, mesoderm and/or endoderm. On MRI, they are relatively circumscribed lesions, most common in decreasing order frequency within the pineal region, suprasellar region, and third ventricle. On MRI, they demonstrate heterogeneous signal intensity on T1WI, T2WI and post-contrast sequences, with suppression of signal on fat-saturated imaging. Marked enhancement of the solid portions of the tumour is a key feature in distinguishing a mature versus a malignant teratoma, with malignant tumours demonstrating enhancement. Additionally, they typically present without perilesional high T2 signal due to intact capsules and an undamaged blood-brain barrier [55]. They may contain calcifications with low signal on T1WI and T2WI.

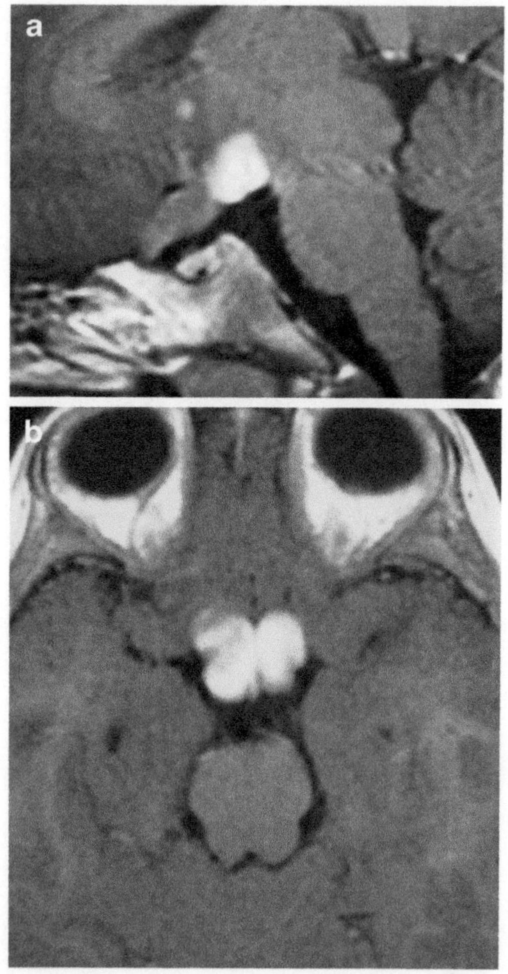

Fig. 21 Glioma in a 2-year-old girl with neurofibromatosis type 1. Sagittal (**a**) and axial (**b**) post contrast T1WI shows a partially enhancing lesion enlarging the optic chiasm and proximal optic nerves

Tuberculous meningitis (Fig. 25) *Mycobacterium tuberculosis* infection remains a major international concern, with increasing burden of disease in developed nations and young children being the most susceptible [56, 57]. MRI is increasingly being used to evaluate patients with suspected tuberculous meningitis, to aid in rapid early diagnosis [58]. MRI findings include basal leptomeningeal enhancement secondary to multiple granulomas and pial tuberculomas. The granulomas can be either non-caseating with homogeneous

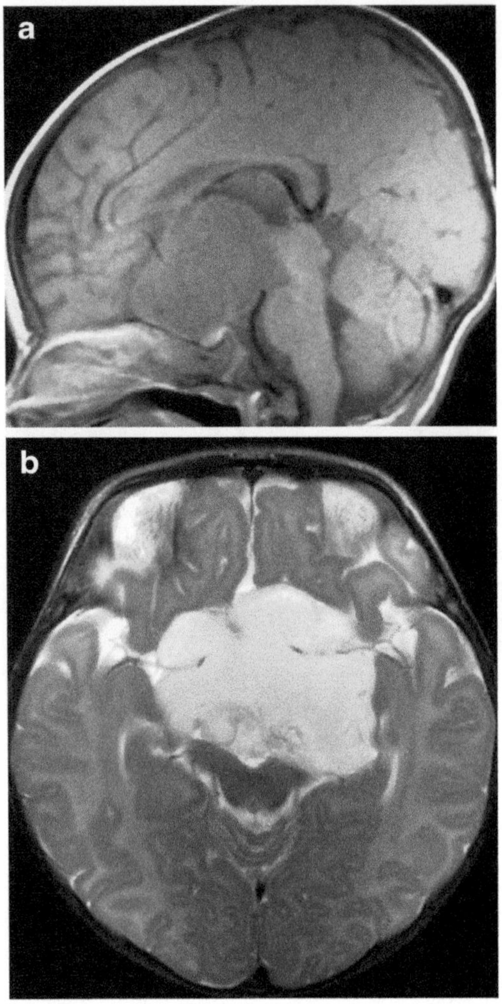

Fig. 22 Pilomyxoid astrocytoma in a 4-month-old baby girl. Sagittal T1WI (**a**) shows a large hypothalamic lesion with intermediate signal which extends superiorly into and filling the third ventricle, and inferiorly into the suparsellar cistern. The tumour has mostly high signal on axial T2WI (**b**)

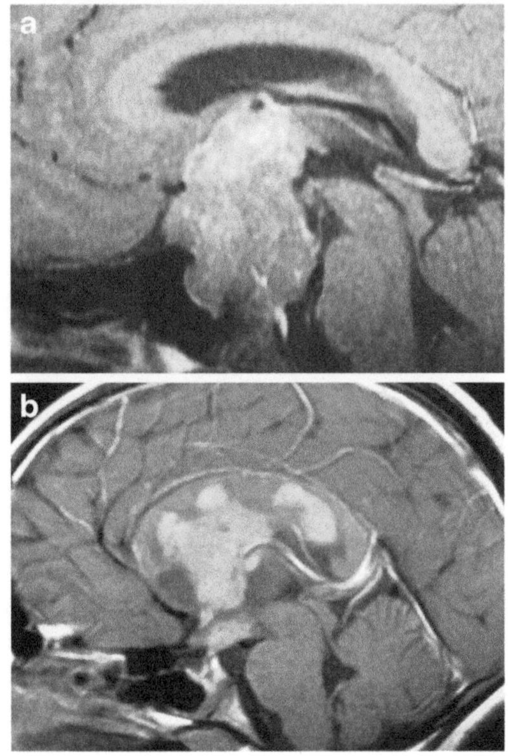

Fig. 23 Germ cell tumours in two different children. Post-contrast T1WI (**a**) shows a large enhancing lesion in the suprasellar cistern extending superiorly into the third ventricle and posteriorly into the prepontine cistern. Sagittal post-contrast T1WI (**b**) in another child shows enhancing, disseminated germ-cell tumour in the suprasellar cistern, third and lateral ventricles, with involvement of the corpus callosum and optic chiasm

enhancement or caseating with rim enhancement (both T1 hypointense and T2 hyperintense) [59].

Osteosarcoma (osteogenic sarcoma) Rare malignant bone tumour comprised of proliferating neoplastic spindle-cells which produce osteoid and/or immature tumoural bone. They usually involve the endochondral bone-forming portions of the skull-base and are locally invasive with high metastatic potential. Over 75 % of osteosarcomas are diagnosed in patients between 8 and 25 years, and account for less than 1 % of all head and neck malignant tumours in the paediatric population [60]. They occur in children as primary tumours and adults associated with Paget's disease, irradiated bone, chronic osteomyelitis, osteoblastoma, giant cell tumour and fibrous dysplasia. MRI will show a destructive lesion involving the skull base, with low-intermediate signal on T1WI, mixed low, intermediate or high signal on T2WI. Usually contains matrix mineralisation/ossification with low signal on T2WI and heterogeneous contrast enhancement.

Ewing sarcoma Bone tumour usually occurring between ages 5 and 30 years, with a greater prevalence in males and is the second most common primary bone malignancy affecting adolescents and young adults. It most commonly arises in the trunk and diaphysis of long bones, with only 4 % of cases within the head and neck region [61]. Tumours are locally invasive with a high metastatic potential. MRI will show a destructive lesion involving the skull base, with low-intermediate signal on T1WI, mixed low, intermediate or high signal on T2WI, with or without matrix mineralisation showing low signal on T2WI and heterogeneous contrast enhancement.

Esthesioneuroblastoma (olfactory neuroblastoma) (Fig. 26) These malignant neoplasms of neuroectodermal origin, arise from olfactory epithelium in the upper nasal cavity and cribiform region. Tumours consist of immature neuroblasts with variable nuclear pleomorphism, mitoses and necrosis. Tumour cells occur in aneurofibrillary intercellular matrix. There is a bimodal age of occurrence in adolescents (11-20 years) and adults (50-60 years) [62], with a

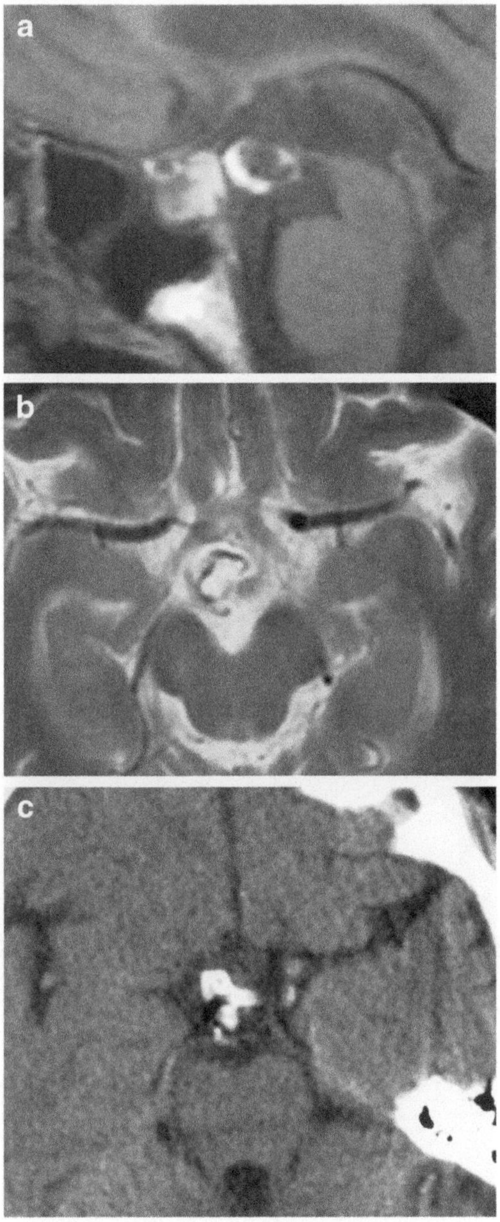

Fig. 24 Teratoma. Sagittal T1WI (**a**) and axial T2WI (b) show a lesion at the undersurface of the hypothalamus which has mixed low, intermediate and high signal. Axial CT image (**c**) shows the lesion to contain zones of calcification, fat and intermediate soft-tissue attenuation

greater prevalence in males. On MRI, they present as a locally destructive lesion with low-intermediate signal on T1WI, intermediate-high signal on T2WI and prominent contrast en-

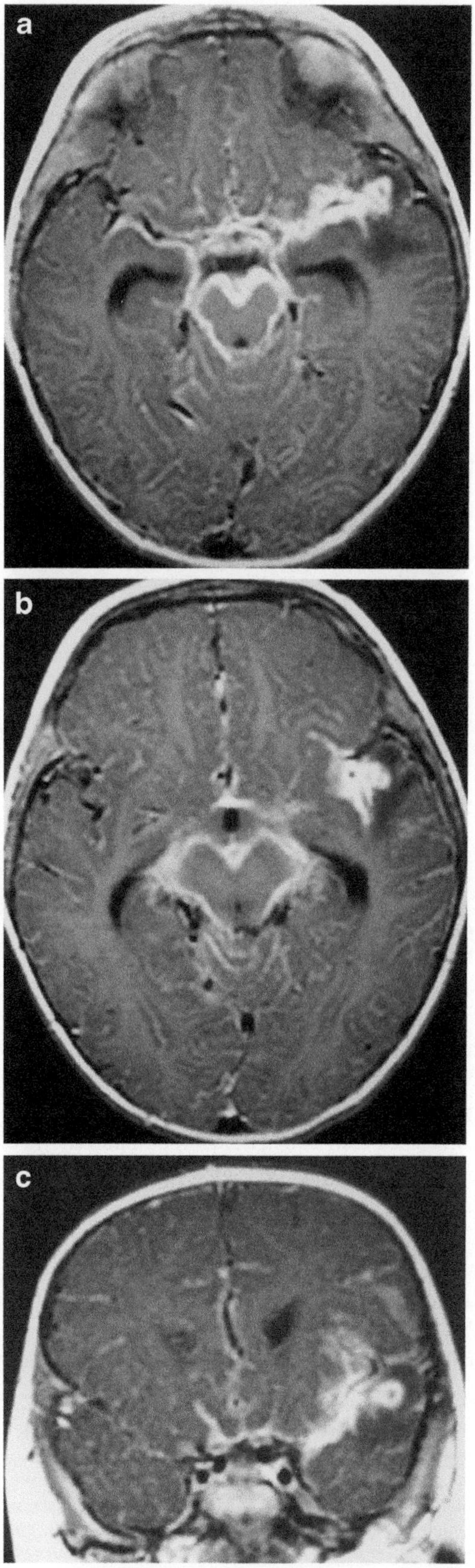

Fig. 25 A 4-month-old baby boy with tuberculous meningitis. Axial (**a**, **b**) and coronal (**c**) post-contrast T1WI shows prominent extra-axial contrast-enhancement in the basal meninges, surrounding the brainstem, cerebellar sulci and Sylvian fissures. The leptomeningeal infection invades the left temporal lobe

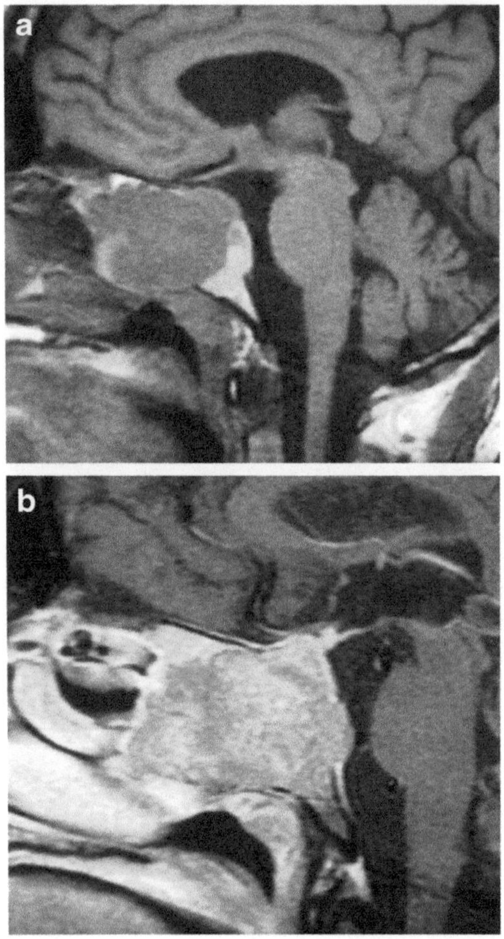

Fig. 26 Enthesioneuroblastoma. Sagittal T1WI (**a**) and post-contrast T1WI (**b**) show a destructive mass lesion involving the sphenoid bone which invades the sphenoid sinus and sella. The tumour shows prominent, mildly heterogeneous contrast enhancement

hancement. They are commonly located within the superior nasal cavity, ethmoid air cells with occasional extension into other paranasal sinuses, orbits, anterior cranial fossa, and cavernous sinuses. Positron emission tomography (PET)/computed tomography (CT) can be useful for staging of disease and detection of metastases [63].

Fibrous dysplasia (Fig. 27) Benign medullary fibro-osseous lesion, which can involve a single site (mono-ostotic) or multiple locations (poly-ostotic), results from developmental failure in the normal process of remodelling primi-

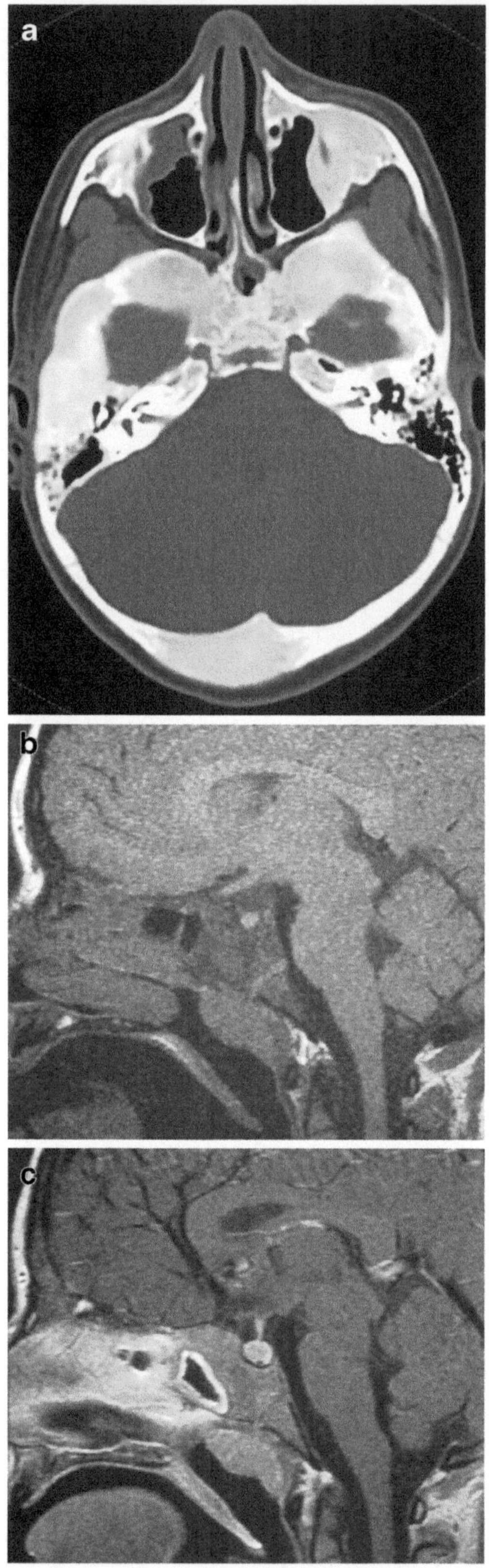

Fig. 27 Fibrous dysplasia in a 5-year-old girl with McCune Albright ▶ syndrome. Axial CT (**a**) shows multiple expansile lesions involving the skull which have a "ground glass" appearance representing sites of polyostotic fibrous dysplasia. Sagittal T1WI shows expansion of the clivus which has diffuse low signal (**b**) with corresponding diffuse enhancement on sagittal post-contrast fat-suppressed T1WI (**c**)

tive bone to mature lamellar bone with zones of immature trabeculae within dysplastic fibrous tissue. Craniofacial bones are involved in 10-20 % of patients with the monostotic disease and in 50 % of patients with the polyostotic form [64]. Patients range in age from <1 year to the eighth or ninth decades of life with 75 % occurring before the age of 30 years. MRI features depend on the proportions of bony spicules, collagen, fibroblastic spindle cells, haemorrhagic and/or cystic changes, and if associated pathological fractures are present. Lesions are usually well-circumscribed and have low-intermediate signal on T1WI and proton-density weighted imaging (PDWI). On T2WI, lesions have variable mixtures of low, intermediate and/or high signal often surrounding by a low signal rim of variable thickness. Internal septations and cystic changes are seen in a minority of lesions. Bone expansion with thickened and/or thinned cortex can be seen. Lesions show contrast enhancement varying in degree and pattern [65].

McCune-Albright syndrome Refers to an uncommon disorder in which polyostotic fibrous dysplasia is associated with pigmented cutaneous macules (café-au-lait spots) with irregular indented borders, precocious puberty, and/or other endocrine disorders such as acromegaly, hyperthyroidism, hyperparathyroidism, and/or Cushing's syndrome. McCune-Albright syndrome is uncommon and occurs in 2-3 % of patients with polyostotic fibrous dysplasia [66].

Langerhans' cell histiocytosis (Fig. 28) Disorder of the reticuloendothelial system in which bone-marrow-derived dendritic Langerhans' cells infiltrate various organs as focal lesions or in diffuse patterns. Langerhans cells have eccentrically located ovoid or convoluted nuclei within pale to eosinophilic cytoplasm. Lesions often consist of Langerhans cells, macrophages, plasma cells and eosinophils. Prevalence of 2 per 100,000 children less than 15 years [67], with only a third of the lesions occurring in adults. Localised lesions (eosinophilic granuloma) can be single or multiple in the skull, usually at the skull base. There is a striking preference for LCH to involve regions without a blood brain barrier, with the hypothalamic-pituitary axis the most frequently involved intracranial region [68], with patients often presenting with diabetes insipidus. MRI will typically show a fusiform or lobulated lesion with intermediate signal on T1WI and T2WI involving the pituitary stalk. The pituitary stalk is usually >3 mm in thickness [69], and is often associated with a loss of high signal on T1WI of the posterior pituitary. Lesions involving the pituitary usually show contrast enhancement [70].

Lymphocytic hypophysitis (Fig. 29) Rare autoimmune inflammatory process involving the pituitary gland confirmed by biopsy showing varying degrees of lymphocytic infiltration and plasma cells with fibrotic changes without multinucleated giant cells. They are more prevalent in women (80 %) who are in late pregnancy or postpartum but can also occur in children. Clinical findings include headaches and pituitary hormonal dysfunction, with deficiency of ACTH in adults and growth hormone in children [71]. Lesions can be associated with Hashimoto thyroiditis, polymyositis, pernicious anaemia, atrophic gastritis, psoriasis, systemic lupus erythematosus, adrenalitis and/or ovarian failure. MRI shows a slightly lobulated lesion with intermediate signal on T1WI, heterogeneous low-intermediate and high signal on T2WI involving the pituitary lobe with thickened pituitary stalk, and prominent homogeneous or heterogeneous contrast enhancement involving the pituitary gland, pituitary stalk and dura. A

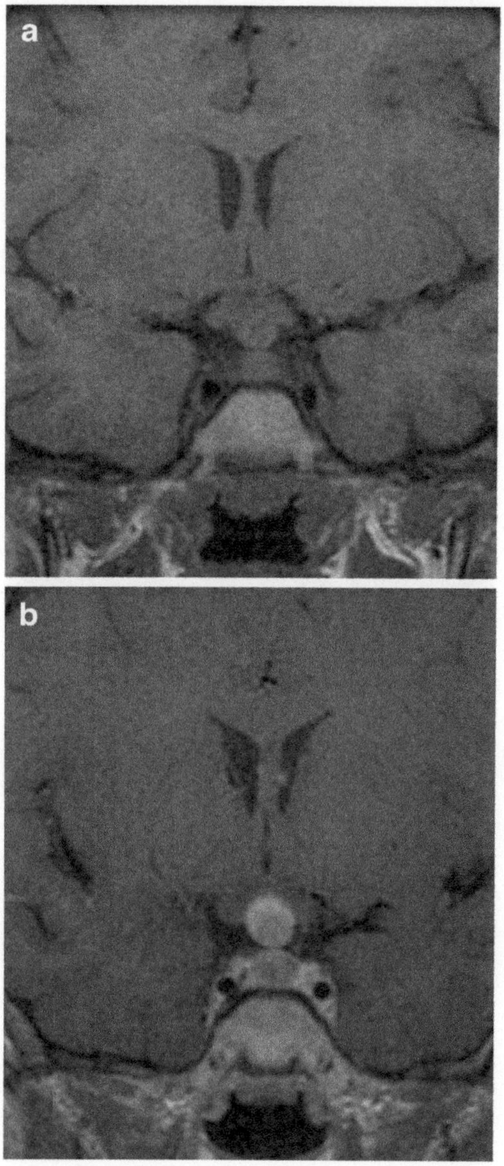

Fig. 28 Langerhans cell histiocytosis in a 6-year-old girl with headaches and diabetes insipidus. Coronal T1WI shows a lesion involving the upper pituitary gland and stalk which has intermediate signal (**a**). The lesion shows prominent enhancement on post-contrast coronal T1WI (**b**)

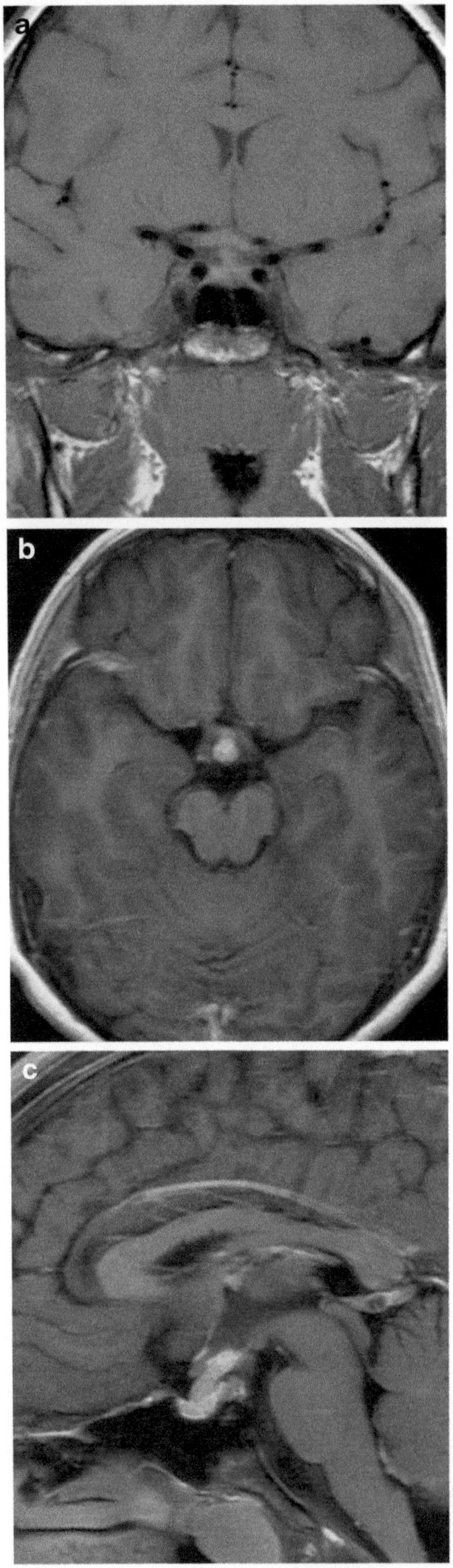

◀ **Fig. 29** Lymphocytic hypophysitis in a 16-year-old boy who presented with frequent urination, which started when he was 9. Coronal T1WI (**a**) shows thickening of the pituitary stalk which has intermdiate signal. Post-contrast axial (**b**) and sagittal (**c**) T1WI shows thickening of the pituitary stalk with homogeneous enhancement

characteristic finding includes a parasellar T2 dark sign, which helps in determining lymphocytic hypophysitis from a pituitary adenoma [72].

Rosai-Dorfman disease A rare benign histiocytosis, also referred to as sinus histiocytosis with massive lymphadenopathy. It usually occurs in children and young adults, with a male-female ratio of 3:2 [73]. Patients may present with painless adenopathy with one or more extranodal sites. When there is intracranial involvement, patients may present with headaches, seizures, visual disturbances, numbness and/or paraplegia. Involvement of the central nervous system (CNS) occurs in 4 % and usually involves the intracranial or spinal dura, rarely occurring in the sella and suprasellar region. On MRI, suprasellar/sellar masses tend to be isointense on T1WI and hypointense/isointense on T2WI with homogeneous enhancement, and may be mistaken as a meningioma. A central hypointensiity on T2WI, thought to be related to free radicals release by inflammatory macrophages, may help distinguish from a meningioma [74, 75].

Lymphomatous leptomeningial metastases (Fig. 30) Primary CNS lymphoma is extremely rare in children, and usually occurs as intra-axial lesions and infrequently as leptomeningeal tumour. Most cases are non-Hodgkin, high-grade B-cell lymphomas. There is a strong link in patients with AIDS or primary immunodeficiency [76]. Leptomeningeal metastases can also be seen with acute lymphoblastic leukaemia, medulloblastomas, germ-cell tumours, ependymomas and malignant gliomas [77].

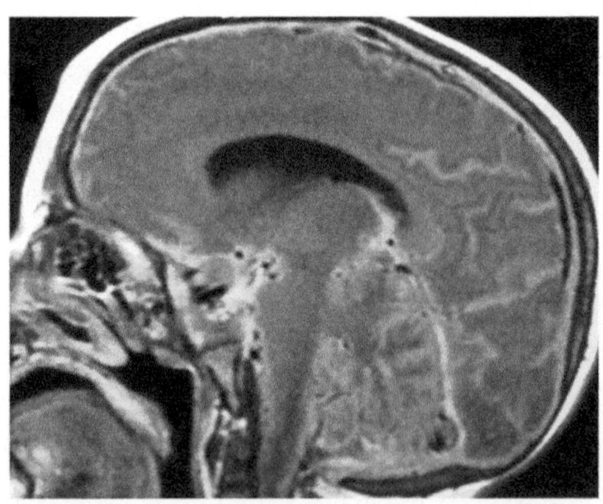

Fig. 30 Leptomeningeal spread of lymphoma. Sagittal post contrast T1WI demonstrates diffuse intracranial and spinal leptomeningeal enhancement in a 22-month-old infant boy with lymphoma including the sella and parasellar subarachnoid space

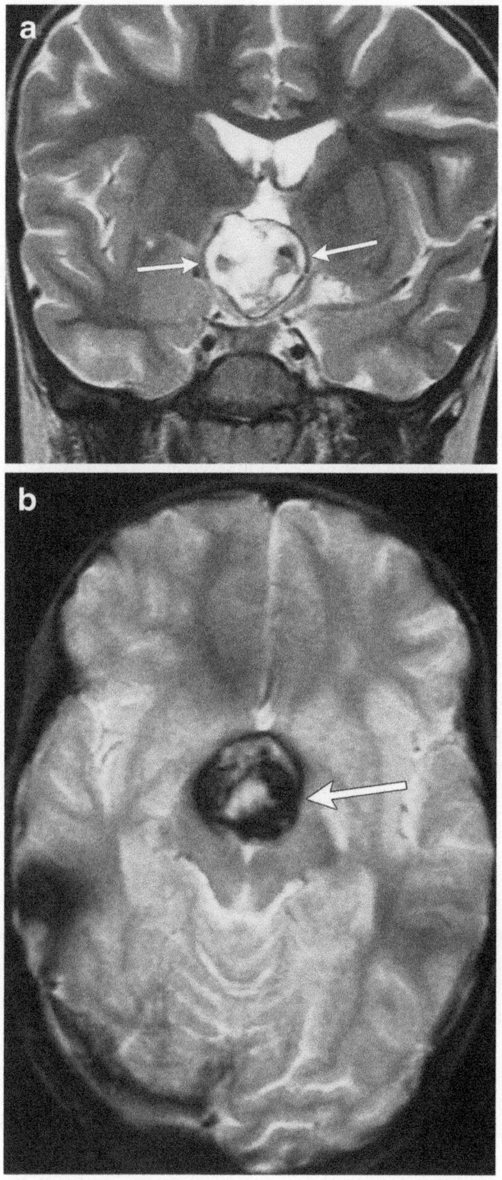

Fig. 31 Cavernous malformation: coronal T2WI (**a**) and axial gradient echo (GRE) (**b**) images in a 5-year-old girl show a large suprasellar lesion with mixed low, intermediate and high signal intensity with a thin rim of low signal on T2WI and foci of low T2* signal from susceptibility effects of blood products on GRE

Vascular malformations (Fig. 31) Numerous vascular malformations can be seen in the sellar/juxtasellar regions, including arterial aneurysms (saccular or giant aneurysms of the internal carotid artery [ICA]), cavernous carotid fistulas, arterial-venous malformations, haemangiomas or cavernous malformations. Cavernous malformations are the most common CNS vascular lesions in children, although the incidence is lower than in adults [78]. Compared to adults, these lesions are more aggressive in children with high rates of growth and haemorrhage, and a mean age of presentation of 9-10 years [79]. MRI findings will show single or multiple multilobulated intra-axial lesions with a peripheral or irregular zone of low signal on T2WI and T2* secondary to haemosiderin, with a central zone of variable signal on T1WI and T2WI depending on ages of haemorrhagic components. Contrast enhancement is usually absent.

Conclusions

Imaging of the sellar and juxtasellar region in the paediatric population is ideally performed with MRI, and relies on a strong fundamental knowledge of the anatomy and signal characteristics of a normal gland and surrounding structures. The knowledge of key differentiating MRI characteristics in common and uncommon disease entities of the paediatric sellar and juxtasellar regions, in conjunction with the clinical findings, undoubtedly aids in alerting and guiding the clinician down the appropriate path of management. It is best to approach a suspected sellar or juxtasellar abnormality with an open mind and a broad differential, with MRI being the "gold standard" of imaging to accurately characterise these lesions.

Disclosures/Conflicts of Interest No funding source was used for this project. There are no relevant financial disclosures or conflicts of interest from any of the authors.

References

1. Delman BN (2009) Imaging of pediatric pituitary abnormalities. Endocrinol Metab Clin N Am 38:673–698
2. Dietrich RB, Lis LE, Greensite FS, Pitt D (1995) Normal MR appearance of the pituitary gland in the first 2 years of life. AJNR Am J Neuroradiol 16:1413–1419
3. Fujisawa I, Asato R, Nishimura K et al (1987) Anterior and posterior lobes of the pituitary gland: assessment by 1.5 T MR imaging. J Comput Assist Tomogr 11:214–220
4. Nishimura K, Fujisawa I, Togashi K et al (1986) Posterior lobe of the pituitary: identification by lack of chemical shift artifact in MR imaging. J Comput Assist Tomogr 10:899–902
5. Fujisawa I, Asato R, Kawata M et al (1989) Hyperintense signal of the posterior pituitary on T1-weighted MR images: an experimental study. J Comput Assist Tomogr 13:371–377
6. Kiortsis D, Xydis V, Drougia AG et al (2004) The height of the pituitary in preterm infants during the first 2 years of life: An MRI study. Neuroradiology 46:224–226

7. Takano K, Utsunomiya H, Ono H et al (1999) Normal development of the pituitary gland: assessment with three-dimensional MR volumetry. AJNR Am J Neuroradiol 20:312–315
8. Cervantes LF, Altman NR, Medina LS (2006) Case 102: pituitary aplasia. Radiology 241:936–938
9. Hamilton J, Blaser S, Daneman D (1998) MR imaging in idiopathic growth hormone deficiency. AJNR Am J Neuroradiol 19:1609–1615
10. Kelly WM, Kucharczyk W, Kucharczyk J et al (1988) Posterior pituitary ectopia: An MR feature of pituitary dwarfism. Am J Neuroradiol 9:453–460
11. Cohen LE, Radovick S (2002) Molecular basis of combined pituitary hormone deficiencies. Endocr Rev 23:431–442
12. Pellegrini-Bouiller I, Bélicar P, Barlier A et al (1996) A new mutation of the gene encoding the transcription factor Pit-1 is responsible for combined pituitary hormone deficiency. J Clin Endicrinol Metab 81: 2790–2796
13. Spampinato MV, Castillo M (2005) Congenital pathology of the pituitary gland and parasellar region. Top Magn Reson Imaging 16: 269–276
14. Hamilton BE, Salzman KL, Osborn AG (2007) Anatomic and pathologic spectrum of pituitary infundibulum lesions. AJR Am J Roentgenol 188:W223–W232
15. Di Iorgi N, Iorgi ND, Allegri AEM et al (2012) The use of neuroimaging for assessing disorders of pituitary development. Clin Endocrinol (Oxf) 76:161–176
16. Slavotinek A, Parisi M, Heike C et al (2005) Craniofacial defects of blastogenesis: duplication of pituitary with cleft palate and orophgaryngeal tumors. Am J Med Genet A 135:13–20
17. Kollias SS, Ball WS, Prenger EC (1995) Review of the embryologic development of the pituitary gland and report of a case of hypophyseal duplication detected by MRI. Neuroradiology 37:3–12
18. Manjila S, Miller EA, Vadera S et al (2012) Duplication of the pituitary gland associated with multiple blastogenesis defects: duplication of the pituitary gland (DPG)-plus syndrome. Case report and review of literature. Surg Neurol Int 3:23
19. Vittore CP, Murray RA, Martin LS (2005) Case 79: pituitary duplication. Radiology 234:411–414
20. Boyko OB, Curnes JT, Oakes WJ, Burger PC Hamartomas of the tuber cinereum: CT, MR, and pathologic findings. AJNR Am J Neuroradiol 12:309–314
21. Saleem SN, Said A-HM, Lee DH (2007) Lesions of the hypothalamus: MR imaging diagnostic features. Radiographics 27:1087–1108
22. Freeman JL, Coleman LT, Wellard RM et al (2004) MR imaging and spectroscopic study of epileptogenic hypothalamic hamartomas: analysis of 72 cases. AJNR Am J Neuroradiol 25:450–462
23. Chen CJ (2001) Suprasellar and infrasellar craniopharyngioma with a persistent craniopharyngeal canal: case report and review of the literature. Neuroradiology 43:760–762
24. Kaushik C, Ramakrishnaiah R, Angtuaco EJ (2010) Ectopic pituitary adenoma in persistent craniopharyngeal canal: case report and literature review. J Comput Assist Tomogr 34:612–614
25. Kucharczyk W, Peck WW, Kelly WM et al (1987) Rathke cleft cysts: CT, MR imaging, and pathologic features. Radiology 165:491–495
26. Nemoto Y, Inoue Y, Fukuda T et al (1988) MR appearance of Rathke's cleft cysts. Neuroradiology 30:155–159
27. Takanashi JI, Tada H, Barkovich AJ et al (2005) Pituitary cysts in childhood evaluated by MR imaging. Am J Neuroradiol 26:2144–2147
28. Byun WM, Kim OL, Kim DS (2000) MR imaging findings of Rathke's cleft cysts: significance of intracystic nodules. AJNR Am J Neuroradiol 21:485–488
29. Binning MJ, Liu JK, Gannon J et al (2008) Hemorrhagic and nonhemorrhagic Rathke cleft cysts mimicking pituitary apoplexy. J Neurosurg 108:3–8
30. Brassier G, Morandi X, Tayiar E et al (1999) Rathke's cleft cysts: surgical-MRI correlation in 16 symptomatic cases. J Neuroradiol 26: 162–171
31. Kim JE, Kim JH, Kim OL et al (2004) Surgical treatment of symptomatic Rathke cleft cysts: clinical features and results with special attention to recurrence. J Neurosurg 100:33–40
32. Jabre A, Tabaddor R, Samaraweera R, Hahn YS (2000) Transsphenoidal meningoencephalocele in adults. Surg Neurol 54: 183–188
33. Ruscalleda J (2005) Imaging of parasellar lesions. Eur Radiol 15: 549–559
34. Pisaneschi M, Kapoor G (2005) Imaging the sella and parasellar region. Neuroimaging Clin N Am 15:203–219
35. Gelabert-González M (1998) Intracranial epidermoid and dermoid cysts. Rev Neurol 27:777–782
36. Smith JK (2005) Parasellar tumors: suprasellar and cavernous sinuses. Top Magn Reson Imaging 16:307–315
37. Venkatesh SK, Phadke RV, Trivedi P, Bannerji D (2002) Asymptomatic spontaneous rupture of suprasellar dermoid cyst: a case report. Neurol India 50:480–483
38. Indulkar S, Hsich GE (2011) Spontaneous rupture of intracranial dermoid cyst in a child. Neurology 77:2070
39. Güzel A, Trippel M, Ostertage CB (2007) Suprasellar arachnoid cyst: a 20-year follow-up after stereotactic internal drainage: case report and review of the literature. Turk Neurosurg 17:211–218
40. Rengachary SS, Watanabe I (1981) Ultrastructure and pathogenesis of intracranial arachnoid cysts. J Neuropathol Exp Neurol 40:61–83
41. Choi JU, Kim DS (1998) Pathogenesis of arachnoid cyst: Congenital or traumatic? Pediatr Neurosurg 29:260–266
42. Di Pietro P, Debbia C, Paola Fondelli M (2004) Pediatric hypothalamic lipoma with hypothermia—case report. Brain Dev 26:61–62
43. Kurt G, Dogulu F, Kaymaz M et al (2002) Hypothalamic lipoma adjacent to mamillary bodies. Childs Nerv Syst 18:732–734
44. Sage MR, Blumbergs PC (2000) Primary empty sella turcica: a radiological-anatomical correlation. Australas Radiol 44:341–348
45. Cacciari E, Zucchini S, Ambrosetto P et al (1994) Empty sella in children and adolescents with possible hypothalamic-pituitary disorders. J Clin Endocrinol Metab 78:767–771
46. Mindermann T, Wilson CB (1995) Pediatric pituitary adenomas. Neurosurgery 36:259–268, discussion 269
47. Partington MD, Davis DH, Laws ER, Scheithauer BW (1994) Pituitary adenomas in childhood and adolescence. Results of transsphenoidal surgery. J Neurosurg 80:209–216
48. Pandey P, Ojha BK, Mahapatra AK (2005) Pediatric pituitary adenoma: a series of 42 patients. J Clin Neurosci 12:124–127
49. Ginat DT, Meyers SP (2012) Intracranial lesions with high signal intensity on T1-weighted MR images: differential diagnosis. Radiographics 32:499–516
50. Rao AA, Naheedy JH, Chen JYY et al (2013) A clinical update and radiologic review of pediatric orbital and ocular tumors. J Oncol. doi: 10.1155/2013/975908
51. Linscott L, Osborn AG, Blaser S et al (2008) Pilomyxoid astrocytoma: expanding the imaging spectrum. AJNR Am J Neuroradiol 29: 1861–1866
52. Fernandez C, Figarella-Branger D, Girard N et al (2003) Pilocytic astrocytomas in children: prognostic factors—a retrospective study of 80 cases. Neurosurgery 53:544–555

53. Derman A, Shields M, Davis A et al (2013) Diseases of the sella and parasellar region: an overview. Semin Roentgenol 48:35–51
54. Jennings MT, Gelman R, Hochberg F (1985) Intracranial germ-cell tumors: natural history and pathogenesis. J Neurosurg 63:155–167
55. Liu Z, Lv X, Wang W et al (2014) Imaging characteristics of primary intracranial teratoma. Acta Radiol 55:874–881
56. Van den Bos F, Terken M, Ypma L et al (2004) Tuberculous meningitis and miliary tuberculosis in young children. Trop Med Int Health 9:309–313
57. Jinkins JR, Gupta R, Chang KH, Rodriguez-Carbajal J (1995) MR imaging of central nervous system tuberculosis. Radiol Clin N Am 33:771–786
58. Janse Van Rensburg P, Andronikou S, Van Toorn R, Pienaar M (2008) Magnetic resonance imaging of miliary tuberculosis of the central nervous system in children with tuberculous meningitis. Pediatr Radiol 38:1306–1313
59. Bernaerts A, Vanhoenacker FM, Parizel PM et al (2003) Tuberculosis of the central nervous system: Overview of neuroradiological findings. Eur Radiol 13:1876–1890
60. Gadwal SR, Gannon FH, Fanburg-Smith JC et al (2001) Primary osteosarcoma of the head and neck in pediatric patients: a clinicopathologic study of 22 cases with a review of the literature. Cancer 91:598–605
61. Cotterill SJ, Ahrens S, Paulussen M et al (2000) Prognostic factors in Ewing's tumor of bone: analysis of 975 patients from the European Intergroup Cooperative Ewing's Sarcoma Study Group. J Clin Oncol 18:3108–3114
62. Broich G, Pagliari A, Ottaviani F (1997) Esthesioneuroblastoma: a general review of the cases published since the discovery of the tumour in 1924. Anticancer Res 17:2683–2706
63. Broski SM, Hunt CH, Johnson GB et al (2012) The added value of 18F-FDG PET/CT for evaluation of patients with esthesioneuroblastoma. J Nucl Med 53:1200–1206
64. Moore AT, Buncic JR, Munro IR (1985) Fibrous dysplasia of the orbit in childhood. Clinical features and management. Ophthalmology 92:12–20
65. Shah ZK, Peh WCG, Koh WL, Shek TWH (2005) Magnetic resonance imaging appearances of fibrous dysplasia. Br J Radiol 78: 1104–1115
66. Bousson V, Rey-Jouvin C, Laredo JD et al (2014) Fibrous dysplasia and McCune-Albright syndrome: imaging for positive and differential diagnoses, prognosis, and follow-up guidelines. Eur J Radiol 83:1828-1842
67. (1996) A multicentre retrospective survey of Langerhans' cell histiocytosis: 348 cases observed between 1983 and 1993. The French Langerhans' Cell Histiocytosis Study Group. Arch Dis Child 75:17–24
68. Prayer D, Grois N, Prosch H et al (2004) MR imaging presentation of intracranial disease associated with Langerhans cell histiocytosis. AJNR Am J Neuroradiol 25:880–891
69. Maghnie M, Cosi G, Genovese E et al (2000) Central diabetes insipidus in children and young adults. N Engl J Med 343:998–1007
70. Louis DN, Ohgaki H, Wiestler OD et al (2007) The 2007 WHO classification of tumours of the central nervous system. Acta Neuropathol 114:97–109
71. Kalra AA, Riel-Romero RMS, Gonzalez-Toledo E (2011) Lymphocytic hypophysitis in children: a novel presentation and literature review. J Child Neurol 26:87–94
72. Nakata Y, Sato N, Masumoto T et al (2010) Parasellar T2 dark sign on MR imaging in patients with lymphocytic hypophysitis. AJNR Am J Neuroradiol 31:1944–1950
73. Rosai J, Dorfman RF (1972) Sinus histiocytosis with massive lymphadenopathy: a pseudolymphomatous benign disorder. Analysis of 34 cases. Cancer 30:1174–1188
74. Wu M, Anderson AE, Kahn LB (2001) A report of intracranial Rosai-Dorfman disease with literature review. Ann Diagn Pathol 5:96–102
75. Lou X, Chen Z, Wang F, Ma L (2012) MR findings of Rosai-Dorfman disease in sellar and suprasellar region. Eur J Radiol 81: 1231–1237
76. Batchelor T, Loeffler JS (2006) Primary CNS lymphoma. J Clin Oncol 24:1281–1288
77. Chamberlain MC (1995) A review of leptomeningeal metastases in pediatrics. J Child Neurol 10:191–199
78. Acciarri N, Galassi E, Giulioni M et al (2009) Cavernous malformations of the central nervous system in the pediatric age group. Pediatr Neurosurg 45:81–104
79. Lena G, Ternier J, Paz-Paredes A, Scavarda D (2007) Central nervous system cavernomas in children. Neurochirurgie 53:223–237

7

Imaging patients with renal colic—consider ultrasound first

Carlos Nicolau · Michel Claudon · Lorenzo E. Derchi · E. Jane Adam · Michael Bachmann Nielsen · Gerhard Mostbeck · Catherine M. Owens · Christiane Nyhsen · Spyros Yarmenitis

Abstract
Renal colic is a common disease in Europe and a common cause of visit to the Emergency Department. Clinical diagnosis is usually confirmed by imaging modalities. Unenhanced computed tomography (CT) is considered the best diagnostic test due to its excellent accuracy detecting ureteral stones. However, ultrasound (US) should be considered as the primary imaging technique. It is a reproducible, non-invasive and non-expensive imaging technique, achieving accurate diagnosis in most cases without the need for radiation. Diagnosis is based on the presence of ureteral stones, but indirect findings such as the asymmetry or absence of ureteric jet, an increase of the resistive index or a colour Doppler twinkling artefact may help to suggest the diagnosis when the stone is not identified.

Main Messages
- *Renal colic diagnosis is usually confirmed by imaging modalities.*
- *Imaging diagnosis of renal colic is based on the detection of ureteral stones.*
- *CT is the most accurate imaging technique to identify ureteral stones.*
- *US allows correct diagnosis in most cases without using radiation.*
- *US should be used as the first imaging modality in patients with renal colic.*

Keywords Computed Tomography · Hydronephrosis · Renal colic · Ultrasound · Ureteral calculi

All authors are members of the ESR Working Group on Ultrasound

C. Nicolau (✉)
Radiology Department, Hospital Clinic, Villarroel 170, 08036 Barcelona, Spain
e-mail: cnicolau@clinic.cat

M. Claudon
Children Hospital, University Hospital-Nancy Brabois, Rue du Morvan, 54511 Vandoeuvre Les Nancy Cedex, France

L. E. Derchi
Emergency Radiology, DISSAL-Radiology, University of Genoa, Genoa, Italy

E. J. Adam
St George's Hospital, Blackshaw Road, SW17 0QT London, UK

M. B. Nielsen
Rigshospitalet-Diagnostisk Center, Blegdamsvej 9, 2100 Copenhagen, Denmark

G. Mostbeck
Department of Radiology, Wilhelminenspital, Montleartstr. 37, 1160 Vienna, Austria

C. M. Owens
Department of Radiology, Great Ormond Street, WC1N 3JH London, UK

C. Nyhsen
City Hospitals Sunderland FT, Kayll Road, Sunderland SR4 7TP, UK

S. Yarmenitis
Department of Radiology, Hygeia Hospital, 4, Erythrou Stavrou St, 15123 Maroussi, Greece

Introduction

Renal stone disease is common in Europe, with a prevalence ranging between 2 and 8 % [1]. It is a condition affecting relatively young individuals with an almost equal sex ratio and high tendency to recur: it is estimated that almost 50 % of stone patients will present recurrence within 10 years [2]. Renal colics are secondary to ureteral obstruction by the stones. They are a common cause of visits to the Emergency Department and frequently require imaging evaluation [1, 2].

In most institutions non-enhanced multidetector computed tomography (MDCT) is considered the gold standard technique to evaluate these patients because of its accuracy in the detection of stones as well as of other pathological conditions mimicking renal colic [3]. It is also considered as the first imaging technique for the evaluation of patients with acute onset of flank pain by The American College of Radiology Appropriateness Criteria [4]. MDCT also allows an overall assessment of the 'stone load', which can help to plan the treatment. However, the vast majority of stones pass spontaneously, and CT imaging in the emergency department rarely alters immediate management [5]. Moreover, concerns about the over-utilisation of CT are growing because of increasing health care costs and, more importantly, exposure to ionising radiation [6, 7]. The use of low-dose techniques can dramatically reduce the radiation dose [8], but these low-dose protocols have not been adopted worlwide [9]. On the other hand, ultrasound (US) is a safe, non-invasive and non-expensive technique able to evaluate patients with renal colic. However, its use remains controversial as it has good capability to identify dilatation of the excretory system even in non-experienced hands [10], but can have difficulties in directly demonstrating the stones, especially in the mid ureters, remaining operator dependent to detect stones and indirect findings that can help in the diagnosis. In addition, the absence of the 'indirect findings' does not exclude ureteral stones. In spite of these difficulties several papers, including a very recent multicentre comparative study between US and CT, have demonstrated the usefulness of US in the diagnosis and management of renal colic patients [11–13].

When to use imaging in renal colic

The diagnosis of renal colic is usually based on clinical grounds and immediate imaging is not always necessary [5, 14]. However, it is now common practice to perform imaging studies in all patients with suspected renal colic admitted to the Emergency Department. This may be due to fear of missing a life-threatening condition mimicking this condition, such as rupture of an aortic aneurysm, ovarian torsion or appendicitis, or to the need for imaging confirmation of the cause of symptoms before deciding on whether a patient may be discharged. At present, additional strong indications for imaging are the desire of patients to know the cause of their symptoms and the fear of litigation. If not in all patients, immediate imaging modalities are necessary in patients without clinical improvement after treatment, in cases with fever or leukocytosis, or in some special circumstances (i.e., patients with a single kidney and/or renal failure) [14, 15]; furthermore, imaging is also recommended in patients with remission of symptoms who do not eliminate the stone within a few days.

CT

CT has become the imaging study of choice for renal colic [2] because of its high sensitivity in the detection of renal and ureteral stones [16]. Moreover, when CT is performed with dual energy, it helps to characterise the composition of the renal stones. However, most hospitals do not have this technology, which in addition has very limited usefulness in case of ureteral stones. CT can identify the presence and size of stones with a very high accuracy of >95 % and is able to detect alternative diagnoses that simulate renal colic in 5–10 % of patients [16, 17]. Nonetheless, in spite of its high accuracy, there is increasing concern about the increase of health care costs and radiation risk that accompanies CT scans, since the use of CT rarely changes the treatment plans of these patients [18]. In this way, in a recent retrospective study, Westphalen et al. determined the proportion of patient visits for flank or kidney pain receiving CT or US and calculated the diagnosis and hospitalisation rates for urolithiasis [19]. From 1996 to 2007, the use of CT to assess patients with suspected urolithiasis increased from 4.0 to 42.5 % over the study period, and the use of US remained low, at about 5 %. However, the diagnosis of kidney stones, identification of significant alternate diagnoses or admission to the hospital did not increase.

The problem of exposure to radiation is very important in these patients, especially because of the possibility of cumulative radiation that is not usually well assessed when multiple CTs are performed in repetitive episodes of renal colic. Thus, the use of dedicated low-dose protocols is essential in these patients. In spite of the advances with dedicated low-dose CT protocols, a recent study evaluated renal colic CT studies conducted in 93 institutions in the USA from May 2011 to January 2013 [9] and demonstrated that reduced-dose renal CT protocols are used infrequently. The overall mean effective institutional dose was 11.2 mSv. Only 2 % of the studies were conducted with a "reduced dose" of 3 mSv, and only 10 % of institutions used an effective dose of 6 mSv or less in at least 50 % of patients. In another study performed in a single institution [6], the mean effective doses for a single study were 6.5 mSv for SDCT and 8.5 mSv for MDCT. Moreover, 4 % of these patients (all with a known history of nephrolithiasis) underwent three or more studies, with estimated effective doses ranging from 19.5 to 153.7 mSv.

US

Ultrasound is an accurate imaging technique to diagnose renal colic [11–13, 20, 21]. Moreover, this technique also allows the diagnosis of other renal diseases or extrarenal conditions that mimic renal colic (Table 1). The diagnosis of renal colic is based on the detection of stones and the consecutive obstruction of the excretory system (Fig. 1) [20]. Although the detection of dilatation of the excretory tract is very useful in the context of renal colic, this sign should be evaluated carefully, as dilatation does not necessarily mean obstruction, and the degree of dilatation does not reflect the severity of obstruction.

1. Features of stones in grey-scale and limitations.

   Stones are identified as hyperechogenic foci with posterior shadowing. The most important limitations of US are the detection of small lithiases (<5 mm), which may be not recognised because of a partial volume effect or the absence of posterior shadowing, and the detection of stones not evaluable whatever the size in the mid ureters, which can be masked by overlying intestinal loops and gas, especially in obese patients. Regarding the detection of small intrarenal stones, one limitation is that hyperechoic foci can also be secondary to vascular or parenchymal calcifications, clots or arcuate arteries. The sensitivity of US in the detection of lithiasis varies greatly depending on the studies, with a wide range of sensitivities that usually depends on the size and location of the stones. Thus, Fowler described a very low sensitivity of 24 % with 73 % of calculi of <3 mm not visualised. Vallone described a sensitivity of 47.57 % in the detection of renal lithiasis smaller than 5 mm [22], and Sheafor reported 61 % sensitivity with 70 % of calculi ≤3 mm not detected [23]. On the other hand, other studies have obtained very high sensitivities, such as 93 % obtained in the study by Patlas performed by three experienced senior radiologists [21], 95 % in the study of Dalla Palma [24] and 96 % in the study of Middleton [12]. The specificity of US detecting ureteral calculi is 100 % [23].

   A complete study should include the kidney, ureterovesical joint (UVJ) and ureters. The presence of

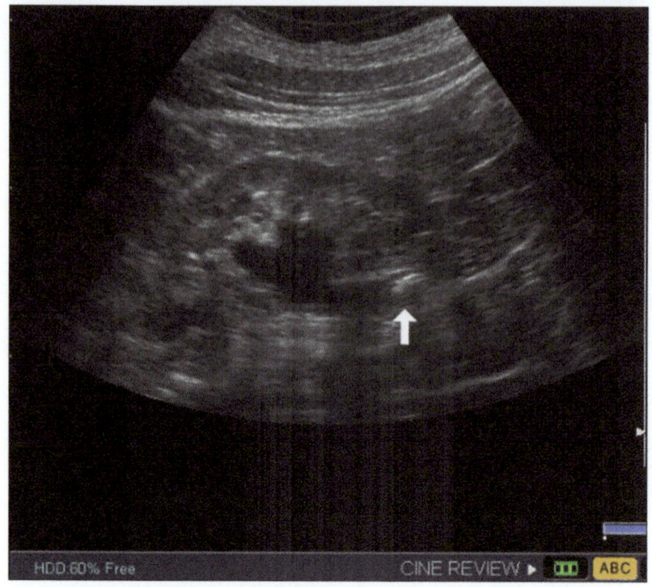

Fig. 1 Left proximal ureteral stone (*arrow*) producing hydronephrosis

Table 1 Alternative diagnoses in patients with renal colic

Entities	Most common US findings
Pyelonephritis	Mild disease may demonstrates no abnormality
	Renal enlargement
	Intra- or extrarenal fluid collections or abscesses may be present
Renal mass	Renal tumour (detection depends on tumour size)
	Spontaneous subcapsular or perinephric bleeds may cause flank pain
Adnexal pathology:	
Hemorrhagic ovarian cysts	Heterogeneous cyst
Pelvic inflammatory disease	Thickened, dilated fallopian tube. Abscesses
Endometriomas	Cyst with diffuse homogenous low-level internal echoes
Ovarian torsion	Enlarged hypo or hyperechoic ovary with little or no intra-ovarian venous flow. In some cases twisted vascular pedicle is observed.
Ovarian neoplasms	Ovarian masses
Appendicitis	Noncompressible appendix with diameter >6 mm
Diverticulitis	Detection of diverticulum
	Signs of inflammation of fat (dirty fat/stranding)
	Thickened bowel wall >4–5 mm
	Pericolic fluid or collections
Dissection/ruptured aneurysms	Thin membrane fluttering in the aortic lumen
	Dilatation of the aorta >3 cm, periaortic fluid collection

UVJ oedema is considered a useful sign of a recent stone evacuation that can help to confirm the diagnosis of renal colic (Fig. 2). Regarding the detection of ureteral stones, the mid ureter is particularly difficult to identify, especially in obese patients or because of interposition of the bowel. However, the visualisation of the mid ureter can be improved by compressing the area with the transducer or changing the patient's position (Fig. 3). The distal part of the ureter far to the vascular cross can also be very difficult to identify even with a well-dilated proximal ureter. In selected patients it can be helpful to perform transrectal or transvaginal US to evaluate the pelvic ureteral segment. Another limitation of US is that in the early phases of renal colic dilatation of the excretory tract is not always identified because there has not been enough time

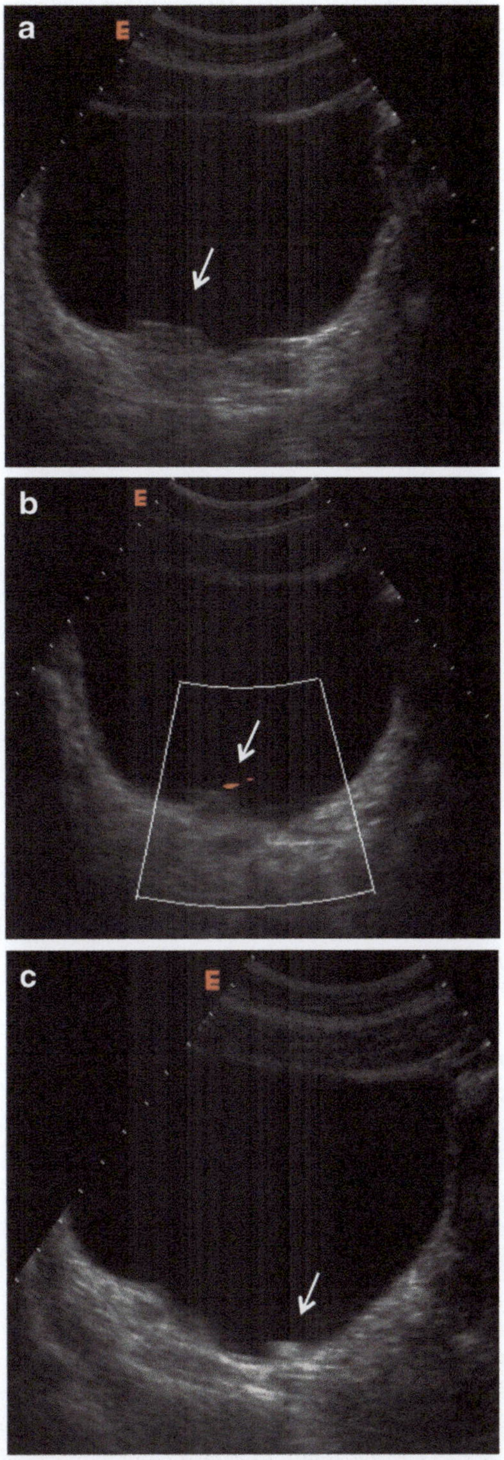

Fig. 2 Patient with right renal colic. **a** US image show an oedematous UVJ (*arrow*). **b** Colour Doppler shows the presence of a small ureteral jet confirming the patency of the ureter (*arrow*). **c** A small stone that moves according to patient decubitus is identified at the urinary bladder (*arrow*)

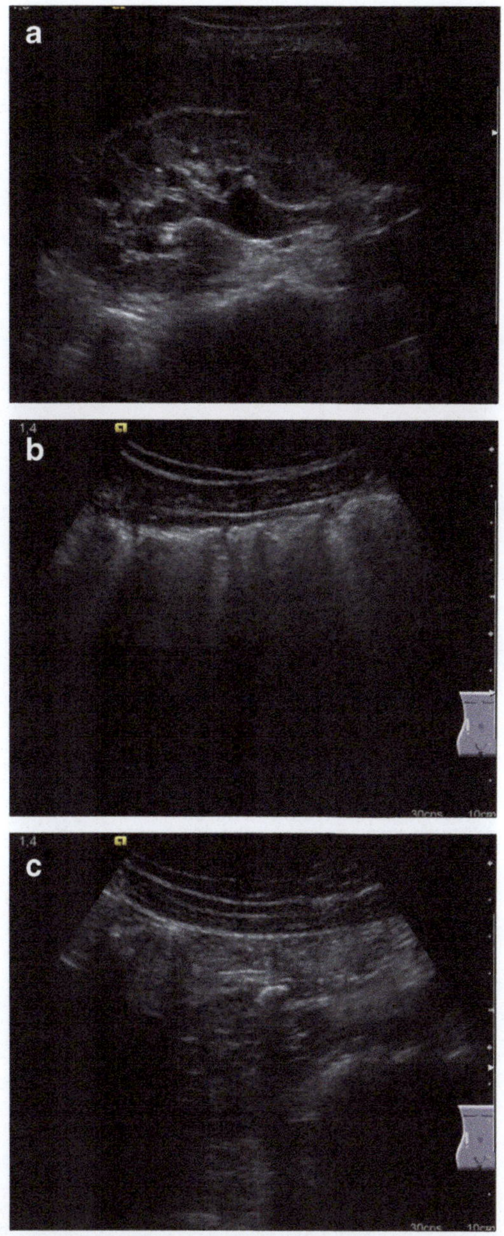

Fig. 3 **a** Right kidney hydronephrosis with ureteral dilatation. **b** Interposition of bowel loops that hampers the identification of the ureter. **c** Correct visualisation of a midureteral stone was obtained after compressing and displacing the bowel loops

for its development; furthermore, dilatation can be minimal in case of small stones (Fig. 4) or can be absent in dehydrated patients. The US study should then be performed following hydration to ensure a distended urinary bladder (thus allowing a good acoustic window to the terminal ureter) as well as visibility of the ureteral jet (produced by the passage of urine from the ureter into the bladder), if there is not complete occlusion. The accuracy of diagnosing renal obstruction and stones improves with the use of Doppler US and colour Doppler identifying secondary signs.

2. Additional sonographic features that can help in the diagnosis.

   – **An absent, asymmetric and/or reduced ureteric jet** from the ureteric orifices evaluated by colour Doppler is an additional indicator of obstruction. However, the presence of a positive ureteral jet does not rule out the presence of ureteral stones [23] since ureteral stones quite often only cause partial obstruction.
   – **Increased resistive index** as a sign of acute obstruction, distinguishing between obstructive and non-obstructive dilatation [25]. A renal RI>0.70 and/or a 10 % difference between the kidneys is considered as diagnostic of obstructive uropathy [25].
   – **Colour Doppler twinkling artefact** [15, 26, 27]. This artefact is a mixture of red and blue pixels on colour Doppler secondary to the "noise" produced from rough interfaces composed of sparse reflectors such as urinary stones. It is very useful to confirm findings of grey-scale, especially in doubtful cases due to small size of the stone [22] or located in difficult-to-visualise ureteral portions [27]. In the study by Moore et al. [15], the sensitivity of US improved from 47.6 to 86 % when the twinkling sign was used. In the recent study by Ripolles et al., [27] which analysed the specific value of the twinkling artefact, the sensitivity of US using the twinkling artefact for detecting lithiasis was 90 % and the specificity 100 %. A total of 78 % of the lithiases showed the twinkling artefact, including three stones not identified by B-mode US, and in 68 % of these stones, the artefact was detected before the stone itself with B-mode.

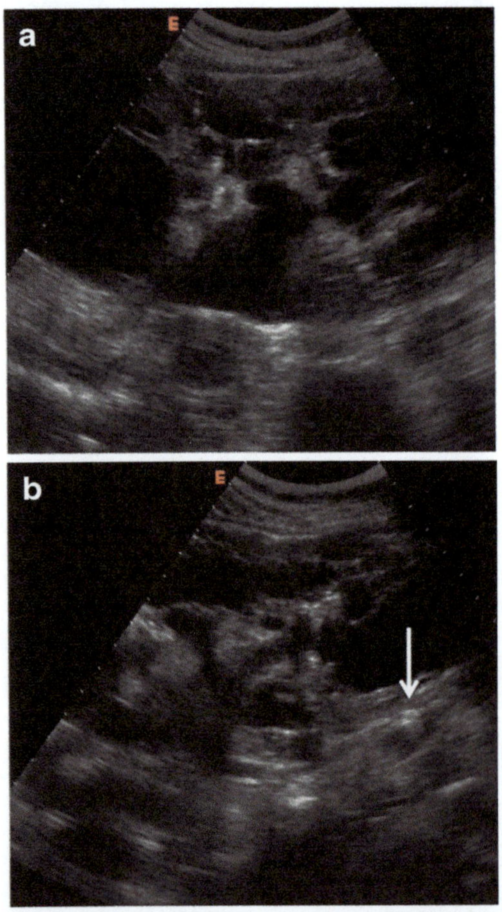

Fig. 4 Patient with known congenital polycystic kidney disease and mild renal impairment with flank pain and acute renal insufficiency. **a** Right kidney with multiple cysts and mild dilatation of the pelvis; **b** minimal dilatation of the ureter due to a small stone (*arrow*) at the upper third of the ureter

Why use US first?

The possibility of obtaining a diagnosis using US in patients with suspected renal colic has several advantages including its widespread availability and reduced cost over the use of CT [10]. Most importantly, the use of an algorithm in which US is used first can avoid radiation exposure in about 70 % of cases [11, 20, 28]. Furthermore, as underlined by Catalano et al. and Ripolles et al., it seems safe to use this diagnostic technique even if it is known to have a lower sensitivity than CT in this field [20, 28]. In fact, in both studies, spontaneous passage of the stone within a few days after the acute episode was observed in all patients with a false-negative US examination. In addition, a recent multicentre study clearly described the primary role of US in the investigation of renal colic today, demonstrating that the initial use of US is not associated with more complications, serious adverse events or hospitalisations than the initial evaluation with CT [13]. It must also be remembered that in patients in whom symptoms are not due to a renal colic US also has the ability to identify alternative diagnoses, albeit with a slightly lower sensitivity than CT, and that most of the important, life-threatening situations that may mimic renal colic can be recognised [29].

Nonetheless, US also has a few disadvantages: it may take longer to perform than nonenhanced CT and must be performed by an experienced examiner. The first of these limitations cannot be justified within the framework of the justification process of diagnostic studies using ionising radiation; radiologists are strongly advised to use alternative, nonionising techniques whenever possible. The second limitation may be difficult to overcome, especially if service is to be provided 24/24 h and 7/7 days. However, Dalla Palma et al. [24] have shown that high sensitivity results can be obtained in well-hydrated patients by general radiologists on call who are not specifically dedicated to US. The performance of US studies by radiologists also has an impact on the need for additional imaging techniques as demonstrated in the multicentre study of Smith-Bindman, in which 40.7 % of the patients initially evaluated with US by emergency physicians, and only 27 % of the patients initially evaluated by radiologists underwent additional CT [13].

Rethinking the imaging strategies in patients with suspected renal colic taking into account radiation protection considerations is possible and it has started both within the radiological community [15, 30] and among emergency physicians [10, 13]. Urologists also agree on this topic: in the 2014 guidelines on urolithiasis of the European Association of Urology it is stated that in patients with renal stone disease US should be used as the primary procedure [31], and CT should be reserved for those patients who do not improve with conservative treatment or on suspicion of a nonurologic process [20].

Conclusion

Ultrasound can achieve a high sensitivity and specificity for the depiction of ureteral calculi and acute obstruction and has several advantages including its availability, lower cost and absence of radiation. Thus, it should be considered the first imaging modality in patients with renal colic. No more complications, serious adverse events, return emergency department visits or hospitalisations are expected using US first instead of CT. CT should be reserved for patients in whom US does not obtain a diagnosis, if symptoms do not resolve or there is a suspicion of alternative diagnoses.

References

1. Johri N, Cooper B, Robertson W et al (2010) An update and practical guide to renal stone management. Nephron Clin Pract 116:c159–c171
2. Teichman JMH (2004) Clinical practice. Acute renal colic from ureteral calculus. N Engl J Med 350:684–693
3. Fulgham PF, Assimos DG, Pearle MS, Preminger GM (2013) Clinical effectiveness protocols for imaging in the management of ureteral calculous disease: AUA technology assessment. J Urol 189: 1203–1213
4. Coursey CA, Casalino DD, Remer EM et al (2012) ACR Appropriateness Criteria® acute onset flank pain—suspicion of stone disease. Ultrasound Q 28:227–233
5. Lindqvist K, Hellström M, Holmberg G et al (2006) Immediate versus deferred radiological investigation after acute renal colic: a prospective randomized study. Scand J Urol Nephrol 40:119–124
6. Katz SI, Saluja S, Brink JA, Forman HP (2006) Radiation dose associated with unenhanced CT for suspected renal colic: impact of repetitive studies. AJR Am J Roentgenol 186:1120–1124
7. Broder J, Bowen J, Lohr J et al (2007) Cumulative CT exposures in emergency department patients evaluated for suspected renal colic. J Emerg Med 33:161–168
8. McLaughlin PD, Murphy KP, Hayes SA et al (2014) Non-contrast CT at comparable dose to an abdominal radiograph in patients with acute renal colic; impact of iterative reconstruction on image quality and diagnostic performance. Insights Imaging 5:217–230
9. Lukasiewicz A, Bhargavan-Chatfield M, Coombs L et al (2014) Radiation dose index of renal colic protocol CT studies in the United States: a report from the American College of Radiology National Radiology Data Registry. Radiology 131601. doi:10.1148/radiol.14131601
10. Dalziel PJ, Noble VE (2013) Bedside ultrasound and the assessment of renal colic: a review. Emerg Med J 30:3–8
11. Dalla Palma L, Stacul F, Mosconi E, Pozzi Mucelli R (2001) Ultrasonography plus direct radiography of the abdomen in the diagnosis of renal colic: still a valid approach? Radiol Med 102:222–225
12. Middleton WD, Dodds WJ, Lawson TL, Foley WD (1988) Renal calculi: sensitivity for detection with US. Radiology 167:239–244
13. Smith-Bindman R, Aubin C, Bailitz J et al (2014) Ultrasonography versus computed tomography for suspected nephrolithiasis. N Engl J Med 371:1100–1110
14. Bultitude M, Rees J (2012) Management of renal colic. BMJ 345: e5499
15. Moore CL, Scoutt L (2012) Sonography first for acute flank pain? J Ultrasound Med 31:1703–1711
16. Smith RC, Verga M, McCarthy S, Rosenfield AT (1996) Diagnosis of acute flank pain: value of unenhanced helical CT. AJR Am J Roentgenol 166:97–101
17. Pernet J, Abergel S, Parra J et al (2014) Prevalence of alternative diagnoses in patients with suspected uncomplicated renal colic undergoing computed tomography: a prospective study. CJEM 16:8–14
18. Zwank MD, Ho BM, Gresback D et al (2014) Does computed tomographic scan affect diagnosis and management of patients with suspected renal colic? Am J Emerg Med 32:367–370
19. Westphalen AC, Hsia RY, Maselli JH et al (2011) Radiological imaging of patients with suspected urinary tract stones: national trends, diagnoses, and predictors. Acad Emerg Med 18:699–707
20. Ripollés T, Agramunt M, Errando J et al (2004) Suspected ureteral colic: plain film and sonography vs unenhanced helical CT. A prospective study in 66 patients. Eur Radiol 14:129–136
21. Patlas M, Farkas A, Fisher D et al (2001) Ultrasound vs CT for the detection of ureteric stones in patients with renal colic. Br J Radiol 74:901–904
22. Vallone G, Napolitano G, Fonio P et al (2013) US detection of renal and ureteral calculi in patients with suspected renal colic. Crit Ultrasound J 5(Suppl 1):S3
23. Sheafor DH, Hertzberg BS, Freed KS et al (2000) Nonenhanced helical CT and US in the emergency evaluation of patients with renal colic: prospective comparison. Radiology 217:792–797

24. Dalla Palma L, Stacul F, Bazzocchi M et al (1993) Ultrasonography and plain film versus intravenous urography in ureteric colic. Clin Radiol 47:333–336
25. Piazzese EMS, Mazzeo GI, Galipò S et al (2012) The renal resistive index as a predictor of acute hydronephrosis in patients with renal colic. J Ultrasound 15:239–246
26. Davran R (2009) The usefulness of color Doppler twinkling artifact in the diagnosis of urinary calculi. Eur J Radiol 71:378
27. Ripollés T, Martínez-Pérez MJ, Vizuete J et al (2013) Sonographic diagnosis of symptomatic ureteral calculi: usefulness of the twinkling artifact. Abdom Imaging 38:863–869
28. Catalano O, Nunziata A, Altei F, Siani A (2002) Suspected ureteral colic: primary helical CT versus selective helical CT after unenhanced radiography and sonography. AJR Am J Roentgenol 178:379–387
29. Van Randen A, Laméris W, van Es HW et al (2011) A comparison of the accuracy of ultrasound and computed tomography in common diagnoses causing acute abdominal pain. Eur Radiol 21:1535–1545
30. Patatas K, Panditaratne N, Wah TM et al (2012) Emergency department imaging protocol for suspected acute renal colic: re-evaluating our service. Br J Radiol 85:1118–1122
31. (2014) Guidelines on urolithiasis. European Association of Urology. In: http://www.uroweb.org/gls/pdf/22%20Urolithiasis_LR.pdf. http://www.uroweb.org/gls/pockets/english/22Urolithiasis_LR.pdf. Accessed 4 May 2014

8

Medical imaging in personalised medicine: a white paper of the research committee of the European Society of Radiology (ESR)

European Society of Radiology (ESR)

Abstract The future of medicine lies in early diagnosis and individually tailored treatments, a concept that has been designated 'personalised medicine' (PM), which aims to deliver the right treatment to the right patient at the right time. Medical imaging has always been personalised and is fundamental to almost all aspects of PM. It is instrumental in solving clinical differential diagnoses. Imaging procedures are tailored to the clinical problem and patient characteristics. Screening for preclinical disease is done with imaging. Stratification based on imaging biomarkers can help identify individuals suited for preventive intervention. Treatment decisions are based on the in vivo visualisation of the location and extent of an abnormality, as well as the loco-regional physiological, biochemical and biological processes using structural and molecular imaging. Image-guided biopsy provides relevant tissue specimens for genetic/molecular characterisation. In addition, radiogenomics relate imaging biomarkers to these genetic and molecular features. Furthermore, imaging is essential to patient-tailored therapy planning, therapy monitoring and follow-up of disease, as well as targeting non-invasive or minimally invasive treatments, especially with the rise of theranostics. Radiologists need to be prepared for this new paradigm as it will mean changes in training, clinical practice and in research.

European Society of Radiology (ESR) (✉)
Neutorgasse 9/2, 1010 Vienna, Austria
e-mail: communications@myesr.org

Key Points

- *Medical imaging is a key component in personalised medicine*
- *Personalised prevention will rely on image-based screening programmes*
- *Anatomical, functional and molecular imaging biomarkers affect decisions on the type and intensity of treatment*
- *Treatment response assessment with imaging will improve personalised treatment*
- *Image-based invasive intervention integrates personalised diagnosis and personalised treatment*

Keywords Individualized medicine · Theranostics · Biomarkers · Radiogenomics · Precision medicine

Introduction

In 2011, the ESR published its first white paper on personalised medicine (PM) [1]. The focus of this article was on the important and essential role of medical imaging in early diagnosis and individually tailored treatment. The article concluded that medical imaging plays a critical role in all aspects of PM: prediction, diagnosis and especially treatment. Thus, for PM to reach its highest potential, medical imaging must play an integral role. As the developments in PM are rapid, it is time to update the original white paper and provide a thorough overview of all areas in PM in which imaging plays a role. Currently, national and European funding agencies as well as public-private collaborations support large research programmes and infrastructures dedicated to PM [2]. It is important that the benefits and contributions of clinical imaging and imaging research to PM are acknowledged and supported in order to fulfil the promises of PM. As PM has already entered the clinical arena, it is also important that the medical imaging community is aware of this concept and is prepared for participating as a relevant partner in PM.

Therefore, the ESR considers it of strategic importance to describe how medical imaging contributes to PM and to delineate major obstacles to the full application of imaging in PM in daily practice. This white paper concludes with recommendations for the medical imaging field.

Definition

Sequencing of the human genome in 2003 opened the way to identifying specific genes that are involved in particular diseases and thus supports the identification of genetic variants that either predispose an individual to a specific disease or regulate that individual's sensitivity to a given treatment [3]. The promise of PM lies in the prediction of disease risk, the choice of the right treatment and the assessment of the treatment response and safety profile based on genomic sequence data. Thus, many consider PM to be synonymous with genomic medicine (Table 1). However, the European Science Foundation (ESF) stated that the range of information that can be used to customise healthcare is far greater than genome sequence data alone. Their definition of PM is broadly described as a customisation of healthcare that accommodates individual differences as far as possible at all stages in the process, from prevention, through diagnosis and treatment, to post-treatment follow-up. In other words, it is about providing the right treatment to the right patient at the right time [3]. The National Academy of Sciences of the USA prefers the term "precision medicine" instead of "personalised medicine" as it does not literally mean the creation of drugs or medical devices that are unique to a patient, but rather the ability to classify individuals into subpopulations that differ in their susceptibility to a particular disease, in the biology and/or prognosis of those diseases they may develop, or in their response to a specific treatment [4].

Genetic differences may determine disease predisposition and therapeutic response in some diseases. However, most diseases are polygenic in nature and highly influenced by environmental factors including climate, social context and behavioural factors such as diet and exercise. The final disease manifestation or phenotype is the result of gene-environment interaction, and it is expected that differences in the biochemical, biological and physiological characteristics (e.g., perfusion, flow, metabolism, diffusion) of diseased lesions are important factors to be taken into account when tailoring personalised treatment. For that reason the ESF stated that "genomics, epigenomics, proteomics, metabolomics, lipidomics and other 'omics technologies, such as analysis of the microbiome, will be required alongside imaging and physiological monitoring to generate biological data. All of this information, along with additional data on environmental exposures and lifestyle, for instance, will need to be integrated, analysed and interpreted" [3].

PM is not only relevant for diagnosis and treatment of cancer, but for most persistent diseases that require aggressive treatment or treatment with considerable side effects. PM not only takes into account disease but also patient characteristics as these may also influence the susceptibility to treatment and side effects [5]. PM is not a totally new approach. Medical care is traditionally delivered at a personal level, and clinicians adapt their therapeutic approach to the individual needs of the patient. In this unique physician-patient relationship, all relevant aspects of a human being and its context are taken into account in both the diagnostic process as well as the subsequent treatment, given the state-of-the-art knowledge at the time of the physician-patient interaction. In the past, personal experience has been the prevailing source of knowledge whilst more recently this knowledge has been amended, sometimes to a greater extent, by the collective experience recorded in scientific publications. This has led to specific guidelines, which are based on diagnostic and treatment outcome in a large number of patients with the same type of disease. PM as perceived today will take into account more in-depth diagnostic information from the patient and its disease for the right treatment allocation.

The promises of PM are better diagnoses, earlier interventions, more efficient drug development, more effective therapies, reduction of side effects of treatment and improved cost effectiveness. Better diagnosis is based on information on genetic variants, gene expression, and biological and physiological description of disease. Earlier intervention is based on better diagnostic tools to identify individuals with a predisposition for the development of a particular condition and to monitor interventions that might prevent it, delay its onset or reduce its impact. More efficient drug development is based on a better understanding of disease, which could help scientists identify new disease subgroups and their associated molecular pathways as well as design drugs that target them. More effective therapies are achieved by selecting the right patients for treatment and by selecting the type of treatment (surgery, radiotherapy, chemotherapy and/or targeted therapy) and the intensity of treatment (the best dosing schedule or radiation dose for a particular patient). Reduction of side effects of treatment is achieved by identification of patients who are at risk for developing side effects, by reduction of the number of patients that are exposed to non-effective treatment. Cost-effectiveness is achieved by pre-selecting patients for treatment or by terminating inefficient treatments early.

There are multiple areas in which medical imaging has and will have a major impact in PM (Table 2).

Table 1 Definitions of terms related to personalised medicine

Personalised medicine
• According to Wikipedia, "Personalized medicine is a medical model that proposes the customization of healthcare using molecular analysis—with medical decisions, practices, and/or products being tailored to the individual patient. In this model, diagnostic testing is often employed for selecting appropriate and optimal therapies based on the context of a patient's genetic content. The use of genetic information has played a major role in certain aspects of personalised medicine and the term was first coined in the context of genetics, though it has since broadened to encompass all sorts of personalization measures" [104]
• The US National Human Genome Research Institute defines personalised medicine as an emerging practice of medicine that uses an individual's genetic profile to guide decisions made in regard to the prevention, diagnosis and treatment of disease. Knowledge of a patient's genetic profile can help doctors select the proper medication or therapy and administer it using the proper dose or regimen [105]
• The US National Cancer institute describes personalised medicine as a form of medicine that uses information about a person's genes, proteins, and environment to prevent, diagnose, and treat disease. In cancer, personalised medicine uses specific information about a person's tumour to help diagnose, plan treatment, find out how well treatment is working, or make a prognosis. Also called precision medicine [106]
• European Science Foundation: Personalised medicine can be broadly described as a customisation of healthcare that accommodates individual differences as far as possible at all stages in the process, from prevention, through diagnosis and treatment, to post-treatment follow-up [3]
• National Academy of Sciences: Precision medicine refers to the tailoring of medical treatment to the individual characteristics of each patient. It does not literally mean the creation of drugs or medical devices that are unique to a patient, but rather the ability to classify individuals into subpopulations that differ in their susceptibility to a particular disease, in the biology and/or prognosis of those diseases they may develop, or in their response to a specific treatment. Preventive or therapeutic interventions can then be concentrated on those who will benefit, sparing expense and side effects for those who will not. Although the term "personalised medicine" is also used to convey this meaning, that term is sometimes misinterpreted as implying that unique treatments can be designed for each individual. For this reason, the Committee thinks that the term "precision medicine" is preferable to "personalised medicine" [4]
Pharmacogenomics
The study of how a person's genes affect the way he or she responds to drugs. Pharmacogenetics is being used to learn ahead of time what the best drug or the best dose of a drug will be for a person [106]
Genomic medicine
The use of genetic information to improve health outcomes
Stratified medicine
The identification of subgroups of patients with a particular disease who respond to a particular drug or, alternatively, are at risk of side effects in response to a certain treatment [3]
Theranostics
The term "theranostics" was coined to define ongoing efforts in clinics to develop more specific, individualised therapies for various diseases and to combine diagnostic and therapeutic capabilities into a single agent [107]
Radiogenomics
Radiogenomics is a relatively recently coined term that describes the relationship between imaging features of a lesion and the underlying genetic/molecular features. It can be helpful for improved personalised diagnosis, prognosis, and assessment of treatment response [72]
Companion diagnostics
A companion diagnostic device can be an in-vitro diagnostic device (IVD) or an imaging tool that provides information that is essential for the safe and effective use of a corresponding therapeutic product. The use of an IVD companion diagnostic device with a particular therapeutic product is stipulated in the instructions for use in the labelling of both the diagnostic device and the corresponding therapeutic product as well as in the labelling of any generic equivalents and biosimilar equivalents of the therapeutic product [108]
Genomic profile
Information about all the genes in an organism, including variations, gene expression, and the way those genes interact with each other and with the environment. A genomic profile may be used to discover why some people get certain diseases while other people do not or why people respond differently to the same drug [106]

Personalised diagnosis

Medical imaging intrinsically enables PM. The first step leading from clinical symptoms and signs to a diagnosis relies on imaging in a substantial number of diseases. Besides imaging, laboratory analysis of body fluids such as blood, serum, urine or stool also play an important role in the diagnostic process. Imaging has played this role for decades by the assessment of the location of disease in individual patients and by characterisation of the structural abnormalities. While classical macroscopic imaging provides some of the most important 'individualised' information on many diseases—namely their localisation and extent—its value for determining the specific aetiology is sometimes limited. Final diagnosis within an acceptable degree of uncertainty is usually possible based on a combination of clinical, biochemical (laboratory) and imaging information. However, pathological diagnosis of lesions detected by imaging is frequently needed.

Recent advances in imaging using specific radiotracers will provide additional tools for better characterisation of a lesion at the molecular level. The combination of different functional and molecular parameters extracted from multimodality imaging techniques will probably reduce the need for pathological diagnosis of lesions.

Key examples of personalised diagnosis include:

- Patients with abdominal pain have a clinical evaluation first and — dependent on the results — additional tests including imaging are performed, which rule out important disease, confirm a clinical diagnosis or narrow a differential diagnosis.
- Patients with an acute neurologic deficit are evaluated with a brain CT and/or MRI to differentiate between ischaemic stroke, intraparenchymal haemorrhage, subarachnoid haemorrhage, sinus thrombosis or a rare cause of stroke.

Table 2 Imaging and personalised medicine

Diagnosis:
From symptoms to underlying diagnosis with the support of imaging
Diagnostic procedure:
Imaging procedures tailored to the clinical problem and patient characteristics
Prevention/screening:
Imaging to improve risk stratification or to detect preclinical disease
Selection of the right treatment with imaging information
Imaging to assess the localisation and extent disease
Imaging for functional and biological characterisation of lesions
Image-guided biopsy to get specimens for genetic/molecular characterisation
Imaging biomarkers to predict response to treatment, recurrence and survival
Agents that can be used for imaging diagnostics and therapeutic purposes (theranostics)
Imaging biomarkers associated with genetic/molecular features (radiogenomics)
Evaluation of treatment response:
Imaging to assess early the effects of treatment in order to adapt treatment
Imaging in drug discovery and drug trials:
Surrogate imaging biomarkers to evaluate the effect of new personalised treatment
Personalised treatment:
Image-guided treatment with surgical, radiotherapeutical, minimally or non-invasive interventional procedures

- Patients with trauma are evaluated with conventional X-ray or CT scans to rule out or confirm and localise fractures, haemorrhage and contusions.
- Patients with angina pectoris are evaluated for underlying coronary artery stenosis by coronary angiography or CT angiography or for underlying myocardial viability by nuclear medicine or cardiac MRI.
- The diagnosis of diabetes mellitus or hyperthyroidism is based on laboratory examinations.
- Patients with symptoms caused by a tumour are biopsied to evaluate the type and aggressiveness of the lesion.

Diagnoses in these examples are based on clinical evaluation, imaging, laboratory examinations or evaluation of tissue specimens. Conceptually, in personalised diagnosis a large group of patients with similar symptoms is subdivided into smaller groups with a specific diagnosis and subsequent treatment allocation.

Personalised diagnostic procedure

Medical imaging procedures are tailored to the clinical problem of the patient and to patient characteristics. The main aims are to perform the right diagnostic procedure for an individual problem, to optimise the quality of the diagnostic examination and to reduce the side effects of the diagnostic procedure. All these aims fit in the concept of PM.

Many radiological organisations provide information about the indications for imaging and the choice of modality in their referral or appropriateness criteria [6, 7]. Specific imaging protocols per modality have been designed to tackle a broad range of clinical problems. These protocols differ for example in the effective patient dose, the amount of contrast injected, injection rate, delay times, image reconstruction algorithms, contrast weightings, slice thicknesses and image orientation.

Examples of tailored protocols for a specific clinical problem are low-dose CT protocols for urinary stone detection [8], CT angiography for detection of arterial stenosis and MRI for spinal cord diseases. Examples of optimisation of a diagnostic procedure based on patient characteristics are contrast media dosing based upon patient weight [9, 10], scan delay in MR or CT angiography based on bolus tracking. Examples of patient characteristics used to reduce side effects of the diagnostic procedure are measures to avoid the use of ionising radiation when imaging children and pregnant women [11, 12], to prevent the use of IV contrast media in patients with eGFR< 30 ml/min/1.73 m^2 [13], and automated tube voltage selection and tube current modulation in CT based on measured attenuation [14, 15].

Imaging in personalised prevention

Many common diseases have a long subclinical history before they become clinically evident. Biomedical imaging allows for the non-invasive assessment of in vivo structural and functional changes that may reflect specific pathologies. This makes it possible to investigate specific pathophysiological substrates of disease in the pre-symptomatic phase and at the population level. Screening a clinically healthy population with imaging to detect and characterise these subclinical abnormalities and to treat the individuals at risk might be an optimal strategy in preventive medicine. Personalised prevention with imaging will result in detection and treatment at the right time and in stratification of the main group into subgroups with low, intermediate and high risk of developing disease. Each group might have its own treatment regime, ranging from discharge, regular follow-up at several years, watchful waiting with an imaging follow-up after several months, or a medical or surgical intervention.

Screening

Screening can be considered as PM as it can provide treatment of disease in a timely fashion before the disease has become clinically manifest with a decreased chance of implementing curative treatment. Imaging-based screening programmes are not only performed in healthy subjects. Patients can also enter an imaging screening programme to detect the progression of disease or development of cancer in an earlier phase (Table 3). The objective of these screening programmes is to start treatment earlier than it would be if based on clinical progression. Well-known examples are the image-based screening programmes for breast, lung, colorectal and prostate cancer [16–18]. Some programmes include all subjects within a certain age range; others identify high-risk categories based on simple algorithms.

The main problem with the detection of asymptomatic disease is the potential for overdiagnosis. Overdiagnosis is the diagnosis of irrelevant diseases or diseases that are sufficiently stable or indolent that they would not have become clinically relevant during the subject's lifetime. Overdiagnosis leads to unneeded treatment with potentially harmful side effects and thus causes both economic and emotional burden. The magnitude of overdiagnosis has been recently estimated to be as much as 25 %–60 % in breast, lung and prostate cancer screening [19]. Fortunately, imaging not only plays a role in the detection of subclinical abnormalities, but can also be used to characterise the lesion as aggressive or indolent. For example, the large number of non-specific nodules detected during lung cancer screening can be addressed by follow-up imaging to assess the change in the volume of the nodule, thereby reducing the number of false-positive diagnoses [20]. A complementary molecular imaging technique allows for better characterisation of incidental findings from screening procedures, such as solitary lung nodules, dense breast lesions and suspected prostate cancer, thus avoiding unnecessary invasive procedures and biopsies in patients with negative molecular scans [21].

Prevention of disease

Currently, prevention of cardiovascular disease and stratification of the healthy population are based on the Framingham risk score or Systematic Coronary Risk Evaluation (SCORE) score. Based on classical risk factors including age, gender, systolic blood pressure, hypertension treatment, smoking, total and HDL cholesterol, an individual is classified as having a low, intermediate or high risk. High-risk individuals are treated with intensive medical treatment while low-risk individuals are helped with lifestyle modifications. The main problem here is the large intermediate-risk group. Extensive research has been performed to better stratify patients within the intermediate risk group. As imaging is able to detect presymptomatic atherosclerotic disease, it is logical to hypothesise that imaging may become the key to identifying people who could benefit from preventive intervention. Candidate imaging biomarkers are the CT-derived calcium score from the coronary arteries [22] or more peripherally located arteries, US-derived intima-media thickness, US- or MRI-derived pulse wave velocity [23], or MRI-based plaque composition [24]. These imaging biomarkers can predict later development of disease, either on their own or by supplementing established risk factors [22]. The development of such new prevention strategies requires imaging at the population level. Population imaging is performed within the context of large population-based, prospective epidemiological studies. Population imaging focusses on finding imaging biomarkers that allow early diagnosis of preclinical disease and prediction of clinical disease. Besides imaging, information about the history of the individual subject, blood and body fluid samples, genetic data and most importantly follow-up data with regard to the development of symptoms and disease are available for correlation.

Imaging in the selection of treatment

Location and extent of disease

Although the question "Where is the disease and what is it?" may have been clearly answered, a clear decision on the optimal treatment cannot always be made without taking into consideration additional imaging data. For example, knowledge of the extent of a disease—a parameter of the severity of disease—is crucial for decisions on the choice of treatment.

Table 3 Examples of screening programmes with imaging

Screening programme	Image modality	Subjects	Biomarker
Breast cancer	Mammography	Females>40 years	BIRADS
Breast cancer	MRI	Females with BRCA1 or BRCA2	Lesion
Lung cancer	CT thorax	People with an increased risk profile	Nodule
Abdominal aortic aneurysm	US	Males>50 years	Maximal diameter
Hepatocellular carcinoma	US	Patients with hepatitis	Lesion
Unruptured cerebral aneurysms	DSA, CTA, MRA	Patients with small intracerebral aneurysm	Diameter (increase)
Meningioma	MRI	Patients with small meningioma	Size (increase)
Ascending aorta	CT thorax	Patients with Marfan's disease	Diameter (increase)

The classical example is tumour staging in which the involvement of adjacent tissues, regional lymph nodes and distant metastasis has an immediate and important impact on prognostic stratification and on the choice of therapeutic options. Improved staging with the use of imaging might help in avoiding unnecessary surgical interventions, which increases the morbidity of disease without a substantial benefit in the reduction of mortality. On the other hand upstaging can lead to the choice of more aggressive therapies, which may reduce the recurrence rate [25, 26].

Tumour staging relies strongly on cross-sectional imaging, with CT and/or MRI information being combined with quantitative metabolic information from PET and SPECT imaging. General consensus criteria and guidelines have been established based on large clinical studies combining multimodality imaging criteria [27–29]. In these guidelines PET/CT is increasingly used in staging. This technique, which visualises specific tracer uptake in normal and abnormal tissue, allows for better localisation of cancer in structurally normal tissue. Moreover, the whole-body approach increases the sensitivity for distant metastases. The improvement in staging with PET/CT compared to PET or CT alone is substantial and has been reported for many cancers and cancers of unknown primary [30, 31]. Cost-effectiveness of preoperative PET has been proven with, for example, prevention of unnecessary surgery in one out of five patients with suspected non-small-cell lung cancer after the addition of [^{18}F]FDG-PET imaging to conventional staging [32]. Recent emergence of combined PET/MR imaging systems is expected to raise the potential for combined criteria in better assessment and tissue characterisation of specific tumour and pathological lesions.

Besides oncology, cardiovascular and cerebrovascular diseases are other areas where severity of disease influences treatment decisions. Specific examples are:

- The decision to treat unruptured intracranial aneurysms is based on the location and maximum diameter of the aneurysm [33].
- Abdominal aneurysms larger than 5.5 cm are treated while smaller aneurysms are monitored during follow-up [34].
- Atherosclerotic stenosis in coronary and peripheral arteries is considered symptomatic and is treated once the diameter stenosis is more than 50 %.
- The benefit of carotid endarterectomy has been proven for symptomatic stenosis of more than 70 %. The carotid endarterectomy trials have used catheter angiography as the modality for the assessment of the severity of stenosis [35]. US, CTA and MRA have replaced this technique after extensive validation as the accurate assessment of the severity of stenosis was crucial in treatment decisions. It is therefore not surprising that carotid stenosis is one of the most evaluated imaging biomarkers in radiology.

Tissue biopsy in interventional radiology

Final diagnosis of specific diseases and subsequent treatment allocation has been based on gross macroscopic, microscopic and/or immunohistochemical evaluation of tissue specimens. The best-known example is a tumour for which the most relevant question is the assessment of the malignant nature of the lesion and the type of malignancy. Collection of tissue samples for diagnosis can been performed by endoscopy or with a surgical procedure. US-, CT- or MRI-guided biopsy sampling is critical and most often represents the least invasive method to obtain relevant material for the in vitro diagnosis of disease in many parts of the body. Specific examples include:

- MRI-guided or contrast-enhanced transrectal US-guided prostate biopsy, which appears to be a useful method for the detection of prostate cancer in patients with prior negative biopsy results [36, 37].
- US- and MRI-guided percutaneous breast biopsy, which has replaced surgical biopsy as the initial method of diagnosis for most breast lesions [38].

Tissue sampling is not only performed for a final pathologic diagnosis, but also for the evaluation of disease spread. Here, the confirmation of potential metastasis through image-guided tissue sampling may change the type of treatment offered, for example from surgery to radiotherapy and/or chemotherapy. Specific examples include:

- US-guided core biopsy of suspicious axillary lymph nodes in patients with breast cancer allows for identification of metastatic nodes preoperatively [38, 39].
- CT-guided bone biopsy in patients with suspected bone metastasis supports a final diagnosis [40].
- US-guided biopsy in sub-centimetre neck lymph nodes improves tumour staging in head and neck cancer [41].

Prognostic and predictive biomarkers

The essence of personalised diagnosis for personalised treatment lies in the use of biomarkers. These can be extracted from tissue, body fluids or medical imaging. In the selection of the right treatment, two different types of biomarkers are of particular importance: prognostic and predictive biomarkers. Prognostic imaging biomarkers predict the likelihood of disease progression in the absence of treatment considerations. Such biomarkers are valuable not only for identifying aggressive disease that requires immediate treatment, but also for identifying indolent disease that can safely be left alone.

- Pre-treatment tumour volume on PET/CT in breast cancer patients predicts tumour recurrence during follow-up [42].

- Baseline lesion glycolysis measured with [^{18}F]FDG-PET predicts progression-free survival in diffuse large B-cell lymphoma [43].

Predictive biomarkers indicate the relative sensitivity or resistance to drug treatment or the success of treatment by surgery, interventional radiology or radiotherapy.

- CT-derived perfusion parameters in metastatic renal cell cancer can predict the biological response to antiangiogenic drugs [44].
- Dynamic contrast-enhanced (DCE) MRI to evaluate the non-enhancing tumour fraction predicts the response to chemo-radiotherapy in advanced cervical cancer [45].

Both types of biomarkers are relevant in PM as they influence the decision for the treatment, type, length and intensity of treatment. A specific application of a prognostic or predictive biomarker is the monitoring of the response after the first cycle of treatment (chemotherapy and/or radiotherapy) in order to predict the final response, progression-free survival, recurrence and overall survival.

- [^{18}F]FDG-PET response after the first cycles of chemotherapy predicts the final response as well as progression-free survival and overall survival [46].
- Diffusion-weighted (DWI) MRI of metastatic ovarian and peritoneal cancer was not able to predict response, while an increase in ADC after the first or third of six cycles of chemotherapy was able to predict tumour response [47].

Multiple prognostic and predictive imaging biomarkers have been identified. The main challenge for PM is the translation of this information in patient management pathways and treatment algorithms.

Molecular imaging

PM implies the identification of the specific genomic and molecular substrate of alterations leading to disease and "medical treatment tailored not just to symptoms, but to the biochemical profile of an individual's disease state (gene expression, proteome, dominant metabolic pathways, etc.)" [48]. This has tremendously changed the evaluation of diseased tissue specimens: from microscopic and/or immunohistochemical evaluation to gene expression profiling.

Parallel to this development, medical imaging has changed. Traditionally, medical imaging has been a tool for non-invasive assessment of anatomy and for detection and localisation of disease processes. Currently, a wide variety of new medical imaging techniques produces important information about physiology, metabolism, molecular biological processes and functional genomics. Multiple methods have been described for imaging the temporal and spatial biodistribution of a molecular probe as well as related biological processes such as cell proliferation, apoptosis, angiogenesis, hypoxia, and gene activation and expression. These new methods combine the ability to measure and quantify biological processes with the ability to localise the measured entities onto a high-resolution anatomical and functional image [49]. In the future, an imaging diagnosis will not only include the location and extent of diseased lesions but also information on the physiological characteristics and biological behaviour of the lesion (e.g., perfusion, flow, metabolism, diffusion).

Molecular imaging is likely to replace several aspects of ex vivo tissue analysis, which will be a key component in PM. It is expected that molecular imaging can be used to detect diseases much earlier because molecular and cellular changes precede anatomical and structural changes on classical imaging modalities such as CT and MRI. As such, it will contribute to PM by treating the patient at the right time. As new therapies will be increasingly based on a foundation of precise understanding of the molecular basis of disease, simultaneous creative probe development will require a deeper understanding of cancer biology [50].

- Hypoxia is common in malignant tumours and increases the resistance to radiation therapy. [^{18}F]-fluoromixonidazole ([^{18}F]-MISO) imaging enables the non-invasive assessment of tumour hypoxia, and its use to predict response and survival benefits from treatment has been demonstrated in oesophageal cancer, lung cancer and renal cell carcinoma [51–53].
- Molecular imaging may help improve staging of malignancies. In a preclinical animal model, detection of prostate cancer and metastasis was possible with the use of an imaging reporter gene under the control of the promoter of astrocyte elevated gene-1 (AEG-1), which is selectively active only in malignant cells. Metastatic lesions were identified through bioluminescence imaging and SPECT with a higher sensitivity than [^{18}F]FDG and [^{18}F]-NaF [54].

Biology-based tissue biopsy in interventional radiology

PM currently requires an in-depth analysis of the genetic expression and molecular and cellular biology of the individual disease. This is based on a more refined evaluation of tissue samples by assessment of molecular and genetic expression patterns. For example, for malignant tumours it is has become relevant to know which of the genetic alterations is functionally relevant for abnormal cell proliferation.

Recent studies have shown that malignant lesions demonstrate intratumoral heterogeneity with regard to genetic alterations and expression patterns, thus indicating the existence of multiple subpopulations of cells. Furthermore, metastatic lesions may have genetic expression patterns that differ from the expression pattern in the primary lesion or from each other, and these lesions can therefore show a different behaviour and response to treatment. For more effective targeted therapy, it is therefore necessary to identify these mutations and confirm them by individual tissue analysis of each subset.

The differences in genetic expression patterns are frequently reflected as differences in imaging appearance. Imaging can thus further play a crucial role in guiding the sampling procedure. For example:

- Contrast-enhanced US in liver tumours not only increases the accuracy of biopsies by improving the visualisation of poorly visible lesions but also helps target the biopsy to the hypervascular areas of a given lesion [55].
- [^{18}F]FDG or [^{11}C]-methionine-PET can detect hypermetabolic areas in brain tumours and improve the diagnostic yield of stereotactic brain biopsy [56].
- PET-directed, US-guided biopsies with a PET/US fusion targeted biopsy system improve prostate cancer detection [57].

Theranostics/companion diagnostics

One of the classical examples of PM is the determination of the status of the human epidermal growth factor receptor 2 (HER2) expression in patients with breast cancer as a prerequisite for treatment with trastuzumab (Herceptin, Genentech). In some cancers, HER2 is over-expressed, causing cancer cells to reproduce uncontrollably [58]. Trastuzumab is a monoclonal antibody that interferes with the HER2 receptor and inhibits the effects of overexpression of HER2. This approach targets one of the core deregulated cellular signalling pathways in cancer, which is totally different from cytotoxic chemotherapy. If the breast cancer does not overexpress HER2, trastuzumab will have no beneficial effect. The coupling of therapy with diagnostic information specific for the intended target is called a theranostic system.

In the HER2-trastuzumab theranostic system, the diagnostic test is a laboratory test on a tissue specimen in vitro, but in vivo imaging can also provide diagnostic tests for theranostic systems. The most common example is ^{123}I/^{131}I for targeted radionuclide radiotherapy in differentiated thyroid cancer. Targeted radionuclide therapy combines "the favourable targeting properties of peptides and antibodies with the effectiveness of radiation-induced cell death. A major advantage is the possibility to determine the selective accumulation in the targeted tissue by molecular imaging studies using structurally identical diagnostic compounds" [59, 60].

Theranostics relying on in vitro testing of small tumour samples does not address the problem of tumour heterogeneity or the phenotypic dedifferentiation of tumour metastases. By using different molecular imaging tracers, we begin to appreciate the heterogeneity of metastatic disease within individual patients. Tumour heterogeneity can often be seen even within the same lesion. Thus, in a patient with metastases of differing biology, a single therapy approach may result in a mixed tumour response. It is not possible to biopsy each and every lesion, so molecular imaging is essential to successfully tailor treatment to the individual tumour biology. A theranostic concept that uses molecular imaging will better address the complexity of tumour biology and will therefore have the potential to enable improved diagnosis, treatment, and monitoring of treatment response all at once [50].

Theranostics provide a unique signature for improved staging of the tumour, for imaging of the biodistribution of the target to predict the biodistribution of the radiation dose and to individually monitor the efficacy of treatment with the same basic compound that is being used to target and treat the disease [60]. Furthermore, the development of new specific biomarkers that can be used for both in-vivo diagnostic imaging and targeted therapy with alpha emitter compounds or carriers of cytotoxic agents will further expand the scope of the application of theranostics in clinical practice. It is even foreseeable that advanced targeted therapy, which is often extremely expensive, would only be applicable if we have a companion diagnostic biomarker that can predict the efficacy of the treatment.

Aside from the targeted therapy with ^{131}I, other examples of image-based theranostics are:

- The norepinephrine analogue metaiodobenzylguanidine (MIBG) conjugated to ^{131}I. MIBG is used for diagnostic purposes, and it is available for targeted therapy of neuroendocrine tumours in adults and neuroblastoma in paediatric patients [61, 62].
- Somatostatin peptide analogues are used in both imaging and radionuclide-based therapy for endocrine tumours [63].
- Numerous other examples of paired molecular imaging therapy are found with other radiopharmaceuticals that are selective for biochemical processes, such as cellular proliferation, steroid synthesis, growth factor receptor expression, catecholamine production, hypoxia-induced gene expression or apoptosis [64–66].

Nanotechnology

The evolving era of nanotechnology will further boost the development and use of theranostics. Nanoparticle-based imaging and therapeutic agents are a specific, advanced and promising form of theranostics. Nanoparticles are synthesised from organic or inorganic materials such as lipids, polymers, metals or semiconductors. Thereafter ligands have to be conjugated to the nanoparticle in order to target cellular receptors (e.g. overexpressed in tumour-induced angiogenesis) or other molecular characteristics of diseased tissue [64]. In addition, visualisation is achieved by conjugation of imaging agents such as radionuclides or paramagnetic/superparamagnetic metals. If the diagnostic scan demonstrates that the lesion is positive for the target, the patient can be treated with the same nanoparticle, which now carries the therapeutic agent. The therapeutic agent can be cytotoxic radionuclides or drugs encapsulated in the nanoparticle structure. In the former case, the nanoparticles have to be engineered with a moiety for chelation of radiometals. Other materials that can be delivered locally are interfering RNAs, genes and peptides. A major advantage of nanoparticles for theranostics would be the high payload of both the therapeutic agent and imaging probe that can be delivered to the target tissue. Specific examples of theranostic agents currently under investigation include:

- liposomal vesicle formulations containing cytostatic drugs and MR contrast agents [67, 68].
- carbon nanotubes as multifunctional carriers for radioisotopes for treatment and imaging [69].

Radiogenomics/integrated diagnostics

Radiogenomics is a new approach in which large sets of complex descriptors of disease are extracted from routine clinical images and related to molecular biology and gene expression patterns of disease [70, 71]. It is based on the assumption that the observed image is the product of mechanisms occurring at a genetic and molecular level. Thus, parameters extracted through image processing and analysis are linked to the genotypic and phenotypic characteristics of the tissue [72].

Like other 'omics techniques, it is not hypothesis-oriented but goal-oriented. In radiogenomics, an a priori hypothesis is not formulated on which imaging technique or feature should be used to reflect a certain biological mechanism. Every imaginable feature is extracted from an image data set, including semantic descriptors (e.g., shape, spiculated patterns, presence of necrosis, localisation) and/or quantitative features. These features are then correlated to gene expression profiles. Radiogenomics is the term used when imaging features are correlated to gene expression. The very large numbers of correlated parameters (usually over a hundred, ideally several hundreds) extracted from the same data sets requires specific statistical methods similar to those used in other 'omics.

One of the first radiogenomics publications linked CT imaging features to gene expression in hepatocellular carcinoma [73]. The expression variation of over 6,000 genes was grouped into 116 gene modules. By combining 28 imaging traits into similar modules, 78 % of gene expression profiles could be predicted. This means that the relative expression of a given gene could be determined in any given liver tumour. This approach has been successfully applied to MRI features of glioblastoma multiforme and gene expression profiles, protein expression [74, 75], microRNAs [75], messenger RNA expression and DNA copy number variation [76]; to MRI features of breast cancer and gene expression profiles [77]; to CT features of renal cell carcinoma and gene mutations [78] and to [^{18}F]FDG features of lung cancer and protein expression [79].

It is clear that medical images inherently contain a wealth of mineable information, which reflects genetic and molecular information of disease in an individual patient. This would potentially allow particular imaging phenotypes to serve as surrogates for the unique molecular programmes that typify a molecular subtype of cancer [80]. Radiogenomics will definitely contribute to personalisation of patient management and help improve existing staging and diagnostic schemes. Imaging can be used to determine the molecular diversity of disease and thereby stratify patients into molecular subclasses with different prognoses [72]. For example, one study demonstrated that imaging features of hepatocellular carcinoma were predictive of a gene expression profile of venous invasion genes and subsequently predictive of a poor outcome [73]. Equally important is the use of imaging to identify patients for whom targeted therapeutic agents will be effective. For example, one study demonstrated that specific imaging traits in GBM were associated with an EGFR protein expression programme and EGFR protein expression [74]. Finally, intratumoral genetic heterogeneity can be reflected in intratumoral imaging heterogeneity, which demonstrates one advantage of imaging over tissue analysis.

Although PM has been boosted by the huge developments in molecular profiling, it is clear that nowadays imaging can provide comparable information. However, competition between the two approaches is not foreseen as each acts on a different level. Michael Kuo, one of the pioneers in radiogenomics, sees a blurring of the traditional lines between the diagnostic sciences and a merging of molecular diagnostics and imaging into a single diagnostic discipline [80]. Integrated diagnostics must include multimodality and multiparametric imaging approaches as well as multiple pathologic, molecular and genetic assays. This integration of the huge diagnostic data from all levels—from genes, molecules, cells, tissues, organs and organ systems—is needed in the era of PM.

Evaluation of treatment response

Imaging plays an important role in the assessment of therapeutic response. Classically decreased morbidity, e.g. relief of symptoms, and mortality have been endpoints for treatment evaluation. In most diseases treatment response can be evaluated more objectively, reproducibly and earlier with imaging than by monitoring symptoms. An early and accurate therapeutic response evaluation is critical in PM as it can influence the decision on discontinuation of treatment, treatment adjustment and/or additional treatment. Imaging can spare patients from prolonged exposure to ineffective treatments and allow alternative therapies to be applied sooner. Imaging not only plays a role in assessing response to chemotherapy, radiotherapy and/or targeted therapies, but also in the monitoring of changes after image-guided intervention.

Timing of response evaluation can differ according to clinical needs. To prevent aggressive treatment — which could be accompanied by severe side effects or expensive treatment in non-responders — it is crucial to evaluate early response in order to discontinue treatment and consider a second-line treatment that is potentially more effective. However, final treatment response evaluation is needed to decide on subsequent surgical treatment or neo-adjuvant treatment after presurgical chemoradiotherapy.

Crucial in the evaluation of treatment is the assumption that early tumour response is related to the final treatment response and that both early and final treatment responses are related to overall survival and/or progression-free survival. Multiple studies have already been performed that demonstrated these relationships. It is now time to integrate and translate these findings into clinical trial design and clinical guidelines, which describe the clinical decisions based on the results of imaging tests. This is especially the case with the further expansion of cancer management based on PET imaging. For example:

- In colorectal cancer, PET of the liver could predict tumour response to chemotherapy in liver metastasis, and PET of the pelvis during or after (chemo)radiotherapy could predict the final tumour response and overall survival [46].
- Patients with advanced oesophageal cancer and no evidence of response to neo-adjuvant chemoradiotherapy on PET imaging, which occurs in 50 % of the patients, have a worse prognosis after surgical resection than patients who respond, even after radical surgical resection [81].
- For both limited stage and advanced stage Hodgkin lymphoma, multiple studies have demonstrated that interim PET imaging has a high negative predictive value and a moderate positive predictive value for progression-free survival. Multiple trials are evaluating the effect of treatment adaption based on early PET evaluation on progression-free survival. These studies will determine whether therapy can be safely escalated or reduced based on treatment response evaluation [31].

How to assess treatment response?

Treatment monitoring in malignant tumours is based mainly on anatomical imaging, frequently still assessed on 2D images, e.g., according to the RECIST criteria. These criteria have been expanded (RECIST 1.1) to include lymph node evaluation and the use of PET [82]. Anatomical imaging detects morphologic changes, which occur relatively late during treatment. Over the last decade, some shortcomings of anatomical imaging with regards to therapy response have become evident [83]. These relate to a poor reproducibility of tumour measurements [84, 85] and inconsistencies between tumour response and survival [86]. Anatomical imaging alone does not support a comprehensive understanding of tumour biology. Furthermore, anatomical imaging falls short of fully assessing the response to targeted therapies that exert a cytostatic rather than a cytotoxic effect as well as the early response assessment to neoadjuvant systemic treatments.

The field of treatment response evaluation is a prime example of the gap between current practice and advances in imaging and image analysis techniques. Three-dimensional display of lesions and volumetric measurements have advanced and may yield advantages in the assessment of tumour response. For example, comparison of both single-diameter and volumetric measurements to assess treatment response demonstrated significant differences in tumour response [87, 88]. In addition, volumetric measurements for response assessment provide more reproducible results [89]. Advances in quantitative imaging and image analysis will contribute to changing the landscape of clinical practice and clinical trials [90, 91].

The development of new imaging techniques such as molecular, metabolic and functional imaging has paralleled the expanding knowledge on tumour biology. These techniques provide additional critical information for care of individual patients when used as a supplement to anatomic imaging, as they expand the ability to biologically characterise tumours and monitor tumour response at a more appropriate level. Cancer is currently seen as a dysregulation of a restricted number of signalling pathways, and treatments that target these pathways will lead to successful therapies. Molecular imaging helps assess changes in the tumour that would indicate the activity of one or more of the key dysregulated pathways. For example, for quantitative analysis of tumour response, [^{18}F]FDG-PET imaging — which assesses the glucose uptake and thus the metabolic activity level of various cancers — has been identified as a reliable indicator of treatment response. PET-based scoring criteria extend the morphological RECIST criteria into a biological dimension with a proposed PERSIST score [92]. This approach was found to be more consistent and showed better prediction of patient response to the treatment in a variety of cancers. A wide range of more specific probes and new imaging biomarkers are currently emerging for assessment of individual types of cancer and monitoring response to treatment.

Advanced imaging can also target the problems related to the use of one single marker for treatment response evaluation. While intratumoral heterogeneity explains the individual response to (targeted) therapy, a monitoring approach based on a single marker is not sensitive to non-response in a heterogeneous lesion or in one of multiple lesions. "This defines the weakness of serum analyses, which provide an average signal of output from all lesions, or of a biopsy program to characterize a tumour—if all can be different, then all must be characterized" [93]. Accurate localisation of regional differences in tumour behaviour and tissue characteristics is the strength of imaging. But even a molecular imaging approach based on a single probe may be insufficient, as alternative dysregulated signal pathways may replace the function of the targeted pathway [93, 94]. Currently, imaging can be performed with different modalities integrated into hybrid systems (SPECT/CT, PET/CT or PET/MRI) and can cover several functional levels. Multi-parametric imaging can potentially better identify heterogeneous and localised response to treatment. By combining imaging markers from different pathways, it may be possible to assess the type of physiological escape mechanisms of a tumour (or other disease) [94, 95], enabling individual treatment to be fitted in real time to the type of response which is, of course, PM in its most basic sense.

- For example, [^{15}O]-labelled water PET to assess blood perfusion and [^{18}F]FDG-PET to assess glucose metabolism was simultaneously applied in females with locally advanced breast cancer treated with neoadjuvant chemotherapy. Changes in PET measures of tumour blood flow and glucose metabolism predicted disease-free survival and overall survival [96].
- Similar evaluation criteria could be expected by combining functional parameters of diffusion and perfusion images combined with metabolic PET data obtained using hybrid PET/MR systems.

Imaging in drug discovery and drug trials

Treatment response is relevant for clinical practice but equally important for pharmacological research, where it can be used to identify and evaluate novel drugs. Indeed, in its Critical Path Initiative, the US Food and Drug Administration (FDA) has recognised the new role of medical imaging in drug development and regulatory approval [97]. Although the Initiative emphasises the role of imaging in the assessment of biomarkers, medical imaging also has other applications in drug discovery: "a molecular imaging probe can be used to determine target occupancy before and after administration of a new drug candidate, which helps to assess binding affinity and to determine correct dosages" [98].

In pharmaceutical research, the demonstration of tumour response is an important element of early drug development. Further investigation is often not performed when antitumour activity and treatment response are not demonstrated. Anatomical imaging is limited to revealing a physical shrinkage of the tumour. With the current molecular and functional imaging techniques all kinds of antitumour activity can be detected such as changes in receptor expression and tumour perfusion. It is expected that these new techniques, which integrate knowledge on the tumour biology, will foster the detection of relevant targeted drugs.

Very important is the increasing use of (imaging) biomarkers as surrogate endpoints for clinical trials. Given that validated surrogate endpoints allow dramatic shortening of clinical trials by shortening the time to the study end point, with associated savings and a faster availability of new treatments, this is an area in which both the pharmaceutical industry and healthcare authorities are pushing for biomarker use. Molecular imaging and radiopharmaceuticals are particularly important within this context as they allow in vivo visualisation of the effect of the treatment.

Personalised treatment

Each intervention on a patient has a personalised approach. This is true for surgery, radiotherapy and interventional radiology. The same disease is treated differently based on disease and patient characteristics provided by imaging before and during the intervention. Imaging helps to plan and guide surgical or minimally invasive individualised therapies. For example, mapping of the anatomy before and during liver surgery is based on imaging. Stereotactic brain biopsy is guided by imaging. Surgical planning of brain tumours is based on fMRI, which maps eloquent areas, and DTI, which visualises relevant brain tracts [99]. In case of complications during an intervention, the solution is even more individualised.

Radiotherapy

Imaging has always been involved in radiotherapy through image-guided radiation therapy planning (RTP), including the verification of treatment delivery. Delineation of primary and metastatic lesions, which helps to optimise target volume definition in radiotherapy, is based on imaging. Initially, the introduction of cross-sectional imaging has tremendously improved the field of radiation oncology [100]. Intensity-modulated radiotherapy, which improves dose delivery to the tumour while reducing exposure of healthy tissue to limit the side effects of treatment, requires a precise delineation of the tumour. For that reason

MRI is increasingly used in treatment planning as it provides better soft tissue contrast, which improves target volume definition. A next step is the application of functional imaging techniques, which can provide information on more aggressive parts or more radiation-resistant parts of the tumour. The target volume definition is then based on the biology of the tumour.

- Hypoxia imaging with [^{18}F]MISO-PET in head and neck cancer can detect regions that are resistant to treatment. Combined [^{18}F]MISO-PET imaging and IMRT planning permit dose painting with delivery of much higher doses to hypoxic regions [101].

Some tumours are located in areas of the body that are prone to movement, such as the lungs, liver and prostate gland, and some tumours are located close to critical organs and tissues. In these patients, image-guided radiation therapy (IGRT) is used in which imaging immediately before or even during a course of radiation therapy is applied to improve the precision and accuracy of the delivery of treatment. In addition, another application of IGRT is the reduction of the target volume during the course of radiation treatment based on the visualisation of tumour shrinkage with imaging.

Interventional Radiology

Image-guided interventions provide the means to deliver therapies locally at the disease site, whether the therapies are based on chemical compounds (including drugs and radiotherapeutics), genes, devices (including stents), cells, sound waves (high-intensity focused ultrasound = HIFU) or induction of ablative temperatures (using hyper- and hypothermia with radiofrequency, microwaves or cryotherapy). Most current interventional image-guided procedures are individually tailored to the local anatomic and functional circumstances as well as the personal needs of the patient. In this way, image-guided interventions are in themselves an important and integral part of PM. For example:

- Embolisation of bronchial arteries in patients with haemoptysis is guided by CT angiography and DSA during interventions.
- Decisions about the treatment of HCC depend on the location, size and number of tumours at each time of presentation, favouring ablation for limited disease and (chemo)embolic techniques for more extensive spread.

Medical imaging is going to play an important role in individualised drug delivery. In the past 30 years, drug delivery research was focussed on targeting carriers such as liposomes, polymeric nanoparticles and micelles to the disease site. New developments now promote the selective release of bioactive compounds after application of a trigger [102]. The trigger mechanism can be applied locally and at specific times, depending on the individual patient's needs, and can be selectively applied with interventional techniques such as HIFU under the guidance of MRI [102]. Although for many reasons most tumour ablations are performed using percutaneous radiofrequency or microwaves, HIFU is the only clinically viable technology that can be used to achieve a local temperature increase deep inside the human body in a non-invasive way. MRI can be used to provide continuous temperature mapping during HIFU for spatial and temporal control of the heating procedure and prediction of the final lesion based on the received thermal dose [103].

Conclusions and recommendations

The future of medicine is in early diagnosis and individually tailored treatments, a concept that has been designated as 'personalised medicine' (PM), which relates to delivering the right treatment to the right patient at the right time. For PM to reach its full potential, medical imaging must be an integral part.

Imaging procedures are tailored to the clinical problem and patient characteristics. Screening for preclinical disease is done with imaging. Stratification based on imaging biomarkers can help identify individuals suited for preventive intervention. Treatment decisions are based on the in vivo visualisation of the location and extent of an abnormality as well as the locoregional physiological, biochemical and biological processes using structural and molecular imaging. Image-guided biopsy provides relevant tissue specimens for genetic/molecular characterisation. In addition, radiogenomics relate imaging biomarkers to these genetic and molecular features. Furthermore, imaging is essential to patient-tailored therapy planning, therapy monitoring and follow-up of disease, as well as targeting non-invasive or minimally invasive treatments, especially with the rise of theranostics. Radiologists need to be prepared for this new paradigm as it will mean changes in training, clinical practice and research.

In order for radiologists to take on these new challenges they must be involved in the following activities:

- Promotion of the use of non-invasive medical imaging as part of PM.
- Integration of anatomical, functional and molecular imaging in one imaging department.
- Validation of quantitative imaging biomarkers for diagnosis and treatment repsonse assessment.
- Implementation of image-guided interventional procedures for providing the most accurate tissue samples for pathology-based biomarkers.
- Integration of personalised diagnostic imaging and therapeutic procedures (theranostics).

- Provision of personalised image-based phenotypic results that complement genomic analysis (radiogenomics).
- Esthablishment of large imaging biobanks that are linked to other -omics data.
- Delivering personalised treatment via a wide range of interventional radiologic procedures.

Acknowledgments This article was kindly prepared by the ESR Working Group on Personalised Medicine (Chair and lead/corresponding author: Aad van der Lugt; members: Thomas Beyer, Laure Fournier, S. Nahum Goldberg, Hans-Ulrich Kauczor, Joachim Lotz, Riccardo Manfredi, Osman Ratib, Pablo Rodriguez-Carnero, Siegfried Trattnig) on behalf of the European Society of Radiology (ESR). It was approved by the ESR Executive Council on 29 January 2015.

References

1. European Society of Radiology (2011) Medical imaging in personalised medicine: a white paper of the research committee of the European Society of Radiology (ESR). Insights Imaging 2:621–630
2. European Commission (2014) Personalising health and care. https://ec.europa.eu/research/participants/portal/desktop/en/opportunities/h2020/topics/2282-phc-24-2015.html. Accessed 29 Dec 2014
3. European Science Foundation (2011) Personalised medicine for the European citizen - towards more precise medicine for the diagnosis, treatment and prevention of disease. http://www.esf.org/fileadmin/Public_documents/Publications/Personalised_Medicine.pdf. Accessed 29 Dec 2014
4. 4 National Academy of Sciences (2011) Toward Precision Medicine: Building a Knowledge Network for Biomedical Research and a New Taxonomy of Disease. http://dels.nas.edu/Report/Toward-Precision-Medicine-Building-Knowledge/13284. Accessed 29 Dec 2014
5. Siegel CA, Melmed GY (2009) Predicting response to Anti-TNF Agents for the treatment of crohn's disease. Therap Adv Gastroenterol 2:245–251
6. The Royal College of Radiologists (2014) iRefer, making the best use of clinical radiology. http://www.irefer.org.uk/. Accessed 29 Dec 2014
7. ACR American College of Radiology (2014) ACR Appropriateness Criteria http://www.acr.org/Quality-Safety/Appropriateness-Criteria. Accessed 29 Dec 2014
8. Sung MK, Singh S, Kalra MK (2011) Current status of low dose multi-detector CT in the urinary tract. World J Radiol 3:256–265
9. Kondo H, Kanematsu M, Goshima S et al (2010) Body size indexes for optimizing iodine dose for aortic and hepatic enhancement at multidetector CT: comparison of total body weight, lean body weight, and blood volume. Radiology 254:163–169
10. Liu J, Gao J, Wu R, Zhang Y, Hu L, Hou P (2013) Optimizing contrast medium injection protocol individually with body weight for high-pitch prospective ECG-triggering coronary CT angiography. Int J Cardiovasc Imaging 29:1115–1120
11. ESR Eurosafe Imaging (2014) Eurosafe Imaging, Together for patient safety. http://www.eurosafeimaging.org/. Accessed 29 Dec 2014
12. Martin L, Ruddlesden R, Makepeace C, Robinson L, Mistry T, Starritt H (2013) Paediatric x-ray radiation dose reduction and image quality analysis. J Radiol Prot 33:621–633
13. European Society of Urogenital Radiology (2014) ESUR guidelines. http://www.esur.org/esur-guidelines/. Accessed 29 Dec 2014
14. May MS, Deak P, Kuettner A et al (2012) Radiation dose considerations by intra-individual Monte Carlo simulations in dual source spiral coronary computed tomography angiography with electrocardiogram-triggered tube current modulation and adaptive pitch. Eur Radiol 22:569–578
15. Frellesen C, Stock W, Kerl JM et al (2014) Topogram-based automated selection of the tube potential and current in thoracoabdominal trauma CT—a comparison to fixed kV with mAs modulation alone. Eur Radiol 24:1725–1734
16. Independent UKPoBCS (2012) The benefits and harms of breast cancer screening: an independent review. Lancet 380:1778–1786
17. Levine MS, Yee J (2014) History, evolution, and current status of radiologic imaging tests for colorectal cancer screening. Radiology 273:S160–S180
18. van Iersel CA, de Koning HJ, Draisma G et al (2007) Risk-based selection from the general population in a screening trial: selection criteria, recruitment and power for the Dutch-Belgian randomised lung cancer multi-slice CT screening trial (NELSON). Int J Cancer 120:868–874
19. Welch HG, Black WC (2010) Overdiagnosis in cancer. J Natl Cancer Inst 102:605–613
20. van Klaveren RJ, Oudkerk M, Prokop M et al (2009) Management of lung nodules detected by volume CT scanning. N Engl J Med 361:2221–2229
21. Evangelista L, Panunzio A, Polverosi R, Pomerri F, Rubello D (2014) Indeterminate lung nodules in cancer patients: pretest probability of malignancy and the role of F-18-FDG PET/CT. American Journal of Roentgenology 202:507–514
22. Kavousi M, Elias-Smale S, Rutten JH et al (2012) Evaluation of newer risk markers for coronary heart disease risk classification: a cohort study. Ann Intern Med 156:438–444
23. Ben-Shlomo Y, Spears M, Boustred C et al (2014) Aortic pulse wave velocity improves cardiovascular event prediction: an individual participant meta-analysis of prospective observational data from 17,635 subjects. J Am Coll Cardiol 63:636–646
24. Saam T, Hetterich H, Hoffmann V et al (2013) Meta-analysis and systematic review of the predictive value of carotid plaque hemorrhage on cerebrovascular events by magnetic resonance imaging. J Am Coll Cardiol 62:1081–1091
25. Arias F, Chicata V, Garcia-Velloso MJ et al (2014) Impact of initial FDG PET/CT in the management plan of patients with locally advanced head and neck cancer. Clin Transl Oncol. doi:10.1007/s12094-014-1204-8
26. Forner A, Bruix J (2013) The size of the problem: clinical algorithms. Dig Dis 31:95–103
27. De Leyn P, Dooms C, Kuzdzal J et al (2014) Revised ESTS guidelines for preoperative mediastinal lymph node staging for non-small-cell lung cancer. Eur J Cardiothorac Surg 45:787–798
28. Silvestri GA, Gonzalez AV, Jantz MA et al (2013) Methods for staging non-small cell lung cancer: Diagnosis and management of lung cancer, 3rd ed: American College of Chest Physicians evidence-based clinical practice guidelines. Chest 143:e211S–250S
29. European Society for Medical Oncology ESMO Clinical Practice Guidelines. http://www.esmo.org/Guidelines. Accessed 29 Dec 2014
30. Czernin J, Allen-Auerbach M, Schelbert HR (2007) Improvements in cancer staging with PET/CT: literature-based evidence as of September 2006. J Nucl Med 48(Suppl 1):78S–88S
31. Kostakoglu L, Cheson BD (2014) Current role of FDG PET/CT in lymphoma. Eur J Nucl Med Mol Imaging 41:1004–1027

32. van Tinteren H, Hoekstra OS, Smit EF et al (2002) Effectiveness of positron emission tomography in the preoperative assessment of patients with suspected non-small-cell lung cancer: the PLUS multicentre randomised trial. Lancet 359:1388–1393
33. Steiner T, Juvela S, Unterberg A et al (2013) European Stroke Organization guidelines for the management of intracranial aneurysms and subarachnoid haemorrhage. Cerebrovasc Dis 35:93–112
34. Moll FL, Powell JT, Fraedrich G et al (2011) Management of abdominal aortic aneurysms clinical practice guidelines of the European society for vascular surgery. Eur J Vasc Endovasc Surg 41(Suppl 1):S1–S58
35. Rothwell PM, Gutnikov SA, Warlow CP, European Carotid Surgery Trialist's C (2003) Reanalysis of the final results of the European Carotid Surgery Trial. Stroke 34:514–523
36. Mowatt G, Scotland G, Boachie C et al (2013) The diagnostic accuracy and cost-effectiveness of magnetic resonance spectroscopy and enhanced magnetic resonance imaging techniques in aiding the localisation of prostate abnormalities for biopsy: a systematic review and economic evaluation. Health Technol Assess 17:1–281
37. Cornelis F, Rigou G, Le Bras Y et al (2013) Real-time contrast-enhanced transrectal US-guided prostate biopsy: diagnostic accuracy in men with previously negative biopsy results and positive MR imaging findings. Radiology 269:159–166
38. Mahoney MC, Newell MS (2013) Breast intervention: how I do it. Radiology 268:12–24
39. Balu-Maestro C, Ianessi A, Chapellier C, Marcotte C, Stolear S (2013) Ultrasound-guided lymph node sampling in the initial management of breast cancer. Diagn Interv Imaging 94:389–394
40. Monfardini L, Preda L, Aurilio G et al (2014) CT-guided bone biopsy in cancer patients with suspected bone metastases: retrospective review of 308 procedures. Radiol Med 119:852–860
41. van den Brekel MW, Castelijns JA (2005) What the clinician wants to know: surgical perspective and ultrasound for lymph node imaging of the neck. Cancer Imaging 5(Spec No A):S41–49
42. Nakajima N, Kataoka M, Sugawara Y et al (2013) Volume-based parameters of 18F-fluorodeoxyglucose positron emission tomography/computed tomography improve disease recurrence prediction in postmastectomy breast cancer patients with 1 to 3 positive axillary lymph nodes. Int J Radiat Oncol Biol Phys 87:738–746
43. Esfahani SA, Heidari P, Halpern EF, Hochberg EP, Palmer EL, Mahmood U (2013) Baseline total lesion glycolysis measured with (18)F-FDG PET/CT as a predictor of progression-free survival in diffuse large B-cell lymphoma: a pilot study. Am J Nucl Med Mol Imaging 3:272–281
44. Fournier LS, Oudard S, Thiam R et al (2010) Metastatic renal carcinoma: evaluation of antiangiogenic therapy with dynamic contrast-enhanced CT. Radiology 256:511–518
45. Mannelli L, Patterson AJ, Zahra M et al (2010) Evaluation of nonenhancing tumor fraction assessed by dynamic contrast-enhanced MRI subtraction as a predictor of decrease in tumor volume in response to chemoradiotherapy in advanced cervical cancer. AJR Am J Roentgenol 195:524–527
46. de Geus-Oei LF, Vriens D, van Laarhoven HW, van der Graaf WT, Oyen WJ (2009) Monitoring and predicting response to therapy with 18F-FDG PET in colorectal cancer: a systematic review. J Nucl Med 50(Suppl 1):43S–54S
47. Kyriazi S, Collins DJ, Messiou C et al (2011) Metastatic ovarian and primary peritoneal cancer: assessing chemotherapy response with diffusion-weighted MR imaging–value of histogram analysis of apparent diffusion coefficients. Radiology 261:182–192
48. Berger M (2006) Molecular imaging as a step towards personalized medicine. http://www.nanowerk.com/spotlight/spotid=1001.php. Accessed 29 Dec 2014
49. European Science Foundation (2007) Science policy Briefing 28, Medical Imaging for Improved Patient Care. http://www.esf.org/fileadmin/links/EMRC/ESF_POLICY28_V09_HD.pdf. Accessed 29 Dec 2014
50. Hricak H (2011) Oncologic imaging: a guiding hand of personalized cancer care. Radiology 259:633–640
51. Thorwarth D, Eschmann SM, Holzner F, Paulsen F, Alber M (2006) Combined uptake of [18F]FDG and [18F]FMISO correlates with radiation therapy outcome in head-and-neck cancer patients. Radiother Oncol 80:151–156
52. Hugonnet F, Fournier L, Medioni J et al (2011) Metastatic renal cell carcinoma: relationship between initial metastasis hypoxia, change after 1 month's sunitinib, and therapeutic response: an 18 F-fluoromisonidazole PET/CT study. J Nucl Med 52:1048–1055
53. Eschmann SM, Paulsen F, Reimold M et al (2005) Prognostic impact of hypoxia imaging with 18 F-misonidazole PET in non-small cell lung cancer and head and neck cancer before radiotherapy. J Nucl Med 46:253–260
54. Bhatnagar A, Wang Y, Mease RC et al (2014) AEG-1 promoter-mediated imaging of prostate cancer. Cancer Res 74:5772–5781
55. Sparchez Z, Radu P, Zaharia T et al (2011) Usefulness of contrast enhanced ultrasound guidance in percutaneous biopsies of liver tumors. J Gastrointestin Liver Dis 20:191–196
56. Pirotte B, Goldman S, Salzberg S et al (2003) Combined positron emission tomography and magnetic resonance imaging for the planning of stereotactic brain biopsies in children: experience in 9 cases. Pediatr Neurosurg 38:146–155
57. Fei B, Nieh PT, Schuster DM, Master VA (2013) PET-directed, 3D Ultrasound-guided prostate biopsy. Diagn Imaging Eur 29:12–15
58. Hudis CA (2007) Trastuzumab–mechanism of action and use in clinical practice. N Engl J Med 357:39–51
59. Wangler C, Buchmann I, Eisenhut M, Haberkorn U, Mier W (2007) Radiolabeled peptides and proteins in cancer therapy. Protein Pept Lett 14:273–279
60. Bouchelouche K, Capala J (2010) 'Image and treat': an individualized approach to urological tumors. Curr Opin Oncol 22:274–280
61. de Kraker J, Hoefnagel KA, Verschuur AC, van Eck B, van Santen HM, Caron HN (2008) Iodine-131-metaiodobenzylguanidine as initial induction therapy in stage 4 neuroblastoma patients over 1 year of age. Eur J Cancer 44:551–556
62. Postema EJ, McEwan AJ (2009) Radioiodinated metaiodobenzylguanidine treatment of neuroendocrine tumors in adults. Cancer Biother Radiopharm 24:519–525
63. van Essen M, Krenning EP, Kam BL, de Jong M, Valkema R, Kwekkeboom DJ (2009) Peptide-receptor radionuclide therapy for endocrine tumors. Nat Rev Endocrinol 5:382–393
64. Lee DY, Li KC (2011) Molecular theranostics: a primer for the imaging professional. AJR Am J Roentgenol 197:318–324
65. Mankoff DA, Link JM, Linden HM, Sundararajan L, Krohn KA (2008) Tumor receptor imaging. J Nucl Med 49(Suppl 2):149S–163S
66. Del Vecchio S, Zannetti A, Fonti R, Pace L, Salvatore M (2007) Nuclear imaging in cancer theranostics. Q J Nucl Med Mol Imaging 51:152–163
67. Kim MJ, Jang DH, Lee YI, Jung HS, Lee HJ, Choa YH (2011) Preparation, characterization, cytotoxicity and drug release behavior of liposome-enveloped paclitaxel/Fe3O4 nanoparticles. J Nanosci Nanotechnol 11:889–893
68. Kono K, Nakashima S, Kokuryo D et al (2011) Multi-functional liposomes having temperature-triggered release and magnetic resonance imaging for tumor-specific chemotherapy. Biomaterials 32: 1387–1395
69. Hong SY, Tobias G, Al-Jamal KT et al (2010) Filled and glycosylated carbon nanotubes for in vivo radioemitter localization and imaging. Nat Mater 9:485–490
70. Kuo MD, Jamshidi N (2014) Behind the numbers: Decoding molecular phenotypes with radiogenomics–guiding principles and technical considerations. Radiology 270:320–325

71. Aerts HJ, Velazquez ER, Leijenaar RT et al (2014) Decoding tumour phenotype by noninvasive imaging using a quantitative radiomics approach. Nat Commun 5:4006
72. Rutman AM, Kuo MD (2009) Radiogenomics: creating a link between molecular diagnostics and diagnostic imaging. Eur J Radiol 70:232–241
73. Segal E, Sirlin CB, Ooi C et al (2007) Decoding global gene expression programs in liver cancer by noninvasive imaging. Nat Biotechnol 25:675–680
74. Diehn M, Nardini C, Wang DS et al (2008) Identification of noninvasive imaging surrogates for brain tumor gene-expression modules. Proc Natl Acad Sci U S A 105:5213–5218
75. Zinn PO, Mahajan B, Sathyan P et al (2011) Radiogenomic mapping of edema/cellular invasion MRI-phenotypes in glioblastoma multiforme. PLoS One 6:e25451
76. Jamshidi N, Diehn M, Bredel M, Kuo MD (2014) Illuminating radiogenomic characteristics of glioblastoma multiforme through integration of MR imaging, messenger RNA expression, and DNA copy number variation. Radiology 270:1–2
77. Yamamoto S, Maki DD, Korn RL, Kuo MD (2012) Radiogenomic analysis of breast cancer using MRI: a preliminary study to define the landscape. AJR Am J Roentgenol 199:654–663
78. Karlo CA, Di Paolo PL, Chaim J et al (2014) Radiogenomics of clear cell renal cell carcinoma: associations between CT imaging features and mutations. Radiology 270:464–471
79. Nair VS, Gevaert O, Davidzon G, Plevritis SK, West R (2014) NF-kappaB protein expression associates with (18)F-FDG PET tumor uptake in non-small cell lung cancer: a radiogenomics validation study to understand tumor metabolism. Lung Cancer 83:189–196
80. Kuo MD, Yamamoto S (2011) Next generation radiologic-pathologic correlation in oncology: Rad-Path 2.0. AJR Am J Roentgenol 197:990–997
81. Salavati A, Basu S, Heidari P, Alavi A (2009) Impact of fluorodeoxyglucose PET on the management of esophageal cancer. Nucl Med Commun 30:95–116
82. Eisenhauer EA, Therasse P, Bogaerts J et al (2009) New response evaluation criteria in solid tumours: revised RECIST guideline (version 1.1). Eur J Cancer 45:228–247
83. Carnaghi C, Sclafani F, Basilico V, Doherty M (2011) Response assessment in oncology: limitations of anatomic response criteria in the era of tailored treatments. Q J Nucl Med Mol Imaging 55: 589–602
84. Ford R, Schwartz L, Dancey J et al (2009) Lessons learned from independent central review. Eur J Cancer 45:268–274
85. Erasmus JJ, Gladish GW, Broemeling L et al (2003) Interobserver and intraobserver variability in measurement of non-small-cell carcinoma lung lesions: implications for assessment of tumor response. J Clin Oncol 21:2574–2582
86. Llovet JM, Ricci S, Mazzaferro V et al (2008) Sorafenib in advanced hepatocellular carcinoma. N Engl J Med 359:378–390
87. Prasad SR, Jhaveri KS, Saini S, Hahn PF, Halpern EF, Sumner JE (2002) CT tumor measurement for therapeutic response assessment: comparison of unidimensional, bidimensional, and volumetric techniques initial observations. Radiology 225:416–419
88. Shah GD, Kesari S, Xu R et al (2006) Comparison of linear and volumetric criteria in assessing tumor response in adult high-grade gliomas. Neuro Oncol 8:38–46
89. Frauenfelder T, Tutic M, Weder W et al (2011) Volumetry: an alternative to assess therapy response for malignant pleural mesothelioma? Eur Respir J 38:162–168
90. Buckler AJ, Mozley PD, Schwartz L et al (2010) Volumetric CT in lung cancer: an example for the qualification of imaging as a biomarker. Acad Radiol 17:107–115
91. Liu F, Zhao B, Krug LM et al (2010) Assessment of therapy responses and prediction of survival in malignant pleural mesothelioma through computer-aided volumetric measurement on computed tomography scans. J Thorac Oncol 5:879–884
92. Wahl RL, Jacene H, Kasamon Y, Lodge MA (2009) From RECIST to PERCIST: Evolving Considerations for PET response criteria in solid tumors. J Nucl Med 50(Suppl 1):122S–150S
93. Nunn AD (2007) Molecular imaging and personalized medicine: an uncertain future. Cancer Biother Radiopharm 22:722–739
94. Eckelman WC, Reba RC, Kelloff GJ (2008) Targeted imaging: an important biomarker for understanding disease progression in the era of personalized medicine. Drug Discov Today 13:748–759
95. Padhani AR, Miles KA (2010) Multiparametric imaging of tumor response to therapy. Radiology 256:348–364
96. Dunnwald LK, Gralow JR, Ellis GK et al (2008) Tumor metabolism and blood flow changes by positron emission tomography: relation to survival in patients treated with neoadjuvant chemotherapy for locally advanced breast cancer. J Clin Oncol 26:4449–4457
97. U.S. Food and Drug Administration (2009) Medical Imaging and Drug Development. http://www.fda.gov/Drugs/DevelopmentApprovalProcess/DevelopmentResources/ucm092895.htm. Accessed 29 Dec 2014
98. Thrall JH (2004) Personalized medicine. Radiology 231:613–616
99. Smits M, Vernooij MW, Wielopolski PA, Vincent AJ, Houston GC, van der Lugt A (2007) Incorporating functional MR imaging into diffusion tensor tractography in the preoperative assessment of the corticospinal tract in patients with brain tumors. AJNR Am J Neuroradiol 28:1354–1361
100. Dawson LA, Jaffray DA (2007) Advances in image-guided radiation therapy. J Clin Oncol 25:938–946
101. Hendrickson K, Phillips M, Smith W, Peterson L, Krohn K, Rajendran J (2011) Hypoxia imaging with [F-18] FMISO-PET in head and neck cancer: potential for guiding intensity modulated radiation therapy in overcoming hypoxia-induced treatment resistance. Radiother Oncol 101:369–375
102. Crommelin DJ, Storm G, Luijten P (2011) 'Personalised medicine' through 'personalised medicines': time to integrate advanced, non-invasive imaging approaches and smart drug delivery systems. Int J Pharm 415:5–8
103. Moonen CT (2007) Spatio-temporal control of gene expression and cancer treatment using magnetic resonance imaging-guided focused ultrasound. Clin Cancer Res 13:3482–3489
104. Wikipedia (2014) Personalized medicine. http://en.wikipedia.org/wiki/Personalized_medicine. Accessed 29 Dec 2014
105. National Institute of Health. National Human Genome Research Institute (2015) Talking Glossary of Genetic Terms. Personalized Medicine. http://www.genome.gov/glossary/index.cfm?id=150. Accessed 29 Dec 2014
106. National Cancer Institute (2015) NCI Dictionary of Cancer Terms. http://www.cancer.gov/dictionary?CdrID=561717. Accessed 29 Dec 2014
107. Xie J, Lee S, Chen X (2010) Nanoparticle-based theranostic agents. Adv Drug Deliv Rev 62:1064–1079
108. U.S. Food and Drug Administration (2015) List of cleared or approved companion diagnostic devices (In Vitro and Imaging Tools). http://www.fda.gov/MedicalDevices/ProductsandMedicalProcedures/InVitroDiagnostics/ucm301431.htm. Accessed 29 Dec 2014

9

The joints in juvenile idiopathic arthritis

Lil-Sofie Ording Muller[1] · Paul Humphries[2] · Karen Rosendahl[3]

Abstract
Juvenile idiopathic arthritis is the most common rheumatic entity in childhood. Imaging has become an important supplement to the clinical assessment of children with JIA. Radiographs still play an important role in the workup, and long-term follow-up in children with JIA, but are not sensitive to findings in the early disease stage. Both ultrasound and MRI are more sensitive to inflammatory changes than clinical assessment alone. However, the differentiation between normal findings and pathology can be challenging, particularly in early disease. The objective of this review is to discuss the role of imaging in JIA, describe the typical findings on different modalities and highlight the challenges we face regarding the reliability and accuracy of the different methods for imaging the joints in children with JIA.

✉ Lil-Sofie Ording Muller
lilmul@ous-hf.no; lilsofie.ording@googlemail.com

Paul Humphries
p.humphries@ucl.ac.uk

Karen Rosendahl
karen.rosendahl@helse-bergen.no

1 Department for Radiology and Intervention, Oslo University Hospital, Oslo, Norway

2 Institute of Child Health, UCL, University College London Hospital NHS Trust and Great Ormond Street Hospital for Children, London, UK

3 Department of Radiology, Haukeland University Hospital, Bergen, Norway

Key Points

- *Imaging is an important supplement to the clinical examination in JIA.*
- *Ultrasound is more sensitive for detecting synovitis than clinical examination alone.*
- *MRI can depict all relevant structures in joint inflammation.*
- *The differentiation between normal variants and pathology is difficult in children.*

Keywords Juvenile idiopathic arthritis · Magnetic resonance imaging · Ultrasound · Paediatrics · Musculoskeletal

Introduction

Juvenile idiopathic arthritis (JIA) is defined as arthritis of unknown cause, with disease duration of more than 6 months, occurring in children under 16 years. It is the most common rheumatic entity in childhood with a prevalence of 0.6–1.9 in 1000 children. The exact pathogenesis is not fully understood but is thought to include both genetic and environmental components. JIA is not one single disease but includes a subset of different childhood arthritides (Table 1). Both clinical presentation and outcome vary with clinical subtype, and persistent oligoarthritis has been shown to have the best prognosis [1–3].

Despite the heterogeneity, it is likely that there is some genetic overlap, as all JIA subtypes share joint inflammation as the most prominent disease feature [1–4].

Joint pathogenesis involves inflammation of the synovial lining, with the potential to cause joint destruction. There is infiltration of the synovium by inflammatory cells. The lining layers of the synovium then become hyperplastic with increased vascularity. The pannus is comprised primarily of invasive cells and the synovium becomes locally invasive at the synovial interface with cartilage and bone. Subsequent

Table 1 Summary of the main features of the six different subtypes of JIA

Subset of JIA	Frequency %	Age at onset	Clinical presentation	Sex
Oligo	27–56	Early childhood, peak 2–4 years	Four or fewer joints involved the first 6 months	F>>M
Poly RF negative	11–28	Early peak 2–4; late peak 6–12 years	Four or more joints involved within the first 6 months, absence of IgM RF. Heterogeneous disease with three subsets. Prognosis varies with the disease subset	
Poly RF positive	2–7	Late childhood-adolescence	Four or more joints involved within the first 6 months, IgM RF positive. Resembles adult RA. Involvement of small joints. Progressive and diffuse joint involvement	F>>M
Ethesitis related	3–11	Late childhood-adolescence	Characterised by enthesitis and arthritis. Often HLA-B27 positive. Commonly hip involvement at presentation. Often a mild and remitting course but may progress with sacroiliac and spinal joint involvement, resembling ankylosing spondylitis	M>>F
Psoriatic	2–11	Early peak 2–4 years; late peak 9–11 years	Arthritis and psoriatic rash or psoriasis in close family. Controversial definition, resembles oligoarthritis but more often with dactylitis and involvement of both small and large joints	F>M
Systemic	4–17	Throughout childhood	Arthritis and quotidian fever plus one or more of the following symptoms: characteristic rash, hepatomegaly, splenomegaly, lymphadenopathy, serositis. Variable course; 5–8 % develop macrophage activation syndrome	F=M

destruction of the bone and cartilage occurs as a result of antibody deposition and degradative enzymes [5]. It is believed that the bone destruction in JIA is a consequence of overlying cartilage degradation. The inflammation may also cause growth disturbances, both systemically and locally in the affected joint. The typical manifestations of the articular and periarticular inflammation in early and late disease are shown in Table 2.

The objective of this review is to discuss the role of imaging in JIA, describe the typical findings on different modalities and highlight the challenges we face regarding the reliability and accuracy of the different methods for imaging the joints in children with JIA.

The role of imaging in JIA

Currently, the diagnosis of JIA is based on clinical and laboratory findings and does not include imaging. However, clinical assessment of children with joint complaints is challenging and laboratory findings are often equivocal. This has led to an increased use of imaging for both diagnosis and follow-up, particularly of joints that are frequently affected but may be asymptomatic, such as the temporomandibular joint (TMJ) [6].

Imaging is used to determine the presence and extension of joint inflammation and can more accurately distinguish between arthritis and tenosynovitis than clinical examination alone. In some cases, it can also help define the subtype of JIA. Imaging has a role in the assessment of differential diagnosis, such as leukaemia, avascular necrosis, trauma or bone tumours, and also shows potential in the evaluation of treatment response.

Table 2 Typical manifestations of the articular and periarticular inflammation of JIA in early and late disease. The order of presentation is not absolute; some of the features may not be present at all or the features may overlap

Periarticular soft tissue change	Early
Synovitis	↓
Tendinitis	
Bursitis	
Periarticular bony change	
Bone oedema	
Periostitis	
Growth disturbances	
Osteoporosis	
Destructive change of bone and cartillage	
Erosive change of bone	
Joint space narrowing, bone fusion, malalignment	Late

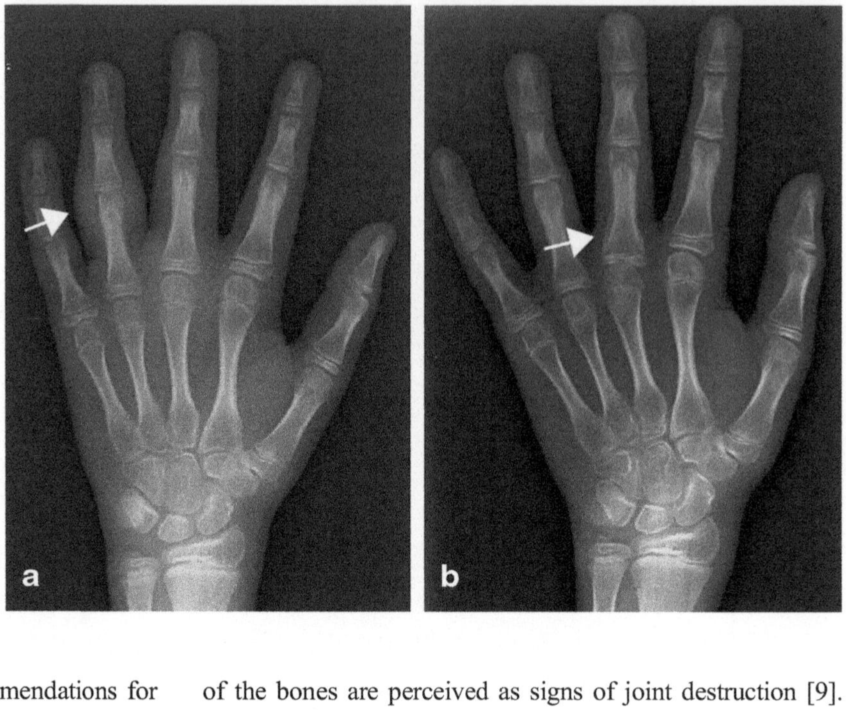

Fig. 1 Plain radiographs of affected joints in JIA may be normal, particularly early in the disease course; however, non-specific soft tissue swelling may be seen (**a**). Periosteal reaction (**b**) may also occur in active synovitis and is most frequently seen in tenosynovitis.

There are no unifying international recommendations for imaging in JIA and both the choice of imaging modality and when and whom to refer for radiological investigations vary between centres. One of the major challenges when interpreting imaging studies is to distinguish between normal findings and pathology in the early stages of the disease, particularly on MRI. Moreover, the lack of standardised scoring systems for all modalities makes the objective evaluation of the degree of inflammation and destruction challenging. Plain radiographs of the affected joint are often not helpful to establish the diagnosis but are advised as a baseline study for longitudinal follow-up and to help narrow the list of differentials or suggest alternative diagnoses, for example an underlying bone tumour or a fracture. Ultrasound and MRI form the basis of more advanced imaging assessment in paediatric arthritis, while cone-beam computed tomography play a role in imaging of the TMJs and conventional CT in imaging of the sacroiliac and facet joint of the cervical spine [7].

Radiographs

Joint malalignment, evaluation of focal growth disturbances and joint damage evaluation in JIA have traditionally been performed by X-ray scoring methods. Radiographs can show soft tissue swelling and periostitis even in the early stages of the disease (Fig. 1) but the findings are not specific for arthritis. Growth disturbances can be seen early as focal accelerated growth or advanced skeletal maturation or later as premature closure of growth plates or squaring of the bones. Radiographs may show bone erosions and may depict cartilage loss indirectly through joint space narrowing [8] (Fig. 2). Joint space narrowing, malalignment and focal concavities or lytic lesions of the bones are perceived as signs of joint destruction [9]. However, the sensitivity is low, particularly for disease in early stages, and the aforementioned features are not sensitive to subtle change over time [10, 11]. Plain radiographs cannot visualise the synovium, joint effusion, articular cartilage, bone marrow, or ligaments and tendons directly. Therefore, in cases of clinical uncertainty or where treatment may be modified on the basis of activity versus quiescent disease, additional imaging modalities may be employed.

Ultrasound

Ultrasound has many advantages in children. It is readily available, non-ionising, dynamic and well tolerated without recourse to anaesthesia or sedation; hence, it is a frequently used radiological examination in a child with JIA. Small

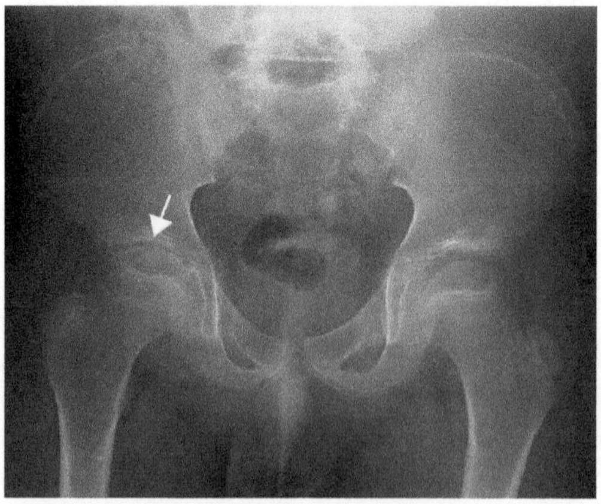

Fig. 2 Erosions and joint space narrowing can be seen on radiographs (arrow) but are normally a late finding in arthritis

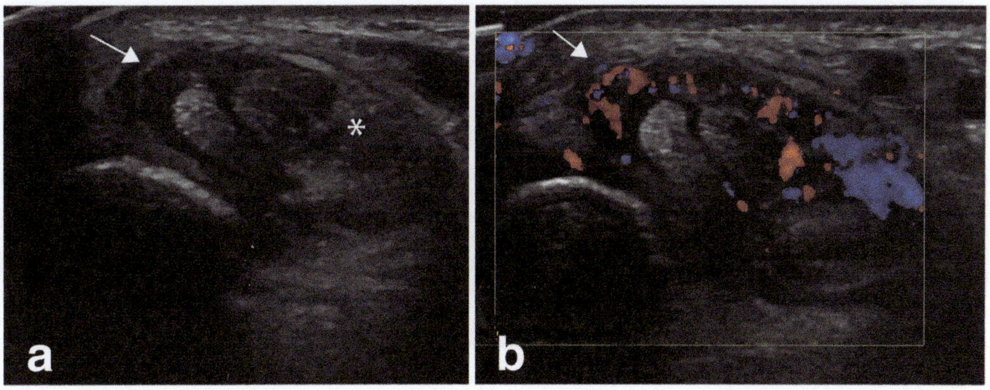

Fig. 3 Ultrasound shows signs of tenosynovitis in the tibialis posterior and flexor digitorum longus tendons with hypertrophic synovium in the tendon sheet (**a**). The hypertrophic synovium can be both hypoechoic (arrow) and hyperechoic (asterisk). Hypervascularity is seen on colour Doppler examination (**b**)

patient size is both an advantage and disadvantage—using modern high-resolution transducers, exquisite detail is possible but requires a meticulous approach and adaptation of scanning equipment. Small "hockey-stick" transducers can be used for small joints but also for larger joints, e.g. ankle scanning in small children. Judicious use of warm jelly, often as a stand-off for small joints, and a child-friendly environment increase the chances of success.

Diagnostic ultrasound may be used to assess for features suggesting acute or active disease, principally joint effusion, synovial thickening, teno-synovial thickening and effusion (Figs. 3, 4 and 5). Ultrasound has a higher sensitivity and specificity for the presence of synovitis than clinical assessment alone and is the most sensitive method for the detection of tenosynovitis [12, 13]. For the less experienced examiner it may be challenging to distinguish between a thickened oedematous synovium and the adjacent cartilage or joint fluid because all these structures may have a similar, hypoechoic appearance. A rule of thumb is that the joint fluid will be compressible and cartilage thickness will not change with the pressure from the ultrasound probe. The synovium will only be partly compressible and may show flow on Doppler examination. Colour and power Doppler may be utilised to assess increased vascularisation, a marker of active inflammation, to differentiate between active and quiescent disease [14]. Chronic disease changes can also be potentially assessed using ultrasound, principally cartilage reduction and bony erosions, particularly in small joints (Fig. 5). Spannow et al. documented normal changes in cartilage thickness with age and sex and described intra- and inter-observer variability of these measurements enabling a clinical assessment of cartilage thickness with reference to normal values [15]. It has been demonstrated that there is reduced cartilage thickness in patients with JIA compared to age- and sex-matched controls, although interestingly this phenomenon is observed in both clinically affected and non-affected joints [16]. The measurements obtained on US correlate with MRI measurements [15] potentially enabling longitudinal US measurements to be used for disease response assessment, with it being recognised that cartilage thickness may increase on treatment.

Ultrasound may also be used in interventional procedures, for both diagnostic purposes, i.e. aspiration of a joint, and treatment, i.e. tendon sheath or joint injection [17]. Despite the stated advantages of ultrasound, there are several limitations. Musculoskeletal ultrasound (MSK US) is not a widespread skill, particularly amongst paediatric radiologists, and there is a learning curve when undertaking these

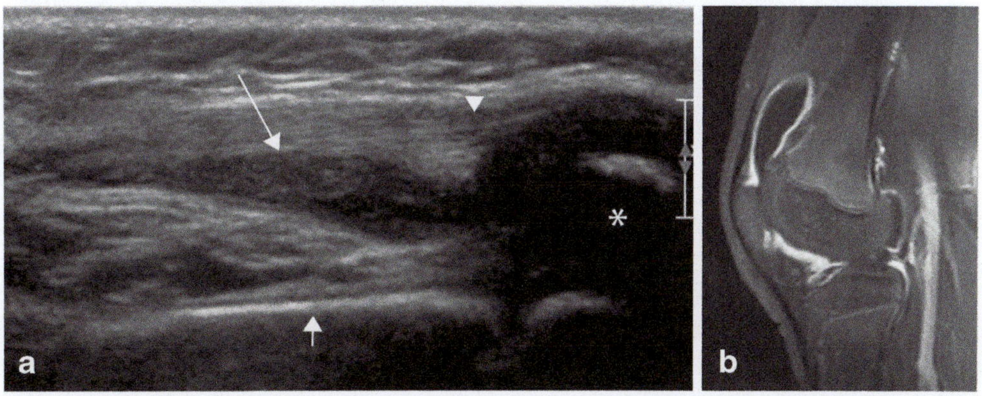

Fig. 4 **a** Ultrasound (panoramic view) of the ventral aspect of the knee shows fluid in the suprapatellar recess (arrow), cranial to the patella (asterisk), under the patellar tendon (arrowhead) and overlying the femur (small arrow) suggestive of synovitis. **b** The findings were confirmed by MRI, which shows slightly hypertrophic, enhancing synovium in keeping with synovitis

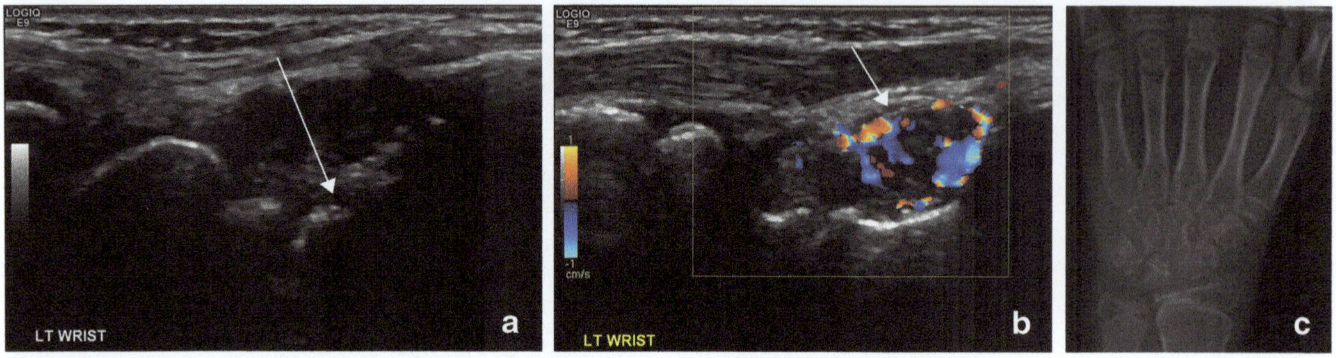

Fig. 5 Ultrasound may depict both synovitis and bone destruction, particularly in small joints. **a** Ultrasound of the dorsal aspect of the wrist shows an irregular surface of the scaphoid (long arrow) suggestive of erosions. **c** There was thickened and hyperaemic synovium over the scaphoid, indicative of active inflammation. **c** Plain radiograph of the wrist confirmed squaring of the carpal bones, carpal crowding and a sclerotic, irregular bony surface

examinations. Ultrasound is an operator-dependent modality, taking time to become proficient. Close collaboration between the clinical team and radiologist, with multidisciplinary discussion where there are discordant findings between the clinical examination and the sonographic assessment, facilitates appropriate management. It is recognised that US will depict more synovitis in JIA than clinically detected [12], but this may represent old inactive changes rather than active disease. Doppler examination may be used to differentiate active from inactive disease, but there is no unifying definition of hyperaemia, and the Doppler appearance will vary with different probes, settings, vendors and the imaging technique (e.g. probe pressure). Therefore the interpretation of the findings, particularly in early disease/subtle findings, is challenging. Comparison with a contra-lateral unaffected joint or the adjacent non-inflamed synovium may help in the evaluation. Furthermore, ultrasound cannot assess changes in the bone marrow. Finally the stages of development and US imaging of the normal growing peri-articular skeletal tissues throughout childhood are in general not well documented (aside from Spannow et al. described above); hence, normal standards for US anatomy are not yet properly established.

Despite the challenges of MSK US in paediatrics there is a growing acceptance of its use and availability. US lends itself to one-stop clinics to establish a diagnosis, formulate a treatment plan and possibly US-guided aspiration or injection.

MRI

MRI is the only diagnostic tool that can assess all relevant anatomical structures in joint inflammation. Contrast-enhanced MRI is able to depict synovial thickening and enhancement, joint fluid, bone marrow oedema as well as damage to cartilage and bone and is therefore potentially a powerful imaging tool in the assessment of joint inflammation and the progression of permanent joint damage. Erosions cannot be assessed clinically and MRI is thought to have greater sensitivity than radiography in early detection of erosions [18]. The standard MRI protocol in arthritis [19] includes a

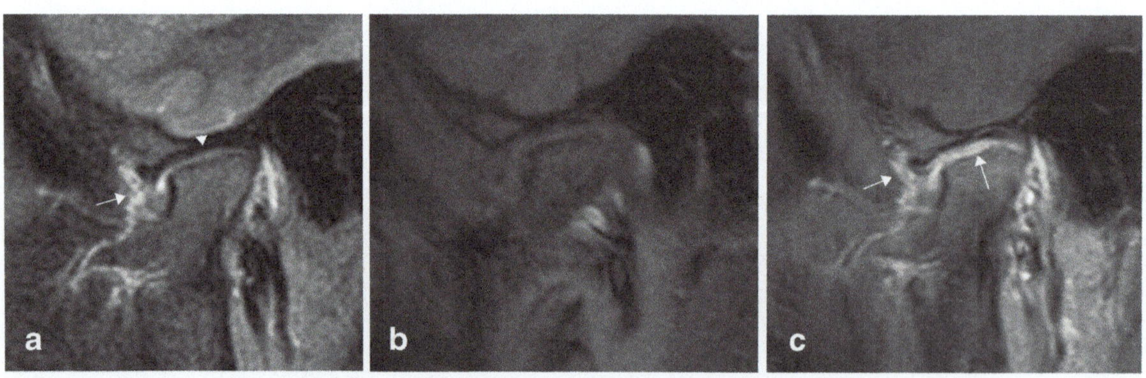

Fig. 6 Sagittal STIR (**a**), T1 f. pre-contrast (**b**) and T1 f. post-contrast image (**c**) of the temporomandibular joint showing thickened, enhancing synovium (arrows) and a sliver of fluid within the joint (arrowhead) indicating active inflammation.

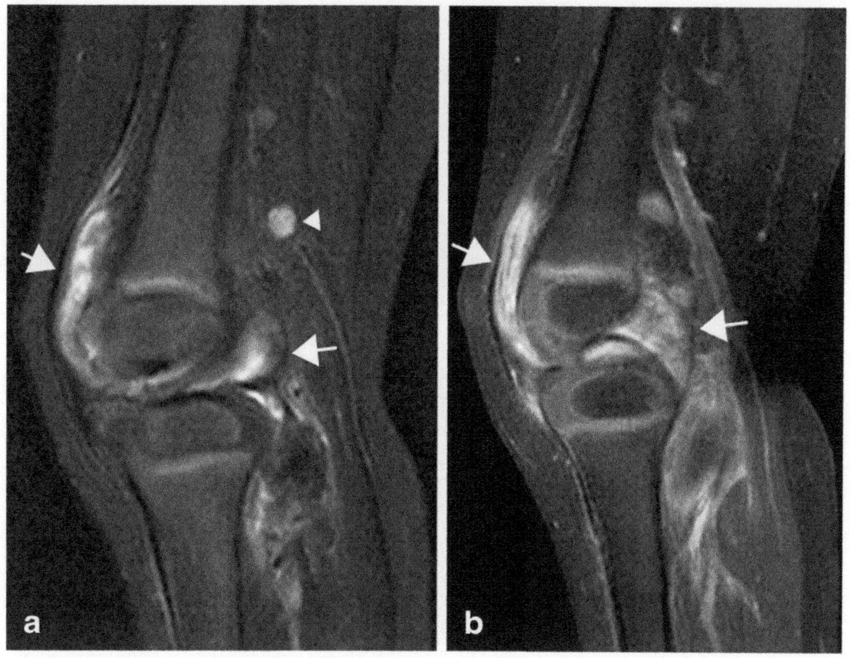

Fig. 7 **a** Sagittal STIR sequence of a knee with long-standing arthritis showing marked synovial hypertrophy (arrows) and marked lymph nodes (arrowheads). **b** On sagittal T1 fat-suppressed sequence post-gadolinium administration inhomogeneous synovial enhancement can be seen (arrows) indicating fibrotic areas within the inflamed synovium. There is no effusion. Soft tissue oedema is seen in the calf

- T1 SE sequence,
- T2 fat-suppressed sequence or a STIR and
- T1 fat-suppressed sequence pre- and post-contrast.

Some may prefer to add a sequence for visualisation of cartilage, such as a proton-weighted or 3D DESS sequence. The DIXON fat-suppression technique is increasingly being used because it gives robust, homogeneous fat suppression and can be combined with high-resolution T2-weighted images, giving a better signal-to-noise ratio compared to the STIR sequence, without increasing the scan time [20]. Contrast administration is necessary for the assessment of synovitis; hence contrast enhanced MRI is part of the standard protocol in JIA. The preferred image planes will vary depending on the joint but the MRI protocol should allow multiplanar reformatting so potential findings, particularly evidence of joint destruction, could be verified in at least two planes.

In active arthritis there will always be pathological enhancement of a thickened synovium (Figs. 4 and 6). In JIA, as opposed to other types of arthritis, the enhancement may be patchy, particularly in chronic disease, due to areas of fibrotic change (Fig. 7). Increased joint fluid is a common finding (Figs. 4 and 6), but may be absent, particularly in small joints such as the wrist, because of compression by the hypertrophic synovium. Sparse fluid may also be seen in larger joints in chronic synovitis where the synovium is thickened and partly

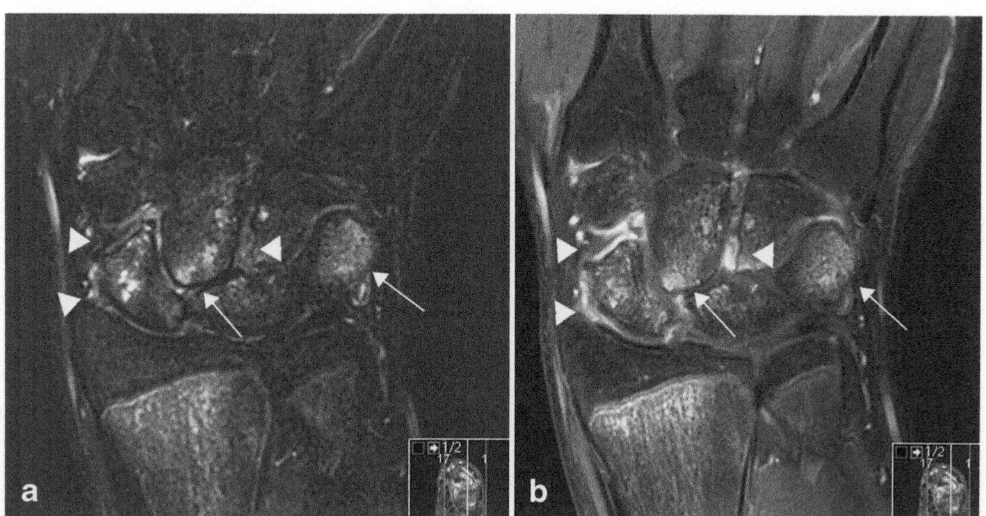

Fig. 8 Coronal images of the wrist in a child with active arthritis at the wrist showing high signal within the carpal bones on STIR sequence (**a**), which enhances on the post-contrast T1 f. sequence (**b**), indicative of inflammation (arrows). There is enhancement of a thickened synovium in the intercarpal and radio-carpal joints but no joint fluid (arrowheads)

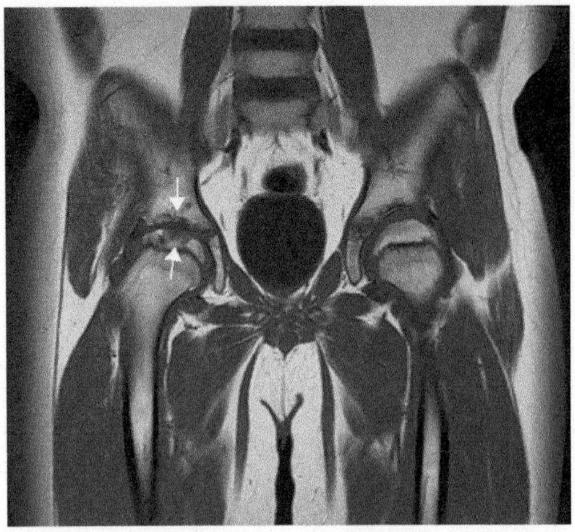

Fig. 9 MRI can be used to depict bone destruction. Coronal T1 TSE of the pelvis shows joint space narrowing and erosions of the right hip; the same case as in Fig. 2 (arrows)

fibrotic (Figs. 7–8). Bone marrow oedema (BMO) in the adjacent skeleton can be caused by reactive osteitis (Fig. 8). Soft tissue oedema and reactive lymph nodes may also be present in long-standing disease or aggressive forms of JIA (Fig. 7). Erosions and/or malalignment of the joint is also depicted on MRI (Fig. 9) and initial studies suggest that MRI has a higher sensitivity to detect erosions than does radiography [18].

Reading of the MRI examinations in children with arthritis may however be difficult, particularly in cases of subtle findings. Recent studies have shown that lesions suggestive of BMO and amounts of joint fluid that in adults would have been defined as pathological, and changes that look like erosions, are frequently seen on MRI of the wrist also in healthy children [21] (Figs. 10, 11 and 12). To date there is no imaging method that can reliably differentiate these normal findings from those caused by disease. There are some studies describing the normal anatomy and contrast enhancement pattern of the temporomandibular joints [22, 23]; otherwise, there is a paucity of age-dependent normal anatomy on MRI. Additional disadvantages of MRI may be the low availability, high costs and the need for sedation in children younger than 4–6 years.

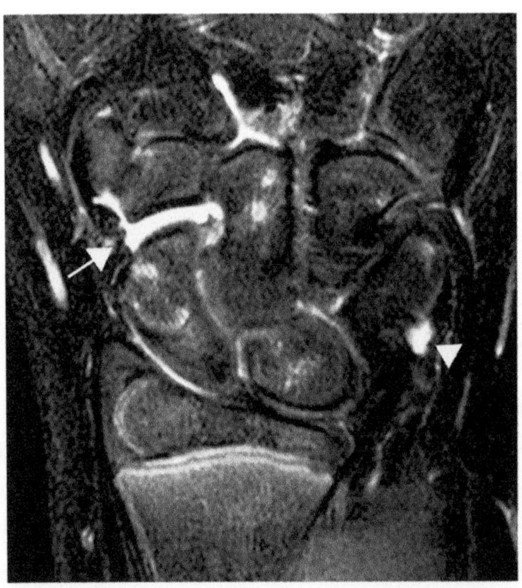

Fig. 10 In adults more than 2 mm of joint fluid is defined as pathologically increased fluid at the wrist. In children this is frequently seen as a normal finding (arrow). Fluid in the pisotriquetral recess is also often seen in healthy children (arrowhead), here seen on a coronal STIR of a 12-year-old healthy, asymptomatic boy

CT

Cone-beam computed tomography (CBCT) is currently accepted as the imaging modality of choice for assessment of permanent bony changes to the TMJs. It can visualise joint space narrowing and erosive change, as well as growth disturbances with a relatively low radiation dose [7].

Computed tomography (CT) may be helpful in the assessment of the facet joints, in particular in the cervical spine. Its use is, however, limited by the relatively high radiation dose.

Validation of imaging markers for active disease and permanent joint damage

There have been major advances in the treatment of JIA during the last decade. The development of new therapeutic agents and new, individually tailored treatment strategies has led to significant improvement in functional outcome in children with JIA [24, 25]. The paramount goal of current treatment in JIA is to achieve inactive disease and remission with or without medication [3]. In order to evaluate the therapeutic response, sensitive and reproducible tools for assessment of change in the severity of inflammation and for bony destruction have become crucial. Of the diagnostic tools currently available, imaging studies are thought best suited for these purposes [26]. The radiological investigations in JIA should ideally be able to determine the presence and degree of (1) active inflammation, (2) precursors of permanent articular damage, (3) established articular damage and (4) complications to treatment.

Synovial contrast enhancement, bone marrow oedema (BMO) and increased joint fluid are all thought to be signs of active inflammation. The presence of bone erosions is a sign of structural joint damage and the presence of BMO may be predictive of later bone erosions [27, 28]. These definitions of active inflammation and destruction are based on research on patients with rheumatoid arthritis and have been adapted for use in children. Recent studies have shown that definitions extrapolated from research in the adult population cannot automatically be used in children and may lead to both over- and under-staging of disease

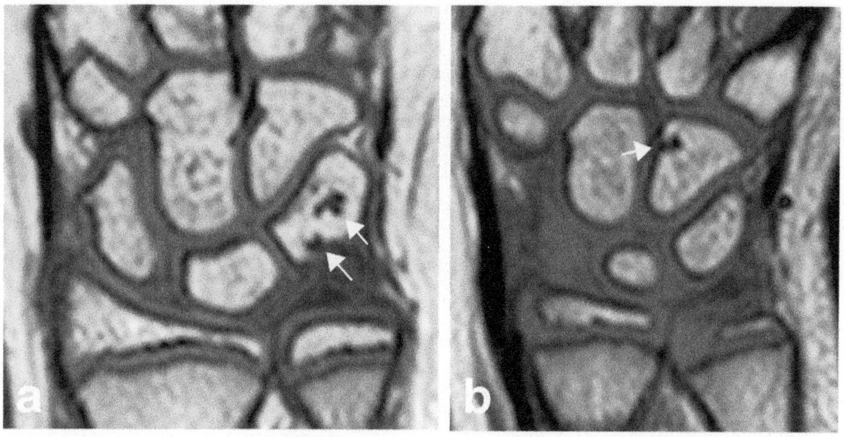

Fig. 11 Bony depressions of the carpal bones and proximal metacarpals (arrows) are a normal finding in children and should not automatically be interpreted as erosions. **a** Coronal T1-weighted image of a 10-year-old healthy girl showing typical normal carpal depressions in the triquetrum. In some areas of the carpal bones bony depressions are more frequently seen in healthy children, e.g. in the radial aspect of the hamate, here shown in an 8-year-old, healthy and asymptomatic girl (**b**)

[21, 29–31]. Therefore separate validation of the different modalities when used in children must be performed in order to provide systems that can reliably quantify the degree of inflammation and destruction in JIA. Large efforts have been made over the last decade to provide objective imaging tools for the quantification of disease activity in children with JIA. A summary of the current status is provided below:

Radiographs

Radiographic scores are only feasible for structural change and not for inflammation. Radiographic scoring systems specific for joint destruction at the wrist in JIA have been devised and show good reproducibility and clinical validity [11]. One initial validation of a scoring system for chronic changes at the hip has been published [32] but validated radiographic scoring systems for other joints are lacking.

Ultrasound

Apart from studies of the age-dependent cartilage thickness [33], normal appearances for the various joints in a growing child throughout childhood are not well documented on ultrasound. In addition, to date there are no unifying definitions of synovial thickening, pathological amounts of joint fluid, hyperaemia or destructive change on ultrasound; hence, no validated scoring systems for disease activity and progression are available and the interpretation of the US findings in JIA remains subjective [12, 34].

MRI

Great efforts have been made by different national and international study groups, e.g. the Health-e-Child Radiology Group and the Outcome Measures in Rheumatology Clinical Trials (OMERACT) Special Interest Group 'MRI in JIA' to create and validate a universal paediatric MRI scoring system [35]. This

Fig. 12 High signal on T2 f. or STIR images (**a**) with corresponding low signal on the T1 TSE sequence (**b**) in the scaphoid suggestive of marrow oedema in a 12-year-old, healthy, asymptomatic boy. Signal changes suggestive of bone marrow oedema can frequently be seen at the wrist in asymptomatic, healthy children

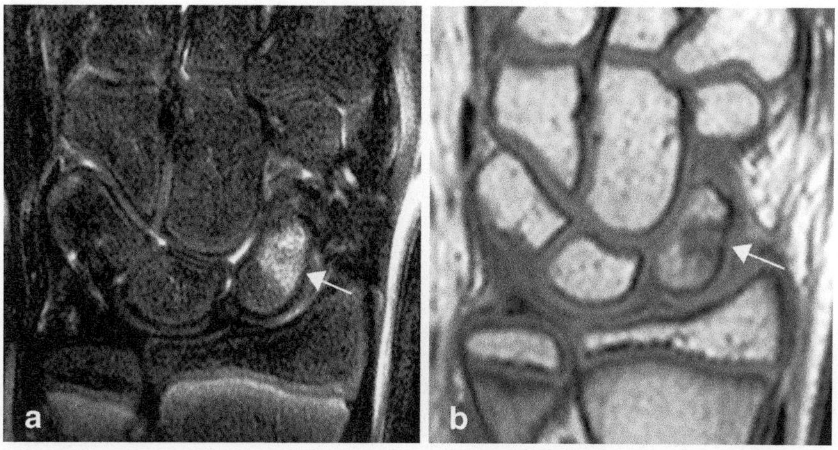

work has shown that in multi-centre studies the assessment and semi-quantification of BMO and tenosynovitis have acceptable repeatability for clinical use, whereas synovial enhancement and overall inflammation can be accurately scored by the same observer while inter-observer agreement was less favourable, but acceptable for the assessment of the radio-ulnar and radio-carpal joints [36, 37]. Moreover, recent studies showing that many of the findings that were previously defined as pathology also appear in healthy children have altered the whole perception of the accuracy of the MRI features included in previous scoring systems and the main challenge we now face is how to differentiate normal findings from disease. Bone erosion is the only feature of destruction included in the suggested scoring systems for JIA on MRI. However, it has previously been suggested, when using radiographs in the assessment, that bone erosions may not even be the most significant sign of bone destruction at the wrist, particularly in younger children, and that carpal crowding or squaring of the carpal bones causing a small and deformed wrist is more characteristic for JIA [10, 38]. This was later confirmed in a study comparing healthy children and those with JIA showing that children with JIA had significantly smaller wrists, but there was no difference in the number of erosion-like changes [30]. Including erosions only in the assessment of bone destruction in children may therefore lead to both over- and understaging of disease. There is ongoing multinational collaboration among several research groups to create accurate and reliable scoring systems for JIA, for both large and small joints, but to date an internationally validated and accepted scoring system for JIA is not yet available for any of the joints on MRI.

Conclusion

Imaging is a useful diagnostic supplement to the clinical assessment of children with JIA. Following the introduction of new, potent biologic drugs, there is an urgent need for accurate markers of disease, both active arthritis and permanent joint damage. Imaging, in particular MRI, has great potential, but more studies addressing the precision and accuracy as well as the clinical validity of the findings should be done.

References

1. Prakken B, Albani S, Martini A (2011) Juvenile idiopathic arthritis. Lancet 377:2138–2149
2. Packham JC, Hall MA, Pimm TJ (2002) Long-term follow-up of 246 adults with juvenile idiopathic arthritis: predictive factors for mood and pain. Rheumatology (Oxford) 41:1444–1449
3. Nordal E, Zak M, Aalto K et al (2011) Ongoing disease activity and changing categories in a long-term nordic cohort study of juvenile idiopathic arthritis. Arthritis Rheum 63:2809–2818
4. Woo P, Colbert RA (2009) An overview of genetics of paediatric rheumatic diseases. Best Pract Res Clin Rheumatol 23:589–597
5. Ravelli A, Martini A (2007) Juvenile idiopathic arthritis. Lancet 369:767–778
6. Cannizzaro E, Schroeder S, Muller LM, Kellenberger CJ, Saurenmann RK (2011) Temporomandibular joint involvement in children with juvenile idiopathic arthritis. J Rheumatol 38:510–515
7. Koos B, Tzaribachev N, Bott S, Ciesielski R, Godt A (2013) Classification of temporomandibular joint erosion, arthritis, and inflammation in patients with juvenile idiopathic arthritis. J Orofac Orthop 74:506–519
8. Babyn P, Doria AS (2007) Radiologic investigation of rheumatic diseases. Rheum Dis Clin N Am 33:403–440
9. Poznanski AK (1992) Radiological approaches to pediatric joint disease. J Rheumatol Suppl 33:78–93
10. Rossi F, Di Dia F, Galipo O et al (2006) Use of the Sharp and Larsen scoring methods in the assessment of radiographic progression in juvenile idiopathic arthritis. Arthritis Rheum 55:717–723
11. Ravelli A, Ioseliani M, Norambuena X et al (2007) Adapted versions of the Sharp/van der Heijde score are reliable and valid for assessment of radiographic progression in juvenile idiopathic arthritis. Arthritis Rheum 56:3087–3095
12. Collado P, Jousse-Joulin S, Alcalde M, Naredo E, D'Agostino MA (2012) Is ultrasound a validated imaging tool for the diagnosis and management of synovitis in juvenile idiopathic arthritis? A systematic literature review. Arthritis Care Res (Hoboken). doi:10.1002/acr.21644
13. Janow GL, Panghaal V, Trinh A, Badger D, Levin TL, Ilowite NT (2011) Detection of active disease in juvenile idiopathic arthritis: sensitivity and specificity of the physical examination vs ultrasound. J Rheumatol 38:2671–2674
14. Terslev L, von der Recke P, Torp-Pedersen S, Koenig MJ, Bliddal H (2008) Diagnostic sensitivity and specificity of Doppler ultrasound in rheumatoid arthritis. J Rheumatol 35:49–53
15. Spannow AH, Stenboeg E, Pfeiffer-Jensen M et al (2011) Ultrasound and MRI measurements of joint cartilage in healthy children: a validation study. Ultraschall Med 32(Suppl 1):S110–S116
16. Pradsgaard DO, Spannow AH, Heuck C, Herlin T (2013) Decreased cartilage thickness in juvenile idiopathic arthritis assessed by ultrasonography. J Rheumatol 40:1596–1603
17. Young CM, Shiels WE 2nd, Coley BD et al (2012) Ultrasound-guided corticosteroid injection therapy for juvenile idiopathic arthritis: 12-year care experience. Pediatr Radiol 42:1481–1489
18. Malattia C, Damasio MB, Magnaguagno F et al (2008) Magnetic resonance imaging, ultrasonography, and conventional radiography in the assessment of bone erosions in juvenile idiopathic arthritis. Arthritis Rheum 59:1764–1772
19. Ostergaard M, Peterfy C, Conaghan P et al (2003) OMERACT Rheumatoid Arthritis Magnetic Resonance Imaging Studies. Core set of MRI acquisitions, joint pathology definitions, and the OMERACT RA-MRI scoring system. J Rheumatol 30:1385–1386
20. Del Grande F, Santini F, Herzka DA et al (2014) Fat-suppression techniques for 3-T MR imaging of the musculoskeletal system. Radiographics 34:217–233
21. Muller LS, Avenarius D, Damasio B et al (2011) The paediatric wrist revisited: redefining MR findings in healthy children. Ann Rheum Dis 70:605–610

22. von Kalle T, Winkler P, Stuber T (2013) Contrast-enhanced MRI of normal temporomandibular joints in children–is there enhancement or not? Rheumatology (Oxford) 52:363–367
23. Karlo CA, Stolzmann P, Habernig S, Muller L, Saurenmann T, Kellenberger CJ (2010) Size, shape and age-related changes of the mandibular condyle during childhood. Eur Radiol 20:2512–2517
24. Hayward K, Wallace CA (2009) Recent developments in anti-rheumatic drugs in pediatrics: treatment of juvenile idiopathic arthritis. Arthritis Res Ther 11:216
25. Ruperto N, Martini A (2011) Emerging drugs to treat juvenile idiopathic arthritis. Expert Opin Emerg Drugs 16:493–505
26. Magni-Manzoni S, Malattia C, Lanni S, Ravelli A (2012) Advances and challenges in imaging in juvenile idiopathic arthritis. Nat Rev Rheumatol. doi:10.1038/nrrheum.2012.30
27. Duer-Jensen A, Horslev-Petersen K, Hetland ML et al (2011) Bone edema on magnetic resonance imaging is an independent predictor of rheumatoid arthritis development in patients with early undifferentiated arthritis. Arthritis Rheum 63:2192–2202
28. Hetland ML, Ejbjerg B, Horslev-Petersen K et al (2009) MRI bone oedema is the strongest predictor of subsequent radiographic progression in early rheumatoid arthritis. Results from a 2-year randomised controlled trial (CIMESTRA). Ann Rheum Dis 68: 384–390
29. Avenarius DM, Ording Muller LS, Eldevik P, Owens CM, Rosendahl K (2012) The paediatric wrist revisited-findings of bony depressions in healthy children on radiographs compared to MRI. Pediatr Radiol. doi:10.1007/s00247-012-2354-x
30. Ording Muller LS, Boavida P, Avenarius D et al (2013) MRI of the wrist in juvenile idiopathic arthritis: erosions or normal variants? A prospective case-control study. Pediatr Radiol 43:785–795
31. Avenarius DM, Ording Muller LS, Eldevik P, Owens CM, Rosendahl K (2012) The paediatric wrist revisited–findings of bony depressions in healthy children on radiographs compared to MRI. Pediatr Radiol 42:791–798
32. Bertamino M, Rossi F, Pistorio A et al (2010) Development and initial validation of a radiographic scoring system for the hip in juvenile idiopathic arthritis. J Rheumatol 37:432–439
33. Spannow AH, Pfeiffer-Jensen M, Andersen NT, Herlin T, Stenbog E (2010) Ultrasonographic measurements of joint cartilage thickness in healthy children: age- and sex-related standard reference values. J Rheumatol 37:2595–2601
34. Magni-Manzoni S, Collado P, Jousse-Joulin S et al (2014) Current state of musculoskeletal ultrasound in paediatric rheumatology: results of an international survey. Rheumatology (Oxford) 53:491–496
35. Damasio MB, Malattia C, Tanturri de Horatio L et al (2012) MRI of the wrist in juvenile idiopathic arthritis: proposal of a paediatric synovitis score by a consensus of an international working group. Results of a multicentre reliability study. Pediatr Radiol 42:1047–1055
36. Tanturri de Horatio L, Damasio MB, Barbuti D et al (2012) MRI assessment of bone marrow in children with juvenile idiopathic arthritis: intra- and inter-observer variability. Pediatr Radiol. doi: 10.1007/s00247-012-2345-y
37. Lambot K, Boavida P, Damasio MB et al (2013) MRI assessment of tenosynovitis in children with juvenile idiopathic arthritis: inter- and intra-observer variability. Pediatr Radiol 43:796–802
38. Poznanski AK, Hernandez RJ, Guire KE, Bereza UL, Garn SM (1978) Carpal length in children–a useful measurement in the diagnosis of rheumatoid arthritis and some concenital malformation syndromes. Radiology 129:661–668

10

The role of MRI in axillary lymph node imaging in breast cancer patients: a systematic review

V. J. L. Kuijs · M. Moossdorff · R. J. Schipper · R. G. H. Beets-Tan · E. M. Heuts · K. B. M. I. Keymeulen · M. L. Smidt · M. B. I. Lobbes

Abstract
Objectives To assess whether MRI can exclude axillary lymph node metastasis, potentially replacing sentinel lymph node biopsy (SLNB), and consequently eliminating the risk of SLNB-associated morbidity.
Methods PubMed, Cochrane, Medline and Embase databases were searched for relevant publications up to July 2014. Studies were selected based on predefined inclusion and exclusion criteria and independently assessed by two reviewers using a standardised extraction form.
Results Sixteen eligible studies were selected from 1,372 publications identified by the search. A dedicated axillary protocol [sensitivity 84.7 %, negative predictive value (NPV) 95.0 %] was superior to a standard protocol covering both the breast and axilla simultaneously (sensitivity 82.0 %, NPV 82.6 %). Dynamic, contrast-enhanced MRI had a lower median sensitivity (60.0 %) and NPV (80.0 %) compared to non-enhanced T1w/T2w sequences (88.4, 94.7 %), diffusion-weighted imaging (84.2, 90.6 %) and ultrasmall superparamagnetic iron oxide (USPIO)- enhanced T2*w sequences (83.0, 95.9 %). The most promising results seem to be achievable when using non-enhanced T1w/T2w and USPIO-enhanced T2*w sequences in combination with a dedicated axillary protocol (sensitivity 84.7 % and NPV 95.0 %).
Conclusions The diagnostic performance of some MRI protocols for excluding axillary lymph node metastases approaches the NPV needed to replace SLNB. However, current observations are based on studies with heterogeneous study designs and limited populations.
Main Messages
- *Some axillary MRI protocols approach the NPV of an SLNB procedure.*
- *Dedicated axillary MRI is more accurate than protocols also covering the breast.*
- *T1w/T2w protocols combined with USPIO-enhanced sequences are the most promising sequences.*

Keywords Breast cancer · MRI · Axilla · Lymph nodes · Neoplasm metastases

V. J. L. Kuijs · R. J. Schipper · R. G. H. Beets-Tan · M. B. I. Lobbes (✉)
Department of Radiology and Nuclear Medicine, Maastricht University Medical Center+, PO Box 5800, 6202 AZ Maastricht, The Netherlands
e-mail: marc.lobbes@mumc.nl

V. J. L. Kuijs · M. Moossdorff · R. J. Schipper · E. M. Heuts · K. B. M. I. Keymeulen · M. L. Smidt
Department of Surgery, Maastricht University Medical Center+, PO Box 5800, 6202 AZ Maastricht, The Netherlands

M. Moossdorff · R. J. Schipper · R. G. H. Beets-Tan · M. L. Smidt · M. B. I. Lobbes
GROW - School for Oncology and Developmental Biology, PO Box 616, 6200 MD Maastricht, The Netherlands

Introduction

Some 15 years ago, sentinel lymph node biopsy (SLNB) replaced axillary lymph node dissection (ALND) for nodal staging in clinically node-negative breast cancer patients. Although less invasive compared to ALND, the SLNB is still associated with non-neglible morbidity. For example, lymph oedema is reported in 5–8 % of patients after an SLNB [1, 2]. Other common complications are pain, paresthesia, decreased arm strength and shoulder stiffness [3]. Sixty percent of newly diagnosed breast cancer patients are pathologically node negative and consequently do not benefit from SLNB. Nonetheless, these patients are at risk of its complications.

As a result, there is a continuous search for novel, non-invasive nodal staging techniques that can accurately identify lymph node-negative breast cancer patients. Hypothetically, a non-invasive technique with high sensitivity and negative predictive value (NPV) could replace SLNB, eliminating its morbidity risk. Very small metastases will be hard to detect with any imaging technique, but recent studies have shown that these small metastases, such as isolated tumour cells (i.e., N0i+, <0.2 mm) and micrometastases (i.e., N1mi, 0.2–2.0 mm), do not influence overall survival. Consequently, sensitivity for detecting very small metastases is less important [4], creating a window of opportunity for (non-invasive) imaging techniques that might be able to perform axillary staging of breast cancer patients.

In recent years, many non-invasive imaging modalities, such as ultrasound or PET-CT, have been suggested for this purpose. We opted to systematically review the current evidence of axillary staging using MRI, since it appears to have several advantages over other imaging modalities, such as the lack of ionising radiation (compared to PET/CT) or less intra- and interobserver variation (common in ultrasound examinations).

The aim of this systematic review is to determine whether the diagnostic performance of MRI is sufficient to confidently exclude axillary lymph node metastasis in breast cancer patients, preventing node-negative patients from undergoing unnecessary invasive staging procedures such as SLNB.

Materials and methods

Search strategy

For this systematic review, the guidelines of Preferred Reporting Items for Systematic Reviews and Meta-Analyses (PRISMA) were followed [5]. A literature search was performed in the Cochrane Library, Embase and PubMed databases up to July 2014. Search terms used were breast or mamma combined with the terms neoplasms, malignancy, cancer, carcinoma and adenocarcinoma. Terms for intervention were magnetic resonance imaging, MRI, MR mammography, MR, and magnetic resonance. Terms for the reference test were axilla, axillary, lymph, node, nodal, stage, status, staging, lymph nodes, lymphatic metastases, sentinel lymph node biopsy, lymph node excision, axillary lymph node dissection, ALND, SLNB, sentinel lymph node, SN and sentinel node. Outcome terms were sensitivity, specificity, negative predictive value, NPV, positive predictive value, PPV and accuracy. A manual search of the reference lists of retrieved articles was performed for any additional publications.

In- and exclusion criteria

To avoid selection bias, in- and exclusion criteria were established prior to the literature search. Inclusion criteria were (1) diagnostic research, (2) newly diagnosed, histologically proven breast cancer patients, (3) at least 15 patients in the final analysis, (4) patients underwent standard breast MRI or dedicated axillary MRI prior to surgery, (5) minimum magnetic field strength of 1.5 T and (6) pathological examination was based on SLNB or ALND.

Additional exclusion criteria were (1) not addressing nodal staging; (2) studies with patients undergoing any type of neoadjuvant chemo-, immune- or endocrine therapy; (3) patients with a history of axillary surgery or treatment; (4) patients with recurrent axillary disease; (5) studies without >3 of the following diagnostic performance parameters: sensitivity, specificity, PPV, NPV or accuracy; (6) editorials, conference publications, surveys, case reports, reviews, meta-analysis, ex vivo studies and animal studies.

Study selection

Two independent reviewers searched for eligible articles and excluded duplicates. First, irrelevant articles based on the abstract and title were excluded by one reviewer and verified by the second one. Second, predefined in- and exclusion criteria were applied. Third, the full text of the remaining articles was obtained and considered by both reviewers. The study selection process did not apply any time or language restrictions. In the last phase, only two articles were additionally excluded (Spanish and Chinese).

Data extraction and quality assessment

Data from the included studies were extracted by both reviewers in consensus, using a standardised extraction form. The following data were collected: first author, year of publication, study design (retrospective or prospective), population size, mean patient age and range, magnetic field strength, breast MRI (i.e., covering the breast and axilla together) or 'dedicated' axillary MRI (i.e., specifically designed for imaging of the axilla), radiofrequency coil used, imaging sequences acquired, contrast agent used, voxel size, imaging analysis, timing of surgery, breast cancer and nodal stage at inclusion, tumour histology, pathological assessment, prevalence of nodal metastases and diagnostic performance parameters such as sensitivity, specificity, NPV, PPV and accuracy.

Both reviewers assessed the quality of the articles using the Quality Assessment of Diagnostic Accuracy Studies 2 (QUADAS-2) checklist [6]. P-values$\leq$0.05 were considered statistically significant. As this is a systematic review, no approval from an institutional review board was required.

Results

A total of 1,372 potentially eligible studies were identified in the primary search. After a first selection 1,220 articles were excluded. Of the remaining 152 studies, duplicates between various searches were removed, leaving 98 studies. During a second selection, abstracts of the remaining 98 studies were read and in- and exclusion criteria were applied, leaving 15 studies to be reviewed. One additional study was found in the references of an included article, and after applying the in- and exclusion criteria, it was included in this review. Therefore, a total of 16 articles were selected for this systematic review [7–22]. The search and selection processes are summarised in Fig. 1.

Publication characteristics

Twelve of the 16 included studies (75 %) had a prospective study design [9–11, 13–19, 21, 22]. The included studies contained a total of 1,591 patients (mean 99 per study, range 18–505). Patient age ranged from 43 to 62 years. Only three articles reported the exact time frame between MRI and surgery (within a mean of 6.7 days, range 1–14 days) [18, 19, 22].

Technical MRI details

In all but one study a 1.5-T MRI was used; in the remaining study both a 1.5- and a 3.0-T MRI system was used [12]. Unenhanced T1w or T2*w imaging was used in three studies [10, 14, 16], seven studies used dynamic contrast-enhanced T1w imaging sequences [7, 9, 11, 12, 17, 20, 21], six studies used diffusion-weighted imaging (DWI) [8–10, 13, 15, 19]

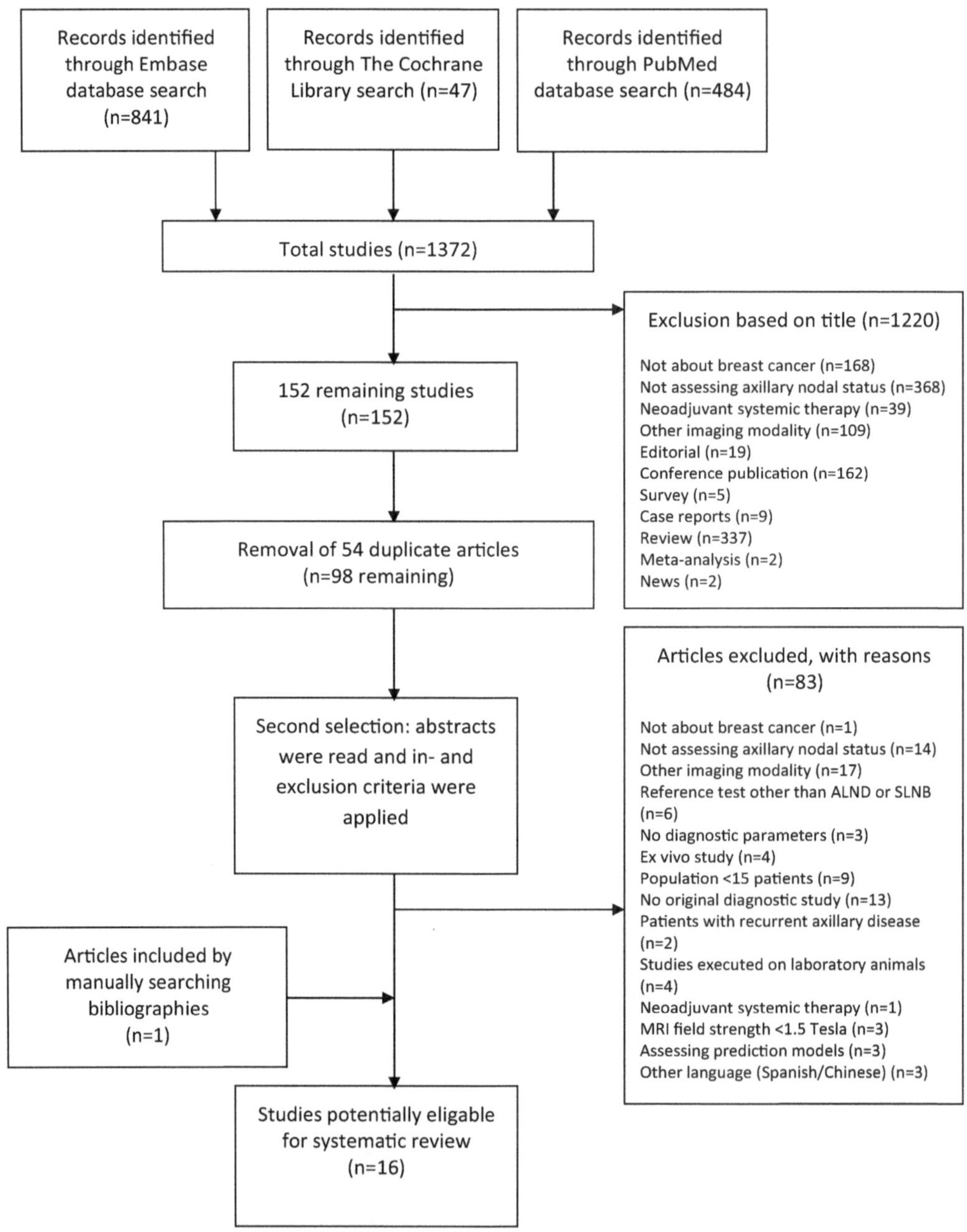

Fig. 1 Flowchart of study selection process according to the Preferred Reporting Items for Systematic Reviews and Meta-Analyses (PRISMA)

and two studies used ultrasmall superparamagnetic iron oxide (USPIO) enhanced T2*w imaging sequences [18, 22]. Only 5 studies used a protocol dedicated to the axilla [11, 14, 16, 18, 22]; the other 11 used a coil covering both the breast and axilla [7–10, 12, 13, 15, 17, 19–21]. Intravenous contrast administration was used in 12 studies; agents used were gadodiamide [11, 21], gadobenate dimeglumine [7–9, 20], gadoterate meglumine [19], gadobutrol [12] and USPIO ferumoxtran-10 [18, 22]. In two studies, the type of contrast was not reported[15, 17]. Criteria for distinguishing positive from negative nodes varied to a large extent; size, short/long axis ratio, lymph nodes >4 mm, short axis diameter >5 or >10 mm, shape, irregular margins, lobulated margins, presence of fatty hilum, cortical thickening, cortical thickness >3 mm, asymmetric cortex, unclear margins, perinodular oedema, matting, anatomical location of the lymph node, signal intensity time curves, heterogeneous uptake of USPIO, lack of USPIO uptake, T2* values, high signal intensity on DWI, early stage enhancement, apparent diffusion coefficient (ADC) values, visual inspection of DWI and ADC and detectability on DWI.

Reference test

Eight studies reported the method of their pathologic analysis of the lymph nodes [7, 9, 12, 14, 16, 18, 19, 22], which consisted of sectioning of the long or short axis or both, sectioning of parallel slices of 2–4 mm thickness, H&E staining, conventional microscopic examination, the position of the lymph nodes, examination of the residual fatty tissue to detect any small lymph nodes and immunohistochemical assay. Five studies did not further specify the used pathologic examination ("histopathological examination", "pathologically confirmed with SLNB or ALND", "pathology was reviewed", "analysed and examined by pathologist" and "histopathologic evaluation") [10, 11, 13, 20, 21], and three studies did not report anything about the used analysis [8, 15, 17].

Pooling of the acquired data in meta-analyses was averted because of the very large heterogeneity of breast cancer stage and subtypes, as well as imaging techniques and pathological assessments used. Instead, descriptive statistics were used. Detailed information of the selected studies is presented in Tables 1 and 2.

Quality of included studies

Quality assessment of the included studies is summarised in Table 3. A significant risk of bias was observed in three included studies [9, 15, 17]. The following items scored poorly or unclear overall: the patient selection, conduct or interpretation of the index test, conduct or the interpretation of the reference standard, and flow and timing of the study.

Diagnostic performance of MRI in axillary lymph node staging: Dedicated to the axilla versus covering the breast and axilla

Of the five studies that used a dedicated axillary coil, the three studies with T1w, T2w or dynamic contrast-enhanced (DCE) imaging sequences had a median sensitivity of 88.4 % (range 79–94.6 %) and NPV of 94.7 % (range 87–95 %) [11, 14, 16]. Two studies using T2*w imaging sequences with USPIO, had a lower median sensitivity (83.0 %; range 73.0–86.4 %), but a slightly higher NPV (95.9 %; range 78.0–98.0 %) compared to the previously mentioned three studies [18, 22]. Overall, the median sensitivity of the five studies together was 84.7 % (range 73–94.6 %) with an NPV of 95.0 % (range 78.0–98.0 %).

A coil covering both the breast and axilla was used in 11 studies [7–10, 12, 13, 15, 17, 19–21], which were divided in two groups that used different imaging sequences. For the studies using T1w, T2w or DCE, median sensitivity was 60.0 % (range 33.3–97.0 %) with an NPV of 80.0 % (range 1.9–99.5 %). For the studies using DWI, median sensitivity was 84.2 % (range 53.8–97.0 %) with an NPV of 90.6 % (range 77.8–99.4 %) [7–10, 12, 13, 15, 17, 19–21]. Overall sensitivity and NPV were 82.0 % (range 33.3–97.0 %) and 82.6 % (range 1.9–95.7 %), respectively. More detailed study results for articles comparing a dedicated axillary coil versus a breast and axillary coil are summarised in Table 4.

Diagnostic performance of MRI in axillary lymph node staging: Studies using T1w/T2w, DCE, DWI and T2*w USPIO imaging sequences

Seven studies using dynamic, contrast-enhanced MR imaging reported a median sensitivity of 60.0 % (range 33.3–97.0 %) and NPV of 80.0 % (range 1.9–99.5 %) [7, 9, 11, 12, 17, 20, 21]. The remaining three imaging sequences reported a more comparable median sensitivity and NPV of 88.4 % (range 79.0–94.6 %) and 94.7 % (range 87.0–95.0 %) for non-enhanced T1w/T2w, 84.2 % (range 53.8–97.0 %) and 90.6 % (range 77.8–99.4 %) for DWI and 83.0 % (range 73.0–86.4 %) and 95.9 % (range 78.0–98.0 %) for T2*w USPIO [8–10, 13–16, 18, 19, 22]. More detailed results for different imaging sequences are summarised in Table 5.

To summarise, the most promising results seem to be achievable when using non-enhanced T1w/T2w and USPIO-enhanced T2*w sequences in combination with a dedicated axillary protocol, sensitivity 84.7 % and NPV 95.0 %.

Discussion

Recent studies have shown that every single axillary metastasis may not require surgery. For example, Giuliano et al. (2011) showed in the ACOSOG Z011 trial that the 5-year overall

Table 1 Study characteristics and MRI technical details

Technical MRI details									
Author	Year	Study design	Field strength	Dedicated vs. covering*	Coil	Imaging sequences	Contrast used	Voxel size	Image analysis
Yoshimura et al.	1999	P	1.5 T	Dedicated	3-Inch circular SC	T1w	None	1.3×0.6×3.0 mm3	Short and long axis ratio and morphology
Kvistad et al.	2000	P	1.5 T	Dedicated	BC and extension to axilla	T1w, dynamic T1w	Gadodiamide	2.0×1.0×4.0 mm3	Normal diameter 2–3 mm, signal intensity time curves, morphology
Michel et al.	2002	P	1.5 T	Dedicated	Cardiac SC	T1w, T2w, T2*w	Ferumoxtran-10	T1w 0.9×0.9×3.5, T2w 0.4×0.4 ×3.5, T2*w 0.9×0.9×2.0 mm3	Size, shape, long-shirt axis ratio, USPIO uptake patterns
Harada et al.	2007	P	1.5 T	Dedicated	Cardiac surface coil	T1w, T2*w, dynamic T2*w	Ferumoxtran-10	0.63×1.25×0.5 mm3	Pre contrast: short axis >5 or >10 mm, replacement fatty hilum, irregular margins. USPIO: heterogeneous uptake or lack of uptake
Orguc et al.	2012	P	1.5 T	Breast and axilla	Not reported	T2w, dynamic T1w	Not reported	Not reported	Size, SI time curves
Fornasa et al.	2012	P	1.5 T	Breast and axilla	4-Channel phased array coil	T1w, T2w, dynamic T1w, DWI (b-value 0/800)	Gadoterate meglumine	T2w 1.3×1.3×4.0; T1w 1.1×1.3 ×4.0; dynamic T1w 1.4×1.4 ×1.8; DWI 5.3 ×5.3×4.0 mm3	Lymph node area, ADC
He et al.	2012	P	1.5 T	Breast and axilla	8-Channel BC	T1w, dynamic T1w, T2w, DWI (b-value 0/500/800)	Gadopente-tate dimeglumine	Dynamic T1w 1.1 ×1.1×2 mm3; DWI 2.7×2.7×4 mm3; T1w not reported (only ST: 5 mm)	SI time curve, shape, margin, diameter, long/short axis ratio, node anatomical location, ADC values, high SI on DWI, early stage enhancement
Scaranelo et al.	2012	P	1.5 T	Breast and axilla	8-Channel BC	T1w, T2w, DWI (b-value 0/50/300/ 700/1000)	None	T1 0.7×0.9×1.2 mm3; (T2 not reported; DWI only ST: 4 mm)	Shape, presence of fatty hilum, cortex irregular, lobulated margins, visual inspection of DWI and ADC
Hwang et al.	2013	R	1.5 T	Breast and axilla	4-Channel BC	T1w, T2w, DWI (b-value 750/1000), Dynamic T1w	Gadopente-tate dimeglumine	Not reported (only ST: T1w 3.4, T2w 2.6, DWI 3.4, Dynamic T1w 2.6 mm)	Cortical thickening, irregular or round shape, loss of fatty hilum
Luo et al.	2013	P	1.5 T	Breast and axilla	8-Channel BC	T1w, T2w, DWI	None	T1w 1.0×0.7×1.0; T2w 1.1×1.1×4.03; DWI 1.0×0.7 ×6.0 mm3	Lymph nodes >4 mm, ADC values

Table 1 (continued)

Technical MRI details

Author	Year	Study design	Field strength	Dedicated vs. covering*	Coil	Imaging sequences	Contrast used	Voxel size	Image analysis
Kamitani et al.	2013	R	1.5 T	Breast and axilla	Body coil	T1w, dynamic T1w, T2w, DWI			
(b-Value 0/1000)	Gadopente-tate dimeglumine	T1w 0.93×0.93 ×4.0 mm3; DWI 2.8×4.1 ×5.0 mm3 (T2w not reported)	Short axis, detectability on DWI						
Basara et al.	2013	P	1.5 T	Breast and axilla	8-Channel BC	CE-T1w, T2w, DWI			
(b-Value 0/600)	Not reported	DWI: 0.2×0.2×5.0 mm3; other sequences not reported	Size, ADC						
Hieken et al.	2013	R	1.5 T	Breast and axilla	BC	Dynamic T1w	Gadobenate dimeglumine	Not reported	Cortical thickness >3 mm, asymmetric cortex, shape, unclear margins, perinodular oedema, loss or displacement of hilum, matting
Abe et al.	2013	P	1.5 T	Breast and axilla	BC	T2w, dynamic T1w	Gadodiamide	1.0×1.0 mm2, ST not reported	Diffuse and asymmetrical cortical thickening, loss of hilum
Li et al.	2014	P	3.0 T	Dedicated	12-Channel body coil	T1w, T2w, T2*w	None	0.8×0.8×3.0 mm3	T2* values
An et al.	2014	R	1.5 or 3.0 T	Breast and axilla	BC	T2w, T1w, dynamic T1w	Gadobutrol	Both 1.5T and 3.0T; T2w ST 3 mm, dynamic unenhanced and CE T1w FOV 320×320, ST 3 mm	Loss of fatty hilum, cortex thickness of >3 mm, irregular or round shape on T2w

Table 2 Patient characteristics

Author	LN imaging analysis	Time to surgery (days)	*n*	Prevalence N+	Mean age in years (range)	T-stage at diag-nosis	Histologic type	Pathologic analysis
Yoshimura et al.	N-N	"Preoperative MRI", n.o.s.	202	40.0 %	55 (30–86)	T1-T3	PT, ST, scirrhous, other	Sectioned long-axis
Kvistad et al.	P-P	"Before surgery",n.o.s	65	37.0 %	59.4 (38–79)	T1-T4	IDC, ILC, MC, tubular, adenocarcinoma	Histopathological examination n.o.s.
Michel et al.	P-P and N-N	2 days (range 1–6 days)	18	61.1 %	53 (22–76)	T1-T4	NR	LN regarded as positive when tumour cells were present at light microscopy, independent from immunohistochemical staining results.
Harada et al.	N-N	Mean 1.2 days	33	19.0 %	58 (36–77)	T1-T4	PT, ST, scirrhous, medullary, MC, apocrien, SC, spindle cell	Sectioned long-axis, H&E staining, conventional microscopic examination
Orguc et al.	N-N	NR	155	25.8 %	43 (28–76)	NR	NR	NR
Fornasa et al.	One LN/ALND/ patient	14 days	43	44.2 %	58 (39–78)	NR	IDC, ILC	Position of the LN and long × short axis
He et al.	N-N	"After MRI", n.o.s.	79	12.0 %	44 (20–67)	NR	DCIS, IDC, ILC, lymphoma	Each LN MRI removed, residual fatty tissue examined, LN sliced 4-mm sections, 3-µm-thick slices cut from each section, stained with H&E
Scaranelo et al.	P-P	"After MRI", n.o.s.	61	43.0 %	53 (33–78)	NR	NR	Embedded in paraffin blocks for histopathologic evaluation n.o.s.
Hwang et al.	P-P	"After MRI", n.o.s.	349	26.4 %	51.3 (25–79)	Only T1	IDC, ILC, MC, others	Intraoperative frozen section, H&E staining. Remaining portions SLNB; sectioning and immunohistological assay
Luo et al.	N-N	"Preoperative MRI", n.o.s.	36	57.0 %	53 (30–63)	T1-T3	DCIS, IDC, ILC, other	Analysed and examined by pathologist n.o.s.
Kamitani et al.	P-P and N-N	NR	108	23.6 %	54.9 (34–84)	Tis-T3	DCIS, IDC,ILC, MC, metaplastic	NR
Basara et al.	P-P and N-N	NR	110	24.0 %	Benign 47 (19–73); malignant 43 (29–70)	NR	IDC, ILC, IDC+ILC, IDC +MC, IDC+pleomorphic, medullary, malignant phyllodes	NR
Hieken et al.	P-P and N-N	'Preoperative MRI", n.o.s.	505	30.1 % with N0i+, 27.3 % without N0i+	62 (24–91)	T1-T4	IDC, ILC, mixed mammary carcinoma, other	Pathology was reviewed and the presence and extent of axillary nodal disease was verified n.o.s.
Abe et al.	P-P	NR	50	32.0 %	59.9 (33–83)	T1-T3	IDC, ILC	Pathologically confirmed with SLNB or ALND n.o.s.
Li et al.	N-N	NR	35	42.0 %	NR (30–58)	T1-T2	IDC, ILC, tubular	Parallel slices 2–3 mm thickness and stained with H&E
An et al.	P-P	'Preoperative MRI", n.o.s.	215	61.4 %	50 (26–83)	T1-T3	IDC, ILC, MC, invasive micro papillary carcinoma, metaplastic, medullary	Sections stained with H&E

P-P patient by patient, *N-N* node by node, *n.o.s.* not otherwise specified, *n* population size, *N+* positive lymph node status, *N0i+* isolated tumour cells, *IDC* invasive ductal carcinoma, *ILC* invasive lobular carcinoma, *DCIS* ductal carcinoma in situ, *PT* papillotubular, *ST* solid tubular *MC* mucinous carcinoma, *SC* squamous carcinoma, *H&E* haematoxylin and eosin, *LN* lymph node, *MRI* magnetic resonance imaging, *SLNB* sentinel lymph node biopsy, *ALND* axillary lymph node dissection, *NR* not reported

Table 3 Presentation for QUADAS-2 results

Study	Risk of bias				Applicability concerns		
	Patient selection	Index test	Reference standard	Flow and timing	Patient selection	Index test	Reference standard
Yoshimura *et al.*, 1999	+	?	?	+	+	+	+
Kvistad *et al.*, 2000	+	+	+	+	+	+	+
Michel *et al.*, 2002	+	+	?	+	+	+	+
Harada *et al.*, 2006	+	+	?	+	+	+	+
Orguc *et al.*, 2012	?	?	?	?	?	?	?
Fornasa *et al.*, 2012	+	?	?	+	+	+	+
He *et al.*, 2012	?	-	-	?	-	+	+
Scaranelo *et al.*, 2012	+	+	+	+	+	+	+
Hwang *et al.*, 2013	+	?	?	+	+	+	+
Luo *et al.*, 2013	?	+	?	?	+	+	+
Kamitani *et al.*, 2013	+	?	+	?	+	+	+
Basara *et al.*, 2013	?	?	-	?	-	+	?
Hieken *et al.*, 2013	+	?	+	?	+	+	+
Abe *et al.*, 2013	?	+	?	?	+	+	+
Li *et al.*, 2014	+	+	+	+	+	+	+
An *et al.*, 2014	+	+	+	+	+	+	+

+ Low risk, - High risk, ? Unclear risk

survival of breast cancer patients with limited sentinel lymph node metastasis, treated with breast conservation and systemic therapy, did not decrease when omitting an ALND [92.5 %; 95 % confidence interval (CI), 90.0–95.1 %] compared to ALND (91.8; 95 % CI, 89.1–94.5 %) [23]. Furthermore, the impact of the true pathological lymph node status on adjuvant systemic treatment recommendations appears limited, thereby eliminating the need to detect every single (extremely small) metastasis [24]. These new insights have created a window of opportunity for many other non-invasive (imaging) modalities to be used in axillary lymph node staging.

In this study we systematically reviewed the available literature on MRI's diagnostic performance for axillary nodal staging in breast cancer patients. We aimed to determine whether MRI could sufficiently exclude axillary lymph node metastasis, thereby replacing SLNB, consequently eliminating the risk of its morbidity. For this purpose, we focused on the sensitivity and NPV, as we are mainly interested in the exclusion of axillary metastases in order to omit SLNB.

Table 4 Diagnostic performance of dedicated vs. standard protocol

First author, year		Sensitivity (95 % CI)	Specificity (95 % CI)	NPV (95 % CI)	PPV (95 % CI)	Accuracy (95 % CI)
Dedicated to axilla						
T1w/T2w/DCE						
Yoshimura et al. 1999		79.0 %	93.0 %	87.0 %	89.0 %	88.0 %
Kvistad et al. 2000		83.0 %	90.0 %	90.0 %	83.0 %	88.0 %
Li et al. 2014		94.6 %	98.5 %	95.0 %	98.2 %	Not reported
	Median	*88.4%*	*93.0%*	*94.7%*	*89.0%*	*86.5%*
	Range	*79–94.6%*	*90–98.5%*	*87–95%*	*83.0–98.2%*	*88.0%*
T2*w USPIO						
Michel et al. 2002	Disease based	82.0 %	100 %	78.0 %	100,0 %	89.0 %
	Two readers lymph node based	73.0–83.0 %	96.0–97.0 %	97.0–98.0 %	71.0–74.0 %	94.0–95.0 %
Harada et al. 2006	Combined study	86.4 %	97.5 %	96.1 %	91.1 %	95.0 %
	Postcontrast alone	84.7 %	96.8 %	95.6 %	88.5 %	94.0 %
	Median	*83.0%*	*97.0%*	*95.9%*	*89.8%*	*94.3%*
	Range	*73.0–86.4%*	*96.0–100%*	*78.0–98.0%*	*71.0–100%*	*89.0–95.0%*
	Median	84.7 %	96.8 %	95.0 %	89.0 %	91.5 %
	Range	*73–94.6%*	*90.0–100.0%*	*78.0–98.0%*	*71.0–100%*	*88.0–95.0%*
Covering breast and axilla						
T1w/T2w/DCE						
Orguc et al. 2012		89.0 %	14.0 %	80.0 %*	21.4 %*	Not reported
He et al. 2012	Overall	33.3–86.5 %	95.2–98.2 %	1.9–16.7 %	66.7–82.6 %	Not reported
	Early stage enhancement rate**	97.0 %	73.5 %	99.5 %*	30.5 %*	Not reported
Scaranelo et al. 2012		88.4 % (76–95)	82.4 % (71–90)	94.7 %*	69.4 %*	85.0 % (77–91)
Hwang et al. 2013		47.8 %	88.7 %	82.6 %	60.2 %	77.9 %
Hieken et al. 2013	N0 with N0i+	54.2 % (46.6–61.6)	78.2 % (73.2–82.5)	75.7 % (70.7–80.1)	57.7 % (49.9–65.2)	69.7 %
	N0 without N0i+	57.2 % (49.1–64.9)	78.2 % (73.2–82.5)	78.9 % (74.0–83.2)	56.2 % (48.2–63.9)	71.3 %
Abe et al. 2013		60.0 %	79.0 %	81.0 %	59.0 %	74.0 %
An et al. 2014		67.5 %	78.0 %	79.2 %	65.9 %	74.0 %
	Median	*60.0%*	*78.6%*	*80.0%*	*59.0%*	*74.0%*
	Range	*33.3–97.0%*	*14.0–98.5%*	*1.9–99.5%*	*21.4–92.6%*	*69.7–85.0%*
DWI						
Fornasa et al. 2012	Cutoff $<1.09\times10^{-3}$ mm²/s	94.7 %	91.7 %	95.7 %	90.0 %	93.0 %
He et al. 2012	Cutoff $<1.35\times10^{-3}$ mm²/s	97.0 %	54.5 %	99.4 %*	20.4 %*	Not reported
Scaranelo et al. 2012	No cutoff value	83.9 % (73–91)	77.0 % (65–86)	90.9 %*	60.5 %*	80.0 % (72–86)
Luo et al. 2013	Cutoff $<0.89\times10^{-3}$ mm²/s	82.2 %	82.4 %	77.8 %	86.1 %	82.3 %
	ADC ratio*** $\leq$1.097	84.4 %	88.2 %	81.1 %	90.5 %	86.1 %

Table 4 (continued)

First author, year		Sensitivity (95 % CI)	Specificity (95 % CI)	NPV (95 % CI)	PPV (95 % CI)	Accuracy (95 % CI)
Kamitani et al. 2013	Cutoff $<1.05\times10^{-3}$ mm^2/s	53.8 %	86.9 %	85.9 %	56.0 %	79.1 %
	Cutoff $<1.22\times10^{-3}$ mm^2/s	75.6 %	71.1 %	90.2 %	54.3 %	Not reported
Basara et al. 2013	Cutoff $<1.49\times10^{-3}$ mm^2/s	95.6 %	30.3 %	95.6 %	30.3 %	Not reported
	Median	*84.2%*	*79.7%*	*90.6%*	*58.3%*	*82.3%*
	Range	*53.8–97.0%*	*30.3–91.7%*	*77.8–99.4%*	*20.4–90.5%*	*79.1–93.0%*
	Median	82.0 %	78.2 %	82.6 %	59.0 %	79.1 %
	Range	*33.3–97.0%*	*14.0–98.5%*	*1.9–95.7%*	*30.3–92.6%*	*69.7–93.0%*

T1w T1 weighted, *T2w* T2 weighted, *T2*w* T2* weighted, *N+* nodal stage positive, *N0* no regional lymph node metastasis, *N0i+* isolated tumour cells, *DCE* dynamic contrast enhanced, *DWI* diffusion-weighted imaging, *T2*w* T2* weighted, *USPIO* ultrasmall superparamagnetic iron oxide, *ADC* apparent diffusion coefficient, *CI* confidence interval

*Calculated parameters, **diagnostic parameter with a combination of the highest senstivity and NPV, ***ADC ratio = ratio of lymph node ADC value to the primary tumour ADC value

Therefore, the NPV should at least be non-inferior to the NPV of SLNB. A recent meta-analysis showed a false-negative rate of 8.61 % (95 % CI: 8.05–9.2 %) of the SLNB [25]. The calculated NPV of the SLNB in a patient group with a prevalence of 40 % of axillary metastasis equals 94.5 %. In our current observation, the most promising results seem to be achievable when using non-enhanced T1w/T2w and USPIO-enhanced T2*w sequences in combination with a dedicated axillary protocol. These protocols turned out to have a sensitivity and NPV of respectively 84.7 and 95.0 %. These results are promising, as the NPV approaches the NPV of SLNB. However, some restraint in the clinical implementation of axillary MRI should be considered because of the study limitations, such as: the heterogeneous study design, overall limited study populations, inclusion of only single-centre studies and lack of 95 % confidence intervals mentioned in studies. To implement axillary MRI in the clinical setting, these promising results should be confirmed in large, multicentre studies and various readers of the examinations. In addition, a protocol that includes non-enhanced T1w/T2w and USPIO-enhanced T2*w sequences in combination with a dedicated axillary protocol need to be considered as they seem to give the most promising results.

In our observations, a dedicated axillary protocol (for example using a surface radiofrequency coil placed on the axilla) was superior to a more standard protocol covering both the breast and axilla in the same field of view. This is only logical, as the use of surface coils and the reduced distance from the axillary to the coil improves signal-to-noise ratios, enabling the use of higher spatial resolutions. More interestingly, DWI has, despite the use of a protocol covering the breast and axilla together, an almost equal sensitivity (84.2 %), but a lower NPV (90.6 %) when compared with studies using a dedicated protocol (84.7 and 95.0 %). Unfortunately, there are no studies that investigated the use of DWI sequences in a dedicated axillary protocol.

However, the clinical implementation of DWI and USPIO-enhanced T2*-weighted imaging might be challenging. Disadvantages of the DWI are high sensitivity to motion artefacts, limited spatial resolution and more pronounced artefacts at higher field strengths. The ADC values used in diffusion-weighted imaging are dependent on scanner and *b*-values. The clinical implementation of USPIO-enhanced imaging is hampered by the necessity of administrating the contrast 24–36 h prior to MRI imaging. Moreover, UPSIO can cause side effects in up to 18 % of the examinations such as rash, pruritus, abdominal and/or lumbar pain, chest pain and an orthostatic reaction[18]. An additional disadvantage of USPIO is that it is not universally available and using USPIO for MR lymphography is 'off-label'. These disadvantages need to be overcome, especially since the NPV approaches the NPV of the SLNB.

Given the evidence from the Z0011 trial, there may be relatively less utility for MRI evaluation of lymph nodal status because a selected number of patients would not necessarily

Table 5 Results of different imaging sequences

First author, year	Prevalence N+%		Sensitivity (95 % CI)	Specificity (95 % CI)	NPV (95 % CI)	PPV (95 % CI)	Accuracy (95 % CI)
Imaging sequences T1w/T2w							
Yoshimura et al. 1999	*40.0%*	T1w	79.0 %	93.0 %	87.0 %	89.0 %	88.0 %
Scaranelo et al. 2012	*43.0%*	T1w	88.4 % (76–95)	82.4 % (71–90)	94.7 %*	69.4 %*	85.0 % (77–91)
Li et al. 2014	*42.0%*	T2*w	94.6 %	98.5 %	95.0 %	98.2 %	Not reported
		Median	*88.4%*	*93.0%*	*94.7%*	*89.0%*	*86.5%*
		Range	*79.0–94.6%*	*82.4–98.5%*	*87.0–95.0%*	*69.4–98.2%*	*85.0–88.0%*
Imaging sequences DCE							
Kvistad et al. 2000	*37.0%*		83.0 %	90.0 %	90.0 %	83.0 %	88.0 %
Orguc et al. 2012	*25.8%*		89.0 %	14.0 %	80.0 %*	21.4 %*	Not reported
He et al. 2012	*12.0%*	Overall	33.3–86.5 %	95.2–98.2 %	1.9–16.7 %	66.7–82.6 %	Not reported
		Early stage enhancement rate**	97.0 %	73.5 %	99.5 %*	30.5 %*	Not reported
Hwang et al. 2013	*26.4%*		47.8 %	88.7 %	82.6 %	60.2 %	77.9 %
Hieken et al. 2013	*30.1%*	N0 with N0i+	54.2 % (46.6–61.6)	78.2 % (73.2–82.5)	75.7 % (70.7–80.1)	57.7 % (49.9–65.2)	69.7 %
	27.3%	N0 without N0i+	57.2 % (49.1–64.9)	78.2 % (73.2–82.5)	78.9 % (74.0–83.2)	56.2 % (48.2–63.9)	71.3 %
Abe et al. 2013	*32.0%*	T1w DCE	60.0 %	79.0 %	81.0 %	59.0 %	74.0 %
An et al. 2014	*61.4%*		67.5 %	78.0 %	79.2 %	65.9 %	74.0 %
		Median	*60.0%*	*78.2%*	*80.0%*	*59.0%*	*74.0%*
		Range	*33.3–97.0%*	*14.0–98.2%*	*1.9–99.5%*	*21.4–83.0%*	*69.7–88.0%*
Imaging sequences DWI							
Fornasa et al. 2012	*44.2%*	Cutoff $<1.09\times10^{-3}$ mm^2/s	94.7 %	91.7 %	95.7 %	90.0 %	93.0 %
He et al. 2012	*12.0%*	Cutoff $<1.35\times10^{-3}$ mm^2/s	97.0 %	54.5 %	99.4 %*	20.4 %*	Not reported
Scaranelo et al. 2012	*43.0%*	No cutoff value	83.9 % (73–91)	77.0 % (65–86)	90.9 %*	60.5 %*	80.0 % (72–86)
Luo et al. 2013	*57.0%*	Cutoff $<0.89\times10^{-3}$ mm^2/s	82.2 %	82.4 %	77.8 %	86.1 %	82.3 %
		ADC ratio*** $\leq$1.097	84.4 %	88.2 %	81.1 %	90.5 %	86.1 %
Kamitani et al. 2013	*23.6%*	Cutoff $<1.05\times10^{-3}$ mm^2/s	53.8 %	86.9 %	85.9 %	56.0 %	79.1 %
		Cutoff $<1.22\times10^{-3}$ mm^2/s	75.6 %	71.1 %	90.2 %	54.3 %	Not reported
Basara et al. 2013	24.0 %	Cutoff $<1.49\times10^{-3}$ mm^2/s	95.6 %	30.3 %	95.6 %	30.3 %	Not reported
		Median	*84.2%*	*79.7%*	*90.6%*	*58.3%*	*82.3%*
		Range	*53.8–97.0%*	*30.3–91.7%*	*77.8–99.4%*	*20.4–90.5%*	*79.1–93.0%*
Imaging sequences T2*w USPIO							
Michel et al. 2002	*61.1%*	Disease based	82.0 %	100 %	78.0 %	100.0 %	89.0 %
		Two readers lymph node based	73.0–83.0 %	96.0–97.0 %	97.0–98.0 %	71.0–74.0 %	94.0–95.0 %
Harada et al. 2006	*19.0%*	Combined study	86.4 %	97.5 %	96.1 %	91.1 %	95.0 %
		Postcontrast	84.7 %	96.8 %	95.6 %	88.5 %	94.0 %
		Median	*83.0%*	*97.0%*	*95.9%*	*89.8%*	*94.3%*
		Range	*73.0–86.4%*	*96.0–100%*	*78.0–98.0%*	*71.0–100%*	*89.0–95.0%*

T1w T1 weighted, *T2w* T2 weighted, *T2*w* T2* weighted, *N+* nodal stage positive, *N0* no regional lymph node metastasis, *N0i+* isolated tumour cells, *DCE* dynamic contrast enhanced, *CI* confidence interval. *DWI* Diffusion-weighted imaging, *T2*w* T2* weighted, *USPIO* ultrasmall superparamagnetic iron oxide, *ADC* apparent diffusion coefficient, *CI* confidence interval

*Calculated parameters

**Diagnostic parameter with a combination of the highest senstivity and NPV

***ADC ratio = ratio of lymph node ADC value to the primary tumour ADC value be managed with ALND. The main gain however is that regional treatment with MRI is based on the true absence or presence of lymph node metastases compared to traditional physical examination and/or ultrasound. Axillary ultrasound was never tested for node-to-node evaluation and is not able to predict 'true' nodal status accurately. In combination with the Z0011 results (in which 27 % of nodal metastases remained) created reluctance among many clinicians to implement these results.

Axillary MRI evaluation with a high NPV could induce omission of the SLNB in case of negative findings, which constitute about 65 % of all breast cancer patients. Axillary MRI with high PPV could result in an SLNB in case of limited nodal metastases. Axillary MRI evaluation with high PPV could further induce two pathways when extended nodal disease is observed: axillary lymph node dissection or neoadjuvant systemic therapy and re-evaluation using MRI after completion of all chemotherapy cycles. All this would result in policy based on the true nodal burden instead of estimating it to the best of our ability using ultrasound and the clinician's opinion regarding the Z0011 trial results.

A subgroup of patients (clinical stage T1-2 and N0 undergoing breast conservative therapy and whole-breast radiation) would not necessarily be managed with ALND: hence the utility of preoperative axillary MRI will depend on whether or not the surgeon has adopted omission of ALND in patients with minimal sentinel node disease. In order to define the importance of MRI evaluation of axillary lymph nodes as a replacement for SLNB, differentiation between minimal and more advanced nodal disease (high nodal disease burden being defined as >3 metastatic nodes in the majority of studies) must be clear. None of the selected papers compared pN status with the number of positive lymph nodes at MRI. Only He et al. mentioned a different diagnostic accuracy for nodes from level I and level III. Future studies should strongly consider the use of node-by-node analyses of the axillary lymph nodes to test whether axillary MRI can replace SLNB.

Previously, other non-invasive techniques that were considered to exclude axillary metastases were axillary physical examination (PE), axillary ultrasound (AUS) and positron emission tomography–computed tomography (PET/CT). However, these methods lack sensitivity and NPV. Sensitivity is 25–35.5 % for PE, 43.5–72.3 % for AUS and 56–62.7 % for PET/CT [12, 26]. The NPV is 81.7 % for PE, 81.6–83.3 % for AUS and 79.1 % for PET/CT [11, 12, 27–29]. Concluding, the diagnostic performance of these techniques is insufficient to exclude lymph node metastases and omit SLNB. At this point, MRI seems to be the most promising non-invasive nodal staging technique with a highest median sensitivity of 84.7 % and NPV of 95.0 %.

Based on the QUADAS-2 tool, there was an overall good quality of studies. Three studies were assessed as studies with a low methodical quality and a high risk of bias. In the study of Orguc et al. (2012), introduction of bias was unclear in all domains: the patient selection, index test, reference test, flow and timing [17]. A high risk of bias of the reference test was observed in the studies of He et al. (2012) and Basara et al. (2013). In the study of He et al. (2012), a physician who was in charge of labelling the lymph node samples took part in every MRI examination and in the surgery of every enrolled patient [9]. Basara et al. (2013) used histopathological examination as a reference test for malignant lymph nodes and clinical examination with imaging findings as reference for benign lymph nodes. Furthermore, Basara et al. (2013) and He et al. (2012) both included patients with various indications for a conventional breast MRI, not just patients with breast cancer. This increased our concerns about whether or not this study population is applicable to our research population.

Along with the more limited methodological quality of the three studies mentioned above, we noticed a great variety in the outcome of these studies compared to other (methodologically stronger) articles. Even when these three studies were excluded, the final conclusions of our review did not change.

Study limitations

First, the included studies were very heterogeneous in their study designs. They used different imaging sequences (T1w, T2w, DCE, DWI and T2*w), different radiofrequency coils and different contrast agents (gadolinium-based and USPIO). This stopped us from pooling data and resulted in a more descriptive analysis of the results.

Second, publication and selection bias is a study limitation in every systematic review. The tendency to not publish studies with negative results might lead to an overestimation of our results. By using the PRISMA approach in combination with an extensive search, selection and inclusion, we think that the influence of publication and selection bias is limited.

Conclusion and outlook

In summary, the diagnostic performance of MRI for assessing axillary nodal staging in breast cancer patients is promising, as the NPV approaches the NPV of the SLNB.

However, current observations are based on (single-centre) studies with heterogeneous study designs and limited populations. Thus, these finding should be interpreted with these limitations in mind.

Based on the current findings, most desirable protocol would be a dedicated axillary coil in combination with T1-weighted, T2-weighted and T2*-weighted USPIO. Additionally, DWI combined with a dedicated coil might create the opportunity to achieve even higher diagnostic values compared to the use of a protocol covering the breast and axilla. However, there are no studies that used one of these specific protocols. Future studies should consider the use of these protocols to see whether the diagnostic performance can be increased by this approach.

In order to further investigate the clinical use of axillary MRI for staging of breast cancer patients, these studies should be performed in a multicentre study comprising a large number of patients, evaluated by multiple radiologists.

References

1. DiSipio T, Rye S, Newman B, Hayes S (2013) Incidence of unilateral arm lymphoedema after breast cancer: a systematic review and meta-analysis. Lancet Oncol 14:500–515
2. Ashikaga T, Krag DN, Land SR, Julian TB, Anderson SJ, Brown AM et al (2010) Morbidity results from the NSABP B-32 trial comparing sentinel lymph node dissection versus axillary dissection. J Surg Oncol 102:111–118
3. Liu CQ, Guo Y, Shi JY, Sheng Y (2009) Late morbidity associated with a tumour-negative sentinel lymph node biopsy in primary breast cancer patients: a systematic review. Eur J Cancer 45:1560–1568
4. Maaskant-Braat AJ, Van de Poll-Franse LV, Voogd AC, Coebergh JW, Roumen RM, Nolthenius-Puylaert MC et al (2011) Sentinel node micrometastases in breast cancer do not affect prognosis: a population-based study. Breast Cancer Res Treat 127:195–203
5. Moher D, Liberati A, Altman DG, PRISMA Group (2009) Preferred reporting items for systematic reviews and meta-analyses: the PRIS MA Statement. Open Med 3:e123–130
6. Whiting PF, Rutjes AW, Westwood ME, Mallett S, Deeks JJ, Reitsma JB et al (2011) QUADAS-2: a revised tool for the quality assessment of diagnostic accuracy studies. Ann Intern Med 155:529–536
7. Hwang SO, Lee SW, Kim HJ, Kim WW, Park HY, Jung JH (2013) The comparative study of ultrasonography, contrast-enhanced MRI, and (18)F-FDG PET/CT for detecting axillary lymph node metastasis in T1 breast cancer. J Breast Cancer 16:315–321
8. Kamitani T, Hatakenaka M, Yabuuchi H, Matsuo Y, Fujita N, Jinnouchi M et al (2013) Detection of axillary node metastasis using diffusion-weighted MRI in breast cancer. Clin Imaging 37:56–61
9. He N, Xie C, Wei W, Pan C, Wang W, Lv N et al (2012) A new, preoperative, MRI-based scoring system for diagnosing malignant axillary lymph nodes in women evaluated for breast cancer. Eur J Radiol 81:2602–2612
10. Scaranelo AM, Eiada R, Jacks LM, Kulkarni SR, Crystal P (2012) Accuracy of unenhanced MR imaging in the detection of axillary lymph node metastasis: study of reproducibility and reliability. Radiology 262:425–434
11. Kvistad KA, Rydland J, Smethurst HB, Lundgren S, Fjosne HE, Haraldseth O (2000) Axillary lymph node metastases in breast cancer: preoperative detection with dynamic contrast-enhanced MRI. Eur Radiol 10:1464–1471
12. An YS, Lee DH, Yoon JK, Lee SJ, Kim TH, Kang DK et al (2013) Diagnostic performance of 18F-FDG PET/CT, ultrasonography and MRI. Detection of axillary lymph node metastasis in breast cancer patients. Nuklearmedizin 53:89–94
13. Luo N, Su D, Jin G, Liu L, Zhu X, Xie D et al (2013) Apparent diffusion coefficient ratio between axillary lymph node with primary tumor to detect nodal metastasis in breast cancer patients. J Magn Reson Imaging 38:824–828
14. Yoshimura G, Sakurai T, Oura S, Suzuma T, Tamaki T, Umemura T et al (1999) Evaluation of axillary lymph node status in breast cancer with MRI. Breast Cancer 6:249–258
15. Basara I, Orguc S, Coskun T (2013) The role of diffusion weighted imaging in the assesment of axillary lymph nodes. J Breast Health 9: 76–81
16. Li C, Meng S, Yang X, Wang J, Hu J (2014) The value of T2* in differentiating metastatic from benign axillary lymph nodes in patients with breast cancer–a preliminary in vivo study. PLoS One 9: e84038
17. Orguc S, Basara I, Pekindil G, Coskun T (2012) Contribution of kinetic characteristics of axillary lymph nodes to the diagnosis in breast magnetic resonance imaging. Balkan Med J 29:285–289
18. Michel SC, Keller TM, Fröhlich JM, Fink D, Caduff R, Seifert B et al (2002) Preoperative breast cancer staging: MR imaging of the axilla with ultrasmall superparamagnetic iron oxide enhancement. Radiology 225:527–536
19. Fornasa F, Nesoti MV, Bovo C, Bonavina MG (2012) Diffusion-weighted magnetic resonance imaging in the characterization of axillary lymph nodes in patients with breast cancer. J Magn Reson Imaging 36:858–864
20. Hieken TJ, Trull BC, Boughley JC, Jones KN, Reynolds CA, Shah SS et al (2013) Preoperative axillary imaging with percutaneous lymph node biopsy is valuable in the contemporary management of patients with breast cancer. Surgery 154:831–838
21. Abe H, Schacht D, Kulkami K, Shimauchi A, Yamaguchi K, Sennett CA et al (2013) Accuracy of axillary lymph node staging in breast cancer patients: an observer-performance study comparison of MRI and ultrasound. Acad Radiol 20:1399–1404
22. Harada T, Tanigawa N, Matsuki M, Nohara T, Narabayashi I (2007) Evaluation of lymph node metastases of breast cancer using ultra-small superparamagnetic iron oxide-enhanced magnetic resonance imaging. Eur J Radiol 63:401–407
23. Giuliano AE, Hunt KK, Ballman KV, Beitsch PD, Whitworth PW, Blumencranz PW et al (2011) Axillary dissection vs no axillary dissection in women with invasive breast cancer and sentinel node metastasis: a randomized clinical trial. JAMA 305:569–575
24. Van Roozendaal LM, Schipper RJ, Van de Vijver KK, Haekens CM, Lobbes MB, Tjan-Heijnen VC et al (2014) The impact of the pathological lymph node status on adjuvant systemic treatment recommendations in clinically node negative breast cancer patients. Breast Cancer Res Treat 143:469–476
25. Pesek S, Ashikaga T, Krag LE, Krag D (2012) The false-negative rate of sentinel node biopsy in patients with breast cancer: a meta-analysis. World J Surg 36:2239–2251
26. Cooper KL, Meng Y, Harnan S, Ward SE, Fitzgerald P, Papaioannou D et al (2011) Positron emission tomography (PET) and magnetic resonance imaging (MRI) for the assessment of axillary lymph node metastases in early breast cancer: systematic review and economic evaluation. Health Technol Assess 15:iii–iv, 1–134
27. Valente SA, Levine GM, Silverstein MJ, Rayhanabad JA, Weng-Grumley JG, Ji L et al (2012) Accuracy of predicting axillary lymph node positivity by physical examination, mammography, ultrasonography, and magnetic resonance imaging. Ann Surg Oncol 19:1825–1830
28. Schipper RJ, Van Roozendaal LM, De Vries B, Pijnappel RM, Beets-Tan RG, Lobbes MB et al (2013) Axillary ultrasound for preoperative nodal staging in breast cancer patients: is it of added value? Breast 22: 1108–1113
29. Houssami N, Ciatto S, Macaskill P, Lord SJ, Warren RM, Dixon JM et al (2008) Accuracy and surgical impact of magnetic resonance imaging in breast cancer staging: systematic review and meta-analysis in detection of multifocal and multicentric cancer. J Clin Oncol 26:3248–3258

11

MDCT of blunt renal trauma: imaging findings and therapeutic implications

M. Bonatti · F. Lombardo · N. Vezzali · G. Zamboni · F. Ferro · P. Pernter · A. Pycha · G. Bonatti

Abstract

Objectives To show the wide spectrum of computed tomography (CT) findings in blunt renal trauma and to correlate them with consequent therapeutic implications.

Methods This article is the result of a literature review and our personal experience in a level II trauma centre. Here we describe, discuss and illustrate the possible CT findings in blunt renal trauma, and we correlate them with the American Association for the Surgery of Trauma (AAST) classification and their therapeutic implications.

Results CT findings following blunt renal trauma can be grouped into 15 main categories, 12 of them directly correlated with the AAST classification and 3 of them not mentioned in it. Non-operative management, which includes the "watchful waiting" approach, endourological treatments and endovascular treatments, is nowadays widely adopted in blunt renal trauma, and surgery is limited to haemodynamically unstable patients and a minority of haemodynamically stable patients.

Conclusions The interpretation of CT findings in blunt renal trauma may be improved and made faster by the knowledge of their therapeutic consequences.

M. Bonatti (✉) · N. Vezzali · F. Ferro · P. Pernter · G. Bonatti
Department of Radiology, Bolzano Central Hospital, 5 Boehler St., 39100 Bolzano, Italy
e-mail: matteobonatti@hotmail.com

F. Lombardo · G. Zamboni
Department of Radiology, University of Verona, Piazzale L.A. Scuro 10, 37134 Verona, Italy

A. Pycha
Department of Urology, Bolzano Central Hospital, 5 Boehler St., 39100 Bolzano, Italy

Teaching Points

- *The majority of blunt renal injuries do not require surgical treatment.*
- *CT findings in blunt renal injury must be evaluated considering their therapeutic consequences.*
- *Some CT findings in blunt renal trauma are not included in the AAST classification.*

Keywords Acute renal injury · Blunt injury · Computed tomography · Kidney · Trauma

Abbreviations

AAST	American Association for the Surgery of Trauma
NOM	Non-operative management
CT	Computed tomography
MDCT	Multidetector computed tomography
CEUS	Contrast-enhanced ultrasound
MPR	Multiplanar reconstruction
MIP	Maximum intensity projection
VR	Volume rendering
HU	Hounsfield units

Introduction

Renal injuries represent a relatively common event, involving 8–10 % of the patients admitted to an emergency department because of abdominal trauma, and the incidence is increasing parallel to the increase in motor-vehicle accidents [1–4]. In 80–95 % of the cases renal injuries occur in the setting of blunt trauma, as a result of a direct trauma to the back, flank, lower thorax or upper abdomen or of a rapid deceleration, whereas penetrating traumas are responsible for the remaining 5–20 % [3, 5–7]. Renal trauma may occur in isolation or in association with other visceral injuries, with the majority of isolated renal injuries represented by low-grade lesions [8–10].

Although gross haematuria is the typical presenting symptom of renal injury, it may be absent in about 5 % of renal injuries, and its presence is not directly correlated with injury severity: for example, haematuria is typically absent in vascular pedicle injuries and ureteral-pelvic injuries [11, 12].

According to the American Association for the Surgery of Trauma (AAST), on the basis of surgical findings renal injuries can be subdivided into five main categories (Table 1), with a progressively poorer prognosis [13]. The suggested treatment options, according to the AAST injury grade, in haemodynamically stable patients affected by renal injuries are reported in Table 2. In the past decades, the indications for surgical treatment of renal trauma have progressively decreased with a consequent drastic reduction in nephrectomy rates, and, nowadays, non-operative management (NOM), which includes the simple watchful waiting ("wait-and-see") strategy, endovascular treatments and endourological treatments, can be considered the most appropriate first line approach for about 90–95 % of renal injuries [14–20]. On the other hand, renal exploration remains mandatory in every case of haemodynamic instability following renal trauma and if a pulsatile or expanding retroperitoneal haematoma is identified during exploratory laparotomy performed for other abdominal injuries.

Indications for renal imaging and imaging modalities

In case of blunt thoraco-abdominal trauma, a clear distinction must be made between haemodynamically unstable and haemodynamically stable or stabilised patients; indeed, the former must immediately undergo surgical exploration in order to try to improve their outcome, whereas the latter should undergo imaging studies in order to better assess the presence of visceral injuries and guide treatment. Although some controversies still exist, in haemodynamically stable (or stabilised) patients who have suffered blunt thoracic and/or abdominal trauma, absolute indications for imaging in the suspicion of renal injuries are gross haematuria, microscopic haematuria associated with hypotension, suspicion of major injuries to other viscera and trauma dynamics strongly associated with renal injury (i.e., rapid deceleration, fall from great height and direct contusion to the flank) [3, 5].

Table 1 American Association for the Surgery of Trauma (AAST) classification of renal trauma

Grade	Type	Description
I	Parenchyma Haematoma	Microscopic or gross haematuria with normal urologic studies (contusion) Non-expanding subcapsular haematoma
II	Parenchyma Haematoma	Laceration <1 cm in depth, without collecting system rupture Non-expanding perirenal haematoma confined to retroperitoneum
III	Parenchyma	Laceration >1 cm in depth without collecting system rupture
IV	Parenchyma Vascular	Laceration with collecting system rupture Main renal artery/vein injury with contained haemorrhage
V	Parenchyma Vascular	Shattered kidney Avulsion of renal hilum that devascularises kidney

Table 2 Treatment options in haemodynamically stable patients affected by renal injury (according to the AAST classification)

Grade	Type	Treatment
I-III	Every	NOM wait and see
IV	Parenchyma Vascular	NOM endourological Debated, surgical vs. NOM interventional radiological
V	Parenchyma Vascular	Debated, NOM is increasingly adopted Surgical. NOM endourological in case of partial pielo-uretheral lacerations
???	Vascular	NOM interventional radiological

NOM non-operative management, ??? = lesions not included in the AAST classification

Several different imaging techniques have been considered as the initial imaging tool in the suspicion of renal injury in haemodynamically stable patients; nowadays, however, thanks to its wide availability, reproducibility, scan speed and high spatial resolution, contrast-enhanced multidetector computed tomography (MDCT) is considered the gold standard imaging modality in case of suspicion of renal injury and has completely replaced intravenous urography for this purpose [3, 5, 21–24]. The great advantage of MDCT is its ability to assess, in an extremely rapid scanning time, the presence of lesions of the parenchyma, vessels and collecting system and of injuries to other abdominal organs.

MDCT of renal trauma: technique and protocols

Multidetector CT systems are nowadays ubiquitously available in trauma centres and represent the minimum requirement for emergency renal imaging. The availability of modern scanners with a high number of detector rows (16 or more) enables shortening acquisition times, therefore reducing the possibility of motion artefacts and increasing image quality.

A correct positioning of the patient on the CT table represents a fundamental prerequisite for performing high-quality MDCT studies. Whenever possible, the patient should lay supine on the table, with the arms bent over the head in order to prevent beam-hardening artefacts; if that position cannot be obtained, the patient's arms should be placed flexed on a large pillow ventrally to the patient's chest [25]. Moreover, all the medical devices that are not strictly necessary should be removed from the scan area.

The MDCT scanning protocol in the setting of suspected renal trauma should always be always tailored according to the clinical conditions of the patient. Most authors sustain that a non-enhanced acquisition should always be performed in order to detect intraparenchymal, subcapsular or perinephric haematomas, which will appear as slightly hyperattenuating areas or collections during this phase, whereas they might be barely recognisable on post-contrast images [26–28]. According to our experience, however, the performance of native scans is not necessary in the setting of renal trauma for two reasons: first, the large majority of the above-mentioned lesions are clearly recognisable also on post-contrast images; second, those lesions that might eventually be missed (i.e., small intraparenchymal or subcapsular haematomas) do not have any therapeutic consequences. In any case, when acquiring post-contrast images using a dual-energy technique, virtual non-enhanced images may be retrospectively generated from post-contrast ones by means of commercially available software and show similar accuracy to true non-contrast ones for the detection of haematomas [29].

On the other hand, post-contrast acquisitions must always be performed in case of suspicion of renal injuries. About 1.7–1.5 ml/kg of 350–370 mgI/ml iodinated contrast material must be administered using a flow rate of at least 3.5 ml/s, followed by a 50-ml saline flush. Contrast-enhanced scans should be acquired cranio-caudally, with thin collimation (0.625 mm). Multi-planar reformats (MPR), maximum intensity projection (MIP) and volume-rendering (VR) reconstructions represent extremely useful tools for imaging interpretation. According to the wide variability of circulatory conditions in trauma patients, post-contrast scans should be always performed using a bolus-tracking technique. A late arterial/corticomedullary phase acquisition should be acquired with a 15-s delay from a 100-HU peak aortic enhancement when using a bolus-tracking technique or with a 30-s fixed delay after injection if bolus-tracking is not available; this phase is mandatory for recognising arterial vascular lesions (i.e., renal artery avulsion or thrombosis, pseudoaneurysms and artero-venous fistulae) and for detecting active arterial contrast material extravasation; moreover, it enables to accurately depict the arterial vascular anatomy and eventual variants. The portal-venous or nephrographic phase, acquired 70-80 s after the start of contrast material injection, represents the best phase for detecting parenchymal lesions (i.e., lacerations and segmental infarctions), venous vascular lesions (i.e., avulsion or thrombosis of the renal vein) and haematomas and should be always performed in case of suspicion of renal injury; moreover, it represents a useful aid for assessing the relevance of an active arterial contrast material extravasation and enables accurately ruling out injuries to other parenchymatous abdominal organs. The decision to acquire a delayed excretory scan is strictly dependent on the patient's clinical conditions and the findings in the previous phases. The timing of the delayed acquisition depends on renal function and may vary from 5 to 15 or more minutes; 8 min may represent a good compromise in the majority of the cases. Delayed acquisitions are fundamental for the detection of collecting system injuries, by showing hyperdense urine extravasation, and may also help in the differential diagnosis between renal contusion and infarction [3].

MDCT findings and therapeutic consequences

MDCT can generate a wide spectrum of findings in renal trauma and the majority of these can be easily categorised into the above-mentioned five AAST grades; moreover, MDCT may also show some findings that are not mentioned in the AAST classification, the latter being based on the kidney appearance at surgery. The AAST classification must be kept in mind when reporting renal injuries, particularly because of its prognostic implications; in any case, subtle differences in AAST grade do often not have practical consequences for patient management. In the following paragraphs we will describe the possible MDCT findings in renal trauma grouped by their therapeutical management and not simply by the AAST grading scale.

Non-operative management: "wait-and-see"

- *Parenchymal contusion (AAST grade I)*. Parenchymal contusions (Fig. 1a–b) appear as ill-defined, irregularly shaped areas of decreased and delayed contrast enhancement within the renal parenchyma. On non-enhanced images their density varies according to the time elapsed from the traumatic event, the patient's haematocrit and the coagulation status: typically they appear isoattenuating to the adjacent cortex, but hyperattenuation may also be observed if blood clots are present. The corticomedullary phase is not useful for identifying renal contusions because of the physiological heterogeneity of parenchymal enhancement. On the other hand, in the majority of the cases renal contusions are clearly recognisable during the nephrographic phase in which they usually appear slightly hypodense in comparison to the adjacent parenchyma; however, a substantial isodensity might be found if blood clots are present. On delayed acquisitions, contusions show persistent contrast retention, and this characteristic may be helpful for differentiating them from renal infarctions (Fig. 1c–d) that remain hypodense. A simple "wait-and-see" management is indicated in case of renal

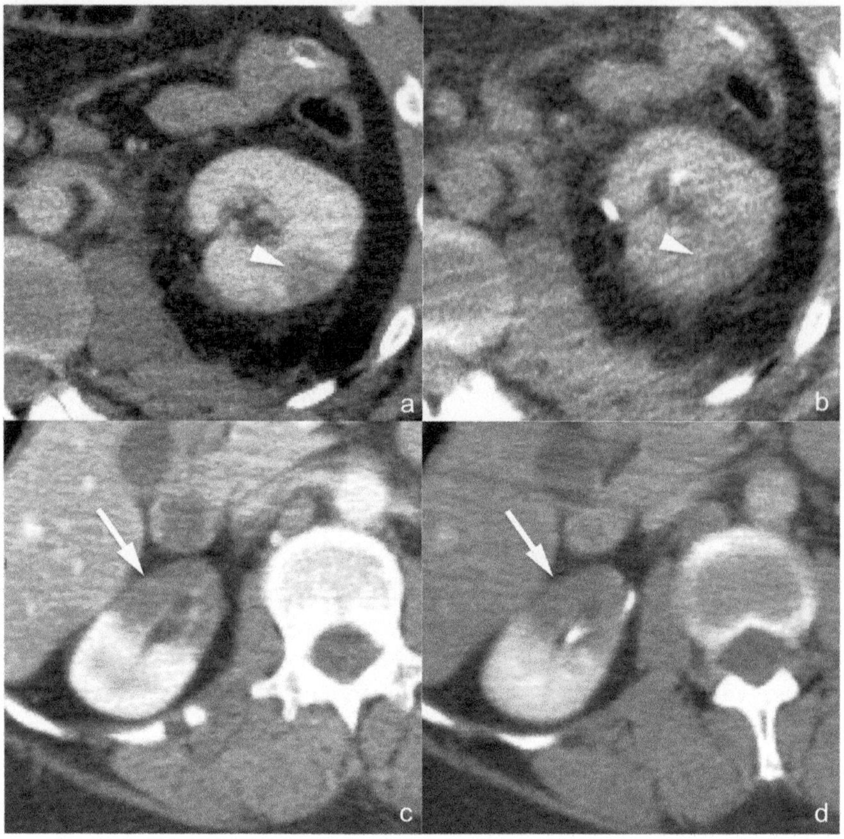

Fig. 1 **a–d** Renal contusion (AAST grade I) (**a** and **b**) and renal infarction (AAST grade IV) (**c** and **d**). Axial multiplanar reconstruction (*MPR*) images (1.5 mm thick **a** and **b**; 3 mm thick **c** and **d**) acquired during the nephrographic phase (**a** and **c**) and the 8-min delayed phase (**b** and **d**) of the study in two different patients. Renal contusion appears as an ill-defined, irregularly shaped area of reduced contrast enhancement during the nephrographic phase (**a**, *arrowhead*) and tends to isodensity in the delayed phase (**b**, *arrowhead*), whereas segmental infarction appears as a wedge-shaped, sharply defined area of reduced/absent contrast enhancement during the nephrographic phase (**c**, *arrow*) and shows marked hypodensity also in the delayed phase (**d**, *arrow*)

contusions, and no follow-up imaging studies are required if the clinical and laboratory data remain stable [30–32].

- *Subcapsular haematoma (AAST grade I)*. Subcapsular haematoma (Fig. 2a–b) appears as a well-delimited, non-enhancing fluid collection located between the renal parenchyma and the renal capsule. Depending on its size, the collection may show a crescent or a biconvex shape; in the latter case, a mass effect is usually exerted on the adjacent parenchyma, which may become flattened or indented. The attenuation of the collection varies according

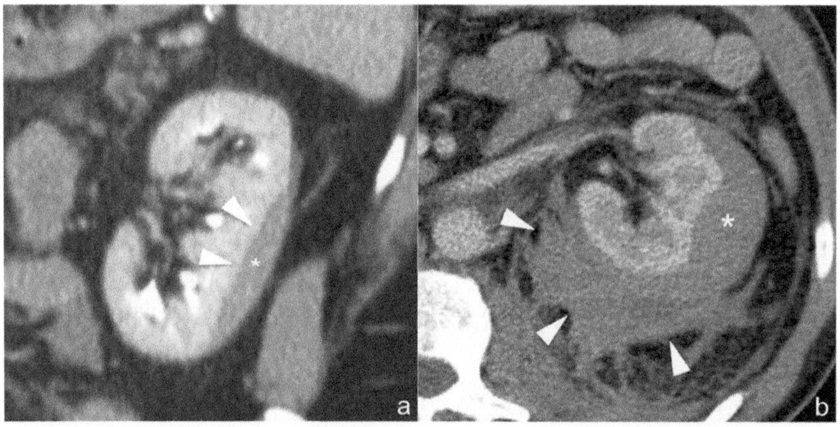

Fig. 2 **a–b** Subcapsular haematoma (AAST grade I) (**a**) and perirenal haematoma (AAST grade II) (**b**). The 3-mm-thick multiplanar reconstruction (*MPR*) coronal image (**a**) acquired during the delayed phase of the study shows a well-delimited hypodense biconvex-shaped collection (*star*), located between the renal parenchyma and renal capsule, which determines the mild mass effect on the adjacent parenchyma (*arrowheads*), representing subcapsular haematoma. A similar finding may also be observed in the 3-mm-thick multiplanar reconstruction (*MPR*) axial image (**b**) acquired during the nephrographic phase in another patient in which, however, an irregularly delimited inhomogenously hypodense collection, representing perirenal haematoma (*arrowheads*), is appreciable between the renal parenchyma and the Gerota fascia. In both cases neither parenchymal lacerations nor active contrast material extravasations can be observed

to its age, and hyperdensity may be seen if blood clots are present. To be classified as a grade I lesion, a subcapsular haematoma must not be associated with parenchymal lacerations and no active contrast material extravasation should be observed; indeed, subcapsular haematomas are often associated with higher grade parenchymal lesions. Moreover, if a capsular lesion coexists, the haematoma often extends to the perirenal space (Fig. 2b). A simple "wait-and-see" management is indicated in case of subcapsular haematoma, and no follow-up imaging studies are required if the clinical and laboratory data remain stable [30–32].

- *Perirenal haematoma* (*AAST grade II*). Perirenal haematoma (Fig. 2b) appears as a poorly delimited, non-enhancing fluid collection located in the fatty area between the renal capsule and Gerota fascia. Its attenuation varies according to the age, appearing inhomogenously hyperattenuating in the acute/subacute stage and becoming progressively iso- or hypoattenuating in the chronic stage. Perirenal haematoma usually does not cause a mass effect on the adjacent renal parenchyma, but large haematomas may displace the kidney and nearby bowel and may also cross the midline, ventrally to the aorta and inferior vena cava, invading the contralateral perirenal space. An extension to the pelvis may also be observed in large perirenal haematomas. Although perirenal haematomas may represent isolated lesions, in most cases they are associated with parenchymal lacerations and the presence of opacified urine extravasation must be accurately ruled out by means of delayed scans. Moreover, particular attention must be paid to collections located medially to the renal hilum: in these cases, the presence of vascular pedicle and uretero-pelvic junction lesions must be ruled out accurately. The tiny perinephric strands that may be observed in patients with impaired renal function should not be misdiagnosed as perirenal haematomas: indeed, these strands are homogeneously hypodense, bilateral and surround the entire kidneys. In case of isolated perirenal haematomas, a simple "wait-and-see" management is indicated and no follow-up imaging studies are required if the clinical and laboratory data remain stable [30–32].
- *Parenchymal laceration not involving the collecting system* (*AAST grade II-III*): Parenchymal lacerations (Fig. 3a–b) appear as irregular or linear clefts of absent contrast enhancement, starting from the renal surface and extending deep into the renal parenchyma, and they are best depicted during the nephrographic phase. Their attenuation varies according to their age and the presence of blood clots, and they are usually associated with perirenal haematomas. If a parenchymal laceration is present, delayed acquisitions should be performed in order to rule out urine extravasation (Fig. 3b). Moreover, it is extremely important to exclude the presence of active contrast material extravasation. The AAST subdivides parenchymal lacerations into grade II if they extend less than 1 cm in depth and grade III if they extend more than 1 cm; in any case, there is no difference in the treatment of grade II and III lesions, which must follow the simple "wait-and-see" management. No follow-up imaging studies are required if the clinical and laboratory data remain stable [30–32].
- *Segmental infarction* (*AAST grade IV*). Segmental infarctions (Fig. 1c–d) appear as sharply demarcated, wedge-shaped areas of absent contrast enhancement, showing a subcapsular basis and apex directed to the hilum, and are the consequence of dissection and/or thrombosis of segmental vessels. Sharp margins and lack of enhancement during the delayed phase are the characteristics that must be identified in order to perform a differential diagnosis with renal contusions (Fig. 1a–b). The coexistence of multiple infarctions is quite frequent. A simple "wait-and-see" management is indicated in the majority of cases, whereas surgical debridement is indicated in case of infarctions involving more than 50 % of the renal parenchyma. No follow-up imaging studies are required if the clinical and laboratory data remain stable [30–32], whereas a CT scan is mandatory in case of pain development in order to exclude colliquation or abscess formation, findings that imply surgical exploration.
- "*Shattered kidney*" (*AAST grade V*). The term "shattered kidney" is used to describe a kidney ruptured in multiple fragments by severe and deep lacerations (Fig. 4a–b). Renal fragments are usually surrounded and subdivided by a fluid collection that occupies the entire renal loggia; some parenchymal fragments may appear devitalised or non-enhancing because of traumatic occlusion of their arterial supply. Particular attention must be paid to excluding the presence of active contrast material extravasation and urine leakage: indeed, if these are ruled out, an increasing number of reports suggest that haemodynamically stable patients can be safely treated conservatively by means of a simple "wait-and-see" treatment, whereas surgical exploration should be reserved for haemodynamically unstable patients and endovascular and/or endourological treatments for patients showing blood and/or urine extravasation [16, 17, 20, 33–38]. Due to the severity of the injury, follow-up CT studies might represent a reasonable option in these patients, also in case of clinical and laboratory stability, in particular in order to detect vascular complications early, such as pseudoaneurysms and artero-venous fistulae, which might have life-threatening effects in an acute setting.

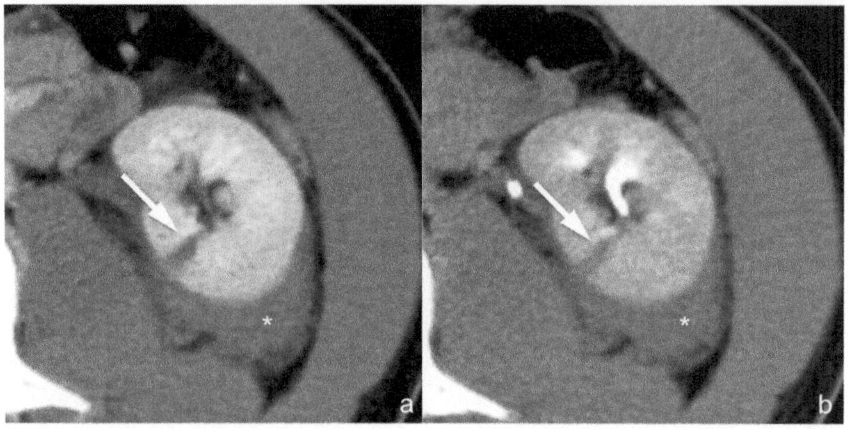

Fig. 3 a–b Parenchymal laceration not involving the collecting system (AAST grade II–III). On these 3-mm-thick multiplanar reconstruction (*MPR*) axial images acquired during the nephrographic (**a**) and 8-min delayed phase (**b**) of the study in the same patient, a linear cleft of absent contrast enhancement (*arrow*) starting from the renal surface and extending deep into the renal parenchyma is clearly appreciable, representing parenchymal laceration. On delayed image (**b**), no lack of hyperdense urine can be seen, excluding collecting system rupture. A perirenal haematoma (*star*) coexists posteriorly to the kidney

Non-operative management: endourological treatment

- *Parenchymal laceration involving the collecting system* (*AAST grade IV*). Parenchymal lacerations involving the collecting system (Fig. 5a–b) extend deep into the medulla and are univocally associated with perirenal fluid collections secondary to blood and urine accumulation. Urine extravasation can be highlighted during the delayed phase of the study as markedly hyperdense material within the perirenal haematoma (Fig. 5b). Ureteral stenting is the treatment of choice in collecting system injuries and at least one follow-up CT examination is indicated in order to assess the evolution of the urinoma and to detect eventual complications early, such as superinfection; attention must be paid to the proximal extremity of the JJ catheter, which should be located within the upper calyceal group in order to maximise its effectiveness in urine drainage.
- *Ureteropelvic junction laceration* (*AAST grade V*). Ureteropelvic junction laceration (Fig. 6a–b) is usually a consequence of fast deceleration traumas and is associated with a large perirenal fluid collection, mostly located medially to the renal hilum and often extending caudally over the psoas. Renal contrast material excretion is normal and the calyceal system is usually intact, while hyperdense urine extravasation can be highlighted in the delayed

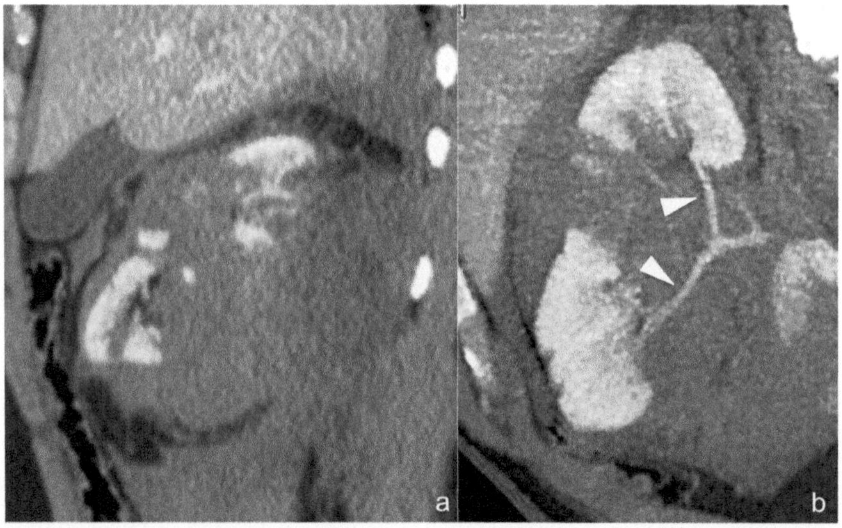

Fig. 4 a–b Shattered kidney (AAST grade V). The 3-mm-thick multiplanar reconstruction (*MPR*) coronal image (**a**) acquired during the nephrographic phase of the study shows a large inhomogenously hypodense collection occupying the renal and perirenal spaces with multiple vascularised kidney fragments within, representing a so-called shattered kidney. On the 10-mm-thick para-coronal maximum intensity projection (*MIP*) of the same series (**b**), the main branches of the *right* renal artery (*arrowheads*) can be accurately delimited and no active contrast material extravasation can be observed

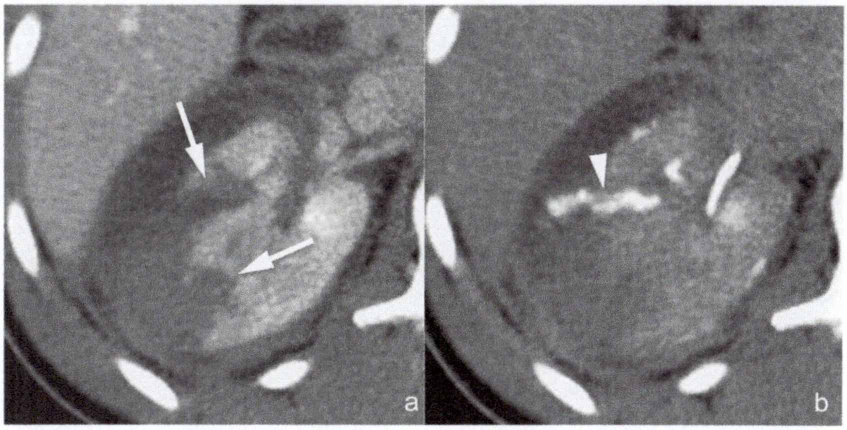

Fig. 5 a–b Parenchymal laceration involving the collecting system (AAST grade IV). On these 3-mm-thick multiplanar reconstruction (*MPR*) axial images acquired during the nephrographic (**a**) and 8-min delayed phase (**b**) of the study in the same patient, multiple irregular clefts of absent contrast enhancement (*arrows*), starting from the renal surface and extending deep into the renal parenchyma, are clearly appreciable, representing parenchymal lacerations. On delayed image (**b**), hyperdense urine leakage (*arrowhead*) is recognisable as a sign of collecting system rupture

phase at the renal hilum. Ureteropelvic junction avulsion, which otherwise shows the same CT findings (Fig. 6c–d), can be excluded if hyperdense urine is seen in the downstream ureter (Fig. 6b). Ureteral stenting is the treatment of choice for ureteropelvic junction laceration, and at least one follow-up CT examination is indicated in order to assess urinoma evolution and detect any complications early; attention must be paid to the proximal extremity of the JJ catheter, which should be located within the upper calyceal group.

Non-operative management: interventional radiology

- *Active contrast material extravasation from branching renal arteries (not included in the AAST classification).*

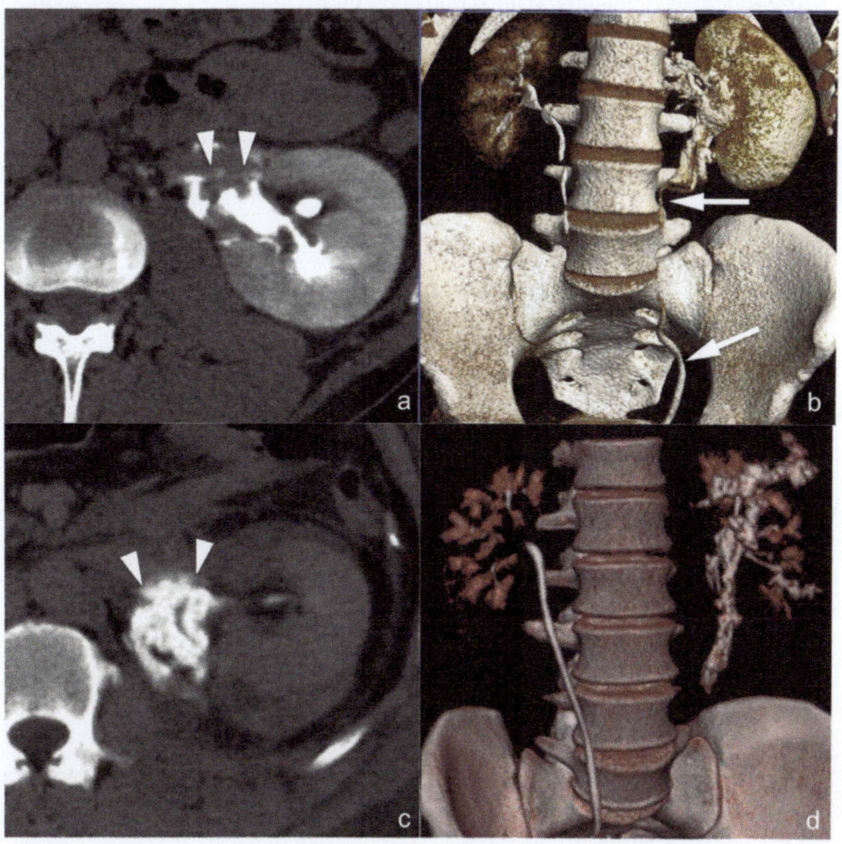

Fig. 6 a–d Laceration of the ureteropelvic junction (**a** and **b**) and avulsion of the ureteropelvic junction (**c** and **d**) (AAST grade V both). On the 3-mm-thick multiplanar reconstruction (*MPR*) axial images acquired during the delayed phase of the study in two different patients (**a** and **c**) a hyperdense urine leakage can be observed medially to the kidney hilum (*arrowheads*), a finding suspicious for a ureteropelvic junction lesion. The volume-rendering technique (*VRT*) reconstructions of the same series (**b** and **d**) show that, in the first case (**b**), the downstream ureter is opacified by hyperdense urine, therefore excluding a complete ureteropelvic disconnection, whereas in the second case (**d**), no opacified urine can be observed in the downstream ureter, indicating therefore a complete ureteropelvic avulsion

Active contrast material extravasation from peripheral arterial branches (Fig. 7a–b) is not directly mentioned in the AAST classification of renal trauma. At CT, small arterial bleedings appear as poorly delimited contrast material extravasations, sometimes flame-shaped, usually located in the setting of a perirenal haematoma, that appear hyperdense in the arterial phase and increase in quantity and density in the following phases. Active arterial contrast material extravasation is often associated with high-grade parenchymal lesions, but occasionally it may also occur in low-grade ones. Non-operative management is indicated in haemodynamically stable patients if no other lesions requiring surgery are detected at CT, and digital subtraction angiography with superselective arterial embolisation represents the treatment of choice [39, 40]; angioembolisation might be avoided in patients with small perirenal haematomas and minimal signs of active bleeding [41]. A CT follow-up should be considered after angioembolisation in order to detect eventual complications, such as pseudoaneurysms and large ischaemic events.

- *Arterial pseudoaneurysm* (*not included in the AAST classification*). Arterial pseudoaneurysm (Fig. 8a–b) appears as a well-delimited ovoid lesion located within the renal parenchyma, enhancing as much as the adjacent arteries during the arterial phase and not increasing in size or density during the subsequent phases in which, indeed, it becomes isoattenuating to the blood pool; these characteristics enable a differential diagnosis with active contrast material extravasation. Digital subtraction angiography (Fig. 8c) with superselective arterial embolisation represents the treatment of choice in order to prevent delayed rupture; surgery may be limited to the few cases in which haemostasis and arterial wall defect repair are required [42].
- *Artero-venous fistula* (*not included in the AAST classification*). Artero-venous fistulae (Fig. 8d–e) usually have the same CT appearance as arterial pseudoaneurysms. An important finding that enables the differential diagnosis between the two lesions is the identification of a dilated renal vein that enhances early during the arterial phase of the study; anyway, a true arterial phase should be acquired in order to appreciate this finding that might be obscured by the physiological venous return during the corticomedullary phase. Digital subtraction angiography (Fig. 8f) with superselective arterial embolisation represents the treatment of choice in order to prevent delayed rupture and arterial hypertension development.

Surgical management

- *Avulsion of the main renal artery or vein* (*AAST grade V*). Avulsions of the main renal artery or vein (Fig. 9a–b) represent extremely dangerous lesions that, in the majority of cases, preclude the patient to undergo CT because of haemodynamic instability. Both lesions are associated with large perirenal haematomas, prevalently located medially to the renal hilum, with abundant contrast material extravasation between the kidney and the aorta in the arterial and/or portal venous phase. Renal artery avulsion in the majority of the cases results in a completely or at least largely devascularised kidney, whereas in case of renal vein avulsion renal enhancement is usually delayed and reduced, but uniformly present. Vascular pedicle avulsion

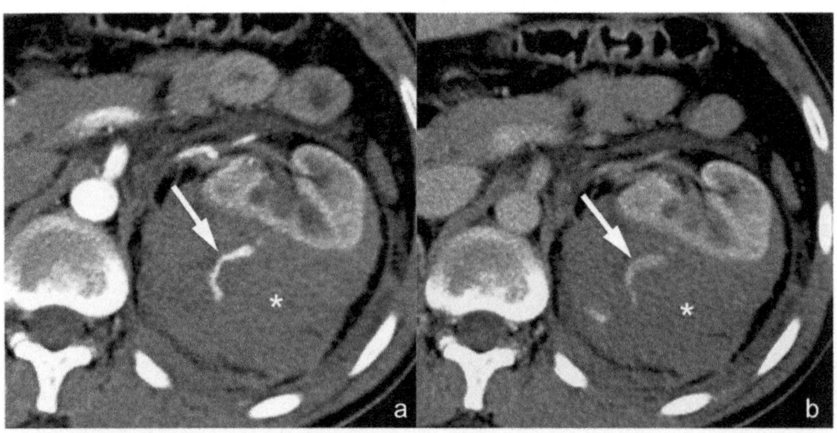

Fig. 7 a–b Active arterial contrast extravasation from a capsular artery (lesion not included in the AAST classification). On these 3-mm-thick multiplanar reconstruction (*MPR*) axial images acquired during the arterial (**a**) and nephrographic (**b**) phases of the study in the same patient, a large perirenal haematoma (*star*) determining a ventral dislocation of the kidney is clearly recognisable. No parenchymal lacerations can be observed, but an active contrast material extravasation (*arrow*) is recognisable within the haematoma during the arterial phase, showing a mild increase in size during the nephrographic phase as a consequence of a capsular artery rupture

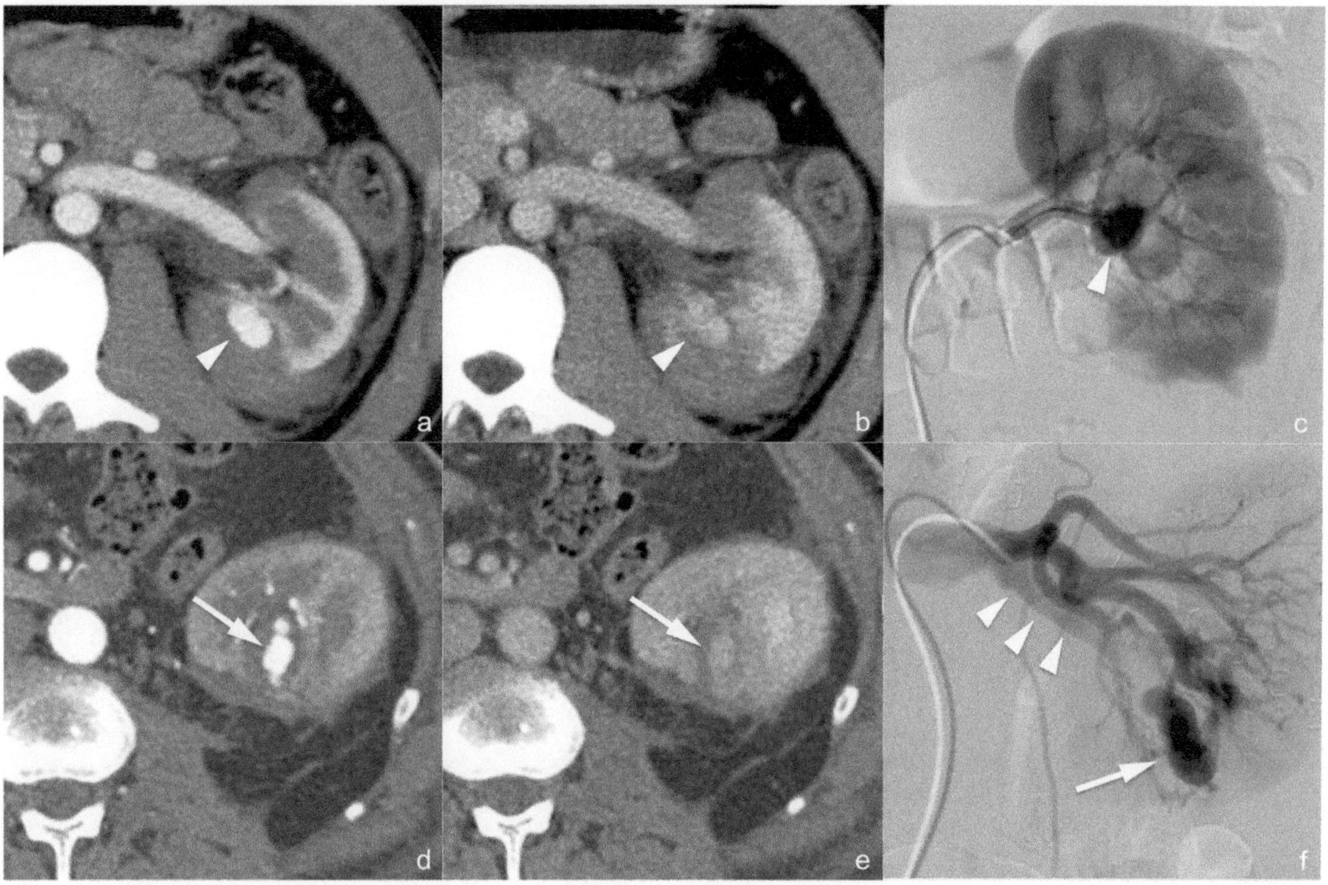

Fig. 8 **a**–**f** Arterial pseudoaneurysm and artero-venous fistula (lesions not included in the AAST classification). On the 3-mm-thick multiplanar reconstruction (*MPR*) axial images acquired during the arterial (**a** and **d**) and nephrographic (**b** and **e**) phases of the study in two different patients, a well-delimited oval lesion (*arrowheads* in the first patient and *arrows* in the second one) with a density that varies parallel to the density of the arterial vessels is clearly recognisable. Digital subtraction angiography characterised these lesions as an arterial pseudoaneurysm in the first patient (**c**) and as an artero-venous fistula in the second one (**f**) in which an early venous output (*arrowheads*) was recognisable

represents a life-threatening emergency: no delayed CT scans must be performed and immediate surgical exploration is mandatory.

- *Avulsion of the ureteropelvic junction* (*AAST grade V*). CT findings in case of complete ureteropelvic junction transection (Fig. 6c–d) are the same as in case of ureteropelvic

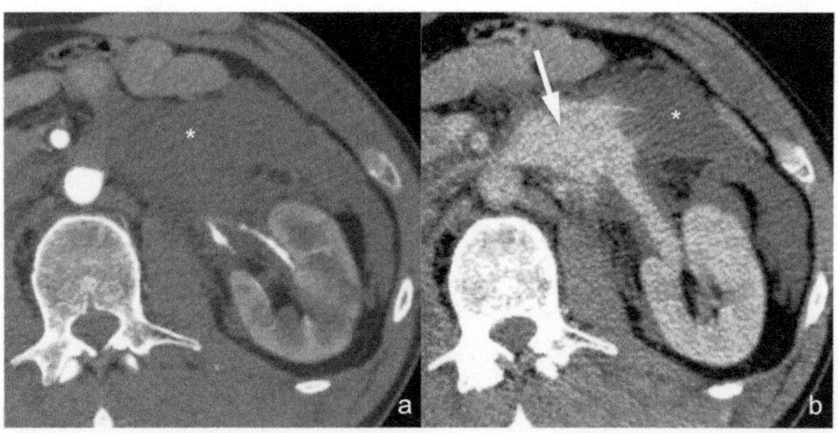

Fig. 9 **a**–**b** Main renal vein laceration (AAST grade V). On these 3-mm-thick multiplanar reconstruction (*MPR*) axial images acquired during the arterial (**a**) and nephrographic (**b**) phases of the study in the same patient, a large perirenal-pararenal haematoma (*star*) is recognisable medially-ventrally to the kidney. No active contrast material extravasation can be observed during the arterial phase of the study, whereas a large contrast material extravasation (*arrow*) appears ventrally to the renal vein in the subsequent nephrographic phase, representing renal vein laceration

junction laceration, with the only important difference a complete absence of opacified urine in the downstream ureter (Fig. 6d). Differently than in case of ureteropelvic junction laceration, ureteropelvic junction avulsion requires surgical repair because endourological treatments are usually ineffective.

Debated management

- *Thrombosis of the main renal artery or vein* (*AAST grade IV*). Arterial thrombosis is usually secondary to traumatic dissection of the main renal artery (Fig. 10a–c), and the resulting occlusion may be complete or partial; consequently, the kidney may appear completely devascularised or hypovascularised. The thrombus, when detectable, appears as an endovascular filling defect, hyperdense on non-enhanced images and hypodense in post-contrast scans. Main renal vein thrombosis is rare and causes delayed enhancement of the kidney in comparison with contralateral renal enlargement and parenchymal oedema. Management of these injuries is extremely controversial: in particular, in case of renal artery dissection both surgical and endovascular revascularisations (Fig. 10b–c) have shown good results [43, 44] and the treatment option should be determined according to the centre's experience. Anyway, in case of complete arterial occlusion the 2-h time limit for revascularisation must be considered: indeed, after 2 h of complete renal ischaemia also a good technical result will bring a poor functional outcome. Nephrectomy is always recommended if conservative treatments fail [45].

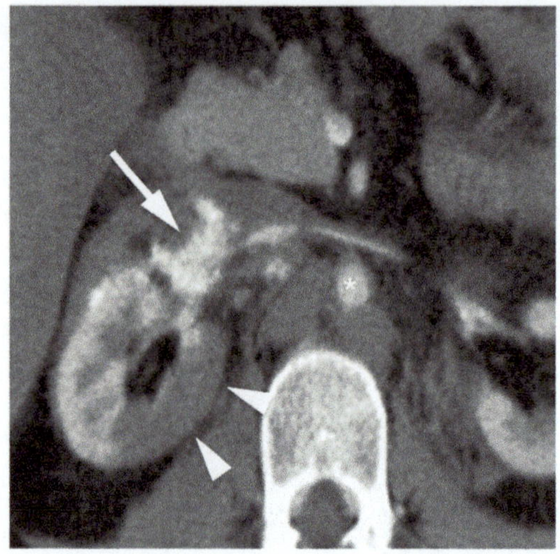

Fig. 11 Main renal artery laceration (AAST grade IV). On this 3-mm-thick multiplanar reconstruction (*MPR*) axial image acquired during the arterial (**a**) phase of the study, a large contrast material extravasation can be observed adjacent to the *right* renal artery (*arrow*) as a consequence of renal artery laceration; to notice, the markedly reduced diameter of the aorta (*star*) as a consequence of the haemodynamic shock status. Moreover, the right renal parenchyma shows a large well-defined hypodense area (*arrowheads*), representing renal infarction

- *Injuries to the main renal artery or vein with a contained haematoma or partial vessel laceration* (*AAST grade IV*). This type of injury manifests with the presence of a perirenal haematoma associated with active arterial or venous bleeding from hilar vessels (Fig. 11). The haematoma is usually located medially to the renal hilum and may extend caudally along the psoas; the kidney is often displaced laterally. Both surgical and endovascular treatments may be considered, also according to the

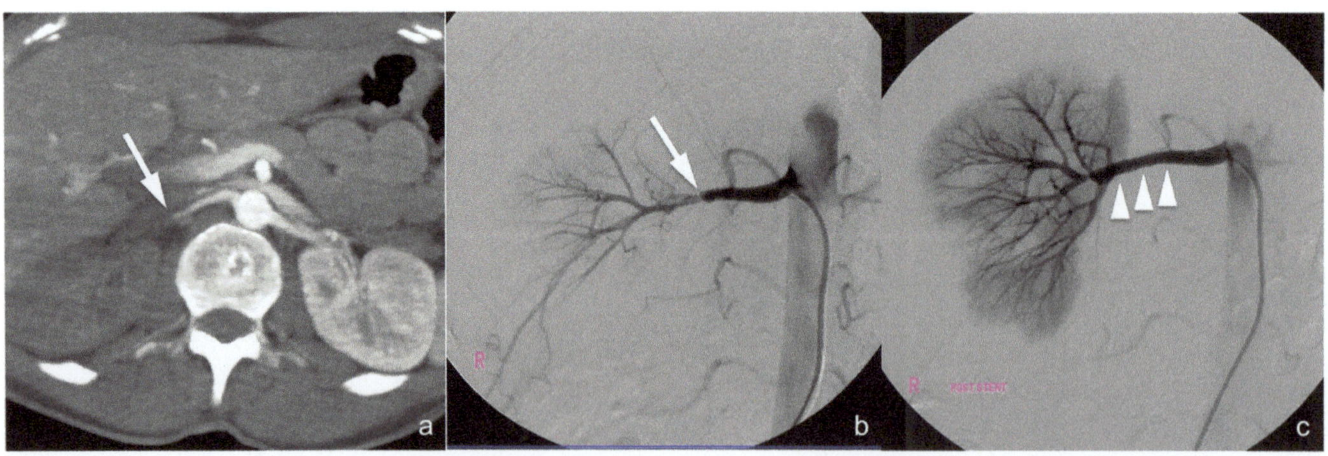

Fig. 10 **a–c** Main renal artery dissection/thrombosis. The 10-mm-thick maximum intensity projection (*MIP*) axial image acquired during the arterial phase of the study (**a**) shows a hypovascularised right kidney as a consequence of renal artery dissection (*arrow*). The finding was confirmed at subsequent digital subtraction angiography (**b**, *arrow*) in which a residual flow was appreciable downstream from the dissection; a stent was placed (**c**, *arrowheads*) with good flow recovery

centre's experience, with the latter associated with lower nephrectomy rates [16].

Conclusions

In case of renal trauma, MDCT can generate a wide spectrum of findings that a radiologist must be able to recognise in order to correctly direct trauma management and allow accurate risk stratification. Anyway, it is important to notice that, in the emergency setting, the differentiation between AAST grade 1, 2 and 3 renal injuries does not result in a change in patient management, the "wait-and-see" approach being the most indicated in all cases of haemodynamic stability. On the other hand, AAST grade 4 and 5 lesions must be promptly recognised and communicated to the clinician because they will shift the treatment to an endourological, endovascular or surgical one; indeed, the simple "wait-and-see" management may be considered only in case of segmental infarctions involving less than 50 % of the renal parenchyma and of shattered kidney without urine or active blood extravasation. Moreover, CT may highlight some peripheral vascular lesions (i.e., active bleedings, pseudoaneurysms and artero-venous fistulae) that are not directly mentioned in the AAST classification, but that must be accurately recognised because of requiring, in the majority of the cases, an endovascular interventional approach.

References

1. Baverstock R, Simons R, McLoughlin M (2001) Severe blunt renal trauma: a 7-year retrospective review from a provincial trauma centre. Can J Urol 8:1372–1376
2. Harris AC, Zwirewich CV, Lyburn ID, Torreggiani WC, Marchinkow LO (2001) Ct findings in blunt renal trauma. Radiographics: a review publication of the Radiological Society of North America, Inc 21 Spec No: S201-214
3. Kawashima A, Sandler CM, Corl FM et al (2001) Imaging of renal trauma: a comprehensive review. Radiogr: Rev Publ Radiol Soc North Am Inc 21:557–574
4. Smith JK, Kenney PJ (2003) Imaging of renal trauma. Radiol Clin N Am 41:1019–1035
5. Alonso RC, Nacenta SB, Martinez PD, Guerrero AS, Fuentes CG (2009) Kidney in danger: CT findings of blunt and penetrating renal trauma. Radiogr: Rev Publ Radiol Soc North Am Inc 29:2033–2053
6. Carpio F, Morey AF (1999) Radiographic staging of renal injuries. World J Urol 17:66–70
7. Pollack HM, Wein AJ (1989) Imaging of renal trauma. Radiology 172:297–308
8. Cass AS, Luxenberg M, Gleich P, Smith CS (1986) Clinical indications for radiographic evaluation of blunt renal trauma. J Urol 136: 370–371
9. Alsikafi NF, Rosenstein DI (2006) Staging, evaluation, and nonoperative management of renal injuries. The Urologic clinics of North America 33:13–19, v
10. Broghammer JA, Fisher MB, Santucci RA (2007) Conservative management of renal trauma: a review. Urology 70:623–629
11. Boone TB, Gilling PJ, Husmann DA (1993) Ureteropelvic junction disruption following blunt abdominal trauma. J Urol 150:33–36
12. Stables DP, Fouche RF, de Villiers van Niekerk JP, Cremin BJ, Holt SA, Peterson NE (1976) Traumatic renal artery occlusion: 21 cases. J Urol 115:229–233
13. Shariat SF, Roehrborn CG, Karakiewicz PI, Dhami G, Stage KH (2007) Evidence-based validation of the predictive value of the American Association for the Surgery of Trauma Kidney Injury scale. J Trauma 62:933–939
14. Hashemzadeh SH, Hashemzadeh KH, Dehdilani M, Rezaei S (2010) Non-operative management of blunt trauma in abdominal solid organ injuries: a prospective study to evaluate the success rate and predictive factors of failure. Minerva Chir 65:267–274
15. McCombie S, Thyer I, Corcoran N et al (2014) The conservative management of renal trauma: a literature review and practical clinical guideline from Australia and New Zealand. BJU Int. doi:10.1111/bju.12902
16. van der Wilden GM, Velmahos GC, Joseph DK et al (2013) Successful nonoperative management of the most severe blunt renal injuries: a multicenter study of the research consortium of New England Centers for Trauma. JAMA Surg 148:924–931
17. Santucci RA, Fisher MB (2005) The literature increasingly supports expectant (conservative) management of renal trauma—a systematic review. J Trauma 59:493–503
18. Santucci RA, Wessells H, Bartsch G et al (2004) Evaluation and management of renal injuries: consensus statement of the renal trauma subcommittee. BJU Int 93:937–954
19. Jacobs MA, Hotaling JM, Mueller BA, Koyle M, Rivara F, Voelzke BB (2012) Conservative management vs early surgery for high grade pediatric renal trauma–do nephrectomy rates differ? J Urol 187: 1817–1822
20. Aragona F, Pepe P, Patane D, Malfa P, D'Arrigo L, Pennisi M (2012) Management of severe blunt renal trauma in adult patients: a 10-year retrospective review from an emergency hospital. BJU Int 110:744–748
21. Heller MT, Schnor N (2014) MDCT of renal trauma: correlation to AAST organ injury scale. Clin Imaging 38:410–417
22. Kawashima A, Sandler CM, Corl FM et al (2002) Imaging evaluation of posttraumatic renal injuries. Abdom Imaging 27:199–213
23. Park SJ, Kim JK, Kim KW, Cho KS (2006) MDCT findings of renal trauma. AJR Am J Roentgenol 187:541–547
24. Razali MR, Azian AA, Amran AR, Azlin S (2010) Computed tomography of blunt renal trauma. Singap Med J 51:468–473, quiz 474
25. Karlo C, Gnannt R, Frauenfelder T et al (2011) Whole-body CT in polytrauma patients: effect of arm positioning on thoracic and abdominal image quality. Emerg Radiol 18:285–293
26. Coppenrath EM, Mueller-Lisse UG (2006) Multidetector CT of the kidney. Eur Radiol 16:2603–2611
27. Foley WD (2003) Renal MDCT. Eur J Radiol 45(Suppl 1):S73–S78
28. Tunaci A, Yekeler E (2004) Multidetector row CT of the kidneys. Eur J Radiol 52:56–66
29. Im AL, Lee YH, Bang DH, Yoon KH, Park SH (2013) Dual energy CT in patients with acute abdomen; is it possible for virtual non-enhanced images to replace true non-enhanced images? Emerg Radiol 20:475–483
30. Breen KJ, Sweeney P, Nicholson PJ, Kiely EA, O'Brien MF (2014) Adult blunt renal trauma: routine follow-up imaging is excessive. Urology 84:62–67

31. Bukur M, Inaba K, Barmparas G et al (2011) Routine follow-up imaging of kidney injuries may not be justified. J Trauma 70:1229–1233
32. Malcolm JB, Derweesh IH, Mehrazin R et al (2008) Nonoperative management of blunt renal trauma: is routine early follow-up imaging necessary? BMC Urol 8:11
33. Altman AL, Haas C, Dinchman KH, Spirnak JP (2000) Selective nonoperative management of blunt grade 5 renal injury. J Urol 164: 27–30, discussion 30-21
34. Hotaling JM, Wang J, Sorensen MD et al (2012) A national study of trauma level designation and renal trauma outcomes. J Urol 187:536–541
35. Eassa W, El-Ghar MA, Jednak R, El-Sherbiny M (2010) Nonoperative management of grade 5 renal injury in children: does it have a place? Eur Urol 57:154–161
36. Salem HK, Morsi HA, Zakaria A (2007) Management of high-grade renal injuries in children after blunt abdominal trauma: experience of 40 cases. J Pediatr Urol 3:223–229
37. Shoobridge JJ, Corcoran NM, Martin KA, Koukounaras J, Royce PL, Bultitude MF (2011) Contemporary management of renal trauma. Rev Urol 13:65–72
38. van der Vlies CH, Olthof DC, Gaakeer M, Ponsen KJ, van Delden OM, Goslings JC (2011) Changing patterns in diagnostic strategies and the treatment of blunt injury to solid abdominal organs. Int J Emerg Med 4:47
39. Charbit J, Manzanera J, Millet I et al (2011) What are the specific computed tomography scan criteria that can predict or exclude the need for renal angioembolization after high-grade renal trauma in a conservative management strategy? J Trauma 70:1219–1227, discussion 1227-1218
40. Hotaling JM, Sorensen MD, Smith TG 3rd, Rivara FP, Wessells H, Voelzke BB (2011) Analysis of diagnostic angiography and angioembolization in the acute management of renal trauma using a national data set. J Urol 185:1316–1320
41. Nuss GR, Morey AF, Jenkins AC et al (2009) Radiographic predictors of need for angiographic embolization after traumatic renal injury. J Trauma 67:578–582, discussion 582
42. Ngo TC, Lee JJ, Gonzalgo ML (2010) Renal pseudoaneurysm: an overview. Nat Rev Urol 7:619–625
43. Lopera JE, Suri R, Kroma G, Gadani S, Dolmatch B (2011) Traumatic occlusion and dissection of the main renal artery: endovascular treatment. J Vasc Int Radiol: JVIR 22:1570–1574
44. Muller BT, Reiher L, Pfeiffer T et al (2003) Surgical treatment of renal artery dissection in 25 patients: indications and results. J Vasc Surg 37:761–768
45. Haas CA, Dinchman KH, Nasrallah PF, Spirnak JP (1998) Traumatic renal artery occlusion: a 15-year review. J Trauma 45:557–561

False positive and false negative diagnoses of prostate cancer at multi-parametric prostate MRI in active surveillance

Jeffrey S. Quon[1] · Bardia Moosavi[1] · Maneesh Khanna[2] · Trevor A. Flood[3] · Christopher S. Lim[1] · Nicola Schieda[1]

Abstract
MP-MRI is a critical component in active surveillance (AS) of prostate cancer (PCa) because of a high negative predictive value for clinically significant tumours. This review illustrates pitfalls of MP-MRI and how to recognise and avoid them. The anterior fibromuscular stroma and central zone are low signal on T2W-MRI/apparent diffusion coefficient (ADC), resembling PCa. Location, progressive enhancement and low signal on b≥1000 mm²/s echo-planar images (EPI) are differentiating features. BPH can mimic PCa. Glandular BPH shows increased T2W/ADC signal, cystic change and progressive enhancement; however, stromal BPH resembles transition zone (TZ) PCa. A rounded morphology, low T2 signal capsule and posterior/superior location favour stromal BPH. Acute/chronic prostatitis mimics PCa at MP-MRI, with differentiation mainly on clinical grounds. Visual analysis of diffusion-weighted MRI must include EPI and appropriate windowing of ADC. Quantitative ADC analysis is limited by lack of standardization; the ADC ratio and ADC histogram analysis are alternatives to mean values. DCE lacks standardisation and has limited utility in the TZ, where T2W/DWI are favoured. Targeted TRUS-guided biopsies of MR-detected lesions are challenging. Lesions detected on MP-MRI may not be perfectly targeted with TRUS and this must be considered when faced with a suspicious lesion on MP-MRI and a negative targeted TRUS biopsy histopathological result.

Keypoints
- *Multi-parametric MRI plays a critical role in prostate cancer active surveillance.*
- *Low T2W signal intensity structures appear dark on ADC, potentially simulating cancer.*
- *Stromal BPH mimics cancer at DWI and DCE.*
- *Long b value trace EPI should be reviewed*
- *Targeted biopsy of MR-detected lesions using TRUS guidance may be challenging.*

Keywords Prostate cancer · Active surveillance of prostate cancer · Multi-parametric MRI · Targeted biopsy · Diffusion-weighted imaging

✉ Nicola Schieda
nschieda@toh.on.ca

Jeffrey S. Quon
jquon@toh.on.ca

Bardia Moosavi
bmoosavi@toh.on.ca

Maneesh Khanna
khanna.maneesh@gmail.com

Trevor A. Flood
tflood@toh.on.ca

Christopher S. Lim
clim@toh.on.ca

1 Department of Medical Imaging, The Ottawa Hospital, The University of Ottawa, 1053 Carling Avenue, Ottawa, ON, Canada K1Y 4E9

2 Department of Radiology, Hamad General Hospital, Doha, Qatar

3 Department of Pathology, The Ottawa Hospital, The University of Ottawa, 501 Smyth Road, Ottawa, ON, Canada K1H 8 L6

Introduction

Prostate cancer (PCa) is the most common cancer among males in North America [1, 2] and the most common solid neoplasm in Europe [3]. PCa is typically diagnosed with non-targeted systematic trans-rectal ultrasound (TRUS)-guided biopsy in patients with an elevated prostate serum antigen (PSA) level and/or abnormal digital rectal examination (DRE). The management of a particular patient with PCa is multi-factorial and patient specific due to the biological heterogeneity of PCa. Traditional treatment of PCa varies from radical prostatectomy (RP) or radiotherapy (RT) to watchful waiting (delayed symptomatic non-curative treatment of apparently localised PCa in males who are not candidates for aggressive local therapy) [1, 3]. Active surveillance (AS) is defined as the expectant management (deferred immediate therapy) of PCa in carefully selected males with localised disease considered to be at low risk for progression [4]. AS differs from watchful waiting because definitive treatment is used in patients managed with AS when there is evidence that the patient is at an increased risk for disease progression [4, 5]. AS has become the treatment of choice for low-grade, low-volume tumours [6, 7] and is heavily reliant on accurate detection of tumour, accurate estimate of tumour volume and accurate Gleason grading of tumour [6, 7].

Non-targeted TRUS-guided biopsy typically obtains 6–12 core biopsies of the peripheral zone (PZ), which harbours approximately 70 % of cancers [1, 8]. The limitations of non-targeted TRUS-guided biopsy are well known [8] with an estimated 20 % false-negative rate [9–11]. Furthermore, non-targeted TRUS-guided biopsy may yield unreliable information regarding the volume, extent and aggressiveness of PCa; it is has been reported that up to 30–45 % of patients are upgraded/upstaged from their initial diagnosis at TRUS-guided needle biopsy after RP [12]. Moreover, certain areas of the prostate gland [i.e., the anterior gland, transition zone (TZ) and apex] are known to be under-sampled or not sampled at all at routine non-targeted TRUS-guided biopsy and are now increasingly being recognised as areas that may contain clinically significant (CS) tumours [13]. These limitations are of critical importance in AS, where treatment decisions are based on risk stratification and dependent on accurate Gleason grading of tumours [4].

Multi-parametric (MP) MRI [diffusion-weighted imaging (DWI)+dynamic contrast enhancement (DCE) and/or MR spectroscopy] has become the reference standard for prostate imaging endorsed by both the American College of Radiology (ACR) and European Society of Uroradiology (ESUR) [14, 15] (Table 1). Two recent meta-analyses concluded that MP-MRI has a high negative predictive value for the detection of CS cancers [16, 17], and it has been shown previously that MP-MRI can estimate grade of PCa compared to histopathology results with a reasonable degree of accuracy [18]. Due to the ability of MP-MRI to detect clinically significant (higher volume Gleason score≥7) tumours with high degrees of accuracy, it has become of tremendous value in AS [19]. Recent studies have demonstrated that MP-MRI can help to determine eligibility for AS [20] and potentially reclassify patients already enrolled in AS before repeat biopsies [21]. In the UK, the National Institute for Health and Care Excellence (NICE) guidelines currently mandate MP-MRI be performed at the onset of AS protocols and that

Table 1 Sequence parameters for multi-parametric MRI of the prostate protocol performed with a pelvic surface coil[a] at 3 T[b]

	Imaging plane	Field of view (mm)	Matrix size	Slice thickness/gap (mm)	TR/TE (ms)	Echo train length	Flip angle	Acceler-ation factor	Receiver bandwidth (Hz/voxel)	Acquisition time (min)	Number of signals averaged
T1 TSE[c]	Axial	350×350	320×320	5.0/1.0	720/8–14	3	111	N/A	244	4 min	2
T1 3D dual-echo GRE[d]	Axial	240×240	292×224	4.0/1.0	4.8/1.1–1.3;TE12.2–2.5; TE2	N/A	12	2	558	Breath hold	1
T2 TSE	Coronal Sagittal Axial	220×220	320×256	4.0/0 3.0/0 3.0/0	3890–5250/105–125	27–35	111	N/A	122	4 min 4 min 4 min	1–2
DWI[e]	Axial	280×280	128×80	5.0/1.0	4200/90	1	90	2	1950	5 min	4–10
T1 GRE[f] dynamic contrast	Axial	220×220	128×128	4.0/0	4.3/1.3	N/A	12	2	488	6 min	1

[a] Integrated pelvic surface coils (4–16 channels) with activated spine coils (8–12 channels)

[b] Clinical 3-T systems: TRIO TIM (Siemens Medical, Malvern, PA) and Discovery 750 W (General Electric, Milwaukee, WI)

[c] Turbo/fast spin echo

[d] Gradient recalled echo

[e] *DWI* Diffusion-weighted imaging performed with spectral fat suppression echo planar imaging with tridirectional motion probing gradients and *b* values of 0, 0, 500, 1000, 1500 mm²/s with automatic apparent diffusion coefficient map generation

[f] Dynamic fast spoiled 2D GRE performed with a temporal resolution of 10 s after injection of 0.2 mmol/kg of gadobutrol (Gadovist, Bayer Inc., Toronto, ON) at a rate of 3 ml/s

MP-MRI be performed in patients while they are enrolled in AS when there is concern about clinical or PSA changes [22].

A variety of interpretive and technical pitfalls may be encountered at MP-MRI of the prostate. A failure to recognise and correct these errors in AS patients can result in suboptimal care. False-positive diagnoses of areas of potential cancers at MP-MRI create clinical uncertainty and often lead to multiple unnecessary biopsies or in certain cases surgical management of low-grade, low-volume disease. Moreover, a failure to recognise clinically significant cancers in males being considered for or treated with AS could result in suboptimal patient outcomes. The purpose of this review is to illustrate both interpretive and technical pitfalls encountered at MP-MRI in the active surveillance population and how to detect, correct and avoid them.

Interpretive pitfalls

(1) Normal anatomic structures can mimic anterior and TZ cancers

A detailed understanding of the normal zonal anatomy of the prostate is essential for interpretation of prostate MRI. In 1981, McNeal [23] described the three distinct prostate zonal regions: (1) the peripheral zone, (2) transition zone and (3) central zone (CZ). The prostatic zonal anatomy is best depicted at T2-weighted (W) MRI (Fig. 1). The PZ is hyperintense on T2W because of abundant glandular tissue, is located at the periphery of the gland and harbours 70 % of PCa [24] (Fig. 1). Previously, it was thought that the TZ [the site of benign prostatic hyperplasia (BPH)] and the CZ (which surrounds the ejaculatory ducts, is located mainly at the base of the prostate, is posterior to the TZ and the urethra, and is proximal to the verumontanum) could not be differentiated at imaging and these areas were collectively referred to as the central gland [25, 26]. The central gland in most adult males consists of hypertrophied TZ that compresses the CZ against the surgical capsule [25]. Currently, it is acknowledged that the CZ can be identified separately from the TZ in up to 4/5 of males and the CZ appears as a symmetric band of homogeneously low signal intensity (SI) on T2W MRI and apparent diffusion coefficient (ADC) maps best seen at the prostate base [25], (Fig. 1).

Accurate identification of the CZ is critical as, in our experience, many false-positive interpretations of PCa occur when mistaking the CZ for PCa. The CZ can be diagnosed by noting its symmetry (particularly on coronal T2W images) and typical location adjacent to the ejaculatory ducts [25, 26]. Functional imaging techniques also aid in the differentiation of CZ

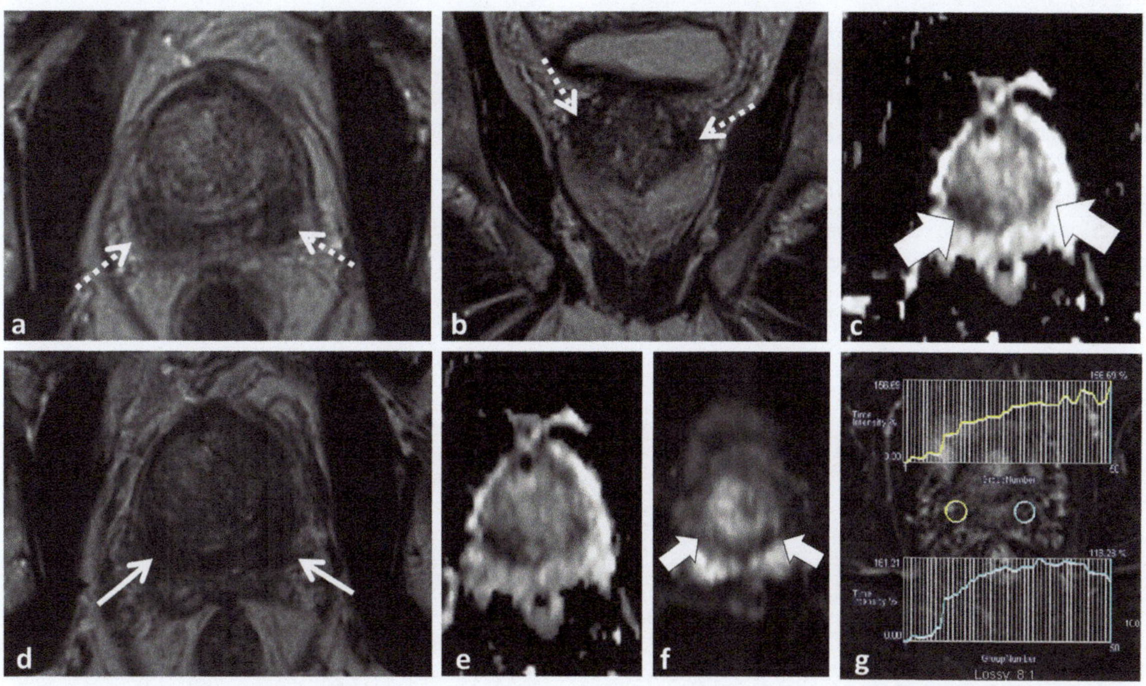

Fig. 1 A 54-year-old male with low volume Gleason score 3+3=6 PCa at TRUS-guided biopsy in the right middle peripheral zone (*PZ*). MP-MRI was performed because of rising PSA to exclude clinically significant (*CS*) tumour. Axial (**a**) and coronal (**b**) T2-weighted (T2W) turbo spin echo (*TSE*) images demonstrate bilateral foci of low T2 signal intensity (SI) at the prostate base (*dotted arrows*) adjacent to the insertion of the vas deferens (not shown). Axial apparent diffusion coefficient (*ADC*) map (**c**) at the same level demonstrates corresponding low SI (*white arrows*). These areas were described as suspicious and repeat targeted TRUS-guided biopsy was suggested. A repeat biopsy with multiple cores through both areas yielded only normal prostatic tissue. A repeat MRI performed 2 years later demonstrates similar findings on the T2W (**d**) and ADC map (**e**), which represent the normal central zone. Corresponding b1000 mm²/s trace echo-planar image (EPI) does not show concordant areas of increased SI (*white arrows* in **f**) and there is benign progressive enhancement on dynamic contrast-enhanced (DCE) imaging (**g**)

from PCa. In the normal CZ, low SI on ADC is due to inherently low T2 SI not true restricted diffusion ("T2 black hole effect"); see Technical Pitfall 2. In the normal CZ, there is no true diffusion restriction; therefore, there should be no increased SI on long (b≥1000 mm²/s) EPI (Figs. 1 and 2). The enhancement pattern of the CZ at DCE has not, to our knowledge, been described; however, in our experience, a progressive type 1 enhancement is typical of the CZ (Fig. 1). CZ PCas are aggressive [26–28], but account for less than 5 % of PCa [26]. An asymmetry of the central zone should raise suspicion for a possible tumour [25]; however, it is more common to observe a slight asymmetry in the thickness of the CZ because of the orientation of the prostate gland and the plane of imaging (Fig. 2). To diagnose the rare CZ PCa, asymmetry at T2W should be confirmed in multiple planes and corresponding functional imaging findings such as increased signal intensity on long b value trace EPIs and/or suspicious contrast kinetics at DCE are helpful, as these latter findings are not expected in the normal CZ (Fig. 2). Ultimately targeted biopsy or MRI follow-up may be necessary for suspicious areas in the CZ.

The anterior fibromuscular stroma (AFMS) is a normal structure at the extreme anterior midline of the prostate gland, which is inseparable from the surrounding normal prostatic stroma [25, 29]. The AFMS contains no glandular tissue and is composed of widely spaced smooth muscle cells. It appears homogeneously hypointense on T2W MRI and because of this inherent low T2W SI will appear as low SI on ADC maps. Differentiation of the AFMS from anterior cancer is established by noting the midline location, well-defined margins, lack of true diffusion restriction (absence of high SI on b≥1000 mm²/s EPI) and a benign progressive type 1 enhancement pattern at DCE (Fig. 3) [25, 30]. PCa arising in the extreme anterior prostate can resemble the AFMS and in many cases anterior tumors can extend up to or invade the AFMS. Both lesions are low SI on T2W; however, anterior PCa is more lenticular or polygonal in shape, has ill-defined or smudged borders, and the bulk of the lesion tends to be off midline (Fig. 4) [31]. The use of functional imaging sequences is contributory (Fig. 4) [30]. DWI increases accuracy for detection of anterior cancers because anterior tumours will be of low SI on ADC because of true restricted diffusion, demonstrating increased SI on trace b≥1000 mm²/s EPI [32]. The utility of DCE in the TZ and anterior prostate is controversial [33]; however, authors have demonstrated more aggressive enhancement patterns in anterior PCa [34–37]. In our experience, DCE can be beneficial to discriminate anterior PCa from AFMS; however, overlap with stromal BPH limits its utility in the TZ (discussed later) [35].

(2) Post-biopsy haemorrhage can mimic PZ PCa on T2W MRI

Detection of PCa on T2W is predicated on the ability to discriminate low T2 SI tumour from the normal adjacent high T2 SI PZ [15, 38–40]. The glandular tissue of the PZ contains high concentrations of citrate, which is a natural anticoagulant; therefore, post-procedural haemorrhage is commonly observed at MRI after prostate biopsies and can persist for up to 4 months after the procedure [41]. Areas of post-biopsy haemorrhage are characteristically hypointense on T2W MRI in up to 80 % of cases and can mimic PCa [41] (Fig. 5). This pitfall is easily avoided by cross-referencing T2W to pre-contrast T1W imaging because areas of haemorrhage will also be characteristically hyperintense on T1W (Fig. 5).

Many institutions continue to defer prostate MRI studies until 3–8 weeks have passed after the biopsy to reduce the amount of post-biopsy haemorrhage and facilitate interpretation. With the advent of functional imaging sequences post-biopsy haemorrhage is, in our experience, much less problematic. Areas of tumour have been shown to be reliably differentiated from haemorrhage using DWI, and DCE analysis can be interpreted through image subtraction [42] (Fig. 5). Moreover, because PCa contains less citrate than the normal PZ,

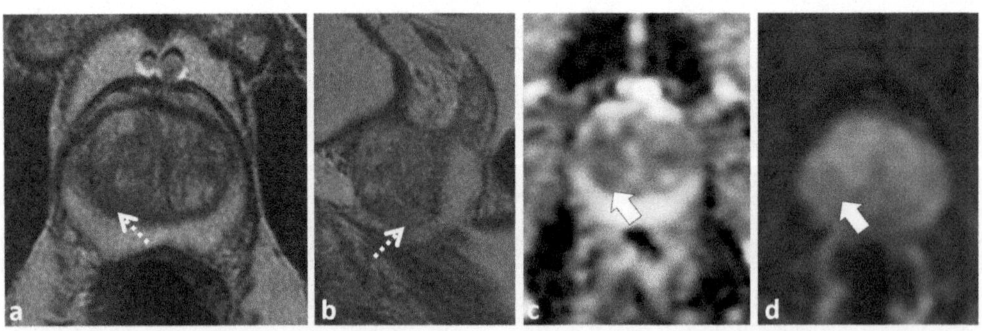

Fig. 2 A 51-year-old patient with low-volume Gleason score 3+3=6 at non-targeted TRUS-guided biopsy. MP-MRI was performed at onset of active surveillance (AS) to exclude higher grade tumour. Axial (**a**) and sagittal (**b**) T2W images demonstrate an ill-defined ovoid lesion of low T2 SI at the junction of the right PZ and transition zone (TZ) (dotted *white arrow*) along the course of the surgical capsule. Axial ADC map image (**c**) at the same level demonstrates corresponding low SI (*white arrow*). This area was considered suspicious for tumour. Targeted TRUS biopsy was performed and yielded only normal prostate tissue. The area did not change on follow-up MP-MRI and represents asymmetry of the normal central zone. In retrospect, corresponding b1000 mm²/s trace EPI (**d**) did not show increased signal (*white arrow*) in this area

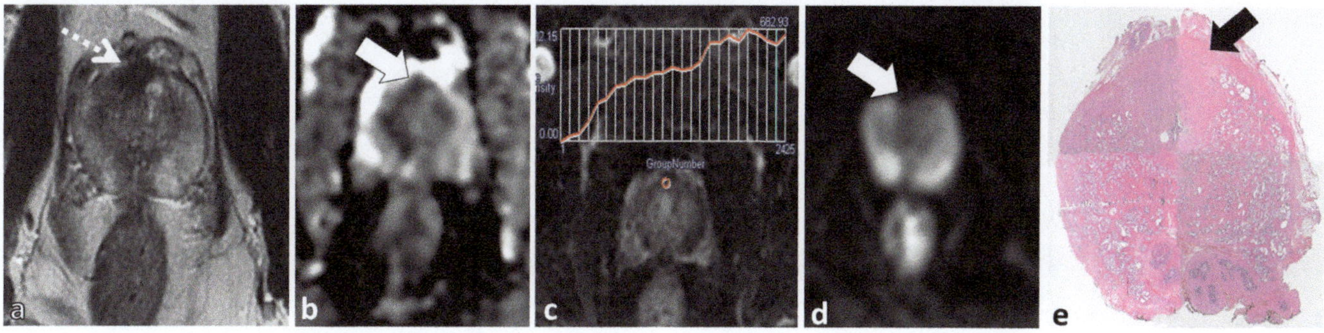

Fig. 3 A 54-year-old patient with elevated and rising PSA. Axial T2W TSE (**a**) demonstrates a low SI focus in the anterior midline (*dotted arrow*) with corresponding low SI (*white arrow*) on the axial ADC map (**b**). This area was reported as suspicious for tumour. Repeat non-targeted biopsies of the PZ revealed Gleason score 3+4=7 tumour in the right PZ (not shown) and the patient underwent radical prostatectomy (RP). The structure highlighted on MRI is the normal anterior fibromuscular stroma (AFMS); note: characteristic midline anterior location on axial T2 (**a**) and benign progressive enhancement on DCE (**c**). Also note that low SI on the ADC (**b**) map is due to inherently low T2 SI rather than restricted diffusion; there is a lack of increased SI on trace b1000 mm²/s EPI (**d**). Whole-mount histopathology image of the RP specimen (**e**) demonstrates the AFMS (*black arrow*), which is predominantly composed of smooth muscle that blends with the overlying prostate stroma

areas that are devoid of haemorrhage in the PZ after biopsy may actually highlight the tumour on T1W imaging ("haemorrhage exclusion sign") [42]. This imaging finding has recently been shown to have >95 % positive predictive value for tumour localisation when combined with characteristic imaging findings at T2W MRI [42].

(3) **Benign prostatic hyperplasia (BPH) resembles TZ PCa**

BPH is extremely common in the TZ and its prevalence increases with age. BPH can be nodular and TZ nodules are commonly encountered at MP-MRI [35], and nodular BPH may mimic TZ PCa [25]. Nodular BPH is categorised into three main subtypes: glandular, stromal and mixed.

Glandular BPH is characterised histologically by hyperplasia of glandular tissue with papillary buds, infoldings and cysts. Glandular BPH is readily differentiated from TZ PCa at MP-MRI [35] and typical features include a well-circumscribed, sharply demarcated and rounded shape, a continuous low T2W SI rim, increased T2W SI often with cystic change, low SI on long≥1000 mm²/s *b* value EPI, "T2 shine-through" on ADC maps and benign/progressive/type I contrast kinetics with a low transfer constant on DCE (Fig. 6) [25, 35].

The presence of increased smooth muscle, lymphocytes and ducts (not associated with prostatitis) and reduced elastic tissue characterises stromal BPH at histopathology. Stromal BPH nodules can be difficult to differentiate from TZ PCa [35] (Figs. 6 and 7). Stromal BPH is typically of low T2W SI, similar to TZ PCa. Stromal BPH is also of low signal intensity on ADC maps because of both inherently low T2W SI and true restricted diffusion (due to compact cellularity) and may or may not have increased SI on long b≥1000 mm²/s trace EPI. Furthermore, ADC values in stromal BPH are low and overlap with TZ PCa [25, 35]. DCE is limited to differentiate stromal BPH from TZ PCa, because enhancement patterns of stromal BPH overlap with TZ PCa [33–35]. Previous authors have reported lower ADC and higher K-trans values in TZ PCa compared to stromal BPH,

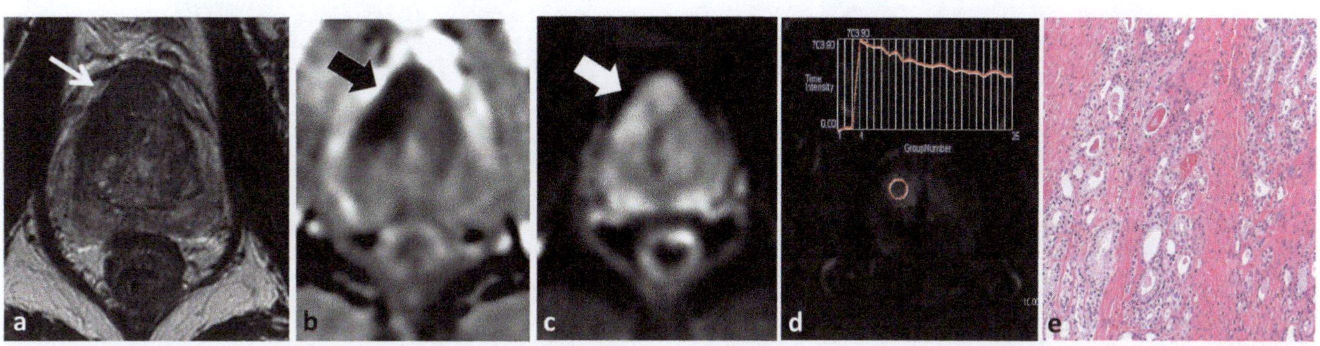

Fig. 4 A 50-year-old patient with rising PSA and a typical anterior tumour involving the right side of the gland. Axial T2W TSE (**a**) demonstrates an amorphous, off midline, lenticular-shaped, ill-defined low T2 SI region (*white arrow*) with low SI (*black arrow*) on the ADC (**b**) map due to restricted diffusion (note increased SI on trace b1000 mm²/s EPI (*white arrow* in **c**) and type III contrast curve kinetics on DCE (**d**). A targeted TRUS biopsy was performed and confirmed Gleason score 4+3=7 tumour anteriorly. Corresponding microscopic image from TRUS biopsy (**e**) demonstrates Gleason pattern 4 tumour

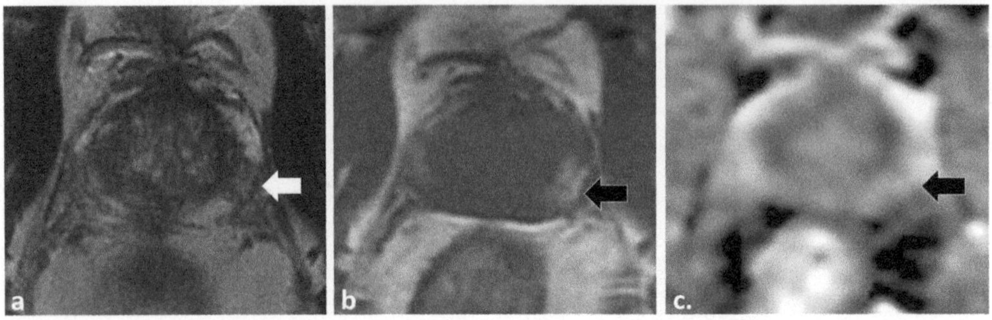

Fig. 5 A 58-year-old male patient with Gleason score 3+3=6 tumour imaged with MP-MRI because of rising PSA. On axial T2W TSE (**a**) there is a low SI focus in the left mid PZ (*white arrow*), which could represent peripheral zone cancer. Corresponding axial T1W TSE (**b**) demonstrates increased T1 SI (*black arrow*) in keeping with post-biopsy haemorrhage. Axial ADC map (**c**) does not reveal the lesion (*black arrow*), which was readily diagnosed as post-biopsy haemorrhage

but substantial overlaps exist (Figs. 6 and 7) [35]. Other differentiating features that are more suggestive of stromal BPH include well-defined sharply demarcated margins, a continuous low T2W SI rim and a rounded shape (Figs. 6 and 7) [31, 33].

At histopathology and MP-MRI, it is more common to identify a TZ BPH nodule with features of both glandular and stromal BPH. Typically one pattern (glandular or stromal) will predominate; however, features of both types of BPH can be seen within the same nodule, which can further complicate the diagnosis. In cases of mixed BPH, a combination of imaging features of glandular and stromal BPH are encountered [31]. Usually, the presence of increased T2W SI and cystic change (from glandular BPH) within a lesion are reassuring findings of BPH (Fig. 7) since these findings are rarely encountered in PCa.

Chesnais et al. previously demonstrated that the majority of TZ cancers involve the anterior and apical third of the gland [43]. At histopathology, Bouye et al. previously demonstrated that anterior tumours tend to grow anteriorly and invade the anterior fibromuscular stroma but rarely extend to the posterior PZ [44]. It should be noted that in some instances, when there is uncertainty at MP-MRI regarding the diagnosis of TZ PCa versus stromal BPH due to overlap in imaging features, a targeted biopsy or follow-up MP-MRI may be suggested (Fig. 6).

(4) **Acute and chronic prostatitis mimics PCa**

Acute bacterial prostatitis (ABP) is commonly encountered in clinical practice and often managed conservatively without imaging or surgical intervention [38]. When patients with ABP are imaged in the acute setting, prostatitis can mimic PCa at MP-MRI, demonstrating low SI on T2WI, restricted diffusion [45] and enhancement patterns that overlap with PCa [25] (Fig. 8). Although PCa has been reported to demonstrate more well-defined borders and nodular appearance compared to prostatitis and lower ADC values [45, 46], aside from the presence of abscess formation in prostatitis, differentiation is mainly based on clinical grounds.

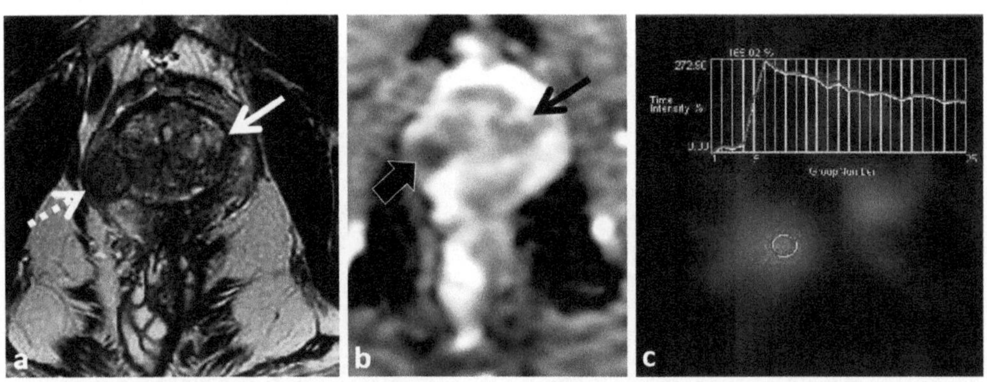

Fig. 6 A 47-year-old patient post-total colectomy for ulcerative colitis and elevated PSA. MP-MRI was performed to evaluate for potential tumour and to plan a biopsy. Axial T2W TSE (**a**) image demonstrates enlargement of the central gland (TZ) consistent with BPH. There is a well-circumscribed, round, mixed but predominantly increased T2W SI nodule with internal cystic change (*white arrow*) and a predominantly homogeneously low T2 SI nodule at the junction of the right middle PZ and central gland (*dotted arrow*). The larger nodule demonstrates T2 shine-through on the ADC map (*black arrow* in **b**) and is characteristic of glandular BPH. The other nodule demonstrates restricted diffusion (*thick black arrow* in **b**) and type III kinetics at DCE (**c**). A diagnosis of prostate cancer was suggested. Targeted biopsy revealed normal prostatic tissue and stromal BPH. Follow-up MRI (not shown) demonstrated no change and the PSA was stable. In retrospect, the nodule is round, well-circumscribed and demonstrates a complete low T2 SI rim (**a**), findings that are more in keeping with stromal BPH rather than cancer

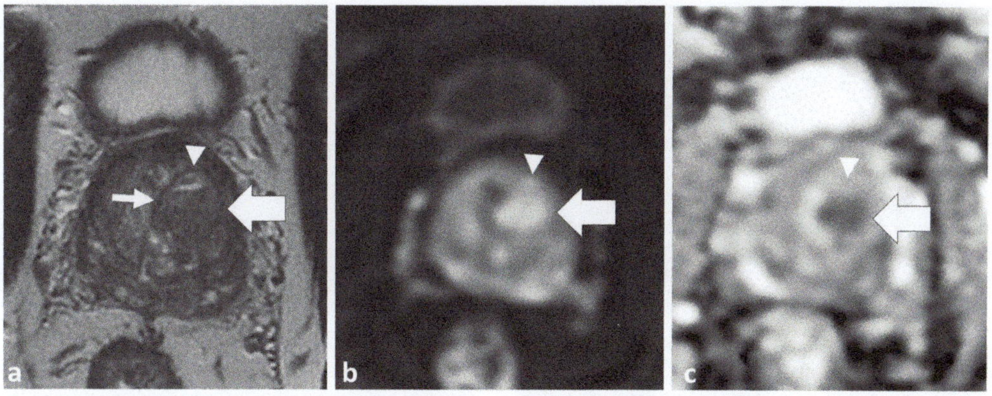

Fig. 7 A 58-year-old patient with low-volume, low Gleason score 3+3=6 tumour in the right mid-peripheral zone undergoing MRI prior to repeat biopsy because of rising PSA. Axial T2W TSE (**a**) image demonstrates a low T2 SI nodule in the left TZ (*thick white arrow*). The nodule is predominantly homogeneously of low T2W SI but demonstrates a small focus of cystic change anteriorly (*arrowhead*). Note that the nodule is round and demonstrates a continuous low T2W SI rim (*thin white arrow*). The nodule demonstrates restricted diffusion, increased SI on trace b1000 mm²/s EPI (**b**) and low SI on the ADC map (**c**) (*thick white arrows*). Note that cystic change demonstrates T2 shine-through (*arrowhead*). Imaging findings are characteristic of a mixed but predominantly stromal BPH nodule

Granulomatous prostatitis (GP) is a benign inflammatory entity that may also be indistinguishable from PCa at MP-MRI, demonstrating low SI on T2W, restricted diffusion and suspicious enhancement at DCE [47]. Moreover, granulomatous prostatitis can involve the periprostatic fat or seminal vesicles, mimicking extraprostatic spread of PCa (Fig. 9). With the correct clinical history [e.g., previous bacille Calmette-Guerin therapy for bladder cancer, tuberculous prostatitis or previous intervention such as transurethral resection of the prostate (TURP)], granulomatous prostatitis may be favoured over PCa [25]; however, histological confirmation is often required [47].

In the chronic setting, areas of prostatitis can mimic PCa because they will demonstrate low T2W SI [48]. Functional imaging techniques can be useful to differentiate areas of chronic prostatitis from cancer (Fig. 10) but there is overlap in imaging features [49, 50] and targeted biopsy or MP-MRI

Fig. 8 Acute prostatitis in a 46-year-old patient with elevated PSA. Axial T2W TSE (**a**) demonstrates an amorphous area of low T2 SI (*dotted arrow*) in the left middle PZ with corresponding low SI on ADC map (*black arrow* in **b**) due to restricted diffusion, note increased SI on trace b1000 mm²/s EPI (*white arrow* in **c**). There is an indeterminate type II contrast curve (plateau kinetics) on DCE in (**d**). A differential diagnosis of prostatitis or cancer was provided, and biopsy or follow-up was suggested. The patient had typical findings of acute bacterial prostatitis clinically and was treated with antibiotics with normalisation of PSA post therapy

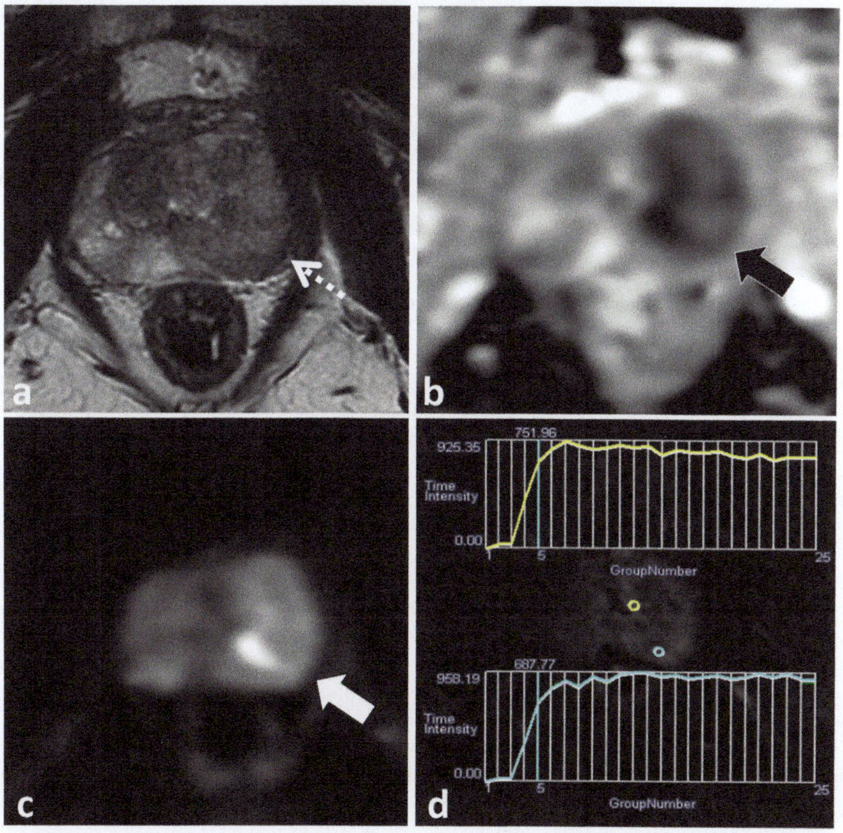

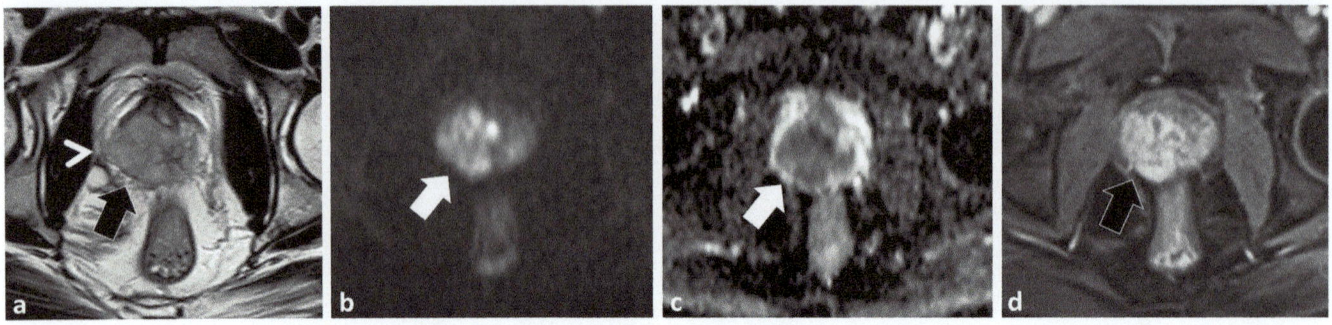

Fig. 9 A 64-year-old patient with rising PSA and history of recurrent urothelial cell carcinoma of the urinary bladder treated with intra-vesical BCG therapy. Axial T2W image (**a**) demonstrates a large mass infiltrating throughout the right prostate (*black arrow*) and breaching the prostate capsule laterally (*arrowhead*) consistent with extra-prostatic spread. Axial b1000 mm²/s (**b**) and ADC map (**c**) demonstrate marked restricted diffusion (*white arrows*) and axial image from DCE shows marked early mass-like hyper-enhancement (type III curve was depicted and is not shown). TRUS biopsy was performed and histology was compatible with diffuse granulomatous prostatitis

follow-up of the suspicion region may be considered depending on the level of suspicion for tumour [47].

(5) **Ductal variant adenocarcinoma may be occult on T2W MRI**

PCa is divided into the most common acinar adenocarcinoma and less common non-acinar subtypes. Ductal adenocarcinoma (DCa) is an aggressive variant of PCa and is the most common of the non-acinar subtypes [51] with a reported incidence of 0.5–6 % [52]. DCa is associated with higher rates of positive surgical margins, extraprostatic extension, vascular invasion, seminal vesicle invasion and metastases [53, 54]. A diagnosis of DCa at needle biopsy requires definitive therapy and is considered an absolute contraindication for AS [55, 56]. Schieda et al. recently demonstrated that DCa is of increased SI on T2W MRI, which can render the tumour occult [39]; however, the same authors demonstrated that DCa resembles Gleason score≥7 or higher tumour on DWI and DCE [57]. Therefore, in a lesion with aggressive imaging findings on DWI/DCE and paradoxical increased T2W SI, DCa should be considered [57] (Fig. 11).

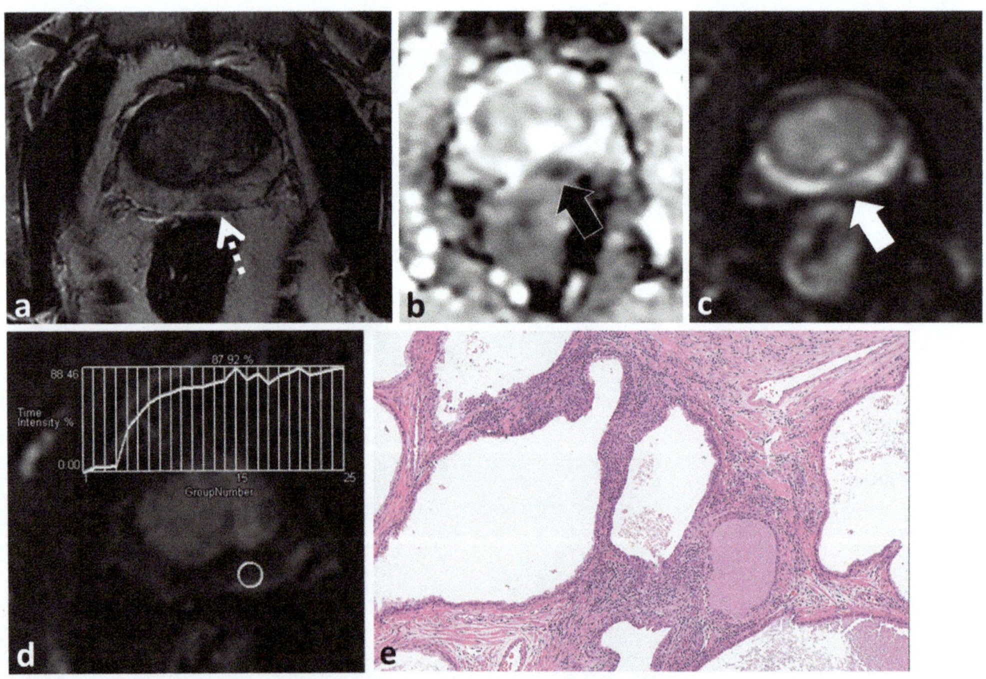

Fig. 10 A 64-year-old patient with Gleason score 3+3=6 in <5 % of one core in the left middle PZ underwent MRI prior to enrolment into active surveillance. Axial T2W TSE image (**a**) demonstrates a low T2 SI focus in the left PZ (*dotted arrow*) with low SI on ADC (*black arrow* in **b**). Based on these findings a diagnosis of potential higher grade tumour was suggested and a repeat biopsy was performed. Saturation biopsies through the left mid PZ revealed only normal prostatic tissue and areas of chronic prostatitis. In retrospect, trace b1000 mm²/s EPI demonstrates low SI (*white arrow* in **c**), which indicates that there is no restricted diffusion in this area. Similarly, there is a benign progressive type I enhancement curve on DCE (**d**), which further argues against a higher grade tumour. Corresponding histopathology slide (**e**) demonstrates areas of chronic inflammation

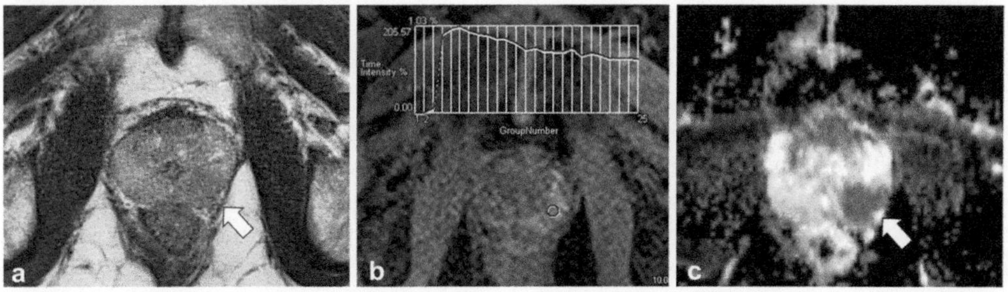

Fig. 11 A 59-year-old patient with Gleason 3+4=7 cancer in the left middle PZ on TRUS biopsy underwent MP-MRI for staging. Axial T2W TSE image shows a subtle lesion in the left middle PZ (*white arrow* in **b**) with type III kinetics on DCE (**b**) and profound restricted diffusion on ADC map (*white arrow* in **c**). Typically with conventional acinar adenocarcinoma T2W signal intensity mirrors findings on ADC map, the discordant findings with only minimally decreased T2W signal and profound restricted diffusion can be seen in ductal variant adenocarcinoma. Final histopathology after RP was Gleason score 4+4=8 tumour with dominant ductal component

Technical pitfalls

(1) **T2W motion correction with radial acquisition obscures some PCa**

As discussed, detection of tumour in the PZ on T2W MRI is based on differentiation of low T2W SI tumour from the high T2W glandular tissue [15, 38–40]. In the TZ, T2W imaging is now recognised as the most important pulse sequence for detection of PCa because of overlap between TZ cancer and stromal BPH on functional imaging (see Interpretive pitfalls, stromal BPH) [58]. T2W imaging is typically performed using turbo/fast spin-echo techniques [39]. Motion correction with radial acquisition (BLADE, Siemens Healthcare, Malvern, PA, USA; PROPELLER, General Electric Healthcare, Milwaukee, WI, USA) sequences are popular for pelvic imaging because they correct for in-plane rotation and translational artefacts and have been shown to result in improved overall image quality when compared to conventional spin echo [59, 60]. A disadvantage of these sequences is decreased image contrast compared to conventional spin echo [59]. Recently, Rosenkrantz et al. demonstrated that a minority of PCa foci may be obscured at T2W MRI when BLADE/PROPELLER is used compared to conventional spin echo [61] (Fig. 12).

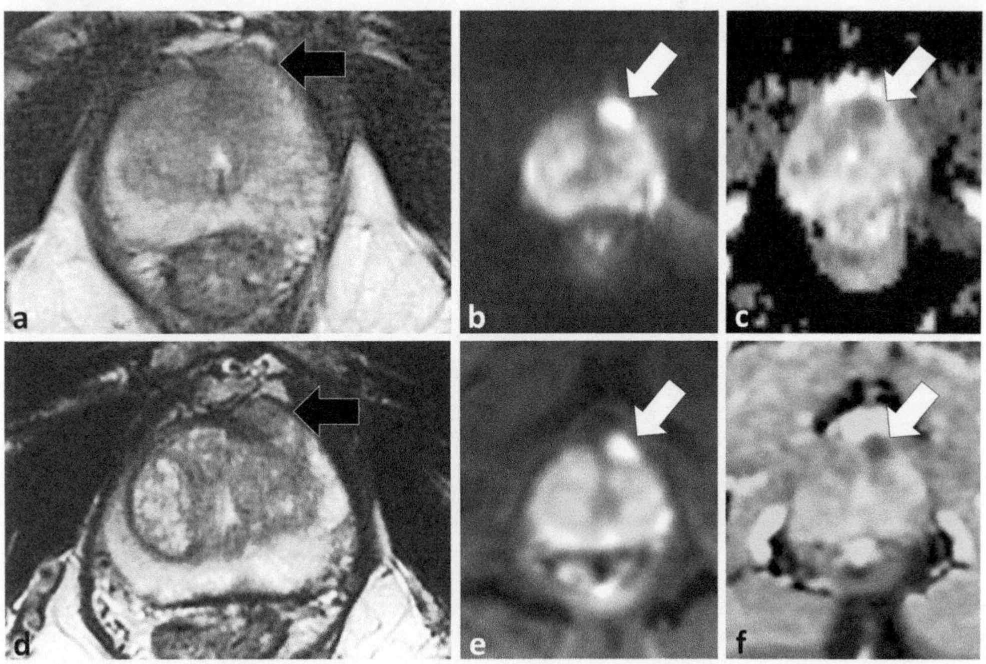

Fig. 12 A 63-year-old patient with elevated PSA and previously negative non-targeted TRUS-guided biopsy with persistent clinical suspicion of prostate cancer underwent MP-MRI in two separate sessions within 3 months demonstrating the loss of contrast with BLADE/PROPELLER imaging. Axial T2W BLADE **a**, b1000 mm²/s EPI **b** and ADC map **c** demonstrate a suspicious focus of restricted diffusion in the left middle anterior horn of the PZ (*white arrows*), which is not visible on axial T2W BLADE (*black arrow* in **a**). Repeat examination performed using T2W FSE (**d**) reveals a T2 hypointense nodule in the same location (*black arrow* in **d**) with persistent restricted diffusion (*white arrows* in **e** and **f**)

(2) **Visual/quantitative analysis of DWI for tumour detection/grading is complex**

DWI improves the detection of cancer foci in the PZ and TZ, and ADC values derived from DWI have been repeatedly shown to inversely correlate with Gleason grade of PCa [18, 38]. DWI is the single best imaging test for analysis of the PZ and is used in conjunction with T2W MRI for evaluation of TZ lesions [58, 62]. The visual analysis of DWI must include assessment of trace EPI and should not rely solely upon review of the derived apparent diffusion coefficient (ADC) map. Structures that are inherently of low T2W SI will appear dark on the ADC map because of an inherently low T2W SI (T2 "black-hole" effect) and not from true restricted diffusion (Figs. 1 and 2). Review of trace EPI is critical to avoid this common pitfall because these structures will not appear bright on long (b≥1000 mm²/s) EPI (Figs. 1 and 2). Conversely, PCa (and as discussed some stromal BPH nodules) is of low SI on ADC and will appear bright on the long (b≥1000 mm²/s) EPI (Figs. 3, 6 and 7). The use of longer b values (b≥1000 mm²/s) facilitates the detection of cancer foci compared to the benign prostatic tissues [63, 64]. Visual analysis of ADC may be further limited by automatic display settings and can result in the failure to detect PCa or an underestimation of tumour grade if not displayed properly (Fig. 13). A previous study demonstrated that by using a window width=1.650 and level=1.675×10–6 mm²/s for display of ADC, higher grade tumours were more likely to appear dark (Fig. 13) [65].

It has been demonstrated repeatedly that ADC values inversely correlate to PCa grade [18]. The use of ADC values across MR systems is problematic because of differences related to magnet strength, vendor system and selection of differing b values [57]. Furthermore, a variety of methods to quantify ADC have been described including single region of interest measurement versus whole lesion analysis and mean, median and complex histogram analysis of ADC. Application of quantitative ADC thresholds may be limited by these factors. A recent study demonstrated that the use of an ADC ratio (normalised to adjacent normal PZ) provided a better inter-scanner comparison than the absolute ADC value [57]. Mean ADC values may also be limited due to the variable composition of prostate cancers and when comparing intermediate prostate cancers (Gleason score 3+4=7 vs. 4+3=7) [66] and studies have demonstrated that the use of the low percentile ADC may be a better reflector of the Gleason score [67, 68]. Regardless of the method used, due to differences across systems, at present, we suggest that the use of quantitative ADC in clinical practice should be applied carefully, derived and validated on an institutional basis.

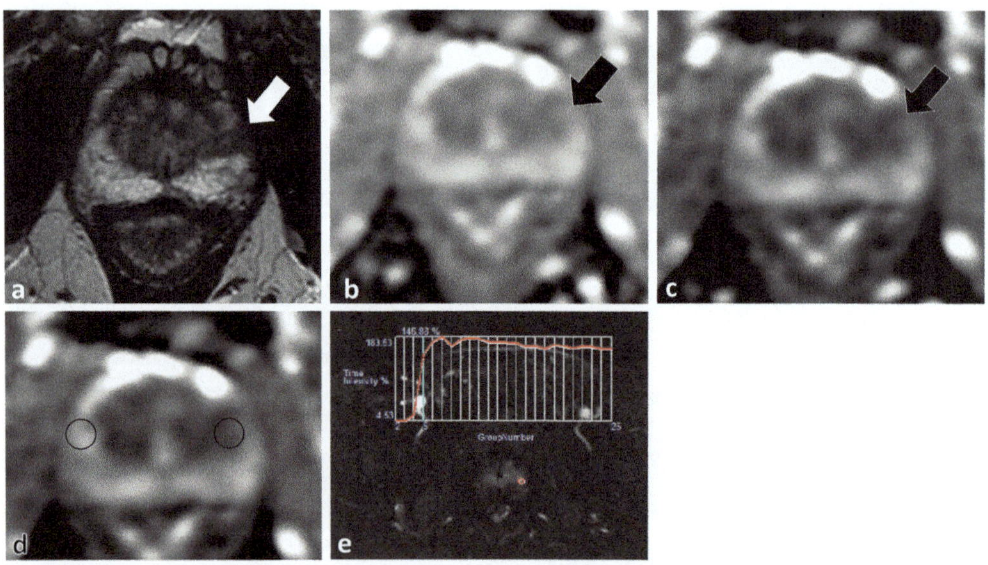

Fig. 13 A 55-year-old patient with low-volume Gleason score 3+3=6 tumour at TRUS biopsy in the left apical PZ underwent MRI prior to consideration for potential AS. Axial T2W TSE image (**a**) demonstrates a low T2 SI focus in the left apical PZ (*white arrow*). Axial ADC map displayed with automatic windowing/levelling shows minimal decreased SI (*black arrow* in **b**). These findings could be considered typical for a 3+3=6 cancer. With modified display of the ADC map using previously validated settings (width=1.650 and level=1.675×10–6 mm²/s) the nodule (*black arrow* in **c**) is noted to be of lower SI than initially displayed in (**b**). Using quantitative data, the ADC value obtained within the tumour (**d**) was 1.462×10^{-3} mm²/s, which would also be considered to be of low (Gleason score 6) grade using previously reported thresholds. Comparing ADC values across systems is challenging due to a lack of standardization, and an ADC ratio has been previously proposed as a better metric to compare ADC. An ADC value from the contralateral normal PZ obtained at the same level was 2.000×10^{-3} mm²/s, which yields an ADC ratio of 0.73, which would be compatible with a Gleason score≥7 tumour based on previously published thresholds. Corresponding DCE image (**e**) from the same level demonstrated a focal enhancing nodule with a type III contrast curve. Based on the imaging findings, a repeat TRUS-guided biopsy was performed, which demonstrated Gleason pattern 4 in the left apical PZ

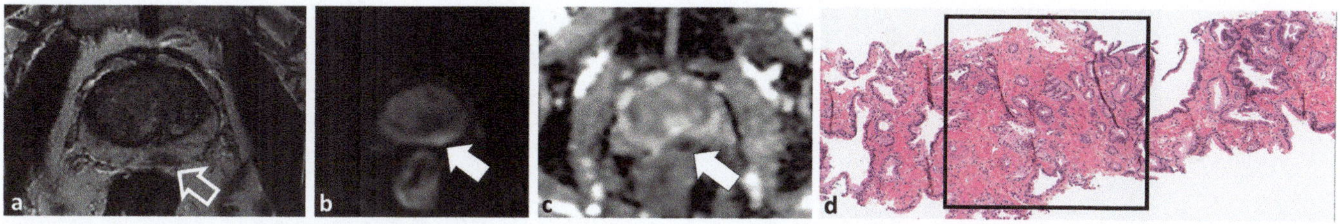

Fig. 14 A 59-year-old patient with low-volume Gleason score 3+3=6 at non-targeted TRUS biopsy underwent MP-MRI to exclude clinically significant cancer after an increase in PSA. Axial T2W TSE image (**a**) demonstrates a low T2 SI focus in the left PZ (*open white arrow*) with restricted diffusion; note increased SI on trace b1000 mm²/s EPI and low SI on ADC (white arrows in **b** and **c**, respectively). Based on the MRI and clinical findings a diagnosis of potential higher grade tumour was suggested and a targeted repeat biopsy was performed. At time of repeat biopsy, which used cognitive registration of MP-MRI and TRUS data, no lesion could be identified at TRUS. Only one core biopsy through the left medial mid peripheral zone sextant was performed. Microscopic image from repeat TRUS-guided biopsy (**d**) demonstrates Gleason pattern 3 tumour. Continued in Fig. 14

(3) **DCE lacks standardisation and is limited in the TZ**

DCE improves the detection of PCa and DCE parameters correlate with PCa grade [69–71]. Currently, there is no established interpretation criteria for DCE analysis which varies from simple visual analysis to semi-quantitative analysis to full quantitative pharmacokinetic modelling [72]. A recent study demonstrated that DCE is underutilised in clinical practice compared to DWI and that semi-quantitative and quantitative analyses were not commonly used [72]. In the revised PI-RADS v2.0 guidelines, DCE analysis has been modified from semi-quantitative curve analysis to a simple visual analysis [58].

Moreover, DCE is very limited for the detection and grading of cancers in the transition zone because of significant overlap with stromal BPH (Fig. 7). Analysis of potential tumour foci in the transition zone should preferentially favour T2W and DWI over DCE. It is currently recognised that the utility of DCE in clinical practice is mainly as a confirmatory sequence for PZ lesions [58]; however, further studies are required to determine the value of DCE in PCa.

(4) **Targeted biopsy of MR-detected lesions using TRUS-guidance is challenging**

MP-MRI for PCa has transformed practice, but has created new challenges. Obtaining accurate histological correlation

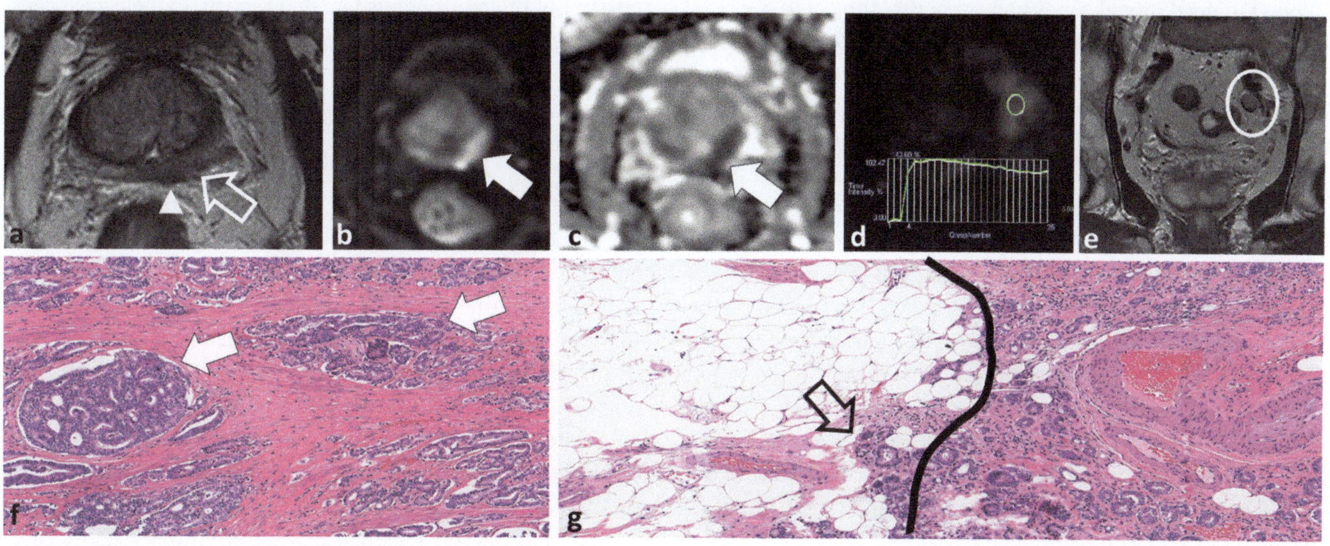

Fig. 15 Although only low-volume Gleason score 3+3=6 was again noted at repeat TRUS biopsy (Fig. 13), a follow-up MP-MRI was performed 3 months later because of interval doubling of PSA to re-evaluate for a focus of higher grade cancer. Axial T2W TSE image (**a**) demonstrates that the small low T2 SI focus in the left PZ has grown substantially (*open white arrow*) with bulging and nodular extension into the peri-prostatic fat (*arrowhead*), which was reported as representing extra-prostatic extension. The lesion again demonstrates restricted diffusion; note increased SI on trace b1000 mm²/s EPI and low SI on ADC (*white arrows* in **b** and **c**, respectively) and demonstrated an aggressive type III contrast curve on DCE (**d**). In the interval, a malignant-appearing lymph node developed along the left pelvic sidewall (**e**). Based on these findings a diagnosis of high-grade tumour with extra-prostatic extension and metastatic adenopathy was provided. The patient underwent RP based on the imaging findings, he declined a repeat biopsy because of previous urosepsis related to prior TRUS biopsy. Corresponding microscopic images (**f** and **g**) demonstrate Gleason pattern 4 tumour (*white arrows* in **f**) and extra-prostatic extension of tumour (*open arrow*), which is beyond the prostate capsule (*black line*) and into the peri-prostatic fat (**g**)

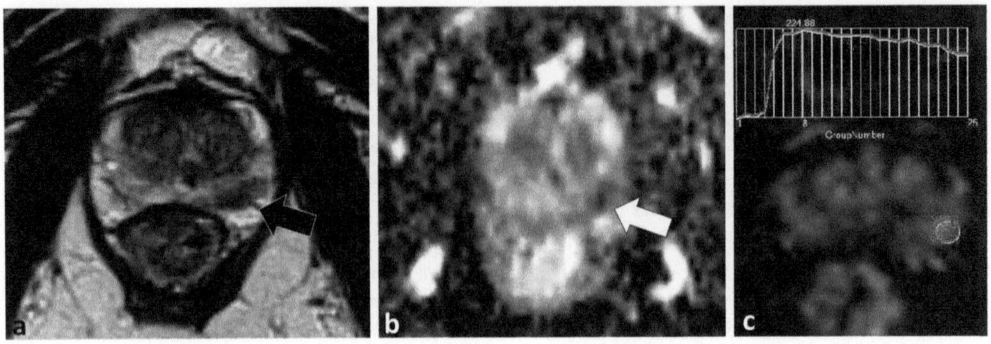

Fig. 16 A 63-year-old patient underwent MP-MRI prior to routine repeat biopsies as part of his active surveillance protocol. Axial T2W TSE (**a**), axial ADC map (**b**) and semi-quantitative contrast curve derived from DCE (**c**) demonstrate a focal low T2W SI lesion (*black arrow*) with restricted diffusion (*white arrow*) and type III kinetics in the left middle peripheral zone. At repeat targeted biopsy using cognitive registration, no corresponding lesion could be identified. With a priori knowledge of the location of the lesion at MP-MRI, the TRUS operator performed three core needle biopsies through the left middle lateral and two core needle biopsies through the left middle medial PZ sextants. Results after targeted biopsies were Gleason 4+3=7 tumour with two out of three core biopsies in the left middle lateral PZ sextant

from lesions detected at MP-MRI may be challenging. MRI guided biopsy is accurate; however, this technique is limited by cost, availability of and access to MRI, prolonged procedure times and patient discomfort [8]. The use of TRUS guidance for biopsy of MP-MRI-detected lesions is currently a preferred option.

Using existing technology, so-called cognitive registration (CR) is performed. CR requires the TRUS operator to mentally integrate MP-MRI with real-time TRUS, identify suspicious MR lesions and, with TRUS guidance, target those lesions for biopsy. Published data regarding the applicability of CR are limited to institutional series and are highly subject to operator experience [8]. TRUS may be limited for the detection of tumours in the PZ and is also limited for assessment of the TZ and the anterior gland in many patients with enlarged glands due to poor ultrasound beam penetration. A failure to recognise the limitations of TRUS when performing CR biopsies can result in a failure to adequately sample suspicious areas on MP-MRI and ultimately result in delayed diagnosis and therapy for clinically significant PCa (Figs. 14 and 15). In our experience, cognitively registered TRUS biopsy of MP-MRI-detected lesions can be successful, provided that the TRUS operator recognises the limitations of TRUS for demonstrating a corresponding lesion to that seen on MP-MRI. It is not uncommon for a lesion detected in the PZ or TZ on mp-MRI to be sonographically occult on TRUS and, in these instances, by oversampling the corresponding location using anatomic landmarks, the diagnostic yield can be significantly improved (Fig. 16).

The use of Fusion software (which automatically integrates MP-MRI data with real-time 3D TRUS images) provides an alternative to cognitive registration [8]. Fusion software is not without its own limitations including mainly errors in fusion that relate to the spatial deformation of the prostate at TRUS compared to mp-MRI [8]. Moreover, this technology is expensive and at the moment is available in a few specialised centres, although availability is increasing. Studies comparing cognitively registered targeted TRUS biopsy to software fused targeted TRUS biopsy are lacking and have shown mixed results. While several studies have shown no difference between CR and Fusion software [73, 74], other studies have shown an improvement in the detection rate of cancer using fusion software systems [75, 76].

It is critical to emphasise that when a targeted TRUS-guided biopsy performed for a suspicious lesion detected on MP-MRI (using either cognitive registration or fusion software) is negative, the MP-MRI should be reviewed in the context of the biopsy results and other clinical factors in order to consider the possibility of an erroneous targeted biopsy. In these instances, repeat MRI or targeted biopsies can be contemplated.

Conclusion

In conclusion, MP-MRI has become a critical component for patients being considered for or enrolled in active surveillance protocols for the management of low-grade and low-volume prostate cancers. MP-MRI is a proven imaging modality that can detect clinically significant foci of prostate cancer with high degrees of accuracy; the high negative predictive value of MP-MRI is particularly well suited for the AS of PCa. A number of pitfalls, both interpretive and technical, may be encountered at MP-MRI of the prostate and a failure to recognise these pitfalls in the AS population can result in suboptimal patient care. Targeted biopsies of MP-MR-detected lesions poses a new challenge and opportunity in clinical practice. The limitations of TRUS-guidance for lesion detection during targeted biopsies should be acknowledged in order to improve the diagnostic yield of targeted biopsies. A thorough understanding of these MP-MRI pitfalls is important for the MR practitioner involved in the management of prostate cancer.

References

1. National Comprehensive Cancer Network NCCN (2012) Clinical practice guidelines in oncology: prostate cancer. Fort Washington, PA. Available via http://www.nccn.com/files/cancer-guidelines/prostate/index.html#/1. Accessed Sept. 13 2013
2. Prostate Cancer Canada (2014) Prostate cancer Canada network. Toronto, ON Canada. Available via http://prostatecancer.ca. Accessed Sept. 2014
3. European Association of Urology (EAU) (2012) Guidelines on prostate cancer. Arnhem, The Netherlands. Available via http://www.uroweb.org/gls/pdf/08%20Prostate%20Cancer_LR%20March%2013th%202012.pdf
4. Thomsen FB, Brasso K, Klotz LH, Roder MA, Berg KD, Iversen P (2014) Active surveillance for clinically localized prostate cancer–a systematic review. J Surg Oncol 109:830–835
5. Heidenreich A, Bellmunt J, Bolla M et al (2011) EAU guidelines on prostate cancer. Part 1: screening, diagnosis, and treatment of clinically localised disease. Eur Urol 59:61–71
6. Cancer Care Ontario CCO (2012) Prostate cancer treatment pathway. Toronto, ON, Canada. Available via http://www.cancercare.on.ca/common/pages/UserFile.aspx?fileID=298448. Accessed Sept. 2014
7. National Institutes of Health NIH (2011) Role of Active surveillance in the management of men with localized prostate cancer. Bethesda, Maryland. Available via http://consensus.nih.gov/2011/prostate.htm. Accessed Sept. 2014
8. Rothwax JT, George AK, Wood BJ, Pinto PA (2014) Multiparametric MRI in biopsy guidance for prostate cancer: fusion-guided. Biomed Res Int 2014:439171
9. Eskew LA, Bare RL, McCullough DL (1997) Systematic 5 region prostate biopsy is superior to sextant method for diagnosing carcinoma of the prostate. J Urol 157:199–202, **discussion 202–193**
10. Presti JC Jr, O'Dowd GJ, Miller MC, Mattu R, Veltri RW (2003) Extended peripheral zone biopsy schemes increase cancer detection rates and minimize variance in prostate specific antigen and age related cancer rates: results of a community multi-practice study. J Urol 169:125–129
11. Babaian RJ, Toi A, Kamoi K et al (2000) A comparative analysis of sextant and an extended 11-core multisite directed biopsy strategy. J Urol 163:152–157
12. Noguchi M, Stamey TA, McNeal JE, Yemoto CM (2001) Relationship between systematic biopsies and histological features of 222 radical prostatectomy specimens: lack of prediction of tumor significance for men with nonpalpable prostate cancer. J Urol 166: 104–109, **discussion 109–110**
13. Bott SR, Young MP, Kellett MJ, Parkinson MC (2002) Anterior prostate cancer: is it more difficult to diagnose? BJU Int 89:886–889
14. Eberhardt SC, Carter S, Casalino DD et al (2013) ACR appropriateness criteria prostate cancer–pretreatment detection, staging, and surveillance. J Am Coll Radiol 10:83–92
15. Barentsz JO, Richenberg J, Clements R et al (2012) ESUR prostate MR guidelines 2012. Eur Radiol 22:746–757
16. Hamoen EH, de Rooij M, Witjes JA, Barentsz JO, Rovers MM (2014) Use of the prostate imaging reporting and data system (PI-RADS) for prostate cancer detection with multiparametric magnetic resonance imaging: a diagnostic meta-analysis. Eur Urol 67:1112–1121
17. de Rooij M, Hamoen EH, Futterer JJ, Barentsz JO, Rovers MM (2014) Accuracy of multiparametric MRI for prostate cancer detection: a meta-analysis. AJR Am J Roentgenol 202:343–351
18. Hegde JV, Mulkern RV, Panych LP et al (2013) Multiparametric MRI of prostate cancer: an update on state-of-the-art techniques and their performance in detecting and localizing prostate cancer. J Magn Reson Imaging 37:1035–1054
19. Schoots IG, Petrides N, Giganti F et al (2015) Magnetic resonance imaging in active surveillance of prostate cancer: a systematic review. Eur Urol 67:627–636
20. Stamatakis L, Siddiqui MM, Nix JW et al (2013) Accuracy of multiparametric magnetic resonance imaging in confirming eligibility for active surveillance for men with prostate cancer. Cancer 119:3359–3366
21. Da Rosa MR, Milot L, Sugar L et al (2014) A prospective comparison of MRI-US fused targeted biopsy versus systemic ultrasound-guided biopsy for detecting clinically significant prostate cancer in patients on active surveillance. J Magn Reson Imaging 41:220–5
22. National Institute for Health and Care Excellence (NICE). CG175 NG (2014) Prostate cancer: diagnosis and treatment. Available via http://www.nice.org.uk/guidance/cg175. Accessed Dec. 2014
23. McNeal JE (1981) The zonal anatomy of the prostate. Prostate 2:35–49
24. McNeal JE, Redwine EA, Freiha FS, Stamey TA (1988) Zonal distribution of prostatic adenocarcinoma. Correlation with histologic pattern and direction of spread. Am J Surg Pathol 12:897–906
25. Rosenkrantz AB, Taneja SS (2014) Radiologist, be aware: ten pitfalls that confound the interpretation of multiparametric prostate MRI. AJR Am J Roentgenol 202:109–120
26. Vargas HA, Akin O, Franiel T et al (2012) Normal central zone of the prostate and central zone involvement by prostate cancer: clinical and MR imaging implications. Radiology 262:894–902
27. Mai KT, Belanger EC, Al-Maghrabi HM, Robertson S, Wang D, Margnean C (2008) Primary prostatic central zone adenocarcinoma. Pathol Res Pract 204:251–258
28. Cohen RJ, Shannon BA, Phillips M, Moorin RE, Wheeler TM, Garrett KL (2008) Central zone carcinoma of the prostate gland: a distinct tumor type with poor prognostic features. J Urol 179:1762–1767, **discussion 1767**
29. Lemaitre L, Puech P, Poncelet E et al (2009) Dynamic contrast-enhanced MRI of anterior prostate cancer: morphometric assessment and correlation with radical prostatectomy findings. Eur Radiol 19:470–480
30. Bonekamp D, Jacobs MA, El-Khouli R, Stoianovici D, Macura KJ (2011) Advancements in MR imaging of the prostate: from diagnosis to interventions. Radiographics 31:677–703
31. Akin O, Sala E, Moskowitz CS et al (2006) Transition zone prostate cancers: features, detection, localization, and staging at endorectal MR imaging. Radiology 239:784–792
32. Lawrentschuk N, Haider MA, Daljeet N et al (2010) 'Prostatic evasive anterior tumours': the role of magnetic resonance imaging. BJU Int 105:1231–1236
33. Hoeks CM, Hambrock T, Yakar D et al (2013) Transition zone prostate cancer: detection and localization with 3-T multiparametric MR imaging. Radiology 266:207–217
34. Yoshizako T, Wada A, Hayashi T et al (2008) Usefulness of diffusion-weighted imaging and dynamic contrast-enhanced magnetic resonance imaging in the diagnosis of prostate transition-zone cancer. Acta Radiol 49:1207–1213
35. Oto A, Kayhan A, Jiang Y et al (2010) Prostate cancer: differentiation of central gland cancer from benign prostatic hyperplasia by

using diffusion-weighted and dynamic contrast-enhanced MR imaging. Radiology 257:715–723
36. Engelbrecht MR, Huisman HJ, Laheij RJ et al (2003) Discrimination of prostate cancer from normal peripheral zone and central gland tissue by using dynamic contrast-enhanced MR imaging. Radiology 229:248–254
37. Turnbull LW, Buckley DL, Turnbull LS, Liney GP, Knowles AJ (1999) Differentiation of prostatic carcinoma and benign prostatic hyperplasia: correlation between dynamic Gd-DTPA-enhanced MR imaging and histopathology. J Magn Reson Imaging 9:311–316
38. Hoeks CM, Barentsz JO, Hambrock T et al (2011) Prostate cancer: multiparametric MR imaging for detection, localization, and staging. Radiology 261:46–66
39. Schieda N, Coffey N, Gulavita P, Al-Dandan O, Shabana W, Flood TA (2014) Prostatic ductal adenocarcinoma: an aggressive tumour variant unrecognized on T2 weighted magnetic resonance imaging (MRI). Eur Radiol 24:1349–56
40. Claus FG, Hricak H, Hattery RR (2004) Pretreatment evaluation of prostate cancer: role of MR imaging and 1H MR spectroscopy. Radiographics 24(Suppl 1):S167–180
41. Barrett T, Vargas HA, Akin O, Goldman DA, Hricak H (2012) Value of the hemorrhage exclusion sign on T1-weighted prostate MR images for the detection of prostate cancer. Radiology 263: 751–757
42. Rosenkrantz AB, Kopec M, Kong X et al (2010) Prostate cancer vs. post-biopsy hemorrhage: diagnosis with T2- and diffusion-weighted imaging. J Magn Reson Imaging 31:1387–1394
43. Chesnais AL, Niaf E, Bratan F et al (2013) Differentiation of transitional zone prostate cancer from benign hyperplasia nodules: evaluation of discriminant criteria at multiparametric MRI. Clin Radiol 68:e323–330
44. Bouye S, Potiron E, Puech P, Leroy X, Lemaitre L, Villers A (2009) Transition zone and anterior stromal prostate cancers: zone of origin and intraprostatic patterns of spread at histopathology. Prostate 69: 105–113
45. Esen M, Onur MR, Akpolat N, Orhan I, Kocakoc E (2013) Utility of ADC measurement on diffusion-weighted MRI in differentiation of prostate cancer, normal prostate and prostatitis. Quant Imaging Med Surg 3:210–216
46. Nagel KN, Schouten MG, Hambrock T et al (2013) Differentiation of prostatitis and prostate cancer by using diffusion-weighted MR imaging and MR-guided biopsy at 3 T. Radiology 267:164–172
47. Bour L, Schull A, Delongchamps NB et al (2013) Multiparametric MRI features of granulomatous prostatitis and tubercular prostate abscess. Diagn Interv Imaging 94:84–90
48. Shukla-Dave A, Hricak H, Eberhardt SC et al (2004) Chronic prostatitis: MR imaging and 1H MR spectroscopic imaging findings–initial observations. Radiology 231:717–724
49. Franiel T, Ludemann L, Rudolph B et al (2008) Evaluation of normal prostate tissue, chronic prostatitis, and prostate cancer by quantitative perfusion analysis using a dynamic contrast-enhanced inversion-prepared dual-contrast gradient echo sequence. Investig Radiol 43:481–487
50. Watanabe Y, Nagayama M, Araki T et al (2013) Targeted biopsy based on ADC map in the detection and localization of prostate cancer: a feasibility study. J Magn Reson Imaging 37:1168–1177
51. Humphrey PA (2012) Histological variants of prostatic carcinoma and their significance. Histopathology 60:59–74
52. Meeks JJ, Zhao LC, Cashy J, Kundu S (2012) Incidence and outcomes of ductal carcinoma of the prostate in the USA: analysis of data from the surveillance, epidemiology, and end results program. BJU Int 109:831–834
53. Seipel AH, Wiklund F, Wiklund NP, Egevad L (2013) Histopathological features of ductal adenocarcinoma of the prostate in 1,051 radical prostatectomy specimens. Virchows Arch 462: 429–436
54. Amin A, Epstein JI (2011) Pathologic stage of prostatic ductal adenocarcinoma at radical prostatectomy: effect of percentage of the ductal component and associated grade of acinar adenocarcinoma. Am J Surg Pathol 35:615–619
55. Montironi R, Hammond EH, Lin DW et al (2014) Consensus statement with recommendations on active surveillance inclusion criteria and definition of progression in men with localized prostate cancer: the critical role of the pathologist. Virchows Arch 465:623–628
56. Amin MB, Lin DW, Gore JL et al (2014) The critical role of the pathologist in determining eligibility for active surveillance as a management option in patients with prostate cancer: consensus statement with recommendations supported by the College of American Pathologists, International Society of Urological Pathology, Association of Directors of Anatomic and Surgical Pathology, the New Zealand Society of Pathologists, and the Prostate Cancer Foundation. Arch Pathol Lab Med 138:1387–1405
57. Coffey N, Schieda N, Cron G, Gulavita P, Mai KT, Flood TA (2014) Multi-parametric (mp) MRI of prostatic ductal adenocarcinoma. J Magn Reson Imaging. doi:10.1002/jmri.24694
58. Weinreb JC, Choyke PL, Cornud F, Haider MA, Katarzyna MJ, Margolis D, Schnall MD, Tempany CM, Thoeny HC, Verma S, Barentsz JO. Prostate imaging and data repording system (PI-RADS) version 2.0. Issued jointly by: American College of Radiology (ACR) and European Society of Urogenital Radiology (ESUR). Website. http://acr.org/~/media/ACR/Documents/PDF/QualitySafety/Resources/PIRADS/PIRADS%20V2.pdf. Accessed April 2015
59. Froehlich JM, Metens T, Chilla B, Hauser N, Klarhoefer M, Kubik-Huch RA (2012) Should less motion sensitive T2-weighted BLADE TSE replace cartesian TSE for female pelvic MRI? Insights Imaging 3:611–618
60. Lane BF, Vandermeer FQ, Oz RC, Irwin EW, McMillan AB, Wong-You-Cheong JJ (2011) Comparison of sagittal T2-weighted BLADE and fast spin-echo MRI of the female pelvis for motion artifact and lesion detection. AJR Am J Roentgenol 197:W307–313
61. Rosenkrantz AB, Bennett GL, Doshi A, Deng FM, Babb JS, Taneja SS (2014) T2-weighted imaging of the prostate: impact of the BLADE technique on image quality and tumor assessment. Abdom Imaging 40:552–9
62. Westphalen AC, Rosenkrantz AB (2014) Prostate imaging reporting and data system (PI-RADS): reflections on early experience with a standardized interpretation scheme for multiparametric prostate MRI. AJR Am J Roentgenol 202:121–123
63. Metens T, Miranda D, Absil J, Matos C (2012) What is the optimal *b* value in diffusion-weighted MR imaging to depict prostate cancer at 3 T? Eur Radiol 22:703–709
64. Wang X, Qian Y, Liu B et al (2014) High-b-value diffusion-weighted MRI for the detection of prostate cancer at 3 T. Clin Radiol 69:1165–1170
65. Haider MA, van der Kwast TH, Tanguay J et al (2007) Combined T2-weighted and diffusion-weighted MRI for localization of prostate cancer. AJR Am J Roentgenol 189:323–328
66. Rosenkrantz AB, Triolo MJ, Melamed J, Rusinek H, Taneja SS, Deng FM (2015) Whole-lesion apparent diffusion coefficient metrics as a marker of percentage Gleason 4 component within Gleason 7 prostate cancer at radical prostatectomy. J Magn Reson Imaging 41:708–714
67. Lawrence EM, Gallagher FA, Barrett T et al (2014) Preoperative 3 T diffusion-weighted MRI for the qualitative and quantitative assessment of extracapsular extension in patients with intermediate- or high-risk prostate cancer. AJR Am J Roentgenol 203:W280–286
68. Donati OF, Mazaheri Y, Afaq A et al (2014) Prostate cancer aggressiveness: assessment with whole-lesion histogram analysis of the apparent diffusion coefficient. Radiology 271:143–152

69. Vos EK, Litjens GJ, Kobus T et al (2013) Assessment of prostate cancer aggressiveness using dynamic contrast-enhanced magnetic resonance imaging at 3 T. Eur Urol 64:448–455
70. Isebaert S, De Keyzer F, Haustermans K et al (2012) Evaluation of semi-quantitative dynamic contrast-enhanced MRI parameters for prostate cancer in correlation to whole-mount histopathology. Eur J Radiol 81:e217–222
71. Langer DL, van der Kwast TH, Evans AJ et al (2010) Prostate tissue composition and MR measurements: investigating the relationships between ADC, T2, K(trans), v(e), and corresponding histologic features. Radiology 255:485–494
72. Quon JKA, Jain R, Schieda N (2015) Assessing the utilization of functional imaging in multi-parametric (mp) prostate MRI in routine clinical practice. Clin Radiol 70:373–378
73. Wysock JS, Rosenkrantz AB, Huang WC et al (2014) A prospective, blinded comparison of magnetic resonance (MR) imaging-ultrasound fusion and visual estimation in the performance of MR-targeted prostate biopsy: the PROFUS trial. Eur Urol 66: 343–351
74. Puech P, Rouviere O, Renard-Penna R et al (2013) Prostate cancer diagnosis: multiparametric MR-targeted biopsy with cognitive and transrectal US-MR fusion guidance versus systematic biopsy–prospective multicenter study. Radiology 268: 461–469
75. Delongchamps NB, Peyromaure M, Schull A et al (2013) Prebiopsy magnetic resonance imaging and prostate cancer detection: comparison of random and targeted biopsies. J Urol 189:493–499
76. Cool DW, Zhang X, Romagnoli C, Izawa JI, Romano WM, Fenster A (2015) Evaluation of MRI-TRUS fusion versus cognitive registration accuracy for MRI-targeted, TRUS-guided prostate biopsy. AJR Am J Roentgenol 204:83–91

13

Multidetector CT imaging of complications after laparoscopic nephron-sparing surgery

Massimo Tonolini[1] · Anna Maria Ierardi[2] · Virginia Varca[3] · Giacomo Piero Incarbone[3] · Marina Petullà[1] · Roberto Bianco[1]

Abstract

Purpose Laparoscopic nephron-sparing surgery (L-NSS) is increasingly performed to treat localised renal lesions. However, the associated morbidity is non-negligible, with a rate of major complications approaching 10 %.

Methods and Results This paper provides an overview of indications, surgical techniques and results of L-NSS; explains the incidence, risk factors and manifestations of postoperative complications; discusses the preferred multidetector computed tomography (CT) acquisition techniques; illustrates the appearance of normal postoperative images following L-NSS; and reviews, with example images, the most common and unusual iatrogenic complications. These include haematuria, haemorrhage, vascular injuries, infections and urinary leaks. Most emphasis is placed on CT, which provides rapid, reliable triage and follow-up of iatrogenic complications after L-NSS, identifying occurrences that require transarterial embolisation or repeated surgery.

Conclusions Multidetector CT allows precise assessment of the surgical resection site; detection of pneumoperitoneum and subcutaneous emphysema; quantification of retroperitoneal blood; and identification of active bleeding, pseudoaneurysms, arterio-venous fistulas, abscess collections and extravasated urine.

✉ Massimo Tonolini
mtonolini@sirm.org

1 Department of Radiology, "Luigi Sacco" University Hospital, Via G.B. Grassi 74, 20157 Milan, Italy

2 Interventional Radiology, Department of Radiology, University of Insubria, Viale Borri 57, 21100 Varese, Italy

3 Department of Urology, "Luigi Sacco" University Hospital, Via G.B. Grassi 74, 20157 Milan, Italy

Teaching Points

- *Laparoscopic nephron-sparing surgery (NSS) is increasingly performed to treat renal lesions.*
- *Radiologists are increasingly requested to investigate suspected post-surgical NSS complications.*
- *Post-NSS complications include haemorrhage, haematuria, vascular injuries, infections and urinary leaks.*
- *Multidetector CT allows choice between conservative treatment, transarterial embolisation or surgery.*

Keywords Laparoscopic nephron-sparing surgery · Haemorrhage · Pseudoaneurysm · Urine leak · Computed tomography (CT)

Introduction

Background

As a result of improved surgical techniques and greater focus on minimising functional impairment over the last decade, the therapeutic approach to localised renal cell carcinoma (RCC) has evolved from the classical radical nephrectomy (RN) towards nephron-sparing surgery (NSS), which was initially performed using an open surgical approach. Compared with RN, open partial nephrectomy (O-PN) achieved a lower rate of postoperative loss of renal function, after adjustment for age, hypertension and diabetes, and similar long-term oncological and quality-of-life outcomes [1, 2].

Meanwhile, the widespread use of ultrasound, computed tomography (CT) and magnetic resonance imaging (MRI) has led to a steady increase in the detection of benign, malignant or indeterminate renal lesions requiring surgery, so that currently almost 50 % of RCCs are diagnosed incidentally, often during imaging studies requested for unrelated reasons.

As a result, conservative surgery is increasingly performed to treat patients with small-sized renal masses. According to the most recent guidelines from the European Association of Urology (EAU) [1, 2], NSS represents the treatment of choice for localised RCC. It can be performed with an open, laparoscopic or robot-assisted approach, based on the surgeon's expertise and skills. Indications for NSS include T1a-b stage RCC and selected masses up to 7 cm, unless contraindicated by unfavourable anatomical location of the tumour or general deterioration of the patient's condition. Absolute indications include tumours in a solitary kidney, impaired renal function and hereditary disorders that predispose to recurrent RCC. Furthermore, laparoscopy is an appealing minimally invasive treatment for indeterminate renal cysts requiring surgery, and benign masses such as angiomyolipoma or oncocytoma. Relative contraindications for laparoscopy include prior surgical procedures (due to the presence of intra-abdominal adhesions), cirrhosis and portal hypertension, marked bowel distension (which increases the risk for bowel injury), ongoing sepsis and cardiopulmonary disease [1–3].

Both O-PN and laparoscopic partial nephrectomy (L-PN) resulted in superior long-term preservation of renal function. After NSS, patients have a much lower (20 %) 3-year probability of developing chronic kidney disease (defined by <60 mL/min per 1.73 m^2 estimated glomerular filtration rate [e-GFR]) compared with RN (65 %). At 10 years, the cumulative incidence of chronic renal failure is 22.4 % and 11.6 % for the RN and NSS groups, respectively [4, 5].

Comparison between O-PN and L-PN revealed shorter operating time and warm renal ischaemia time with the open approach, and lower blood loss and shorter hospital stay in the laparoscopic group. No differences were reported in long-term impact on renal function (mean E-GFR decrease 4.1 vs 1.1 mL/min), overall postoperative morbidity and mortality, or progression-free and overall survival (91–94 % 5-year cancer-specific survival) [6–16].

However, L-PN is a technically demanding surgical procedure, with a steep learning curve and potentially serious complications particularly in elderly patients with comorbidities. The overall complication rate in a European multi-institutional series was reported to be 23 %, while a worldwide literature review reported a rate of major complications approaching 10 % [8, 9].

Alternatively, localised renal masses may be treated by laparoscopic or imaging-guided ablative techniques. Although no definite conclusions can be drawn from available studies, surgically treated patients show lower local recurrence rate and cancer-specific mortality; therefore the EAU recommends cryoablation and radiofrequency ablation in elderly and/or comorbid patients with limited life expectancy [1, 2, 17]. However, percutaneous cryoablation and radiofrequency ablation were recently shown to be effective in the treatment of T1 stage RCC, offering excellent preservation of kidney function and similar clinical efficacy and oncological outcome (5-year survival exceeding 90 %) compared with surgery, with a limited incidence of major (4.3–5.6 %) and minor complications and no significant differences between the two modalities [18–21].

Purpose

Owing to the increasing use of laparoscopy, in hospitals with active surgical practices urologists increasingly request imaging studies to assess patients with suspected postoperative complications following L-PN. This paper provides an overview of the indications, results and technical principles of laparoscopic NSS (L-NSS), and describes the postoperative radiological outcome following L-NSS [22–25].

Laparoscopic nephron-sparing surgery

Preoperative assessment

The RENAL (Radius, Exophytic, Nearness, Anterior, Location) nephrometry score (Table 1) was recently introduced as a reproducible means to describe the relevant tumour anatomy, stratify the complexity of renal masses, and objectively compare perioperative and long-term outcomes. The RENAL score includes the five most reproducible features—namely, diameter, exophytic or endophytic growth, proximity to the collecting system, anterior versus posterior location and relationship to the polar lines, which should be assessed on volumetric contrast-enhanced multidetector CT including renal vascular, parenchymal and excretory imaging (Fig. 1) [26, 27]. Tumour staging and complexity dictate the urologist's therapeutic choice: increasing RENAL scores were found to be strongly associated with RN and O-PN rather than L-NSS [28].

Laparoscopic surgical technique

In the majority of patients, L-NSS is performed via the transperitoneal (TP) route; conversely, posterior and posterolateral renal tumours are best managed with a retroperitoneal approach [9, 11, 29, 30]. Preoperative ureteral catheterisation may be used, particularly when access to the collecting system is necessary. According to some authors, intraoperative ultrasonography for assessment of renal perfusion, tumour location and borders may prove beneficial and result in a change of procedure in a minority (2.5 %) of patients [31]. After laparoscopic access to the retroperitoneum and opening of Gerota's fascia, en bloc or selective arterial clamping of the renal hilar vascular pedicle is performed to decrease bleeding and ensure a clear surgical field: the acceptable warm ischaemia time is limited to 30 min or less. Depending on the tumour's size and

Table 1 RENAL nephrometry score (adapted from Parsons et al. [26])

	Score		
Renal lesion feature	1 point	2 points	3 points
R—Radius (maximal diameter)	≤4 cm	4–7 cm	≥7 cm
E—Exophtic vs endophytic	≥50 % Exophytic (projecting outside the renal cortex)	<50 % exophytic	Completely endophytic
N—Nearness to the collecting system/renal sinus	≥7 mm	4–7 mm	≤4 mm
A—Anterior vs posterior location)	Descriptive (no numeric score) "a", ventral; "p", dorsal; "x", others		
L—Location relative to polar lines	Entirely below lower or above upper polar line	Crosses polar line	50 % of mass across polar line Entirely between polar lines Crosses the axial midline
	Additional suffix "h" if tumour reaches hilar vessels		
Renal lesion complexity		RENAL nephrometry score range	
Low		4–6	
Intermediate		7–9	
High		10–12	

location, NSS options include segmental polar nephrectomy, wedge resection, transverse resection and enucleation, to obtain complete tumour excision with a proper margin of normal tissue, and preservation of the maximum possible amount of functioning renal parenchyma. After removal of the resected renal portion, surgery requires suture repair of collecting system defects, filling of the parenchymal defect with peri-renal fat or bioabsorbable bolster agents, renal parenchymal

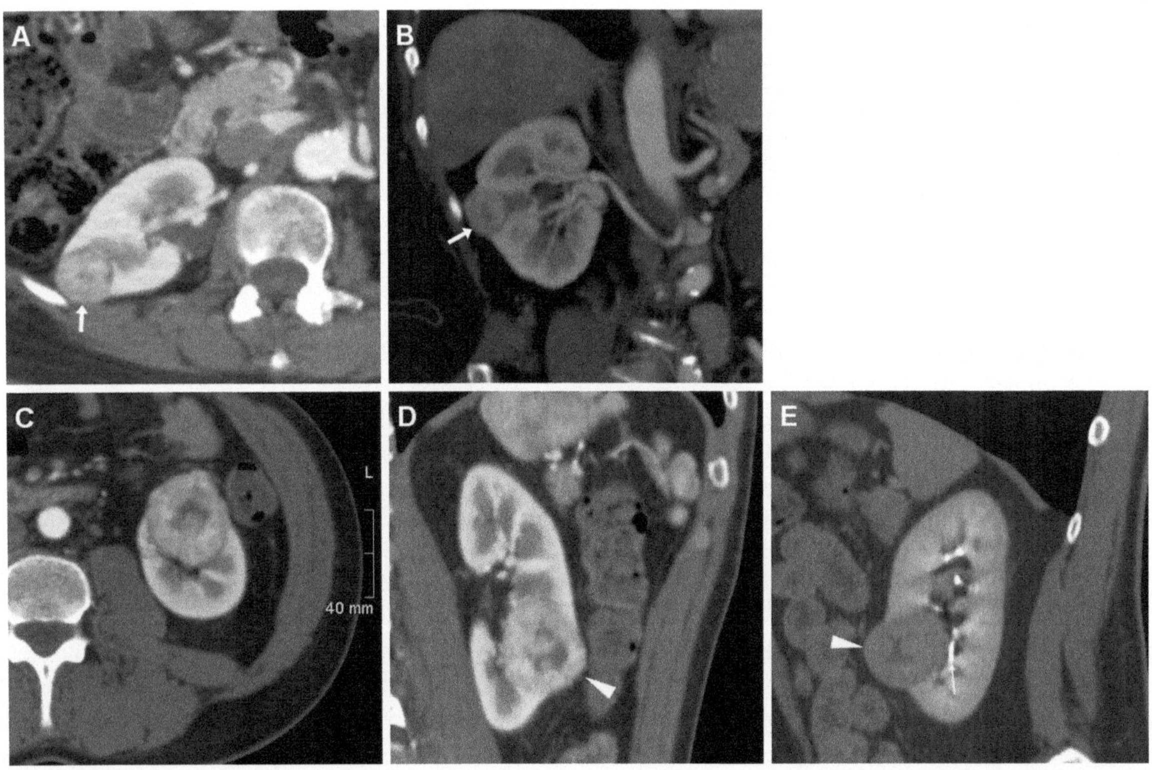

Fig. 1 Examples of RENAL nephrometry scores. Total body contrast-enhanced multidetector CT (**a**, **b**) performed for clinical suspicion of systemic lymphoproliferative disease in a healthy 61-year-old woman led to incidental detection of a 2.5-cm, vascularised, partially (<50 %) exophytic mass at the middle third of the right kidney (*arrows*), consistent with T1 stage renal cell carcinoma (RCC). Nephrometry resulted 1+2+2+p+3 (8p). The patient underwent laparoscopic nephron-sparing surgery (L-NSS) complicated by haematoma (*see* Fig. 5). Multiphase CT-urography (**c**–**e**) in a 55-year-old man confirmed ultrasound detection of a 43-mm, inhomogeneously enhancing, left-sided RCC. The lesion appeared partially exophytic, crossed the inferior polar line (**d**) and touched the lower pole calyx (**e**). Nephrometry score was 2+2+3+a+2 (9a). The patient successfully underwent laparoscopic partial nephrectomy (L-PN)

reconstruction and closure with a combination of absorbable sutures, argon-beam coagulation and haemostatic agents. Finally, after reconstruction is finished, the vascular clamp is released to restore circulation. Hilar masses, multiple and/or infiltrating tumours with pelvicalyceal involvement pose specific and significant technical challenges for NSS. In selected patients, conversion to laparoscopic RN or O-PN may be necessary when L-NSS is deemed unfeasible by the surgeon after renal exploration [9, 11, 29, 30].

Postoperative complications: manifestations, incidence and risk factors

The spectrum of non-urological complications after L-NSS includes cardiovascular (deep venous thrombosis, congestive heart failure, atrial fibrillation), pulmonary (pleural effusion, atelectasis/pneumonia, thromboembolism) and gastrointestinal issues (ileus, colonic segmental ischemia, bowel injury, splenic haemorrhage); sepsis; wound infection; and incisional hernias. Specific (urological) complications include massive subcutaneous emphysema, persistent haematuria, haemorrhage, renal vascular injuries, urine leak, renal failure and infections (such as urinary infection, peri-renal abscess and sepsis) [6–12]. Clinically, complications are usually graded by urologists according to the validated Clavien–Dindo system, including, in ascending order of severity, grades I (any deviation from usual postoperative course limited to treatment with anti-emetics, antipyretics, analgesics, diuretics and electrolytes), II (requiring other medical therapies including blood transfusions), III (surgical, endoscopic or interventional treatment), IV (life-threatening complication necessitating intensive care support) and V (death) [32, 33].

Overall, adverse events after L-NSS occur in 23 % of patients: almost two-thirds of cases are minor occurrences (Clavien grades I–II). Despite favourable preoperative patient features and lower objective complexity of tumours, laparoscopic surgery is associated with more major (grade III or higher) overall (6.2-9 % versus 3–6.3 %) and urological (particularly urine leak) complications compared with O-PN [6–12].

The RENAL score is an objective assessment of the complexity of a tumour and may provide a consistent basis for comparing perioperative and long-term outcomes after L-NSS [26, 27]. According to several studies, patients with highly complex tumours are more likely to experience postoperative complications. Posterior location and proximity to the renal sinus seem to have the greatest association with overall complications and haemorrhage [34–39]. Nephrometry scores have been shown to correlate with increased postoperative hospital stay, blood loss, duration of renal ischaemia risk of conversion to open surgery and postoperative renal function loss [35–41].

Conversely, other studies failed to confirm the predictive value of the RENAL score for complications. Apart from tumour size and central growth, other risk factors are reported, including advanced age and comorbidities, limited surgeon's experience, intraoperative blood loss and opening of the collecting system [40–43].

Postoperative CT imaging: indications and techniques

Postoperative imaging following L-NSS is generally indicated when clinical features such as hypotension, flank or abdominal pain, gross or persistent haematuria, bleeding from the drainage tube or laboratory abnormalities (particularly blood loss, leucocytosis and increased C-reactive protein levels) suggest a possible complication. Emergency investigation is warranted when signs and symptoms of haemodynamic impairment or sepsis are present [1, 2, 22–25, 29].

In most cases multidetector computed tomography (CT) represents the mainstay imaging technique to comprehensively investigate the abdomen and pelvis in search of possible iatrogenic complications. Experience with blunt body trauma has established that CT is by far the preferred, most rapid and robust technique to depict and grade renal lesions, thus providing the anatomic and functional information necessary for appropriate injury staging and therapeutic choice [22–25, 44]. Intravenous contrast medium (CM) should be administered, unless contraindicated. Since patients that have recently been operated upon are often dehydrated, with limited urine output, the European Society of Urogenital Radiology (ESUR) guidelines recommend special care in ensuring adequate hydration before and after CT, in order to improve urinary tract opacification and to prevent CM nephrotoxicity [45, 46].

In most postoperative urology patients, initial investigation requires a comprehensive multiphase CT acquisition protocol, including: (1) preliminary unenhanced acquisition to demonstrate the postoperative anatomy and detect hyperattenuating blood and abnormal air collections; (2) corticomedullary phase and (3) nephrographic-phase images after CM injection to assess the operated kidney structure and perfusion of the operated kidney, and to identify CM extravasation indicating active bleeding; (4) excretory phase imaging obtained 8–10 min after CM, which demonstrates the opacified urinary cavities and may detect iodinated urine leaks and urinomas. Postoperative CT studies are reviewed interactively on dedicated workstations and complemented with multiplanar reconstructions as necessary, to better depict postoperative anatomy and relevant findings [22–25].

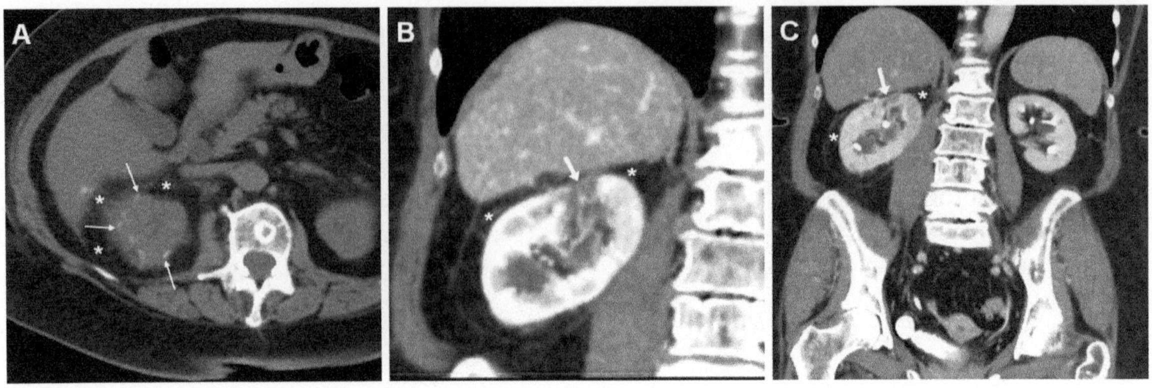

Fig. 2 Normal early postoperative imaging appearance in a 77-year-old woman investigated with multidetector CT 4 days after laparoscopic enucleation of a 2-cm RCC of the right kidney. Unenhanced axial image (**a**) showed hyperattenuating linear structures (*thin arrows*) corresponding to surgical sutures at the upper renal pole, and normal peri-renal fat (*). Axial nephrographic (**b**) and coronal excretory-phase (**c**) images showed a focal, wedge-shaped, non-enhancing portion of the renal cortex (*arrows*) with continuous renal contour corresponding to the resection site, and confirmed normal peri-renal fat planes (*) without extravasated blood and urine. Despite postoperative pain and blood loss, the patient had an uneventful postoperative course and was discharged without further treatment

The main drawback of classical multiphase CT protocol is the high radiation dose, which poses a serious concern, particularly considering that these patients usually require serial studies and long-term imaging follow-up. Currently, most institutions are increasingly adopting split-bolus CT-urography acquisitions, which provide combined corticomedullary, nephrographic and excretory imaging with reduced effective radiation dose. In our experience, the time- and dose-efficient triple-bolus protocol described by Kekelidze et al. [47] has proved very useful in the investigation of iatrogenic urinary tract injuries. This technique includes an initial 30-mL CM bolus injected at a flow of 2 mL/s for urinary

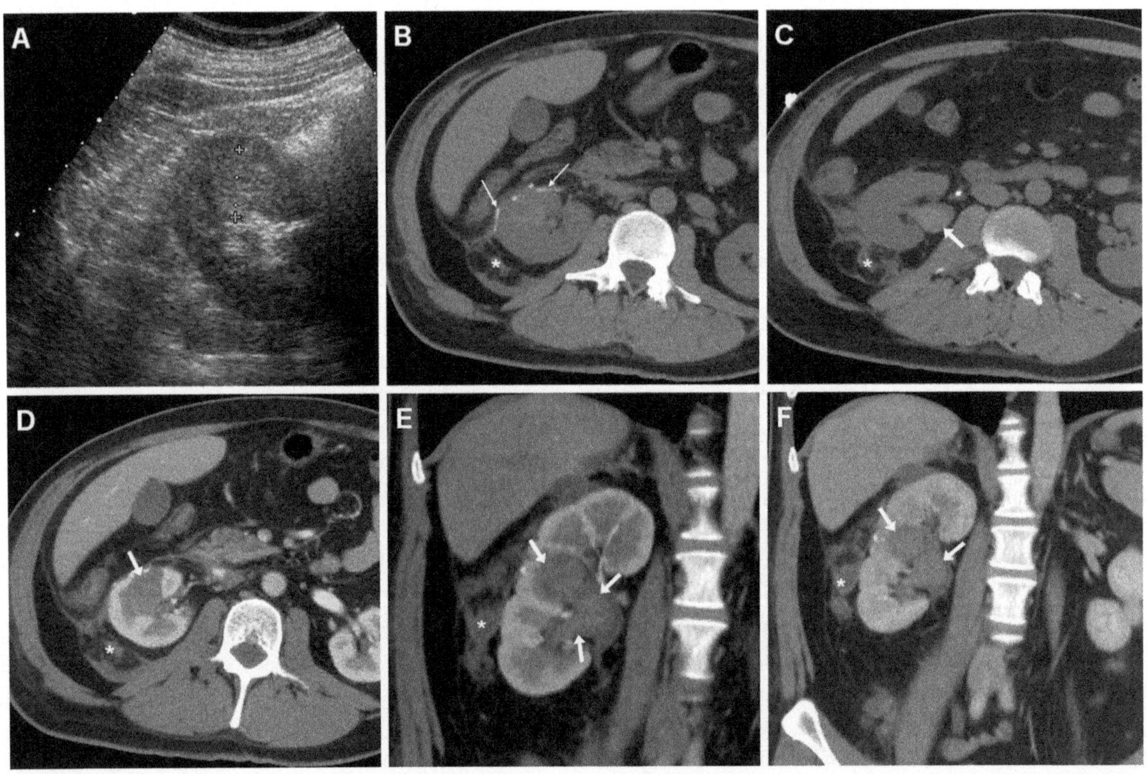

Fig. 3 Gross haematuria with hypotension, moderate leucocytosis and blood loss (12 g/dL haemoglobin) in a 32-year-old man shortly after L-PN for a 2.5-cm, hyperechoic RCC (sonographic image in **a**). Unenhanced axial CT images (**a, b**) showed hyperattenuating linear structures (*thin arrows*) corresponding to surgical sutures along the ventral renal contour, minimal fluid and blood in the ipsilateral peri-renal space and retroperitoneal fasciae (*), hyperattenuating blood (*arrow*) in the renal pelvis. Corticomedullary (**d, e**) and nephrographic (**f**) phase images confirmed blood (*arrows*) occupying most of the renal collecting system. The lack of CM extravasation indicating active bleeding allowed conservative treatment including prolonged vesical catheterisation and lavage

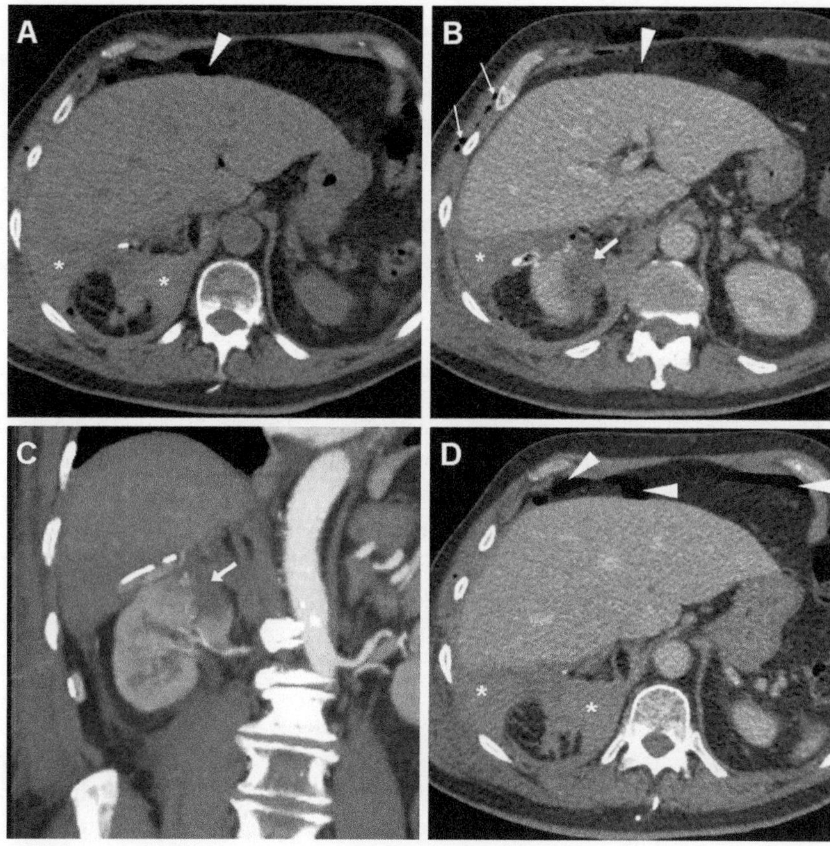

Fig. 4 Haematoma in a 74-year-old man with diabetes, cardiac pacemaker, and progressive postoperative blood loss after L-PN. Unenhanced (**a**) and post-contrast (**b, c**) Multidetector CT images showed residual intraperitoneal gas bubbles (*arrowheads*) and minimal emphysema of the abdominal wall (*thin arrows* in **b**). Hyperattenuating blood collection (*) with the distal end of the drainage tube was seen along the posterior aspect of the right liver lobe, abutting the upper right renal pole with the hypoenhancing resection site (*arrows* in **b, c**) without CM extravasation indicating active bleeding in the corticomedullary phase (**b, c**) or urine leak in the excretory phase (**d**). The patient recovered with transfusion support

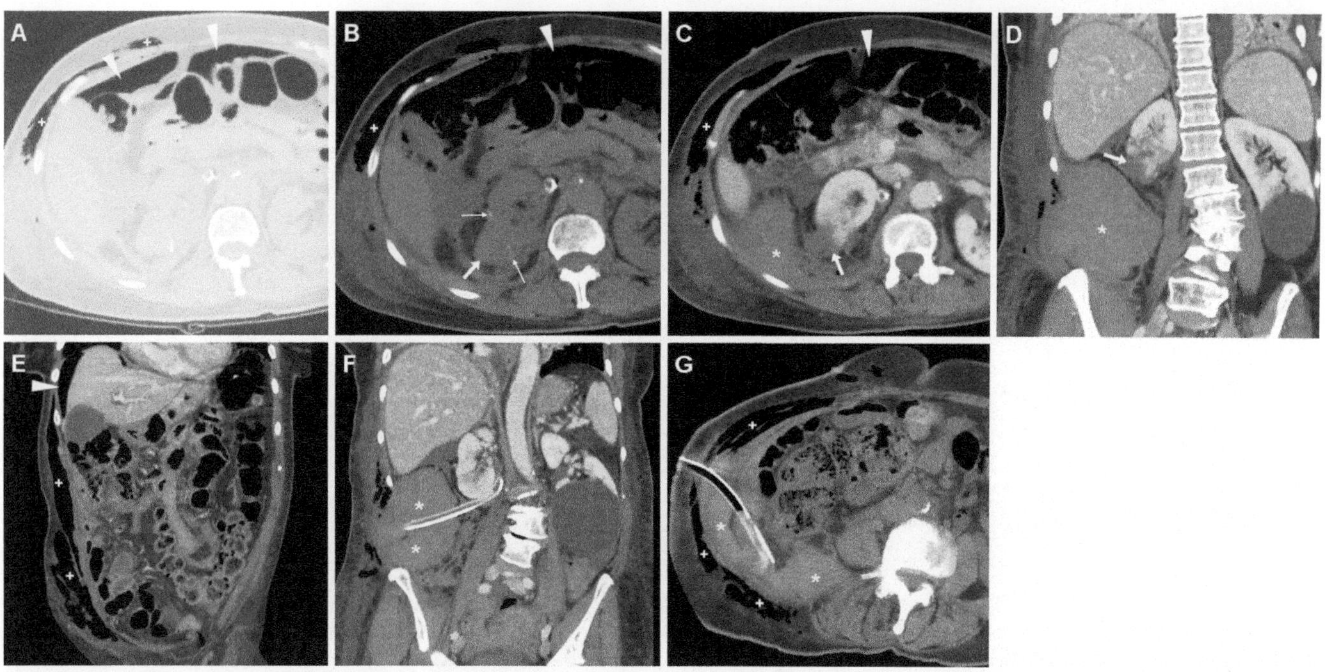

Fig. 5 Two days after L-NSS for T1N0M0 RCC of the right kidney, the same patient as in Fig. 1a, b suffered from abdominal pain and progressive blood loss (nadir haemoglobin 11.5 g/dL), with stable vital signs. Urgent CT images viewed at lung window settings (**a**) showed moderate pneumoperitoneum (*arrowheads*) and subcutaneous emphysema of the abdominal wall (+). Unenhanced (**b**) and post-contrast (**c–f**) image showed the renal resection site (*arrows* in **b–d**) with sutures (*thin arrows*), a sizeable haematoma centred in the posterior para-renal space (*) causing kidney displacement, without active bleeding. Coronal CT reformation (**f**) confirmed massive subcutaneous emphysema (+) and pneumoperitoneum (*arrowhead*). Following conservative treatment and drainage tube repositioning, repeated CT 5 days later (**g**) showed persistent subcutaneous emphysema (+), decreased retroperitoneal blood collection (*)

opacification, followed by a 7-min delay, then a second (50 mL at 1.5 mL/s) CM injection, with a third one (65 mL at 3 mL/s) 20 s later, to provide parenchymal and vascular visualisation respectively, followed by a single volumetric CT acquisition. Alternatively, a combined nephrographic–excretory phase may be obtained by administration of an initial 30–45 mL CM bolus followed, after a 6– to 8-min delay, by a second 75– to 100-mL injection, which may be useful when bleeding or vascular injuries are not suspected, and during follow-up. Furthermore, we recommend repeated (ultra-delayed) excretory acquisition 45–50 min after CM administration in all patients with urinary leak suspected on the basis of surgical, clinical or laboratory data. If available, dual-energy CT may be beneficial to limit the radiation dose, by allowing reconstruction of a virtual unenhanced dataset from CM-enhanced acquisition [47, 48]. Finally, repeated CT provides consistent monitoring of injuries after conservative or interventional treatment [47–49].

Normal postoperative CT imaging appearances

Following tumour resection or limited PN, the surgical site of resection (SSR) may be recognised as a wedge-shaped hypoattenuating portion of the renal cortex, sometimes demarcated by thin linear hyperattenuating sutures (Figs. 2, 3). The SSR generally does not enhance, closely resembles a traumatic laceration and may sometimes tend to shrink or form linear or stellate parenchymal scars in the long-term. After PN, the operated kidney commonly has a more posterior location, and abuts or adheres to the posterior aspect of Gerota's fascia. Dense thickening of the peri-renal septa, corresponding to fluid or haemorrhagic stranding, is commonly observed in the ipsilateral peri-renal and para-renal spaces (Fig. 3) [22–25].

Sometimes, to improve haemostasis, surgeons may pack the SSR intraoperatively with perinephric fat, which should not be mistaken for a fatty mass. Localised non-enhancing fluid collections corresponding to seroma (sometimes with fat-fluid level) may be visualised. In some patients, biologically absorbable haemostatic agents such as Gelfoam (absorbable gelatine compressed sponge; Pfizer, NY, USA) or Surgicel (oxydised cellulose polymer; Ethicon, Somerville, NJ, USA) may be used to control intraoperative bleeding. Within a few weeks, these bolster agents may show near-water attenuation with interspersed gas foci and can potentially be confused with an abscess; differentiation should rely on knowledge of surgical details, visualisation of gas bubbles arranged in linear fashion and stable appearance or regression on serial scanning. Conversely,

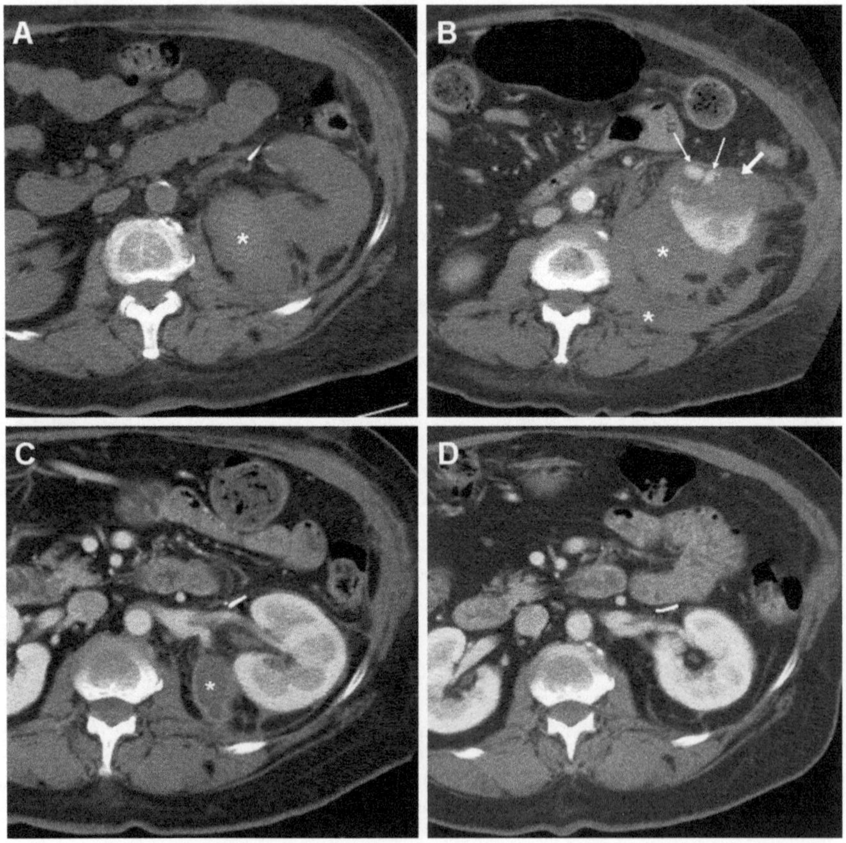

Fig. 6 Abdominal pain and hypotension in a 62-year–old woman 24 h after laparoscopic enucleation of an early-stage RCC. Unenhanced CT acquisition (**a**) showed renal displacement by hyperattenuating medial peri-renal and posterior para-renal haematoma (*). Post-contrast corticomedullary-phase images (**b**) depicted foci of active extravasation (*thin arrows*) near the site of resection (*arrow*) at the resected inferior renal pole. The haematoma (*) become progressively liquefied and demarcated during CT follow-up (**c**) and eventually resolved 1 year later (**d**). (Partially reprinted with permission from Tonolini et al. [52])

abscess should be suspected if a localised fluid collection shows a CM-enhancing rim and contains a gas-fluid level or moving bubbles [22–25].

Subcutaneous emphysema (Figs. 4, 5) is a common finding after laparoscopic surgery, and results from prolonged insufflation with the Trocar displaced into the abdominal wall. Emphysema is always non-dependent and most prominent immediately after surgery, and should not be misinterpreted as necrotising fasciitis, which usually occurs later and is associated with erythema, foul-smelling drainage from the wound, fever and pain [3].

In patients operated on through a TP laparoscopic approach, air-fluid levels of the small bowel consistent with adynamic ileus and minimal or moderate pneumoperitoneum (Figs. 4, 5) are commonly observed during the early postoperative period. If unknown, the type of laparoscopic access used may be guessed by searching for port access sites, in either the anterior ipsilateral abdomen (TP) or flank (retroperitoneal) [3]. Owing to the small incisions and the rapid absorption of CO_2 from the perfusion gas, relative to that of room air, variable amounts of residual intraperitoneal free air are commonly observed following laparoscopy (in at least one-third of patients) within the first 3 days, and may sometimes last up to 9 days after surgery. However, postoperative pneumoperitoneum after laparoscopy is generally more limited than with open surgery, and decreases on serial imaging. Conversely, persistent or increasing intra-abdominal gas should raise concern for hollow viscus injury [3, 50, 51].

Haemorrhagic and vascular complications

Bleeding

Resulting from inadequate suturing or coagulation of transacted blood vessels, early postoperative haemorrhage with or without radiologically identifiable active bleeding represents the most common complication after L-NSS, with a reported incidence approaching 6–8 % of procedures. Blood transfusions are required in 5–21 % of patients and constitute a Clavien grade II complication [6–12].

As mentioned above, minimal or moderate degrees of peri- and para-renal blood are generally apparent after L-PN and should not be reported as abnormal. However, intra-luminal blood is closely related to gross haematuria and is identified

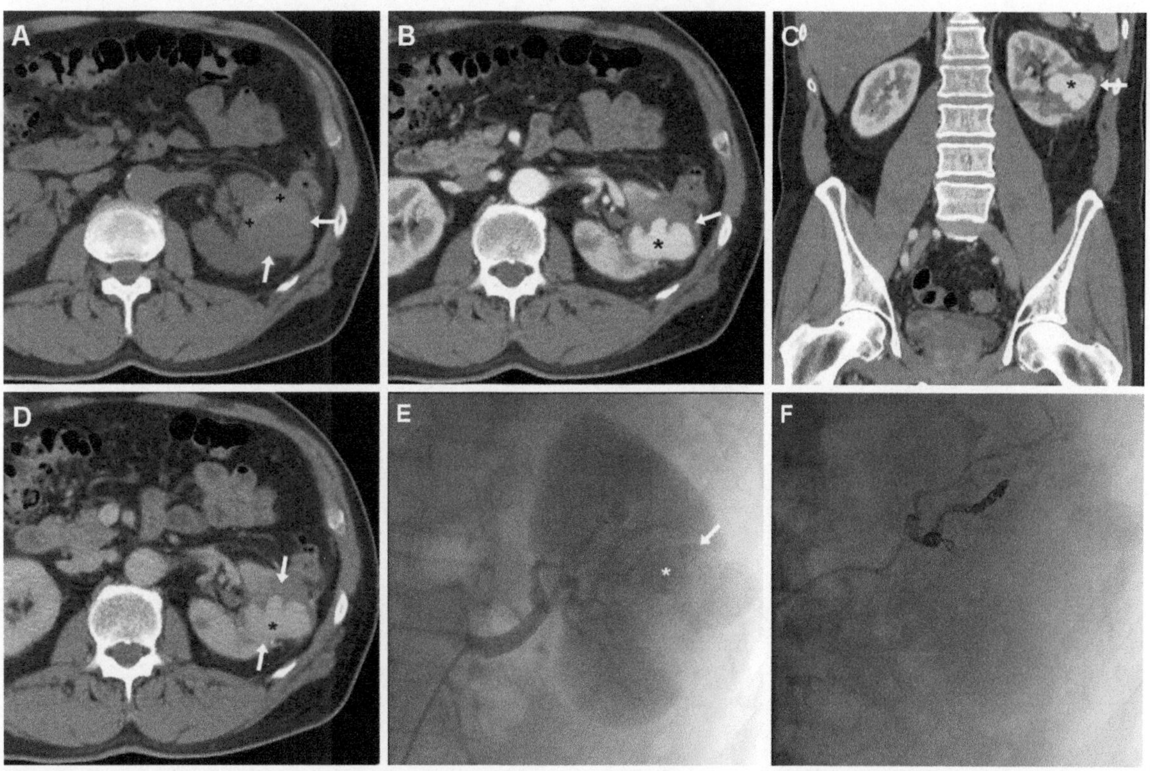

Fig. 7 Postoperative gross haematuria in a 55-year-old man 5 weeks after enucleation of a left-sided, 3.7-cm, pT1a clear-cell RCC including the calyceal opening. Unenhanced CT images revealed a 4.5-cm, inhomogeneous, roundish renal mass (*arrowheads*) with non-dependent hyperattenuating material (+), suggesting thrombus. After intravenous contrast, corticomedullary (**b**, **c**) and nephrographic (**d**) CT images showed perfusion (*) synchronous to arterial vessels of most of the same lesion, consistent with pseudoaneurysm. Renal angiography (**e**) confirmed roundish lesion (*arrow*) occupied by haemorrhagic focus (*) from the distal portion of the anteromedial branch, corresponding to the site of recent tumour excision. Super selective catheterisation and embolisation with coils (**f**) allowed the bleeding to be stopped

on unenhanced CT scans as hyperattenuating content of the pelvicalyceal system (Fig. 3). In our experience, clinically significant iatrogenic haematomas after L-NSS appear as hyperattenuating collections compared to the renal parenchyma, which measure between 45 and 90 Hounsfield units (HU) depending on their stage, and mostly occupy the peri- and para-renal spaces (Figs. 4, 5, 6). Indicated by strongly hyperattenuating (85–370 HU, isodense to enhanced arterial vessels) foci corresponding to CM extravasation in the vicinity of the SSR, active bleeding at CT (Fig. 6) indicates a high risk of failure of conservative management and thus represents the strongest indication for interventional or surgical treatment. In addition, multidetector CT provides consistent follow-up of conservatively treated lesions (Figs. 5, 6) showing progressive demarcation, size reduction and decreasing attenuation of haematomas [22–25, 44, 52].

Renal vascular complications

According to the EAU guidelines, iatrogenic renal vascular injuries (IRVI) rank among the rarest (less than 1 % overall), yet most feared complications after percutaneous biopsy, nephrostomy, nephroureterolithotomy, renal artery angioplasty or stenting, and NSS. The IRVI spectrum encompasses arterio-venous fistulas (AVFs), renal pseudoaneurysms (R-PA), vascular thrombosis and renal infarction. IRVIs can lead to significant morbidity, including massive haemorrhage, life-threatening haematuria, need for nephrectomy or deterioration of renal function [24, 32, 37].

Renal artery and intra-parenchymal pseudoaneurysms occur after 0.43–1.3 % of L-NSS procedures, and result from partial or complete injury to an intra-renal artery at the SSR, the main renal artery or one of its main branches. Specifically, R-PA may form when the combined effect of hypotension, coagulation and pressure from the adjacent structures leads to temporary cessation of the bleeding, followed by recanalisation from clot degradation. R-PAs may sometimes grow, become unstable from restorated blood flow, and eventually erode into the pelvicalyceal system or the surrounding perinephric tissues. Most cases are diagnosed during the first 2–3 weeks after surgery, occasionally after a few months' delay. Diagnosing R-PA requires a high level of suspicion, since clinical manifestations are often vague or non-specific such as flank

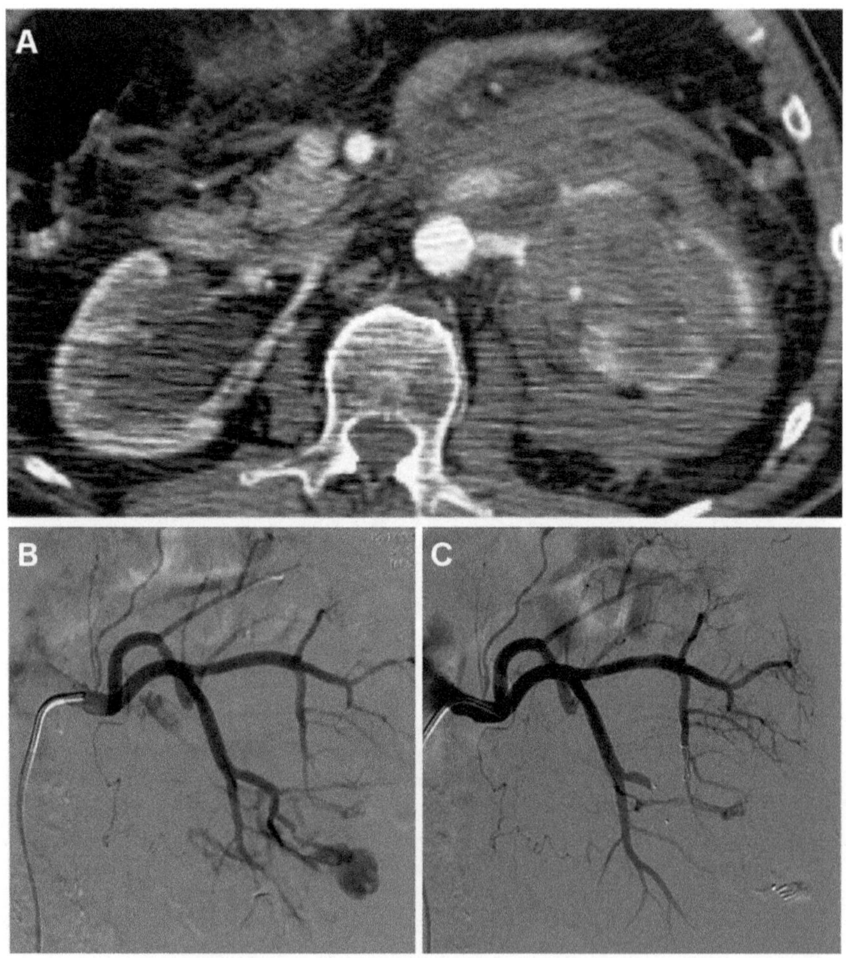

Fig. 8 Progressive blood loss, haematuria and ipsilateral flank pain in a 75-year-old man 3 days following enucleation of a left-sided RCC. Arterial-phase CT acquisition (**a**) revealed a small pseudoaneurysm plus arterio-venous fistula suggested by early opacification of the left renal vein, which were confirmed by urgent angiography (**b**). After selective embolisation with a 4-mm Amplatzer vascular plug and 2-mm microcoil, repeated angiogram (**c**) demonstrated complete exclusion of both lesions

pain, gross haematuria, dizziness and fever [11, 32, 53, 54].

Ultrasound may detect R-PA as a cystic mass or liquefied haematoma, with the characteristic "to-and-fro" internal flow at colour-Doppler sonography. On unenhanced CT images, a haematoma is commonly seen near to the surgical site, often associated with hyperattenuating blood clots in the renal pelvis, but the pseudoaneurysm itself is usually not visible. Conversely, arterial-phase CT-angiography acquisition shows a roundish, well-circumscribed lesion (usually measuring 1–3 cm) with contained arterial phase enhancement that appears isodense to the adjacent arterial vessels and becomes isoattenuating relative to the blood pool during the nephrographic phases (Fig. 7). Coronal CT-angiographic maximum intensity projection (MIP) reconstructions allow visualisation of the R-PA with its relationship to the renal vasculature. A R-PA may be missed in the excretory phase, owing to CM wash-out from the cavity [22–25, 44, 53, 55].

AVFs are most commonly iatrogenic rather than congenital; they are indicated by macro- or micro-haematuria from rupture within the collecting system, and may cause variable degrees of blood loss. The CT hallmark of AVF includes tortuous arteries and early or simultaneous opacification of one or more intra-parenchymal arteries and veins during the corticomedullary phase (Fig. 8) [55, 56].

Occasionally, arterial clamping may injure the vessel intima, thus leading to thrombosis, infarction and atrophy. CT-angiography depicts arterial thrombosis as abrupt vessel cut-off, and renal infarction (Fig. 8) as a peripheral wedge-shaped non-enhancing area in the renal parenchyma, with a rim of enhancement at the periphery of the cortex (rim sign) due to preserved capsular blood flow [22, 24].

Selective angiography evaluates the lesion dynamically and allows planning for trans-arterial embolisation (TAE) and super-selective catheterisation [56]

Treatment

In the past, severe bleeding and IRVIs required laparotomy. Currently, the therapeutic approach is increasingly conservative, provided that clinical and laboratory parameters remain stable and CT excludes active bleeding. Although haematomas and IRVI may heal spontaneously with conservative management, selective TAE (Figs. 7, 8, 9) is recommended as the established minimally invasive treatment of choice for life-threatening occurrences with persisting or massive bleeding, severe haematuria from communication to the pelvicalyceal system, or progressively deteriorating renal function. Notably, the need for interventional treatment such as TAE constitutes a major (Clavien grade III) complication. Arteriography confirms R-PA as an ovoid CM pool close to

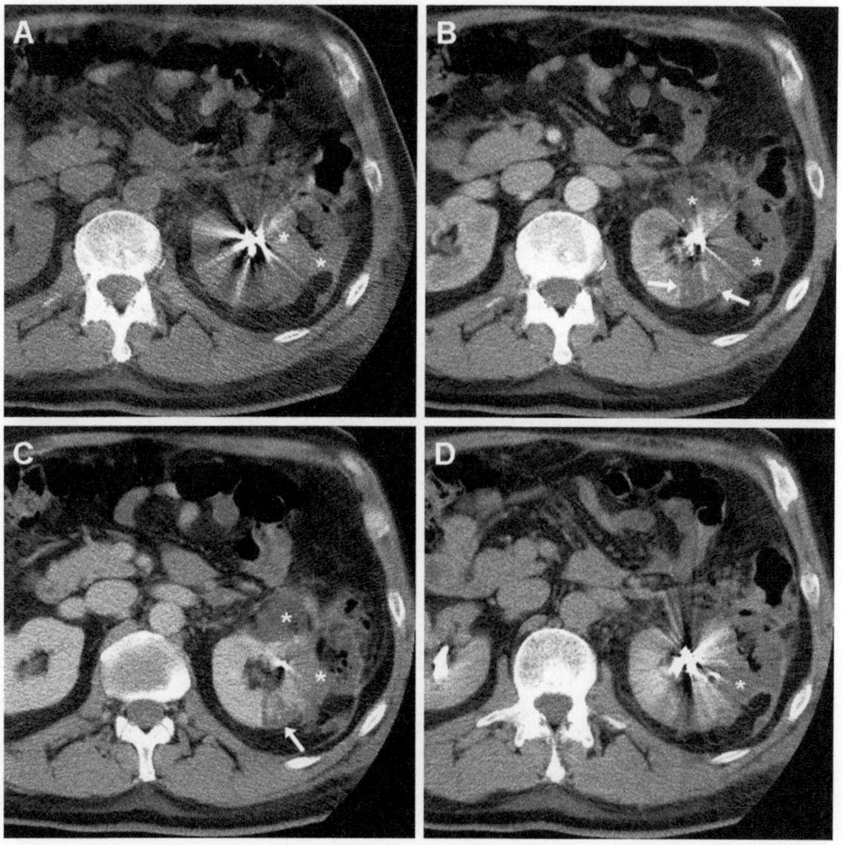

Fig. 9 Post-embolisation status in a 53-year-old man with acute haemorrhage after L-PN. Selective embolisation of arterial branches with Embozene particles and metallic coils achieved bleeding control and prompt clinical improvement. Five days later, unenhanced (**a**), corticomedullary (**b**) and nephrographic (**c**) phase multidetector CT acquisitions showed strongly hyperdense coils at the renal sinus causing beam-hardening artefacts, some residual peri-renal blood (*) without persistence of active bleeding, and a wedge-shaped non-enhancing parenchymal area (*arrows*) consistent with focal infarction. Excretory (**d**) phase images excluded urine leak from the collecting system

the SSR (Fig. 7). In patients with post-surgical IRVI, TAE using coils or other embolisation agents proved to be safe and effective treatment with a low rate of complications, rapid recovery and short hospital stay, and excellent (nearly 100 %) technical and clinical success rates, respectively corresponding to complete angiographic exclusion of bleeding and haemodynamic stabilisation without the need for blood transfusion. Super-selective embolisation, carried out as distally as possible is recommended to minimise parenchymal loss and avoid long-term impairment of renal function [32, 55, 56].

Miscellaneous complications

Postoperative infections

Occasionally, fluid collections (seroma, haematoma or urinoma) forming close to the SSR after L-PN may become infected. Differentiation of non-infected collections from an abscess requires correlation of clinical signs and laboratory data with imaging appearances, mostly represented by enlarging intra- or peri-renal hypoattenuating collections with a peripheral, thickened enhancing capsule (Fig. 10). Alternatively, the residual renal parenchyma may show the characteristic "striated nephrogram" appearance consistent with pyelonephritis [22–25, 57, 58].

Urine leaks and urinomas

Surgical access to the collecting system is necessary to ensure an adequate margin of resection for tumours extending deeply into the renal parenchyma: if the subsequent pelvicalyceal repair is not watertight, urine may leak into the surgical bed leading to a peri-renal urinoma or collection of a mixture of blood and urine. Urine leakage has been estimated to occur in 1.3-3.6 % of L-PN interventions [6–12].

The characteristic appearance of leakage seen on CT relies on identification of CM-opacified urine (80–200 HU) extravasated from the collecting system into the peri-renal space, visualised on excretory phase acquisitions (Fig. 11). Urinomas appear as more or less homogeneous collections, with progressive opacification over repeated delayed acquisitions [22–25, 49, 52].

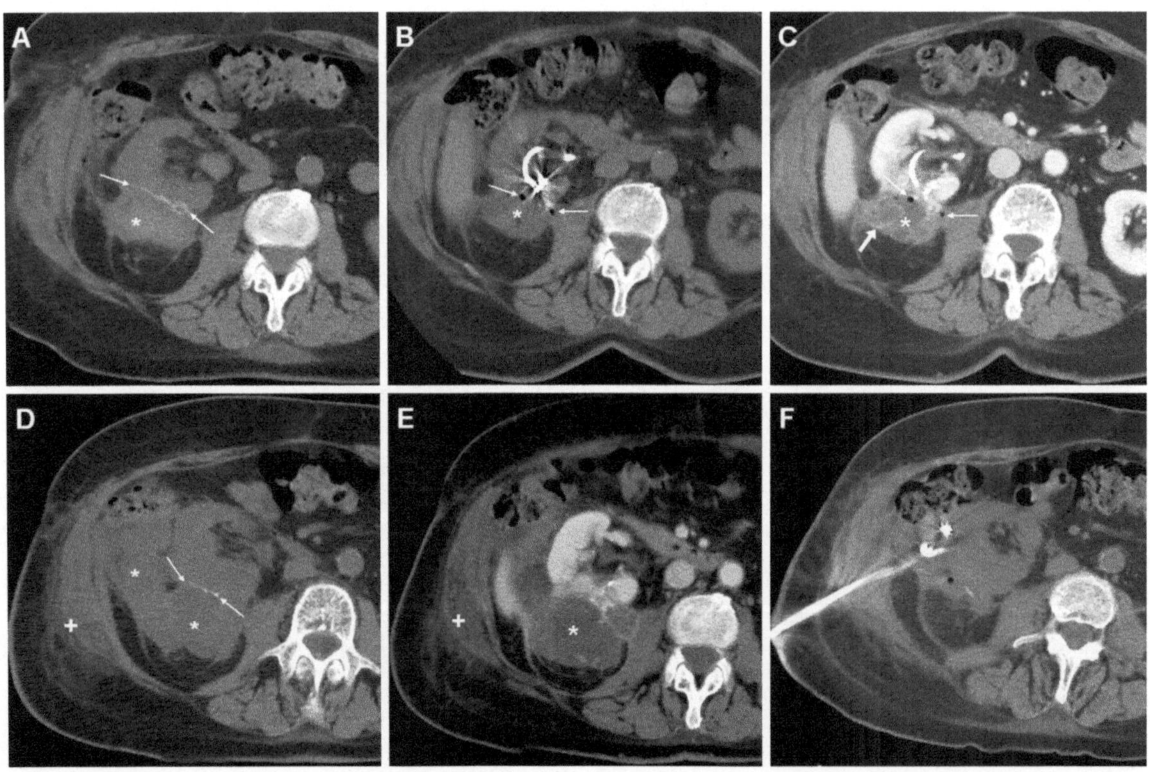

Fig. 10 A 69-year-old woman suffering from persistent pain and haematuria 10 days after right renal tumour resection had evidence of confined peri-renal haematoma (*) abutting the site of resection indicated by sutures (*thin arrows*) on unenhanced (**a**) CT. After conservative treatment repeated CT (**b**, **c**—note positioning of ureteral stent) the collection (*) showed decreased attenuation, appearance of non-dependent gas bubbles (*thin arrows*) and rim-like enhancement (*arrow* in **c**) suggesting infection. Abscessualisation (*) was confirmed by significant size increase despite antibiotic treatment at follow-up CT (**d**, **e**) with persistent peripheral enhancement, by appearance of oedematous inflammatory thickening of the ipsilateral abdominal wall (+), and was relieved by percutaneous drainage (**f**)

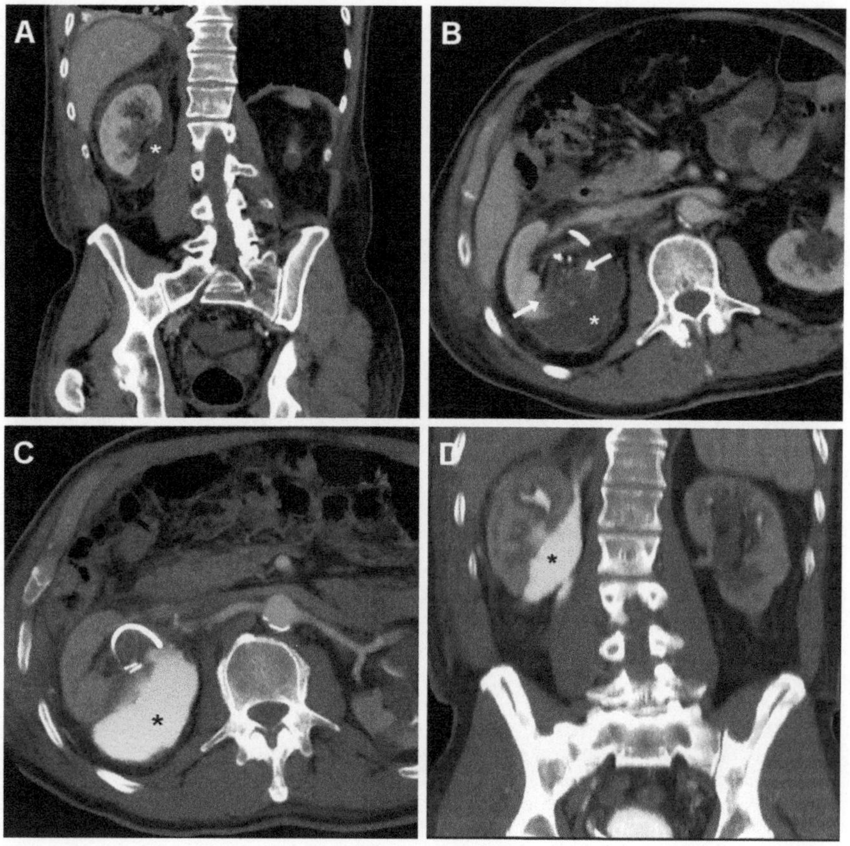

Fig. 11 Peri-renal urinoma in a 73-year-old man investigated with multidetector CT after laparoscopic resection of right-sided renal tumour because of progressive blood loss and acute flank pain. Contrast-enhanced coronal (**a**) and axial (**b**) images showed a medial peri-renal fluid collection (*), ureteral stent in place and clips at the renal hilum, and a 2.5-cm hypoenhancing portion of the posterior renal cortex (*between arrows*) corresponding to the resection site. Forty-eight hours later, follow-up split-bolus CT-urography (**c**, **d**) showed minimally enlarged collection filled with enhanced urine consistent with urinoma from injured renal pelvis. Postoperative course included prolonged ureteral stenting and blood transfusions. (Partially reprinted with permission from Tonolini et al. [52])

Most urine leaks resolve spontaneously over time and are generally managed conservatively with ureteral stenting, Foley catheter or percutaneous nephrostomy. Endourological fulguration and percutaneous imaging-guided drainage may be required to treat persistent leaks and urinomas, respectively [29, 49].

Conclusions

In most patients with suspected postoperative complications after L-NSS, urgent multidetector CT imaging allows detection of intraluminal and peri-renal haemorrhage, active bleeding, vascular injuries, extravasated urine and infections. Therefore, CT findings usually provide a consistent basis for assessment of the severity of injury and a correct choice between conservative treatment, TAE, repeated surgery, nephrostomy and/or ureteral stenting [44, 49].

References

1. Ljungberg B, Bensalah K, Bex A et al (2014) Guidelines on Renal Cell Carcinoma. European Association of Urology (EAU). Available at: http://www.uroweb.org/gls/pdf/10%20Renal%20Cell%20Carcinoma_LR.pdf. Accessed 2015/02/10
2. Ljungberg B, Cowan NC, Hanbury DC et al (2010) EAU guidelines on renal cell carcinoma: the 2010 update. Eur Urol 58:398–406
3. Hindman NM, Kang S, Parikh MS (2014) Common postoperative findings unique to laparoscopic surgery. Radiographics 34: 119–138
4. Huang WC, Levey AS, Serio AM et al (2006) Chronic kidney disease after nephrectomy in patients with renal cortical tumours: a retrospective cohort study. Lancet Oncol 7:735–740
5. Lau WK, Blute ML, Weaver AL et al (2000) Matched comparison of radical nephrectomy vs nephron-sparing surgery in patients with unilateral renal cell carcinoma and a normal contralateral kidney. Mayo Clin Proc 75:1236–1242
6. Campero JM, Ramos CG, Valdevenito R et al (2012) Laparoscopic partial nephrectomy: a series of one hundred cases performed by the same surgeon. Urol Ann 4:162–165
7. Dominguez-Escrig JL, Vasdev N, O'Riordon A et al (2011) Laparoscopic partial nephrectomy: technical considerations and an update. J Minim Access Surg 7:205–221
8. Gill IS, Kavoussi LR, Lane BR et al (2007) Comparison of 1,800 laparoscopic and open partial nephrectomies for single renal tumors. J Urol 178:41–46
9. Reifsnyder JE, Ramasamy R, Ng CK et al (2012) Laparoscopic and open partial nephrectomy: complication comparison using the Clavien system. JSLS 16:38–44

10. Springer C, Hoda MR, Fajkovic H et al (2013) Laparoscopic vs open partial nephrectomy for T1 renal tumours: evaluation of long-term oncological and functional outcomes in 340 patients. BJU Int 111:281–288
11. Touma NJ, Matsumoto ED, Kapoor A (2012) Laparoscopic partial nephrectomy: the McMaster University experience. Can Urol Assoc J 6:233–236
12. Wheat JC, Roberts WW, Hollenbeck BK et al (2013) Complications of laparoscopic partial nephrectomy. Urol Oncol 31:57–62
13. Liu Z, Wang P, Xia D et al (2013) Comparison between laparoscopic and open partial nephrectomy: surgical, oncologic, and functional outcomes. Kaohsiung J Med Sci 29:624–628
14. Minervini A, Siena G, Antonelli A et al (2014) Open versus laparoscopic partial nephrectomy for clinical T1a renal masses: a matched-pair comparison of 280 patients with TRIFECTA outcomes (RECORd Project). World J Urol 32:257–263
15. Xu H, Ding Q, Jiang HW (2014) Fewer complications after laparoscopic nephrectomy as compared to the open procedure with the modified Clavien classification system—a retrospective analysis from southern China. World J Surg Oncol 12:242
16. Becker A, Pradel L, Kluth L et al (2014) Laparoscopic versus open partial nephrectomy for clinical T1 renal masses: no impact of surgical approach on perioperative complications and long-term postoperative quality of life. World J Urol 33:421–426
17. Klatte T, Shariat SF, Remzi M (2014) Systematic review and meta-analysis of perioperative and oncologic outcomes of laparoscopic cryoablation versus laparoscopic partial nephrectomy for the treatment of small renal tumors. J Urol 191:1209–1217
18. Kapoor A, Wang Y, Dishan B et al (2014) Update on cryoablation for treatment of small renal mass: oncologic control, renal function preservation, and rate of complications. Curr Urol Rep 15:396
19. Atwell TD, Schmit GD, Boorjian SA et al (2013) Percutaneous ablation of renal masses measuring 3.0 cm and smaller: comparative local control and complications after radiofrequency ablation and cryoablation. AJR Am J Roentgenol 200:461–466
20. Schmit GD, Thompson RH, Kurup AN et al (2013) Usefulness of R.E.N.A.L. nephrometry scoring system for predicting outcomes and complications of percutaneous ablation of 751 renal tumors. J Urol 189:30–35
21. El Dib R, Touma NJ, Kapoor A (2012) Cryoablation vs radiofrequency ablation for the treatment of renal cell carcinoma: a meta-analysis of case series studies. BJU Int 110:510–516
22. Israel GM, Hecht E, Bosniak MA (2006) CT and MR imaging of complications of partial nephrectomy. Radiographics 26:1419–1429
23. Lee MS, Oh YT, Han WK et al (2007) CT findings after nephron-sparing surgery of renal tumors. AJR Am J Roentgenol 189:W264–W271
24. Saddala P, Ramanathan S, Tirumani SH et al (2015) Complications of minimally invasive procedures of the abdomen and pelvis: a comprehensive update on the clinical and imaging features. Emerg Radiol 22:283-294
25. Sarwani NI, Motta Ramirez GA, Remer EM et al (2007) Imaging findings after minimally invasive nephron-sparing renal therapies. Clin Radiol 62:333–339
26. Parsons RB, Canter D, Kutikov A et al (2012) RENAL nephrometry scoring system: the radiologist's perspective. AJR Am J Roentgenol 199:W355–W359
27. Chapin BF, Delacroix SE Jr, Wood CG (2011) Renal cell carcinoma: what the surgeon and treating physician need to know. AJR Am J Roentgenol 196:1255–1262
28. Canter D, Kutikov A, Manley B et al (2011) Utility of the R.E.N.A.L. nephrometry scoring system in objectifying treatment decision-making of the enhancing renal mass. Urology 78:1089–1094
29. Mucksavage P, McDougall EM, Clayman RV (2011) Laparoscopic transperitoneal nephrectomy for renal cancer: the University of California, Irvine, technique. J Endourol 25:195–200
30. Haber GP, Gill IS (2006) Laparoscopic partial nephrectomy: contemporary technique and outcomes. Eur Urol 49:660–665
31. Kang N, Niu Y, Zhang J et al (2012) Intraoperative ultrasonography: a useful tool in retrolaparoscopic nephron-sparing surgery. Urol Int 88:338–342
32. Summerton DJ, Kitrey ND, Lumen N et al (2012) EAU guidelines on iatrogenic trauma. Eur Urol 62:628–639
33. Mitropoulos D, Artibani W, Biyani CS et al (2014) Quality assessment of partial nephrectomy complications reporting using EAU standardised quality criteria. Eur Urol 66:522–526
34. Simhan J, Smaldone MC, Tsai KJ et al (2011) Objective measures of renal mass anatomic complexity predict rates of major complications following partial nephrectomy. Eur Urol 60:724–730
35. Reddy UD, Pillai R, Parker RA et al (2014) Prediction of complications after partial nephrectomy by RENAL nephrometry score. Ann R Coll Surg Engl 96:475–479
36. Yang CM, Chung HJ, Huang YH et al (2014) Standardized analysis of laparoscopic and robotic-assisted partial nephrectomy complications with Clavien classification. J Chin Med Assoc 77:637–641
37. Fardoun T, Chaste D, Oger E et al (2014) Predictive factors of hemorrhagic complications after partial nephrectomy. Eur J Surg Oncol 40:85–89
38. Ellison JS, Montgomery JS, Hafez KS et al (2013) Association of RENAL nephrometry score with outcomes of minimally invasive partial nephrectomy. Int J Urol 20:564–570
39. Liu ZW, Olweny EO, Yin G et al (2013) Prediction of perioperative outcomes following minimally invasive partial nephrectomy: role of the R.E.N.A.L nephrometry score. World J Urol 31:1183–1189
40. Long JA, Arnoux V, Fiard G et al (2013) External validation of the RENAL nephrometry score in renal tumours treated by partial nephrectomy. BJU Int 111:233–239
41. Hayn MH, Schwaab T, Underwood W et al (2011) RENAL nephrometry score predicts surgical outcomes of laparoscopic partial nephrectomy. BJU Int 108:876–881
42. Mathieu R, Verhoest G, Droupy S et al (2013) Predictive factors of complications after robot-assisted laparoscopic partial nephrectomy: a retrospective multicentre study. BJU Int 112:E283–E289
43. Kruck S, Anastasiadis AG, Walcher U et al (2012) Laparoscopic partial nephrectomy: risk stratification according to patient and tumor characteristics. World J Urol 30:639–646
44. Cano Alonso R, Borruel Nacenta S, Diez Martinez P et al (2009) Kidney in danger: CT findings of blunt and penetrating renal trauma. Radiographics 29:2033–2053
45. Thomsen HS, Webb JAW (eds) (2009) Contrast media: safety issues and ESUR guidelines. Springer, New York
46. Stacul F, van der Molen AJ, Reimer P et al (2011) Contrast induced nephropathy: updated ESUR Contrast Media Safety Committee guidelines. Eur Radiol 21:2527–2541
47. Kekelidze M, Dwarkasing RS, Dijkshoorn ML et al (2010) Kidney and urinary tract imaging: triple-bolus multidetector CT urography as a one-stop shop—protocol design, opacification, and image quality analysis. Radiology 255:508–516
48. Van Der Molen AJ, Cowan NC, Mueller-Lisse UG et al (2008) CT urography: definition, indications and techniques. A guideline for clinical practice. Eur Radiol 18:4–17
49. Titton RL, Gervais DA, Hahn PF et al (2003) Urine leaks and urinomas: diagnosis and imaging-guided intervention. Radiographics 23:1133–1147

50. Hope WW, Heniford BT, Norton HJ et al (2009) Duration and clinical significance of radiographically detected "free air" after laparoscopic nephrectomy. Surg Laparosc Endosc Percutan Tech 19:415–418
51. Borofsky S, Taffel M, Khati N et al (2015) The emergency room diagnosis of gastrointestinal tract perforation: the role of CT. Emerg Radiol 22:315-327
52. Tonolini M, Campari A, Bianco R (2012) Common and unusual diseases involving the iliopsoas muscle compartment: spectrum of cross-sectional imaging findings. Abdom Imaging 37: 118–139
53. Cohenpour M, Strauss S, Gottlieb P et al (2007) Pseudoaneurysm of the renal artery following partial nephrectomy: imaging findings and coil embolization. Clin Radiol 62:1104–1109
54. Albani JM, Novick AC (2003) Renal artery pseudoaneurysm after partial nephrectomy: three case reports and a literature review. Urology 62:227–231
55. Ierardi AM, Floridi C, Fontana F et al (2014) Transcatheter embolisation of iatrogenic renal vascular injuries. Radiol Med 119:261–268
56. Hatzidakis A, Rossi M, Mamoulakis C et al (2014) Management of renal arteriovenous malformations: a pictorial review. Insights Imaging 5:523–530
57. Stunell H, Buckley O, Feeney J et al (2007) Imaging of acute pyelonephritis in the adult. Eur Radiol 17:1820–1828
58. Craig WD, Wagner BJ, Travis MD (2008) Pyelonephritis: radiologic-pathologic review. Radiographics 28:255–277, **quiz 327–258**

14

ESR Position Paper on Imaging Biobanks

European Society of Radiology (ESR)

Abstract In March 2014 the European Society of Radiology (ESR) established a dedicated working group (ESR WG on Imaging Biobanks) aimed at monitoring the existing imaging biobanks in Europe, promoting the federation of imaging biobanks and communication of their findings in a white paper. The WG provided the following statements: (1) Imaging biobanks can be defined as "organised databases of medical images and associated imaging biomarkers (radiology and beyond) shared among multiple researchers, and linked to other biorepositories". (2) The immediate purpose of imaging biobanks should be to allow the generation of imaging biomarkers for use in research studies and to support biological validation of existing and novel imaging biomarkers. (3) A long-term scope of imaging biobanks should be the creation of a network/federation of such repositories integrated with the already-existing biobanking network. The aim of the WG was to investigate the existence, consistency, geographical distribution and type of imaging biobanks in Europe. A survey among ESR members resulted in the identification of 27 imaging biobanks, mostly disease-oriented and designed for research and clinical reference. In 80 % access to imaging biobanks is restricted.

Key points

- *Imaging biobanks are "shared databases of imaging biomarkers, linked to biorepositories".*
- *Exploitation of traditional and imaging biobanks is meaningful for "personalised medicine".*
- *A European imaging biobank network would significantly boost research in the imaging domain.*

✉ European Society of Radiology (ESR)
communications@myesr.org

1 Neutorgasse 9/2, 1010 Vienna, Austria

Keywords Biomarker · Biobank · Personalised medicine · Quantitative imaging

Introduction

Biobanks are repositories for the storage and retrieval of biological samples of a large number of subjects. A major goal of biobanks is the organised collection of biological material and associated information to spread access among scientists requiring this information [1].

The first biobank project, established in 1948, collecting blood samples and data, was the Framingham Heart Study (FHS), funded by the National Institute of Health-National Heart, Lung, and Blood Institute (NIH-NHLBI) [2]. A recent review performed by Kang et al. reported that 70 % of the world's biobanks are located in Europe and that the top six countries with biobanks are the UK ($n=15$), USA ($n=14$), Sweden ($n=12$), France ($n=9$), The Netherlands ($n=8$) and Italy ($n=8$) [3].

Until recently, imaging data coming from sources such as magnetic resonance imaging (MRI) or computed tomography (CT) were not included in such biobanks. Over the past 3–4 years, projects have been launched that plan to acquire large repositories of image data, including the UK Biobank and the German National Cohort [4–6].

With the rise of these efforts it is of utmost importance to register and document all existing and new imaging biobanks and provide a structured unified approach for storage of and access to these data from distributed databases. The next challenge will be to reliably connect the available imaging biobanks to tissue biobanks to explore possible imaging biomarkers and provide access to deep phenotypes.

Due to the vast amount of data, imaging biobanks need specific requirements, which have to be considered when setting up the database. Furthermore, imaging data have to be processed to extract *quantitative* information, which might evolve into a so-called "*imaging biomarker*" [7].

Due to the variety of image acquisition methods and sequences, especially in MRI, it is crucial to store detailed image acquisition parameters along with the image data. The large variability in the selection of imaging acquisition parameters in MRI provides a considerable challenge in connecting data from multiple imaging biobanks worldwide. Harmonising data-acquisition protocols as well as standardising image processing methods to extract reliable information will be of great value. The need for harmonisation, validation and standardisation of quantifiable imaging biomarkers in medical imaging has been the motivation to establish the Quantitative Imaging Biomarkers Alliance (QIBA^{TM}) initiative of the Radiological Society of North America (RSNA) and the European Imaging Biomarkers Alliance (EIBALL), initiative of the European Society of Radiology (http://www.myesr.org/cms/website.php?id=/en/membership/statutory_committees_working_groups/research_committee/european_imaging_biomarkers_alliance_-_eiball.htm). [8, 9].

In March 2014, the European Society of Radiology also established a dedicated working group (ESR WG on Imaging Biobanks) aimed at monitoring the existing imaging biobanks in Europe, promoting the federation of such imaging biobanks, and elaborated a white paper [10]. Therefore, as part of the working group's objectives, this article aims to explicate the ESR's position on the establishment and development of imaging biobanks.

Imaging biobanks: definition and rationale

Imaging biobanks are defined as organised databases of medical images, and associated imaging biomarkers (radiology and beyond), shared among multiple researchers, linked to other biorepositories [10].

Already existing biobanks are designed to give researchers access to large collections of patient/subject samples and data. Biobanks group biological material of healthy subjects (population-based) and/or patients with specific pathologies (disease-oriented), of which the most frequent are cancer-related. Most biobanks focus only on the collection of genotype data, but do not simultaneously come with a system to collect related clinical or phenotype data. In particular, most biobanks do not include or are not linked to any kind of imaging information, neither primary images nor imaging biomarkers. Comprehensive exploitation of biobanks that also include imaging (genotype and phenotype) is an important cornerstone in diagnostics in the era of "personalised medicine" [10–14].

Personalised medicine describes the intent to provide individual patients with state-of-the-art diagnostic tests, tailored interventions and specific treatments, whenever clinically indicated. Personalised medicine proposes the adjustment/customisation of health care from a one-size-fits-all approach to a patient-specific diagnosis and treatment [15]. As such, personalised medicine can be described as an evidence-supported pre-selection and assignment of tests and therapy selections to patients in need. Quantitative medical imaging, potentially resulting in the discovery of imaging biomarkers, is an essential part of personalised medicine providing a priori selection criteria and a posteriori follow-up strategies, tailored to a given patient with a specific clinical need. Obviously, development of such strategies will be greatly enhanced by the availability of large data repositories [16–19].

Biobanks give researchers access to large repositories of biomaterials for a broad spectrum of further and future analysis, e.g., genetic, genomic, epigenetic, mRNA, proteomics and transcriptomics. The large scale and the broad spectrum of data allow the detection and validation of relevant biomarkers for personalised medicine. Moreover, biobanking in European networks will result in harmonisation of health, lifestyle and other exposure data as well as the development and implemention of harmonised definitions of diseases by increased consensus on the criteria for clinical endpoints.

The classical biobanking activities are to be mirrored by a similar network of imaging biobanks. Modern radiology and nuclear medicine can also provide multiple imaging biomarkers of the same patient, using quantitative data derived from all sources of digital imaging, such as CT, MRI, PET, SPECT, US, x-ray, etc. [20, 21]. Imaging biobanks are infrastructures with massive storage and computing capacity. High-performance computing resources are needed to facilitate image processing comparison, standardisation and validation. Integration of resources and services through a platform that manages the information flow and image processing is a step needed in the development of imaging biobanks.

Other types of images can also be collected from endoscopy, microscopy, surgery, etc., also providing measurable personalised data. All this imaging information should be considered as the phenotypic expression of a patient and can be linked to the genotype. Such data should be available to the research community [22, 23].

A European imaging biobanks network would significantly boost European research in the imaging domain by stimulating the design and validation of new imaging biomarkers, as well as improving our understanding of their biological significance.

This requires standardisation, validation and benchmarking of the data in imaging biobanks. This activity will further stimulate the linking and integration of existing (national and regional) image data repositories as well as the link between imaging biobanks and traditional biobanks.

Standards will have to be developed and implemented. Innovative solutions that promote fair access to high-quality data sets with regard to image-based phenotypes and imaging biomarkers will provide support to users for its utilisation.

Finally, the economic and ethical/legal issues for the management of imaging biobanks have to be explored. These will advance insights and yield benefits to enhance collaborative research, utilise limited resources effectively and share data, technology and expertise. Research on image data management and analysis plays a key role in improving the performance of protocols, software-based analysis and further methodologies for imaging biobanks and the development and validation of imaging biomarkers. All these aspects will surely foster high-level multicenter collaboration.

Imaging informatics of imaging biobanks

An imaging biobank is a data repository supporting the gathering, querying and dissemination of imaging data for primary or secondary use in research, education and training. It comprises a repository of images and a database to support indexing based on the organ, modality or pathology, etc.

An imaging biobank may be used for different research purposes, for example, defining and validating new imaging biomarkers for diagnosis or prognosis, by comparing them with existing proven (imaging) biomarkers. It may also be used to identify the genetic origin of a disease or factors (including environmental factors) favouring disease development (cohort studies). The images may also be used to build high-quality anatomical templates, tailored to specific populations, e.g., young subjects between 15 and 20 years or patients with Parkinson's disease above 65 years.

General requirements with respect to the data collection are therefore a database facilitating storage of image data and metadata, storage of derived image-based measurements and storage of associated non-imaging data, taking into account the need to deal with longitudinal data and to cope with multiple file formats (DICOM, of course, but also formats used in research and post-processing settings such as NifTI) [24]. With respect to security, functional and technical requirements should be defined with respect to data transformation (including de-identification and encryption), infrastructure (e.g., user identity management, audit log) and data access and movement (including authorisation and transmission protection) [25]. International collaboration will require the advance of both technological and organisational matters (incorporation, procedures, protocols, data sharing, boards and access criteria). This new environment can be considered as a framework on top of a set of computing and data-intensive infrastructures that will provide researchers with tools, protocols, data and expertise to improve medical imaging research and patient health care.

Three main scenarios currently exist in terms of setup:

1. imaging biobanks of clinical research data
2. imaging biobanks with disease-specific data (not necessarily connected to a precise clinical research question)
3. imaging biobanks with general population data

First scenario: In this scenario, imaging biobanks are envisaged as infrastructure to archive, share and disseminate (for secondary use) image data that were originally used in the context of clinical research projects, such as clinical trials. In this scenario, the images may have undergone some image processing in order to extract one or more imaging biomarkers relevant to the scientific question that motivated the study. It is natural to store such biomarkers as well as related provenance metadata in the imaging biobank database.

Second scenario: In this scenario, imaging biobanks are envisaged as resources to receive, archive, share and disseminate images in specific clinical domains, e.g., Alzheimer's disease or multiple sclerosis. Such systems aim at collecting the clinical images of patients with a given pathology on a broad scale (e.g., national scale). They usually address common specific image acquisition protocols and ensure quality control at the time of image importation to ensure optimal image use. These imaging biobanks can also be based on a regional or national screening initiative collecting image data of a group of persons with specific characteristics such as habits, previous disease or a genetic profile. Breast cancer, lung cancer and colon cancer screenings are examples of image-based screening with subsequent storage of images in an imaging biobank.

Third scenario: In this scenario, imaging biobanks are composed of data collections obtained from the general population without a specific research goal or disease-oriented approach. Longitudinal data are collected over a long period of time with as much data collected of as many subjects as possible. Research projects may gain paid access to this data upon request for a specific research question. The technical setup of this scenario is similar to the second scenario, but the data collection is not performed for clinical purposes and will in many cases be acquired by entities established especially for the data collection of the population study.

Services provided by imaging biobanks

(1) **Management of image collections**: This involves several aspects: (a) negotiating the conditions of image acceptance and conservation: duration of conservation, formats, image quality, sharing with owners, sharing with other parties, general and specific (i.e., collection-dependent) metadata, ability to link to external data (clinical information, biological information, biological specimen); (b) defining metadata associated with a new image collection; (c) applying workflow when a new image is added to a collection (receiving images from a source and assessing image quality, recording information about data acquisition and acquisition devices, assessing proper data selection according to the specific research project, recording additional information besides the images such as measurements, functional data).

(2) **Supporting image collections' consultation**: This includes sending study requests to a review committee that determines the scientific merit and checks for similar requests that were previously granted. If approved, the committee sets up access rights at the desired level to the selected subset of the data and supports query/retrieval processes, i.e., processing queries from external parties, verifying access rights, querying the database, providing references of images and related metadata, and downloading images.

(3) **Relating image cases to external data (data, specimen)**: This involves: (a) receiving notifications from external parties, (b) cross-referencing identifiable information to connect the two databases and determine subjects for which this is feasible and reliable enough, and (c) updating the database with the references of external data.

(4) **Production of imaging biomarkers**: This service requires the prior definition of a process to validate the imaging biomarker to guarantee to the requesting party that the measurements performed are accurate. Standardisation and registration of the process should also be part of this. The biomarkers' calculation service includes: (a) applying the relevant image-processing workflow, (b) recording the calculated values in the database as well as (c) the detailed provenance data (by whom, how and when such data were obtained).

Federated access to imaging biobanks

A key feature is to provide end-users with large federated systems (e.g., through a web portal or a set of web services), facilitating data query from multiple imaging biobanks. This avoids users querying all the imaging biobanks successively that they believe might contain the kind of data they are looking for. Providing such service involves:

(1) setting up a catalogue of image collections provided by multiple imaging biobanks;
(2) striving towards a "federated data model" for databases querying (e.g., using common data schemas, standard nomenclatures, reference to common ontologies);
(3) receiving queries from external parties;
(4) querying the distributed databases according to the "federated data model";
(5) providing image metadata matching the query, including references to image data. These federated systems will improve health care through studies of quality control, such as image quality and radiation dose, technical and protocol comparisons, follow-up assessment of clinical guidelines, fast translation of research findings into image-guided management, assessment of image biomarker prognostic factors and early assessment of treatment response.

Clinical focus

Imaging biobanks should be focussed on collecting data from healthy subjects or—disease-oriented—from patients (oncologic imaging, rare diseases, other). In the case of healthy subjects (as in the UK Biobank), it should be considered how these data can be collected to ensure participant safety and identity protection. In principle, the imaging acquisition should minimise or avoid the use of ionising radiation with greater dependence on US and MRI in healthy subjects. In contrast, disease-related IB can also be collected by x-ray and (ultra) low-dose CT, represented by data derived from screening programmes for breast cancer (x-ray mammography) and colon and lung cancer (CT colonography and low-dose lung CT) [26–30]. Furthermore, developments in CT imaging with ultra-low-dose acquisitions could open the possibility of CT imaging in population screening for subjects above a certain age.

Oncologic imaging seems to be the easier setting for the collection of imaging biomarkers from multiple imaging modalities. Oncology patients routinely undergo multiple imaging studies for staging and follow-up of the disease to evaluate the TNM and the treatment response. The same patients undergo multiple laboratory tests, pathologic specimen analysis (which provides further imaging data), genetic sequencing, etc. In this setting it seems highly relevant to link imaging biomarkers derived from clinical investigation with those collected by traditional biobanking [31].

Clinical research will benefit from the increased production of scientific researchers' contributions from the field of radiology.

Economics, standards, security, legal issues

Economic

The creation and realisation of biobanks is a very expensive process because of the involvement of a large number of participants, e.g., the UK Biobank with about 500,000 participants or the nationwide biobank in Iceland. Imaging procedures as part of prospective cohort studies will contribute to the overall costs in a relevant portion, especially if MR imaging is necessary because of the research focus and radiation exposure, contrast media or medication with other modalities (e.g., cardiac CT).

In large studies, dedicated imaging centres have been established or are in planning. Based on the example of the UK, it has been shown that the costs per participant would be approximately €500; however this would end up at about €50 M for the imaging part based on the assumption of 100, 000 participants [32].

Standards

Standards are relevant for different levels, e.g., legal regulation, organisational issues for the institution, standard operating procedures for handling of data and samples, but also for the syntax and semantic (ontologies) representation in information systems.

In the context of medical imaging, there are three major topics:

Reporting: there is a common trend to structured reporting worldwide [33]. Automated evaluation of information in databanks would work best with standardised documentation of findings and measurements. There are relatively mature solutions providing the platform for such efforts. The Integrating the Healthcare Enterprise (IHE) profile, "Managing Radiology Report Templates", describes the use of appropriate templates. Recommendations for workflows and implementations are available, while first implementations are under evaluation [33].

Semantic Interoperability: Imaging procedures for imaging biobanks will very often rely on quantitative imaging biomarker data, to be exchanged between systems. Suitable models should therefore be defined to describe them in an explicit and consistent way, ideally using semantic models such as ontologies (e.g., SNOMED, RadLex, ICD).

Imaging and communication formats: due to the worldwide acceptance of DICOM there are minor issues in the topic of imaging formats. DICOM has ongoing revised and new requirements, e.g., new imaging techniques or ontologies will be included into the standard. Workflows and communication across institutions are almost covered by IHE profiles. Based on the IHE Cross-Enterprise-Communication concept (IHE-XDS family), which is the core of many regional and national eHealth concepts, there is already a logical approach for connecting imaging centres with imaging biobanks. These IHE-XDS concepts would allow decentral storage of primary data, but also the aggregation of data, and also communication across different imaging biobank domains (www.ihe.net). Actually, there is a missing link between the imaging world and the information about biobanks. The description of requirements and workflows should be followed by the development of an appropriate IHE profile for these use cases [34, 35].

Security and legal issues

Security and legal issues are two of the most challenging tasks in building large research databases in general. This is due to the requirements for the probable long-term aggregation of medical data from different sources linked with personal information on one side and the request for patient privacy and security aspects on the other. Such databases might contain personal data and information, and also digitised collections of specimens such as tissues or blood, genomic and imaging data.

Many of such research-oriented databases are built as legacy systems with proprietary regulations, regulated by different levels of privacy rules, for example [36, 37].

There are some examples of concepts for the legal frameworks for biobanking; one of these is from the German "Telematics Platform of Medical Research Network" (TMF) [38]. One of the relevant requirements is a solution for interdisciplinary and active collaboration between different institutions, for which the property rights and privacy of the "donors" (information data and/or biological material from volunteers and patients) have to be protected, even for scientific and also possible commercial use by third parties.

Therefore different legal requirements have to be considered [39]:

- *Legal status of the institution* organising and maintaining the databank.
- *Property rights* of samples and information, will often require explicit transfer of rights by the donor.
- *Relevance of medico-legal and professional regulations*, e.g., the acquisition of samples is usually a medical act, which requires interaction with a physician, even in a research setting. Another topic is a regulation about the communication on new findings while in research or data analysis, which might impact the health of the donor.
- *Continuity* of databanks in case of ending projects or insolvence of the institution;
- *Secure transfer* of samples or information and *secure storage*;
- *Confiscation protection and research secrecy.*

Table 1 Results of the ESR survey on imaging biobanks

Purpose of the biobank	Number (percentage)
Research	14 (82.4)
Clinical reference	12 (70.6)
e-learning	9 (52.9)
Other	1 (5.9)
Types of cases available	
Oncologic	13 (76.5)
Cardiovascular	8 (47.1)
Healthy volunteers	7 (41.2)
Rare diseases	6 (35.3)
Other	6 (35.3)
Number of cases available	
Less than 300	5 (29.4)
300–500	3 (17.6)
500–1000	3 (17.6)
1000–2000	1 (5.9)
More than 2000	5 (29.4)
Kind of imaging data available	
Computed tomography	14 (82.4)
Magnetic resonance	15 (88.2)
Hybrid imaging	5 (29.4)
Ultrasound	9 (52.9)
Other	5 (29.4)
Availability of follow-up image examinations	
Not available	5 (29.4)
Available	12 (70.6)
Availability of publications based in the image biobank	
Not available	12 (70.6)
Available	5 (29.4)
Accessibility to the biobank	
Fully open on the Internet	1 (6.3)
Open to any registered user (free registration)	2 (12.5)
Restricted to users involved in predefined projects	5 (31.3)
Restricted to the personnel of the local department/hospital	8 (50.0)
Imaging data supported	
Strictly limited to acquired images	5 (31.3)
Also contains processed images (segmentation, registration, etc.)	8 (50.0)
Also contains imaging biomarkers	3 (18.8)
Image formats	
Strictly limited to DICOM	13 (81.3)
DICOM and other common formats used in research (such as NIFTI, Analyze)	1 (6.3)
Also contains imaging biomarkers	2 (12.5)

The complexity in building large databanks for international collaboration may increase in case of different national regulations. The actual development at the European level with the preparation of a General Data Protection Regulation (COM (2012) 0011) will also be relevant for the future of imaging biobanks [40].

There is an interest in unified worldwide legislation regarding privacy issues and ownership, also to require mandatory registration of biobanks.

Imaging biobanks in Europe: results of the ESR survey

One of the aims of the working group was to investigate the existence, consistency, geographical distribution and type of imaging biobanks in Europe.

A survey was carried out, using a free online poll service (www.surveymonkey.com), inviting heads of radiology departments across Europe to answer the following nine questions: purpose of the biobank, types of cases, number of cases, kind of imaging data, presence of follow-up image examinations, already existing publications on the image biobank, accessibility of the image biobank (open, restricted to user), imaging data supported and image format.

The results of the questionnaire are summarised in Table 1.

Twenty-seven responses were received from Austria, Finland, France, Germany, Kazakhstan, Italy, Russia, Slovenia, Spain, Sweden, Switzerland, The Netherlands, Turkey and the UK.

Most biobanks are for research and clinical reference and are disease-oriented (oncologic and cardiovascular type of cases); the number of cases included is extremely variable, but mostly less than 1000, and most biobanks contain CT and MR images.

Of note, the accessibility of the biobanks is in the vast majority (80 %) restricted to registered users involved in predefined projects or personnel of the local department/hospital.

Conclusion

Medical imaging biobanks are virtual biobanks recently emerging for advancing the study of rare, cardiovascular, oncologic and neurological diseases, the identification of early biomarkers and surrogates, and the development of population studies. These biobanks will evaluate the impact of new quantitative biomarkers in early disease diagnosis, disease phenotyping, disease grading, targeting therapies and evaluation of disease response to treatment.

Such imaging biobanks are currently at an early stage of development and dissemination within Europe. The survey carried out among heads of radiology departments across Europe proved the existence and operation of some disease-oriented patient- or healthy population-based image databases. Most of them were developed within institutional projects and are not freely accessible. The working group elaborated the rationale, definition, technical, clinical, economics, management, legal and ethical issues related to the setup, development, federation and maintenance of imaging biobanks. As the imaging biobanks are focussing on the phenotype expression, there is an unmet need to link the information to other biomarkers from other sources of information, especially all biobanks. Therefore the working group endorsed the integration of imaging biobanks with already traditional biobanks (genomic, tissue and other type of "omics"), since the joint exploitation of both biobanks is an important cornerstone for diagnosis and targeted therapies in the era of personalised medicine.

Acknowledgments This article was kindly prepared by the ESR Working Group on Imaging Biobanks (Chair and lead/corresponding author: Emanuele Neri, Members: Bernard Gibaud, Matthias Guenther, Alan Jackson, Hans-Ulrich Kauczor, Luis Marti-Bonmati, Peter Mildenberger, Osman Ratib, Siegfried Trattnig, Aad van der Lugt, Peter Van Ooijen) on behalf of the European Society of Radiology (ESR). It was approved by the ESR Executive Council on 26 March 2015.

References

1. Hewitt R, Watson P (2013) Defining biobank. Biopreserv Biobank 11:309–315
2. Dawber TR, Kannel WB (1966) The Framingham study, an epidemiologic approach to coronary heart diseas. Circulation 34:553–555
3. Kang B, Park J, Cho S, Lee M, Kim N, Min H et al (2013) Current status, challenges, policies, and bioethics of biobanks. Genomics Inform 11:211–217
4. Woodbridge M, Fagiolo G, O'Regan DP (2013) MRIdb: medical image management for biobank research. J Digit Imaging 26:886–890
5. Petersen SE, Matthews PM, Bamberg F et al (2013) Imaging in population science: cardiovascular magnetic resonance in 100,000 participants of UK Biobank—rationale, challenges and approaches. J Cardiovasc Magn Reson 15:46
6. Starkbaum J, Gottweis H, Gottweis U et al (2014) Public perceptions of cohort studies and biobanks in Germany. Biopreserv Biobank 12:121–130
7. Prescott JW (2013) Quantitative imaging biomarkers: the application of advanced image processing and analysis to clinical and preclinical decision making. J Digit Imaging 26:97–108
8. Kessler LG, Barnhart HX, Buckler AJ, QIBA Terminology Working Group et al (2014) The emerging science of quantitative imaging biomarkers terminology and definitions for scientific studies and regulatory submissions. Stat Methods Med Res 24(1):9–26
9. Raunig DL, McShane LM, Pennello G, QIBA Technical Performance Working Group et al (2014) Quantitative imaging biomarkers: a review of statistical methods for technical performance assessment. Stat Methods Med Res 24(1):27–67
10. Mission Statement of the ESR Working Group on Imaging Biobanks (2014) https://www.myesr.org/cms/website.php?id=/en/research/esr_wg_on_imaging_biobanks/esr.htm
11. Olson JE, Bielinski SJ, Ryu E, Winkler EM, Takahashi PY, Pathak J et al (2014) Biobanks and personalized medicine. Clin Genet 86:50–55
12. Watson PH, Barnes RO (2011) A proposed schema for classifying human research biobanks. Biopreserv Biobank 9:327–333
13. Terry SF, Horn EJ, Scott JA, Terry PF (2011) Genetic alliance registry and biobank: a novel disease advocacy-driven research solution. Pers Med 8:207–213
14. Asslaber M, Zatloukal K (2007) Biobanks: transnational, European and global networks. Brief Funct Genomic Proteomic 6:193–201
15. European Society of Radiology (ESR) (2015) Medical imaging in personalised medicine: a white paper of the research committee of the European Society of Radiology (ESR). Insight Imaging. doi:10.1007/s13244-015-0394-0
16. Hewitt RE (2011) Biobanking: the foundation of personalized medicine. Curr Opin Oncol 23:112–119
17. Fiore LD, D'Avolio LW (2011) Detours on the road to personalized medicine: barriers to biomarker validation and implementation. JAMA 306:1914–1915
18. Hamburg MA, Collins FS (2010) The path to personalized medicine. N Engl J Med 363:301–304
19. European Society of Radiology (2011) Medical imaging in personalised medicine: a white paper of the research committee of the European Society of Radiology (ESR). Insights Imaging 2: 621–630
20. European Society of Radiology (2013) ESR statement on the stepwise development of imaging biomarkers. Insights Imaging 4:147–152
21. European Society of Radiology (2010) White paper on imaging biomarkers. (ESR). Insights Imaging 1:42–45
22. Ko KH, Kown CI, Park JM, Lee HG, Han NY, Hahm KB (2014) Molecular imaging for theranostics in gastroenterology: one stone to kill two birds. Clin Endosc 47:383–388
23. Croce AC, Bottiroli G (2014) Autofluorescence spectroscopy and imaging: a tool for biomedical research and diagnosis. Eur J Histochem 58:2461
24. Marcus DS, Erickson BJ, Pan T, (CTSA Imaging Informatics Working Group) (2012) Imaging infrastructure for research. Part 2: data management practices. J Digit Imaging 25:566–569
25. Pan T, Erickson BJ, Marcus DS, (CTSA Imaging Informatics Project Group) (2012) Whitepapers on imaging infrastructure for research. Part 3: security and privacy. J Digit Imaging 25: 692–702
26. Regge D, Iussich G, Senore C, Correale L, Hassan C, Bert A et al (2014) Population screening for colorectal cancer by flexible sigmoidoscopy or CT colonography: study protocol for a multicenter randomized trial. Trials 15:97
27. Sali L, Grazzini G, Carozzi F et al (2013) Screening for colorectal cancer with FOBT, virtual colonoscopy and optical colonoscopy: study protocol for a randomized controlled trial in the Florence district (SAVE study). Trials 14:74
28. Grannis FW Jr (2014) National lung screening trial limitations and public health policy. Oncology 28(11):956–63
29. Black WC, Gareen IF, Soneji SS et al (2014) National lung screening trial research team. Cost-effectiveness of CT screening in the national lung screening trial. N Engl J Med 371: 1793–1802
30. Horeweg N, van Rosmalen J, Heuvelmans MA et al (2014) Lung cancer probability in patients with CT-detected pulmonary nodules: a prespecified analysis of data from the NELSON trial of low-dose CT screening. Lancet Oncol 15(12):1332–41

31. Rezai P, Pisaneschi MJ, Feng C, Yaghmai V (2013) A radiologist's guide to treatment response criteria in oncologic imaging: functional, molecular, and disease-specific imaging biomarkers. AJR Am J Roentgenol 201:246–255
32. Scholtes VP, de Vries JP, Catanzariti LM, de Kleijn DP, Moll FL, de Borst GJ et al (2014) Biobanking in atherosclerotic disease, opportunities and pitfalls. Curr Cardiol Rev 7: 9–14
33. Bosmans JM, Neri E, Ratib O, Kahn CE Jr (2015) Structured reporting: a fusion reactor hungry for fuel. Insights Imaging 6: 129–132
34. IHE Radiology Technical Committee (2014). IHE Radiology Technical Framework V13.0. Supplement. Management of Radiology Report Templates (MRRT). IHE International, Inc. http://www.ihe.net/uploadedFiles/Documents/Radiology/IHE_RAD_Suppl_MRRT.pdf
35. Dogac A, Laleci GB, Aden T, Eichelberg M (2007) Enhancing IHE XDS for federated clinical affinity domain support. IEEE Trans Inf Technol Biomed 11:213–221
36. Virani AH, Longstaff H (2014) Ethical considerations in biobanks: how a public health ethics perspective sheds new light on old controversies. J Genet Couns
37. Platt J, Bollinger J, Dvoskin R, Kardia SL, Kaufman D (2014) Public preferences regarding informed consent models for participation in population-based genomic research. Genet Med 16:11–18
38. Platt J, Kardia S (2015) Public trust in health information sharing: implications for biobanking and electronic health record systems. J Pers Med 5:3–21
39. Simon J, Paslack R, Robienski J, Cooper DN, Goebel JW, Krawczak M (2007) A legal framework for biobanking: the German experience. Eur J Hum Genet 15:528–532
40. Regulation of the European Parliament and of the Council on the Protection of Individuals with Regard to the Processing of Personal Data and on the Free Movement of Such Data (General Data Protection Regulation) (2012): http://ec.europa.eu/justice/data-protection/document/review2012/com_2012_11_en.pdf

15

Summary of the European Directive 2013/59/Euratom: essentials for health professionals in radiology

European Society of Radiology (ESR)

Abstract The aspects of the new European Directive 2013/59/Euratom most relevant to diagnostic imaging and intervention are summarised. The Directive, laying down basic safety standards for protection against the dangers from exposure to ionising radiation, emphasises the need for justification of medical exposure (including asymptomatic individuals), introduces requirements concerning patient information and strengthens those for recording and reporting doses from radiological procedures, the use of diagnostic reference levels, the availability of dose-indicating devices and the improved role and support of the Medical Physics Experts in imaging. Relevant changes include new definitions, a new dose limit for the eye lens, non-medical imaging exposures, procedures in asymptomatic individuals, the use and regular review of diagnostic reference levels (including interventional procedures), dosimetric information in imaging systems and its transfer to the examination report, new requirements on responsibilities, the registry and analysis of accidental or unintended exposure and population dose evaluation (based on age and gender distribution). These changes will require Member States, the radiology community and the industry to adapt regulations, practices and equipment for a high standard of radiation safety. By 6 February 2018, the Directive has to be transposed into the national legislation of the Member States of the European Union.

Main messages

- *The new European Basic Safety Standards Directive impacts radiology departments*
- *Changes in justification, patient information, responsibilities and dose reporting are most significant*
- *Diagnostic reference levels and the role of medical physics experts are clarified*
- *Dose limits to the eye lens are lower than in the previous directive*
- *Responsibilities in radiation safety have been defined*

Keywords Protection · Radiation · Legislation · Medical · European Union · Government regulations

Introduction

The new European Directive 2013/59/Euratom [1], laying down basic safety standards (BSS) for protection against the dangers arising from exposure to ionising radiation and repealing Directives 89/618/Euratom, 90/641/Euratom, 96/29/Euratom, 97/43/Euratom and 2003/122/Euratom, is expected to have a relevant and positive impact on European radiology.

The basic safety standards take into account the new recommendations of the International Commission on Radiological Protection (ICRP) [2, 3] and are revised in the light of new scientific evidence and operational experience.

The Directive was unanimously adopted by the Council of the European Union (EU) on 5 December 2013 after 4 years of work by different European scientific and technical committees.[1] The press release after the Council meeting held in Brussels on 5 December 2013 highlighted that the new Directive, under which the Member States will establish legal requirements and an appropriate regime of regulatory control,

[1] The Council of the EU is the institution representing the member states' governments. Also informally known as the EU Council, it is where national ministers from each EU country meet to adopt laws and coordinate policies.

✉ European Society of Radiology (ESR)
communications@myESR.org

[1] Neutorgasse 9/2, 1010 Vienna, Austria

reflects a system of radiation protection based on the principles of justification, optimisation and dose limitation for all exposure situations. Dose limits shall not apply to medical exposures.

According to the new Directive, a high level of competence and a clear definition of responsibilities and tasks among all professionals involved in medical exposure are fundamental to ensure adequate protection of patients undergoing medical radiodiagnostic and radiotherapeutic procedures. This applies to medical doctors, dentists and other health professionals entitled to take clinical responsibility for individual medical exposures, to medical physics experts and to other professionals carrying out practical aspects of medical radiological procedures, such as radiographers and technicians in radiodiagnostic medicine, nuclear medicine and radiotherapy.

Furthermore, the Directive provides radiation protection education, training and provision of information. The Member States will have 4 years to transpose this Directive into national legislation.

The most relevant changes in the new Directive in comparison to the existing ones—96/29/Euratom [4] on the protection of workers and the general public and 97/43/Euratom [5] on medical exposures—are summarised in Tables 1 and 2.

The Directive distinguishes between existing, planned and emergency exposure situations. Taking into account this new framework, the Directive covers all exposure situations and all categories of exposure, namely occupational, public and medical.

Table 1 Most relevant changes for radiology imaging in Directive 2013/59/Euratom

1. New set of definitions
2. New dose limit for the lens of the eyes
3. Consideration of occupational doses in justification and optimisation
4. Regulation for radiological procedures in asymptomatic individuals
5. Use and regular review of diagnostic reference levels (including interventional)
6. Education and training (out of the chapter on medical exposures)
7. Responsibilities (the full Art. 57 should be analysed)
8. Role of medical physics experts in diagnostic and interventional procedures
9. New requirements for equipment in use
10. Procedures: optimisation process, clinical protocols and clinical audit
11. Registry and analysis of accidental or unintended exposures
12. Population dose evaluation taking into account age distribution and gender
13. Old "medico-legal" and new "non-medical imaging exposures"

Chapter VII in the new Directive deals with medical exposures but other chapters contain articles relevant to radiology imaging (see Table 2).

Table 2 Other requirements of Directive 2013/59/Euratom with high relevance to imaging

Dose constraints for occupational, public and medical exposure (Art. 6)
Dose limits for occupational exposure including the new limit for the lens of the eyes of 20 mSv in a single year (Art. 9)
Pregnant worker protection (Art. 10)
Education, information and training in the field of medical exposure (Art. 18)
Chapter VI on occupational exposures, in particular:
• Operational protection of exposed workers (Art. 32)
• Operational protection of apprentices and students (Art. 33)
• Consultations with radiation protection experts (Art. 34)
• Controlled and supervised areas (Arts. 37-38)
• Radiological surveillance of the workplace (Art. 39)
• Categorisation of exposed workers (Art. 40)
• Individual monitoring and access to the results (Arts. 41 and 44)
• Medical surveillance of exposed workers (Art. 45)

The new Directive provides minimum rules, and Member States should be free to adopt or maintain more stringent measures in the subject matter covered by the Directive, without prejudice to the free movement of goods and services in the internal European Union market.

New set of definitions

The definition of "medical exposure" in the new Directive is similar to the previous one, but excludes the "medico-legal", now called "non-medical imaging exposure". The relevant definitions (with some changes in comparison to the previous Directives) are included in the Annex.

Occupational dose limits and new limit for the lens of the eye

New scientific information on tissue reactions calls for better protection of the eye lens and, following the ICRP guidance, the new Directive modifies the occupational dose limit for the eye lens to 20 mSv/year from the previous value of 150 mSv/year.

Articles 9 and 11 on dose limits for occupational exposure and dose limits for apprentices and students indicate that:

- Dose limits for occupational exposure apply to the sum of annual occupational exposures of a worker from all authorised practices.
- The limit on the effective dose shall be 20 mSv in any single year (in special circumstances 50 mSv if the

average annual dose over any 5 consecutive years does not exceed 20 mSv).

- The limit on the equivalent dose for the lens of the eye shall be 20 mSv in a single year or 100 mSv in any 5 consecutive years subject to a maximum dose of 50 mSv in a single year.
- The limit on the equivalent dose for the skin and extremities shall be 500 mSv in a year.
- Apprentices and students (aged 16–18 years) have more restrictive dose limits: an effective dose of 6 mSv in a year and equivalent doses of 15 mSv in a year to the lens of the eye as well as of 150 mSv in a year to the skin and the extremities.
- In addition, Art. 40 establishes the categorisation of exposed workers. Workers are required to be classified as 'category A' (i.e., subject to individual monitoring and medical surveillance) if (a) an effective dose greater than 6 mSv per year or (b) an equivalent dose greater than 15 mSv per year for the lens of the eye or (c) greater than 150 mSv per year for the skin and extremities might be expected.

Article 10 deals with pregnant and breastfeeding workers:

- As soon as a pregnant worker informs the employer of the pregnancy the employment conditions shall assure that the equivalent dose to the unborn child is as low as reasonably achievable and unlikely to exceed 1 mSv during at least the remainder of the pregnancy.
- As soon as workers inform the employer that they are breastfeeding an infant, they shall not be employed in work involving a significant risk of intake of radionuclides or of bodily contamination.

Consideration of occupational doses in justification and optimisation

Articles 55 and 56 in Chap. VII on Medical Exposures maintain most of the requirements of the previous 97/43/Euratom Directive, but the explicit consideration of occupational doses in justification and optimisation (as made by ICRP) in some previous articles should be noted.

Article 19.4. Practices involving medical exposure shall be justified both as a class or type of practice, taking into account medical and, where relevant, associated occupational and public exposures, and at the level of each individual medical exposure.

Article 32.b. Member States shall ensure that the operational protection of exposed workers is based on optimisation of radiation protection in all working conditions, including occupational exposures as a consequence of practices involving medical exposures.

Regulation for radiological procedures in asymptomatic individuals

A new article (55.2.h) on justification has been added, concerning medical radiological procedures on asymptomatic individuals, to be performed for early disease detection. Such procedures should either be part of a health screening programme or require specific documented justification for that individual by the practitioner, in consultation with the referrer, following guidelines from relevant medical scientific societies and the competent authority. Special attention shall be given to the provision of information to the individual subject to medical exposure.

Use and regular review of diagnostic reference levels (including interventional)

The new Directive strengthens and expands the previous requirements regarding diagnostic reference levels.

Article 56.2. Member States shall ensure the establishment, regular review and use of diagnostic reference levels for radiodiagnostic examinations, having regard to the recommended European diagnostic reference levels where available, and where appropriate, for interventional radiology procedures and the availability of guidance for this purpose.

Article 58.f. underlines the need for appropriate local reviews whenever diagnostic reference levels are consistently exceeded and requires that the corresponding corrective action is taken without undue delay.

Education, information and training in the field of medical exposure

Article 18 of the new Directive deals with education, information and training in the field of medical exposure. This article is now part of Chap. VII (Medical Exposures) and its content is the same as in the previous 97/43/Euratom Directive. Article 59 on "training and recognition" in the new Directive refers to this Art. 18.

- Member States shall ensure that practitioners and the individuals involved in the practical aspects of medical radiological procedures have adequate education, information and theoretical and practical training for the purpose of medical radiological practices, as well as relevant competence in radiation protection.
- For this purpose Member States shall ensure that appropriate curricula are established and shall recognise the corresponding diplomas, certificates or formal qualifications.

- Individuals undergoing relevant training programmes may participate in practical aspects of medical radiological procedures.
- Member States shall ensure that continuing education and training after qualification are provided and, in the special case of the clinical use of new techniques, training is provided on these techniques and the relevant radiation protection requirements.
- Member States shall encourage the introduction of a course on radiation protection in the basic curriculum of medical and dental schools.

Responsibilities

Article 57 deals with responsibilities and contains new requirements regarding the optimisation process and the provision of information to patients.

1. Member States shall ensure that:

   (a) Any medical exposure takes place under the clinical responsibility of a practitioner;
   (b) The practitioner, the medical physics expert and those entitled to carry out practical aspects of medical radiological procedures are involved, as specified by Member States, in the optimisation process;
   (c) The referrer and the practitioner are involved, as specified by Member States, in the justification process of individual medical exposures;
   (d) Wherever practicable, prior to the exposure taking place, the practitioner or the referrer, as specified by Member States, ensures that the patient or his/her representative is provided with adequate information relating to the benefits and risks associated with the radiation dose from the medical exposure. Similar information as well as relevant guidance shall be given to carers and comforters, in accordance with point (b) of Art. 56(5).
2. Practical aspects of medical radiological procedures may be delegated by the undertaking or the practitioner, as appropriate, to one or more individuals entitled to act in this respect in a recognised field of specialisation.

Role of the medical physics expert in imaging

Article 58 (procedures), part d, indicates that a medical physics expert shall be involved in radiodiagnostic and interventional radiology practices involving high doses as referred to in point (c) of Art. 61(1) (i.e. interventional radiology and computed tomography). For other medical radiological practices, a medical physics expert shall be involved as appropriate, depending on the radiological risk posed by the practice, for consultation and advice.

Article 83 defines the responsibilities of the medical physics expert:

Member States shall require the medical physics expert to act or give specialist advice as appropriate on matters relating to radiation physics for implementing the requirements set out in Chap. VII and in point (c) of Art. 22(4) of the Directive (i.e. "Practices involving the deliberate exposure of humans for non-medical imaging purposes").

Member States shall ensure that depending on the medical radiological practice, the medical physics expert takes responsibility for dosimetry, including physical measurements for evaluation of the dose delivered to the patient and other individuals subject to medical exposure, give advice on medical radiological equipment and contribute in particular to the following:

(a) Optimisation of the radiation protection of patients and other individuals subject to medical exposure, including the application and use of diagnostic reference levels;
(b) The definition and performance of quality assurance of the medical radiological equipment;
(c) Acceptance testing of medical radiological equipment;
(d) The preparation of technical specifications for medical radiological equipment and installation design;
(e) The surveillance of the medical radiological installations;
(f) The analysis of events involving, or potentially involving, accidental or unintended medical exposures;
(g) The selection of equipment required to perform radiation protection measurements;
(h) The training of practitioners and other staff in relevant aspects of radiation protection;

It is also required that the medical physics expert shall, where appropriate, liaise with the radiation protection expert.

New requirements for equipment in use

Article 60.3 (equipment) underlines the responsibility of Member States to ensure that:

(a) The use of fluoroscopy equipment without a device to automatically control the dose rate, or without an image intensifier or equivalent device, is prohibited.
(c) Any equipment used for interventional radiology has a device or a feature informing the practitioner and those carrying out practical aspects of the medical procedures of the quantity of radiation produced by the equipment

during the procedure. Equipment installed prior to 6 February 2018 may be exempted from this requirement.

(d) Any equipment used for interventional radiology and computed tomography and any new equipment used for planning, guiding and verification purposes have a device or a feature informing the practitioner, at the end of the procedure, of relevant parameters for assessing the patient dose.

(e) Equipment used for interventional radiology and computed tomography has the capacity to transfer the information required under 3(d) to the record of the examination. Equipment installed prior to 6 February 2018 may be exempted from this requirement.

(f) Without prejudice to points (c), (d) and (e) of paragraph 3, new medical radiodiagnostic equipment producing ionising radiation has a device, or an equivalent means, informing the practitioner of relevant parameters for assessing the patient dose. Where appropriate, the equipment shall have the capacity to transfer this information to the record of the examination.

Procedures

Article 58.a now requires the establishment of written protocols for every type of standard medical radiological procedure and for each piece of equipment, but also "for relevant categories of patients".

Article 58.b (procedures) indicates that Member States shall ensure that "Information relating to patient exposure forms part of the report of the medical radiological procedure".

In Art. 58.c the previous term "recommendations concerning referral criteria" has been replaced with "referral guidelines for medical imaging" to better reflect the European practice.

Article 58.e maintains the requirements on clinical audits as in the previous Directive 97/43/Euratom [5], stating that "clinical audits are carried out in accordance with national procedures".

Registry and analysis of the accidental or unintended irradiations

Article 63 introduces a new set of requirements for registration and analysis of accidental and unintended medical exposures.

Member states shall ensure that:

(c) For all medical exposures the undertaking implements an appropriate system for the record keeping and analysis of events involving or potentially involving accidental or unintended medical exposures, commensurate with the radiological risk posed by the practice;

(d) Arrangements are made to inform the referrer and the practitioner, and the patient or their representative, about clinically significant unintended or accidental exposures and the results of the analysis;

(e) (i) The undertaking declares as soon as possible to the competent authority the occurrence of significant events as defined by the competent authority;
(ii) The results of the investigation and the corrective measures to avoid such events are reported to the competent authority within the time period specified by the Member State;

(f) Mechanisms are in place for the timely dissemination of information relevant to radiation protection in medical exposure regarding lessons learned from significant events.

Population dose evaluation taking into account the age distribution and the gender

Article 64 states that Member States shall ensure that the distribution of individual dose estimates from medical exposure for radiodiagnostic and interventional radiology purposes are determined, taking into consideration where appropriate the distribution by age and gender of the exposed.

Old medico-legal and new non-medical imaging exposures

The "medico-legal" exposures introduced in Directive 97/43/Euratom have been replaced in the new Directive by the "non-medical imaging exposures" defined as deliberate exposure of humans for imaging purposes where the primary intention of the exposure is not to bring a health benefit to the individual being exposed. The Directive adopts a different approach for procedures using medical radiological equipment and for procedures not using such equipment.

The practices using medical radiological equipment, as defined in Annex V, include:

1. Radiological health assessment for employment purposes;
2. Radiological health assessment for immigration purposes;
3. Radiological health assessment for insurance purposes;
4. Radiological evaluation of the physical development of children and adolescents with a view to a career in sports, dancing, etc.
5. Radiological age assessment;

6. Use of ionising radiation for the identification of objects concealed within the human body.

The Directive requires practices using medical radiological equipment to be placed under appropriate regulatory control and to be justified at three levels: before being generally adopted, for each particular application and for the particular exposed individual. The Directive also requires reviews of the general and particular justification of such practices.

Article 22.3 indicates that Member States may exempt justified practices involving non-medical imaging exposure using medical radiological equipment from the requirement for dose constraints according to point (b) of Art. 6(1) (i.e. dose constraint shall be set for the individual dose that members of the public receive from the planned operation of a radiation source) and from the dose limits set out in Art. 12 (i.e. dose limits for public exposure).

Article 22.4.c requires that for procedures using medical radiological equipment, the relevant requirements identified for medical exposure as set out in Chap. VII (Medical Exposures) are applied, including those for equipment, optimisation, responsibilities, training and special protection during pregnancy and the appropriate involvement of the medical physics expert.

Conclusion

The changes introduced with Council Directive 2013/59/Euratom will require Member States, the radiology community (including medical physics experts) and the industry to adapt their regulations, procedures and equipment to the new high standards of radiation safety.

Member States will have 4 years for the transposition of the Directive into national legislation (by 6 February 2018).

Acknowledgments This paper was prepared by Eliseo Vano (Madrid/ES), Reinhard Loose (Nuernberg/DE) and Peter Vock (Berne/CH) on behalf of the ESR Radiation Protection Subcommittee (chairperson: P. Vock; members: D. Akata, E.J. Adam, J. Damilakis, H. Ducou le Pointe, R. Loose, C. Owens, G. Frija, F. Kainberger, L. Oleaga, M. Prokop; advisers: E. Vano, A. Meghzifene, G. Paulo, observers: D. Koff, W. Stiller, D. Sheppard). It was approved by the ESR Executive Council on 14 April 2015.

The authors thank Georgi Simeonov, Policy Officer, European Commission, Directorate-General for Energy, Unit D.3 Radiation Protection, for proof-reading and completing the final draft.

Appendix: Relevant definitions

Accidental exposure	An exposure of individuals, other than emergency workers, as a result of an accident.
Carers and comforters	Individuals knowingly and willingly incurring an exposure to ionising radiation by helping, other than as part of their occupation, in the support and comfort of individuals undergoing or having undergone medical exposure.
Clinical audit	A systematic examination or review of medical radiological procedures that seeks to improve the quality and outcome of patient care through structured review, whereby medical radiological practices, procedures and results are examined against agreed standards for good medical radiological procedures, with modification of practices, where appropriate, and the application of new standards if necessary.
Clinical responsibility	Responsibility of a practitioner for individual medical exposures, in particular, justification; optimisation; clinical evaluation of the outcome; cooperation with other specialists and staff, as appropriate, regarding practical aspects of medical radiological procedures; obtaining information, if appropriate, on previous examinations; providing existing medical radiological information and/or records to other practitioners and/or the referrer, as required; and giving information on the risk of ionising radiation to patients and other individuals involved, as appropriate.
Diagnostic reference levels	Dose levels in medical radiodiagnostic or interventional radiology practices, or, in the case of radiopharmaceuticals, levels of activity, for typical examinations for groups of standard-sized patients or standard phantoms for broadly defined types of equipment.
Dose constraint	A constraint set as a prospective upper bound of individual doses, used to define the range of options considered in the process of optimisation for a given radiation source in a planned exposure situation.
Interventional radiology	The use of X-ray imaging techniques to facilitate the introduction and guidance of devices in the body for diagnostic or treatment purposes.
Medical exposure	Exposure incurred by patients or asymptomatic individuals as part of their own medical or dental diagnosis

	or treatment, and intended to benefit their health, as well as exposure incurred by carers and comforters and by volunteers in medical or biomedical research.
Medical physics expert	An individual or, if provided for in national legislation, a group of individuals, having the knowledge, training and experience to act or give advice on matters relating to radiation physics applied to medical exposure, whose competence in this respect is recognised by the competent authority.
Medical radiological	Pertaining to radiodiagnostic and radiotherapeutic procedures and interventional radiology or other medical uses of ionising radiation for planning, guiding and verification purposes.
Medical radiological installation	A facility where medical radiological procedures are performed.
Medical radiological procedure	Any procedure giving rise to medical exposure.
Non-medical imaging exposure	Any deliberate exposure of humans for imaging purposes where the primary intention of the exposure is not to bring a health benefit to the individual being exposed.
Practitioner	A medical doctor, dentist or other health professional who is entitled to take clinical responsibility for an individual medical exposure in accordance with national requirements.
Radiodiagnostic	Pertaining to in-vivo diagnostic nuclear medicine, medical diagnostic radiology using ionising radiation and dental radiology.
Radiotherapeutic	Pertaining to radiotherapy, including nuclear medicine for therapeutic purposes.
Referrer	A medical doctor, dentist or other health professional who is entitled to refer individuals for medical radiological procedures to a practitioner, in accordance with national requirements
Unintended exposure	Medical exposure that is significantly different from the medical exposure intended for a given purpose.

References

1. European Council Directive 2013/59/Euratom on basic safety standards for protection against the dangers arising from exposure to ionising radiation and repealing Directives 89/618/Euratom, 90/641/Euratom, 96/29/Euratom, 97/43/Euratom and 2003/122/Euratom. OJ of the EU. L13; 57: 1–73 (2014).
2. International Commission on Radiological Protection (2007) ICRP Publication 103. The 2007 Recommendations of the International Commission on Radiological Protection. Ann. ICRP 37(2–4):1–332
3. International Commission on Radiological Protection (2012) ICRP statement on tissue reactions and early and late effects of radiation in normal tissues and organs–threshold doses for tissue reactions in a radiation protection context. ICRP publication 118. Ann ICRP 41(1–2):1–322
4. European Council Directive 96/29/Euratom laying down basic safety standards for the protection of the health of workers and the general public against the dangers arising from ionizing radiation. OJ of the EU. L 159; 1-114 (1996)
5. European Council Directive 97/43/Euratom on health protection of individuals against the dangers of ionizing radiation in relation to medical exposure and repealing Directive 84/466/Euratom. OJ of the EU. L 180; 22-27 (1997)

16

A practical approach to imaging the axilla

V. Dialani • D. F. James • P. J. Slanetz

Abstract Imaging of the axilla typically occurs when patients present with axillary symptoms or newly diagnosed breast cancer. An awareness of the axillary anatomy is essential in order to generate an accurate differential diagnosis and guide patient management. The purpose of this article is to review the indications for axillary imaging, discuss the logistics of the scanning technique and percutaneous interventions, and present the imaging findings and management of a variety of breast diseases involving the axilla.

Teaching points

- *Knowledge of normal axillary anatomy aids in determining the aetiology of an axillary mass.*
- *The differential diagnosis of an axillary mass is broad and can be subdivided by the location of the lesion.*
- *Imaging evaluation of the axilla usually entails diagnostic mammography and targeted ultrasound.*
- *FNA or core needle biopsies are safe and accurate methods for diagnosis and guiding management.*

Keywords Mammography · Axilla · Targeted ultrasound

V. Dialani (✉) · P. J. Slanetz
Department of Radiology, Beth Israel Deaconess Medical Center, 330 Brookline Avenue, Boston, MA 02215, USA
e-mail: vdialani@bidmc.harvard.edu

P. J. Slanetz
e-mail: pslanetz@bidmc.harvard.edu

D. F. James
Jefferson Radiology, 85 Seymour Street, Suite 200, Hartford, CT 06106, USA
e-mail: djames@jeffersonradiology.com

Introduction

Over the past several decades, coinciding with the introduction of ultrasound, radiologists have increasingly imaged the axilla in females presenting with axillary symptoms and newly diagnosed breast cancer. In addition, image-guided axillary procedures have been embraced as a means to diagnose findings and guide patient management. The purpose of this article is to review the indications for axillary imaging, discuss the logistics of the scanning technique and percutaneous interventions, and present the imaging findings and management of a variety of breast diseases involving the axilla.

Basic anatomy

The axilla is composed of the axillary artery and vein, brachial plexus, lymph nodes, fat, accessory breast tissue, skin and subcutaneous glands. The anatomic boundaries are as follows: superior: the clavicle, scapula and first rib; posterior: subscapularis, teres major and latissimus dorsi muscles; anterior: pectoralis major and minor muscles; medial: serratus anterior and first four ribs; lateral: coracobrachialis and short head of the biceps muscle. Generally, the breast imager is primarily concerned with the lymph nodes located in the axilla (Fig. 1). The lymph node-bearing area is divided into three regions:

Level I: Lymph nodes lateral and inferior to the pectoralis minor muscle
Level II: Lymph nodes beneath the pectoralis minor muscle
Level III: Lymph nodes deep and medial to the medial border of the pectoralis minor muscle

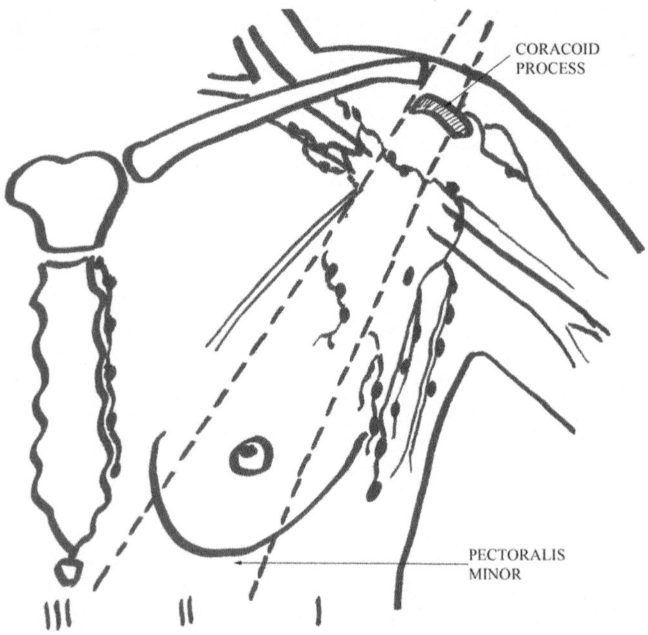

Fig. 1 The axilla is composed of the axillary artery and vein, brachial plexus, lymph nodes, fat, accessory breast tissue, skin and subcutaneous glands. The lymph node-bearing area is divided into three regions: level I: lymph nodes lateral and inferior to the pectoralis minor muscle; level II: lymph nodes under the pectoralis minor muscle; level III: lymph nodes deep and medial to the medial border of the pectoralis minor muscle

Scanning technique, logistics and image-guided interventions

The standard imaging evaluation of a palpable axillary lump for females over the age of 30 years in most of the USA typically includes a mammogram with a "skin marker" overlying the palpable finding followed by a focussed ultrasound of the area of concern. This may vary in different countries and typically in the UK, for example, mammographic evaluation begins at age 40 years. In younger patients, imaging begins with ultrasound. For patients with a focal lump, scanning is typically targeted over the area of concern; however, if there is a suspicious finding, it is important to cover the entire axillary region to evaluate for any associated findings. When the study is being performed in a female newly diagnosed with breast cancer, imaging should be performed broadly to include the entire extent of the axillary contents. Examination of level I lymph nodes necessitates visualising the axillary vessels as well as scanning the entire fatty contents from the margin of the pectoralis muscles anteromedially to the latissimus dorsi and teres major margin posterolaterally. The lateral thoracic and thoracodorsal arteries and smaller branches will be seen variably along each margin, respectively. Although node groups typically follow these vessels, lymph nodes are frequently found in isolation within the axillary fat. It is also very important to scan inferiorly, down through the axillary tail, because abnormal nodes are frequently found in this location as well. Levels II and III are not routinely scanned, although large level II nodes can sometimes be seen [1].

Axillary ultrasound should be performed using a high-frequency (7.5–17-MHz) linear-array transducer. A lower frequency (5–7.5-MHz) setting may be needed for larger patients or for patients with a large axillary fat pad; however, the spatial resolution will be compromised. The patient should lie in a supine oblique position, with her hand above her head with the arm abducted and externally rotated ("bathing beauty" position). All findings should be documented in orthogonal planes with and without calipers and a lesion's largest dimension should also be recorded. Some facilities employ grey-scale and colour Doppler US or power Doppler US during the study, especially when assessing lymph nodes. When colour Doppler US is used, it is important to use low wall filter settings and low velocity settings (higher pulse repetition frequency) to detect abnormal blood flow. The colour gain should be increased high enough to detect

Table 1 Axillary findings

	Benign	Malignant
Skin and subcutaneous tissues	Seborrheic keratosis, sebaceous cyst, epidermoid inclusion cyst	Skin metastases, melanoma
Accessory breast tissue	Fibroadenoma, pseudoangiomatous stromal hyperplasia (PASH), fibrocystic change	Breast cancer
Lymph node enlargement	Hyperplasia/reactive node, HIV/ immunocompromised state, granulomatous disease-sarcoidosis, lymphoma/ leukaemia, Castleman's disease	Primary breast malignancy, metastatic disease (breast, lung, ovarian, gastric, melanoma)
Lymph node calcifications/punctuate densities	Granulomatous disease, gold therapy (rheumatoid arthritis treatment)	Ductal carcinoma in situ (DCIS), metastatic disease [thyroid (papillary), ovarian]
Post-operative findings	Skin thickening, lymphoedema, post-operative fluid collections/lymphocele, fat necrosis, abscess, haematoma	Primary or metastatic recurrence
Neoplasms	Granular cell tumour, schwannoma	Primary breast cancer

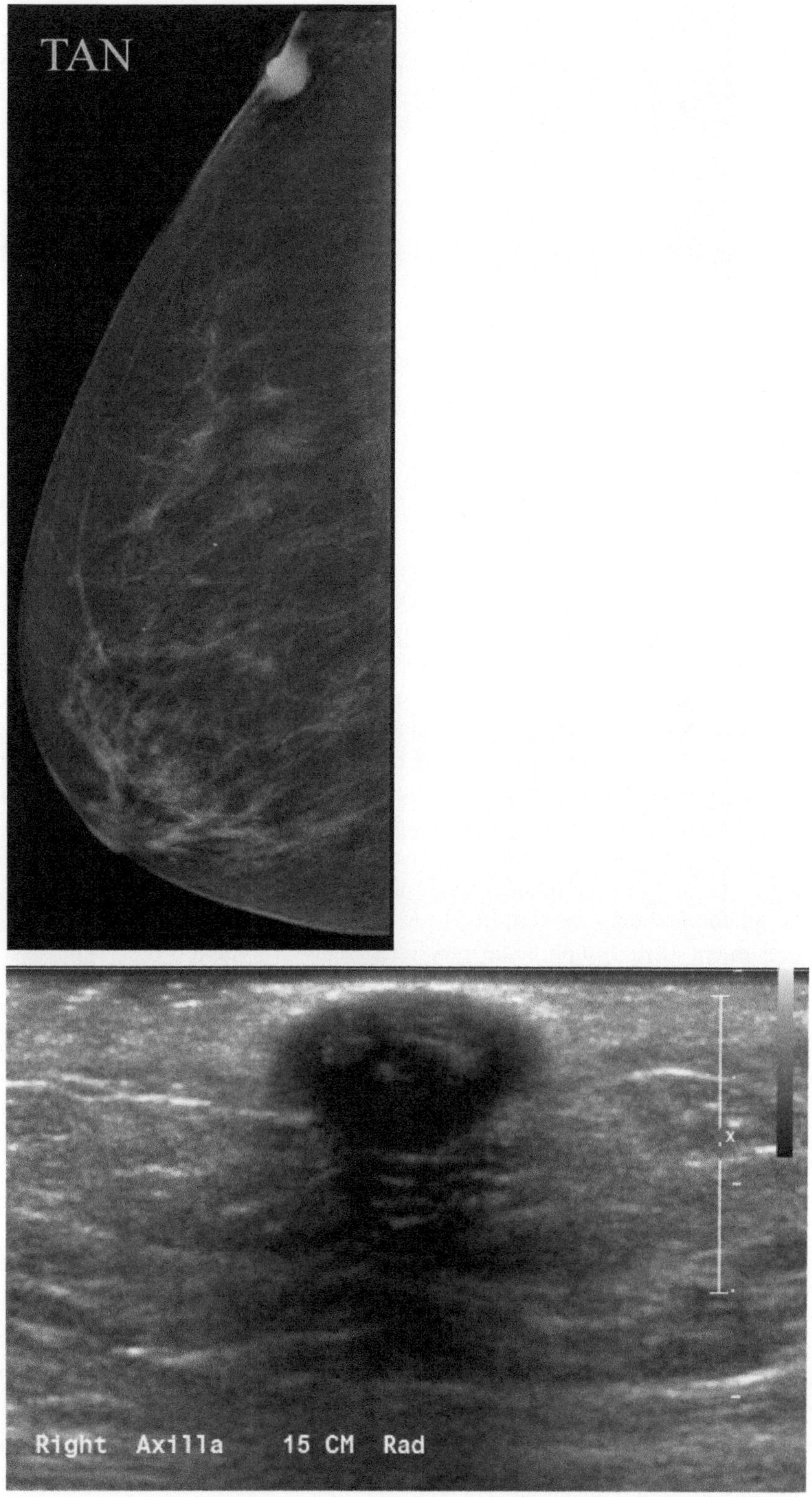

Fig. 2 Sebaceous cyst or epidermal inclusion cyst. **a** Tangential view reveals that this lesion is located within in the skin. **b** Ultrasound confirms a hypoechoic mass within the skin

subtle flow without causing a colour noise artefact. When evaluating lymph nodes, ultrasound is 94 % sensitive and 72 % specific in characterising nodes as suspicious or benign based on size and morphologic features [2].

If the initial imaging evaluation of the axilla reveals a suspicious finding, percutaneous procedures, such as ultrasound-guided fine-needle aspiration (FNA) or ultrasound-guided core biopsy, may be performed. At

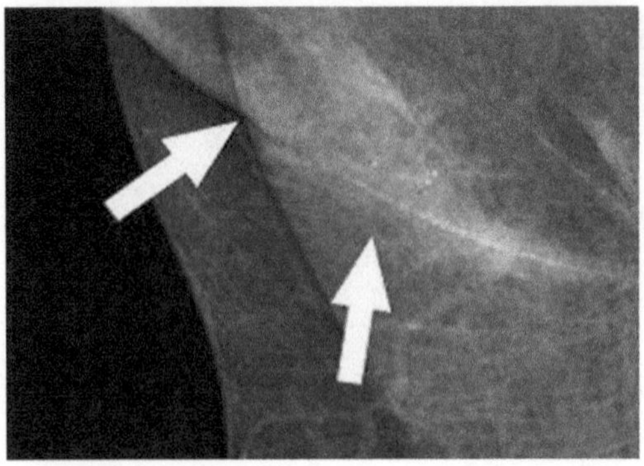

Fig. 3 Antiperspirant artefact: magnified view shows radiopaque densities overlying the axilla

most institutions, FNA is currently the preferred approach as the procedure is usually diagnostic and potential complications are minimal (bleeding, infection, non-diagnostic sample). FNA is typically performed using 22–25-gauge needles with aspirates sent to cytology. In most cases, at least three passes are made, especially if the cytologist is not on site during the procedure. If lymphoma is of clinical concern, additional aspirates should be obtained for flow cytometry. However, limitations do exist for FNA as it can be operator dependent, requires access to reliable cytology and carries a relatively high false-negative rate of 12–23 % [3] . Most commonly performed for suspicious lymphadenopathy, the confirmation of metastatic involvement in a lymph node precludes sentinel lymph node biopsy in females with newly diagnosed breast cancer leading to full axillary node dissection. In one study of 224 patients, the sensitivity of ultrasound-guided FNA for suspicious, indeterminate and normal-appearing axillary nodes was 93, 44 and 11 %, respectively, with an overall sensitivity of 59 % and overall specificity of 100 % [2]. The likelihood of a positive FNA correlated directly with the size of the primary breast malignancy, being 29 % for tumours <1 cm, 50 % for tumours 1–2 cm, 69 % for tumours 2–5 cm and 100 % for tumours >5 cm [2]. Alternatively, percutaneous core needle biopsy using 12–18 gauge spring-loaded or vacuum-assisted devices can safely be performed [4–7]. The risks of axillary core biopsy are similar to other image-guided procedures, namely bleeding and infection. However, given the presence of axillary vessels and nerves coursing through the axilla, a "no-throw" technique is preferred as this minimises the risk of haematoma or unintended nerve damage. If a spring-loaded device is used, this most commonly is performed on masses that exceed the throw of the device so that the needle does not pass into unaffected axillary tissue, thereby minimising the risk of unintended complications. In one study of 39 patients with suspicious lymphadenopathy, axillary core biopsy revealed 90 % sensitivity, 100 % specificity and 92 % accuracy [8] without any clinically significant complications. By recognising that the nerves course alongside the axillary vessels, the risk of bleeding and untoward nerve injury can easily be avoided in almost all cases. Although core biopsy may yield a benign aetiology, there is conflicting evidence concerning whether this approach is substantially better than FNA as the upgrade rate on surgical excision ranges from 0 to 36 % in several studies, possibly related to the small cohort size and inherent sampling error [8].

Differential diagnosis of axillary findings

There are a wide variety of imaging findings that can be seen while scanning the axilla. Ranging from skin lesions to abnormal lymphadenopathy to posterior chest wall masses, the astute radiologist must apply their anatomic and medical knowledge to recommend the most appropriate management. Findings typically fall into six categories: skin lesions, congenital and developmental anomalies, infectious, inflammatory and metastatic lymphadenopathy, post-operative changes, benign neoplasms and extra-axillary masses (Table 1). Each of these categories is covered in greater detail below.

Skin lesion/glands

The most common skin lesion is seborrheic keratosis, a raised benign skin lesion with a verrucoid appearance. Epidermal inclusion cysts and sebaceous cysts (Fig. 2) are located at the junction of the dermis and subcutaneous fat and present on imaging as circumscribed masses often with a visible tract to the skin surface [9]. Epidermal inclusion cysts may occur anywhere but tend to be more common in the axilla and the inframammary fold. In addition, antiperspirant can appear as radiopaque densities overlying the axilla seen on mammographic imaging (Fig. 3).

Congenital developmental anomaly-accessory breast tissue

Breast tissue develops from the mammary ridges that extend from the base of the forelimb bud along the ventral surface of the embryo to an area medial to the base of the hind limb bud, which is the primitive inguinal region. Typically, the milk line regresses, leaving the middle portion of the upper third of the mammary ridge from

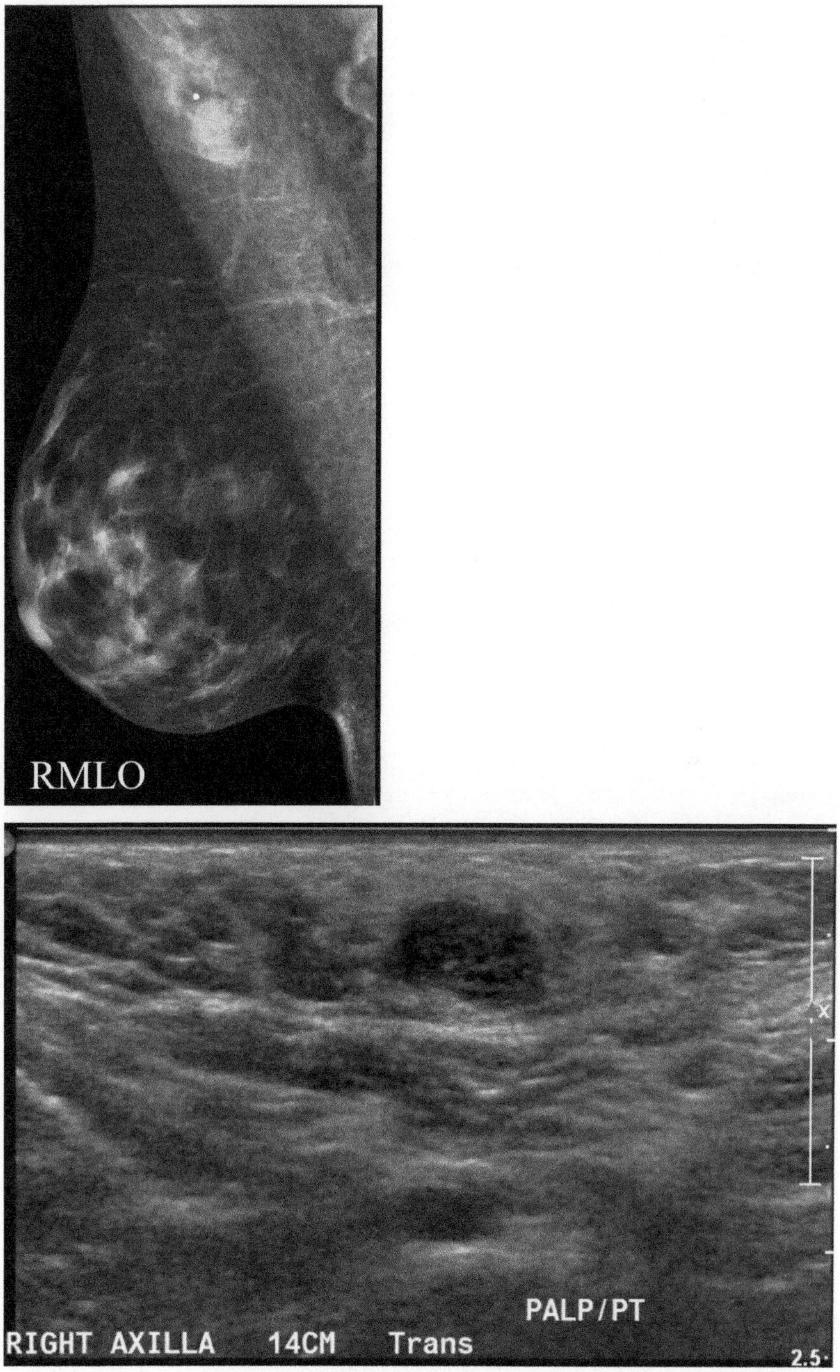

Fig. 4 Accessory breast tissue with fibroadenoma: **a** BB placed on the skin in the area of concern to the patient. MLO views show hetereogeneously dense 4 cm asymmetry of similar density and morphology to breast tissue. **b** Targeted sonographic evaluation of the right axilla in the area of concern demonstrates fibroglandular breast tissue and a hypoechoic 8-mm solid mass. Biopsy of the nodule using a no-throw vacuum-assisted biopsy device revealed fibroadenoma

which the breast is formed. Failure of involution of the milk line results in accessory breast tissue, most commonly in the axilla, but it can occur anywhere from the axilla to the inguinal region. Accessory breast tissue occurs in 2–6 % of women (Fig. 4) [9, 10] and can be appreciated on mammography, ultrasound and MRI. When accessory tissue occurs, both benign and malignant breast lesions can be seen (i.e. cysts, fibroadenomas, PASH, breast cancer).

Lymph nodes

Although the axilla is partially imaged on mammography, axillary lymph nodes can often be seen. Classically, benign axillary lymph nodes typically are smaller than 2 cm in maximal size and have a hilar radiolucent notch. Increased size and/or increased density of a node on mammography raises concern for pathology. However, ultrasonography provides the best means to assess the axillary nodes given its

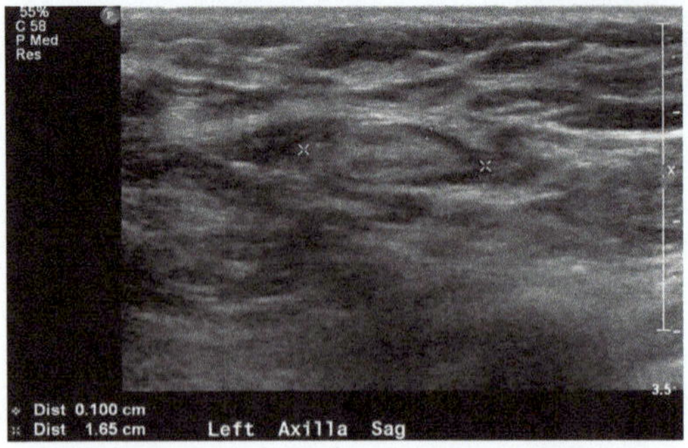

Fig. 5 Normal lymph node: On ultrasound, lymph nodes typically are smooth, gently lobulated ovals with a hypoechoic cortex measuring less than 3 mm in thickness with a central echogenic hilum

relatively sensitive and highly specific capabilities. A normal or benign-appearing axillary lymph node should have an oval or lobulated shape and a smooth, well-defined margin. The lobulated shape is because of concurrent constrictions and bulges of both the cortex and fatty hilum. The cortex should be slightly hypoechoic and uniformly thin, measuring 3 mm or less (Fig. 5). Nodes that meet this description have a very high negative predictive value for excluding metastases [11]. The echogenic hilum should constitute the majority of the node. Arterial flow in the hilum can be demonstrated with colour Doppler imaging. Morphologic criteria, such as cortical thickening, hilar effacement and non-hilar cortical blood flow, are more important than size criteria in the identification of metastases. Characteristics of lymph nodes that are concerning for malignancy besides overall size include round shape, absence of the fatty hilum, and increased concentric or focal cortical thickness greater than 3 mm, all being predictors of malignancy (Fig. 6) [12–16].

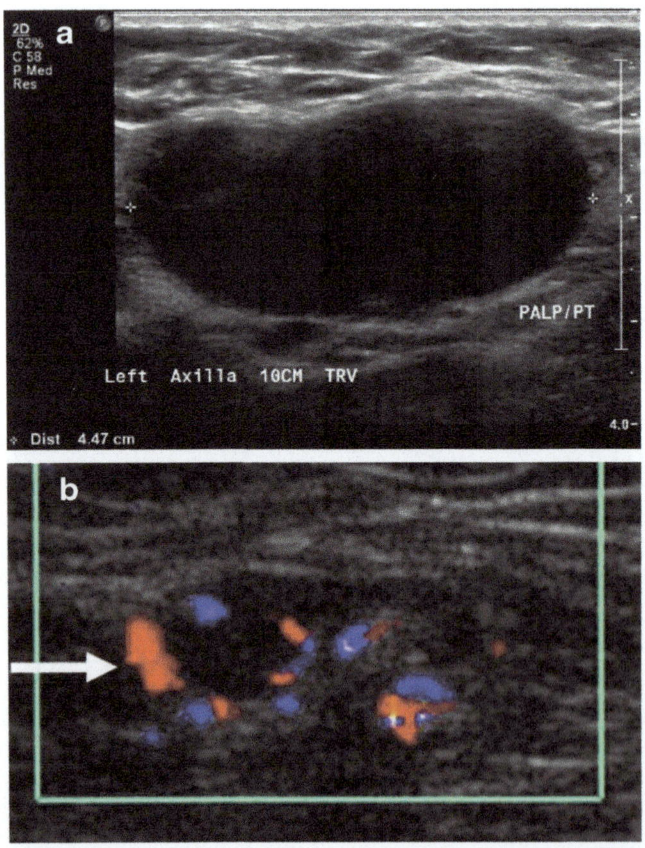

Fig. 6 Abnormal lymph nodes: characteristics concerning for malignancy: **a** absence of the fatty hilum and **b** increased focal cortical thickness greater than 3 mm with colour Doppler US that shows hyperaemic blood flow in the hilum and central cortex or abnormal (non-hilar cortical) blood flow

A focal cortical bulge (Fig. 7) or thickening is considered the earliest detectable morphologic change in the presence of metastasis, but this criterion is difficult to apply and has a low positive predictive value because it is non-specific. This finding is therefore considered indeterminate. A true abnormal cortical bulge is seen as focal thickening of the cortex that does not follow the margin of the echogenic hilum and should be distinctly hypoechoic, and this sign is more accurate if associated with another finding such as the presence of cortical in addition to hilar blood flow. Diffuse cortical thickening can also be seen with metastasis, but this finding is even more non-specific, more often being associated with a reactive node. Eccentric cortical thickening is more suspicious than diffuse thickening, but both are non-specific and concerning enough to warrant intervention in most cases (Fig. 8). Findings seen in cases with more advanced nodal involvement, such as effacement of the fatty hilum or a rounded hypoechoic mass, have a higher positive predictive value in patients with invasive breast cancer. Replacement of the entire node or a portion of the node by an ill-defined mass is highly suspicious for malignant involvement. Occasionally, nodal microcalcifications can be seen on imaging (Fig. 7).

Contrast-enhanced ultrasonography has been used with some success to visualise enhancing abnormal nodes after periareolar injection of microbubbles. Server et al. in their study showed that sentinel lymph node can be successfully identified and biopsied using microbubble contrast-enhanced ultrasound, thereby avoiding surgical biopsy in some patients [17].

Ultrasound and axillary core biopsy enable adequate pretreatment staging in patients with breast cancer and has a positive impact on their management [18, 19]. The benefit of pre-operative identification of axillary metastases is that it allows the surgeon to proceed directly to full axillary lymph node dissection and to avoid an unnecessary sentinel lymph node biopsy,

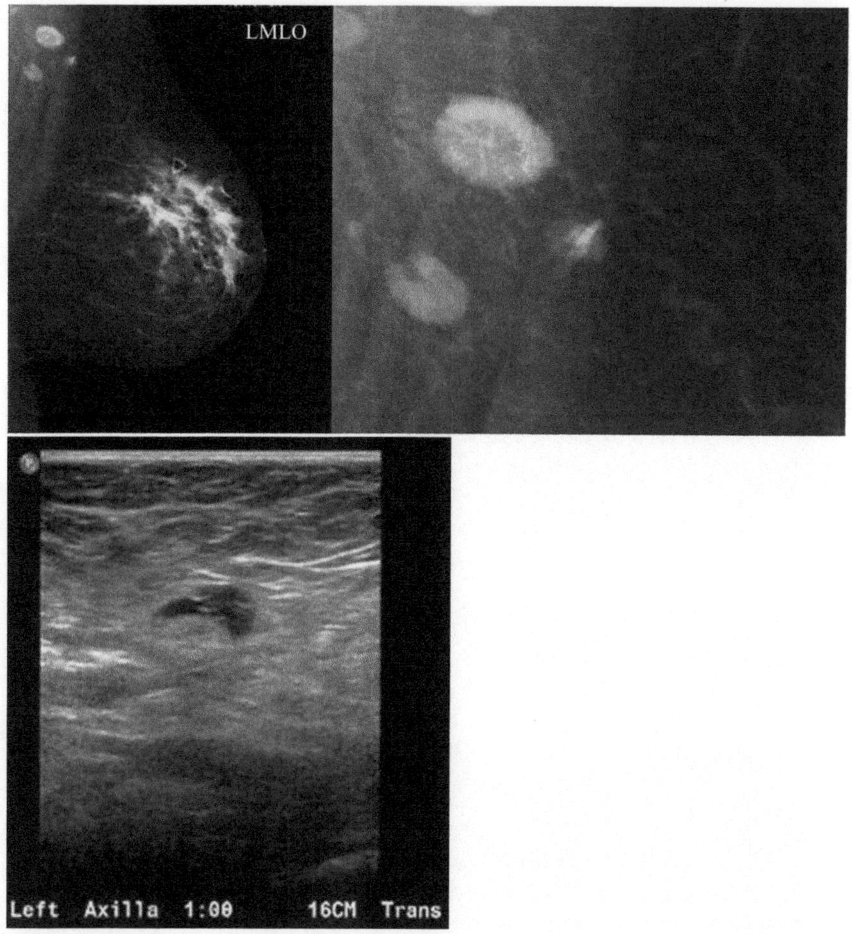

Fig. 7 A 47-year-old female with a palpable left breast lump. **a** Left MLO view with magnified image of the left axilla demonstrates a 1.4×1-cm lymph node with eccentric cortical thickening and cortical calcifications. **b** Transverse image of left axillary lymph node confirms echogenic foci within the thickened cortex suspicious for malignancy. FNA was performed with aspirates sent for routine cytology and flow cytometry. Final diagnosis: metastatic carcinoma

thereby avoiding a second surgical procedure involving the axillary nodes. Houssami et al. in their meta-analysis found that axillary ultrasound-guided needle biopsy (UNB) had better utility in females with average or higher underlying risk of nodal metastases [20] and found that a median proportion of 18.4 % (interquartile range = 13.3 %–27.4 %) from 7,097 patients can be effectively triaged to axillary treatment and avoid sentinel node biopsy (SNB). However, the changing algorithm of axillary surgical treatment means that ultrasound-guided FNA will have relatively less utility where surgeons omit axillary lymph node dissection (ALND) for minimal nodal metastatic disease. Research that allows enhanced application of ultrasound and UNB to specifically identify and biopsy sentinel nodes and to discriminate between patients with minimal versus advanced nodal metastatic involvement is likely to have the most impact on future management of the axilla in patients newly diagnosed with breast cancer [21].

Recently, the field of breast cancer surgery has seen a dramatic shift with the results of the American College of Surgeons Oncology Group Z0011 trial [22]. This study, which randomly assigned patients with sentinel lymph node (SLN)-positive breast cancer to SNB and (ALND) or to SNB alone, reported that ALND was not associated with any survival benefit and that both groups had an extremely low regional recurrence rate (0.9 % for SNB alone and 0.5 % for ALND). This was despite the fact that 27.3 % of the patients who received ALND had additional positive non-sentinel lymph nodes. This study confirmed what many surgical oncologists had suspected: that ALND provided minimal benefit while exposing a substantial number of patients to long-term morbidity, specifically lymphoedema. Therefore, there was great interest in shifting away from routine ALND for patients with SLN-positive disease, instead reserving this operation for patients who did not meet the Z0011 criteria (i.e. patients undergoing neoadjuvant chemotherapy, patients with palpable nodes, patients having mastectomy or patients with more than three involved nodes). With the results of Z0011, there has been some shift in the approach to staging the axilla. Some surgeons have

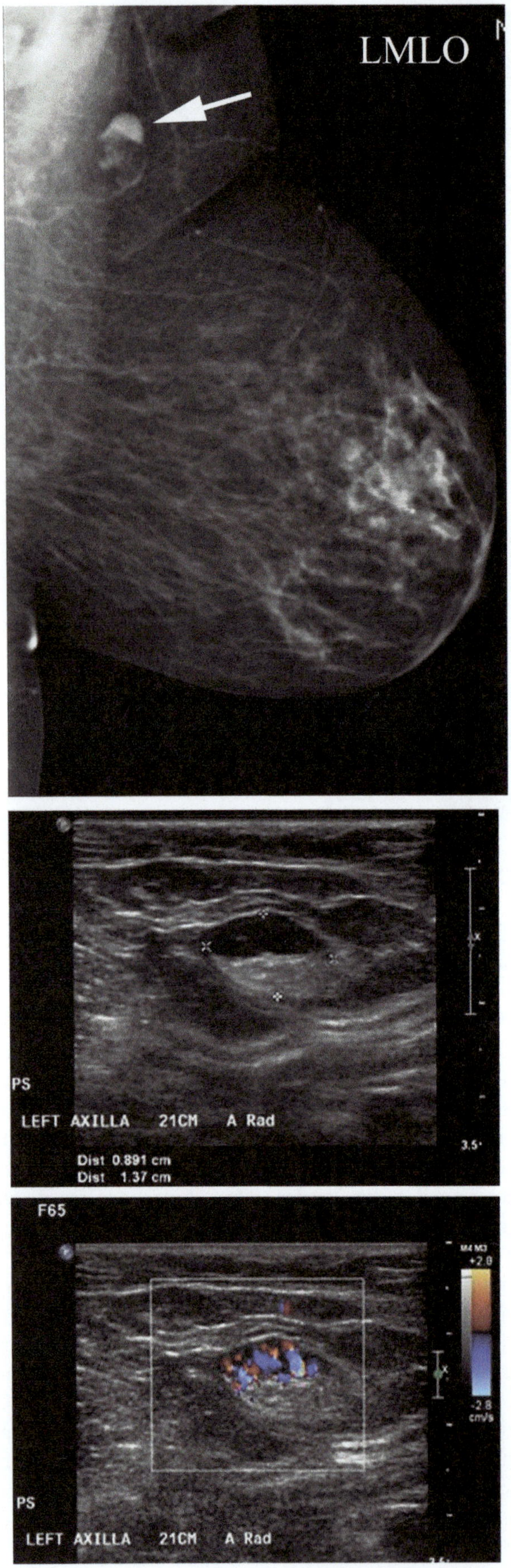

◀ **Fig. 8** A 54-year-old female with remote history of right breast cancer and a left knee sarcoma now for screening. **a** MLO view demonstrates a focally thickened non-enlarged left axillary lymph node. **b** Ultrasound confirms a 1.4-cm lymph node with focal cortical thickening of 6 mm and (**c**) internal vascular flow. FNA was performed for diagnosis. Aspirates were sent for routine cytology and flow cytometry. Final diagnosis: reactive lymph node

advocated to no longer obtain axillary ultrasound and fine-needle aspiration (FNA) biopsy of suspicious nodes because this practice identifies women with "clinically evident" disease who, in the absence of

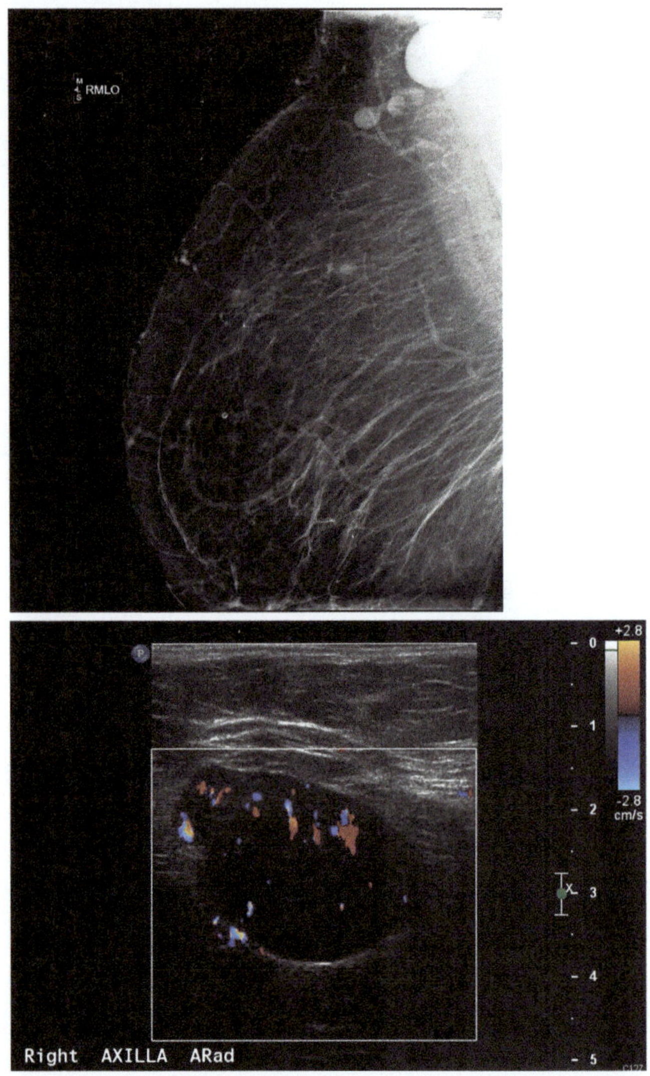

Fig. 9 A 55-year-old African American female for screening. **a** MLO views of the breasts demonstrate a dense enlarged right axillary lymph node and several abnormal-appearing intramammary lymph nodes. Right axillary ultrasound confirms a large fatty replaced lymph node with non-hilar internal vascular flow. This is highly suspicious for malignancy in a patient with breast cancer; however this patient had a negative mammogram and so an ultrasound-guided core biopsy was performed for diagnosis. Final diagnosis: sarcoidosis

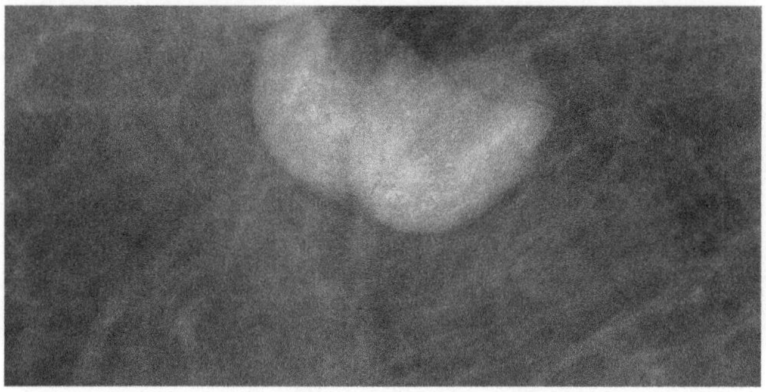

Fig. 10 A 56-year-old female treated with gold therapy for rheumatoid arthritis. Right MLO (magnified image) of two right axillary lymph nodes reveals fine punctate radiopaque densities secondary to previous gold therapy for rheumatoid arthritis

the ultrasound, would have been "SLN positive" and thus eligible for avoidance of the ALND. However, a point to remember is that pre-operative ultrasound of the axilla is still an extremely useful staging test as nodal disease identified by ultrasound and FNA biopsy is strongly correlated with tumour burden and the number of involved nodes [23, 24].

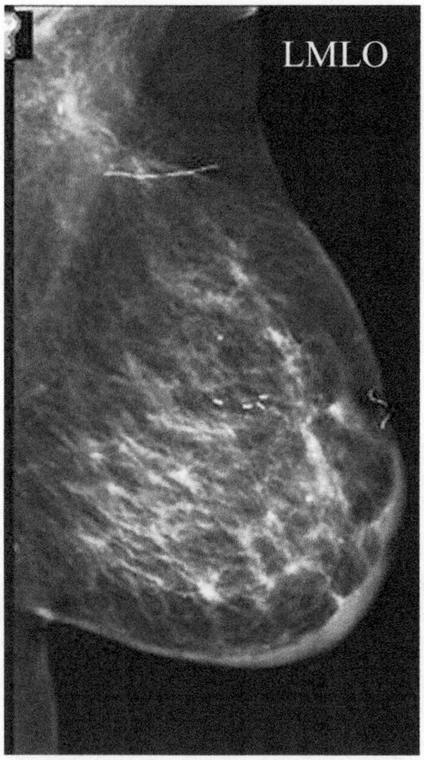

Fig. 11 A 66-year-old female, 7 months out from lumpectomy, sentinel lymph node biopsy and radiation therapy, presents for first post-treatment mammogram. Diffuse left breast skin and trabecular thickening accompanied by post-surgical distortion in the breast and axilla are visible. Final diagnosis: Expected post-treatment changes following breast cancer diagnosis

Additionally abnormal appearing lymph nodes may be seen related to both benign (Figs. 8 and 9) and neoplastic processes (Figs. 6 and 7). In general, the differential diagnosis for an enlarged axillary lymph node includes reactive hyperplasia, HIV/immunocompromised state, sarcoidosis or other granulomatous diseases, lymphoma/leukaemia and metastatic disease (most commonly breast cancer, lung cancer, ovarian cancer, gastric cancer or melanoma). Calcifications involving lymph nodes within the axilla can be seen because of either benign or malignant causes. The differential diagnosis for calcified lymph nodes includes prior granulomatous infection, gold therapy in patients with rheumatoid arthritis (Fig. 10), collagen vascular disease, and metastasis from breast, thyroid or ovarian cancer. However, if high-density particles are seen in the axilla, the first step is to confirm that they are indeed located within a lymph node and not related to antiperspirant on the skin surface. This can readily be accomplished by recalling the patient for a repeat MLO view after cleaning the axilla to show that the densities are no longer present on the image.

Post-operative axilla

Following axillary surgery, an array of findings can be seen in the axilla. The most common findings include skin and trabecular thickening (Fig. 11), post-operative fluid collections/lymphoceles (Fig. 12), fat necrosis and recurrence.

Benign neoplasms

There are several rare benign neoplasms that can occur in the axilla, which also can mimic breast cancer in the axillary tail of Spence. These tumours are most frequently are neural in origin and asymptomatic. Therefore, they are most commonly encountered on screening mammography. As these tumours are almost always benign, percutaneous biopsy to confirm a benign entity is sufficient and most often surgery is avoided.

Granular cell tumour (GCT) GCT is a rare neoplasm of neural origin arising from perineural cells, accounting for less than 1 % of breast lesions and more commonly seen in African American women. Clinically, GCTs manifest as firm, palpable masses and average 1 to 2 cm in size. Histologically, they arise from the intralobular breast stroma and tend to form cords that extend into adjacent normal breast parenchyma, a characteristic that simulates the growth pattern of

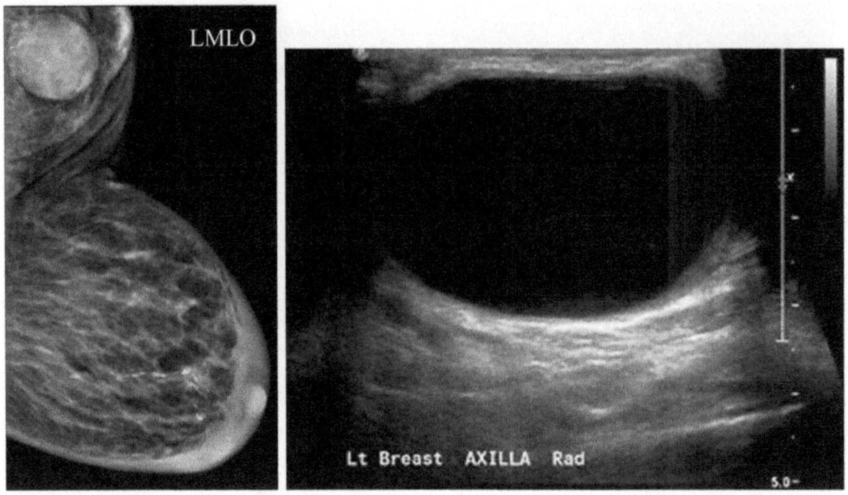

Fig. 12 A 80-year-old female with a history of sarcoidosis presenting with a left axillary mass 1 year following axillary surgery of a benign node. **a** MLO view and (**b**) ultrasound of the left axilla demonstrates a 4.1×2.7×3.5-cm well-circumscribed predominantly anechoic structure with internal debris consistent with a complicated cyst. Aspiration was performed for symptomatic relief. Final diagnosis: lymphocele of the left breast demonstrates extensive skin and trabecular thickening and a well-circumscribed left axillary mass

infiltrating carcinoma [25–27]. On mammography, granular cell tumour of the breast is difficult to distinguish from carcinoma and may have irregular or spiculated margins. On ultrasound it may be solid hypoechoic with irregular margins (Fig. 13). GCTs are usually benign neoplasms [28]. Despite the fact that most cases occur in pre-menopausal women, GCTs have been shown to be non-dependent on oestrogen and progesterone [25]. The most widely accepted theory supports a Schwann cell origin because of similarities in ultrastructural features and the positivity of the tumour for the S-100 protein, which is found in peripheral nerves. Diagnosis is confirmed by special staining for S-100 protein, NSE and CEA [28]. Less than 1 % of all GCTs, including mammary lesions, are malignant. Malignant GCTs are considered high-grade sarcomas with a high rate of metastasis and short survival. Features suggestive of malignancy include large size (>4 cm), increased mitotic rate (>2 mitosis/10 high-power fields at × 200 magnification), rapid growth, local invasion, and variation in cell size and shape. The main histological element that distinguishes GCTs from more ominous lesions is the presence of a granular cytoplasm. Current treatment is wide surgical excision. To date, there is no role for radiation or chemotherapy [26, 28]. Local recurrence has been reported after incomplete excision as late as 10 years following removal, especially when the margins are irregular or inadequate. GCTs pose a real diagnostic challenge for physicians. Pre-operative diagnosis with core needle biopsy is important because treatment is with wide surgical excision rather than mastectomy given the infiltrative pattern of growth [27].

Schwannoma There are scattered case reports in the literature citing examples of breast schwannomas [29]. Schwannomas arise from Schwann cells of the peripheral nerve sheath. The most common locations include the head, neck and extensor surfaces of the extremities. Intramammary schwannomas account for only 2.6 % of schwannomas. Mammographically, schwannomas are most commonly described as a well-defined round or oval mass, but sometimes may be ill defined (Fig. 14). Sonographically, more variation in appearance has been reported; however, it is most commonly described as a solid hypoechoic well-defined mass with variable posterior acoustic enhancement [29]. Microscopically, classic schwannoma is an encapsulated neoplasm having two components known as Antoni A and B tissue, in variable proportions. Antoni A tissue is cellular and consists of monomorphic spindle-shaped Schwann cells, with a poorly defined eosinophilic cytoplasm and pointed basophilic nuclei, set in a variable collagenous stroma [30]. These cells commonly show nuclear palisading and parallel arrays of such palisades with intervening eosinophilic cell cytoplasm (processes) are known as Verocay bodies [31]. Breast schwannomas show no definite worrisome mammographic or ultrasonographic features, and diagnosis on imaging alone is not possible. A diagnosis of schwannoma of the breast may be suggested on core needle biopsy if there is a cytologically bland spindle cell lesion with areas of palisading and lack of epithelial elements, especially if the cells show immunostaining for S-100 protein [31]. However,

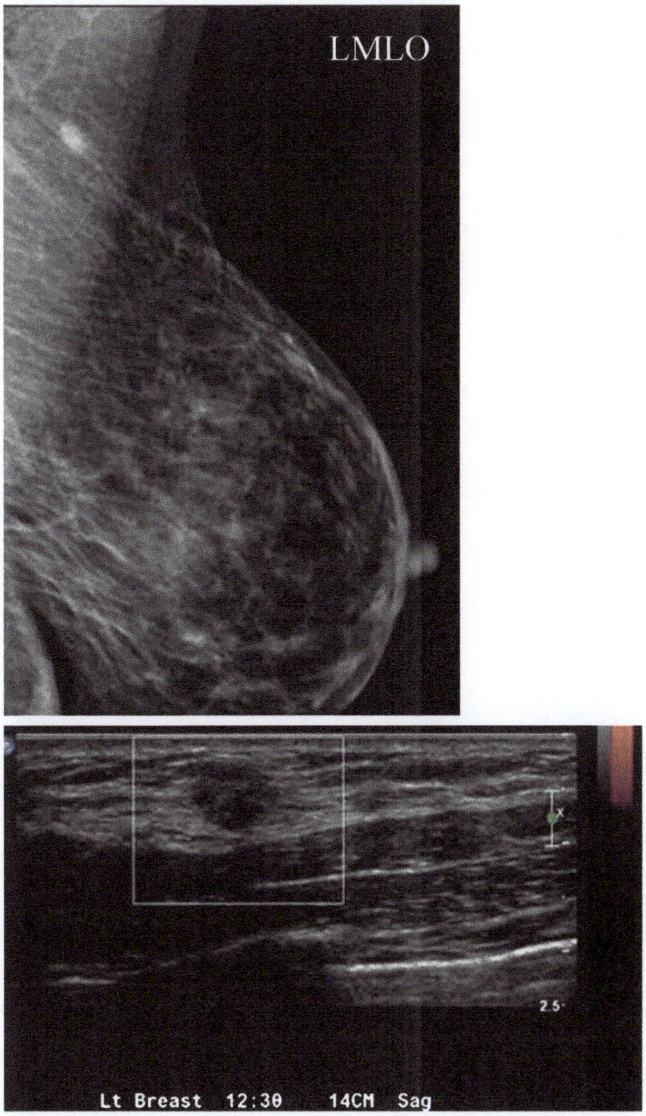

Fig. 13 A 50-year-old female with focal 1-cm asymmetry in the left axilla region. **a** MLO views demonstrate left axillary irregular asymmetry, which persisted on spot compression. **b** Ultrasound of the left axilla demonstrated a 12-mm irregular hypoechoic hypovascular mass in the left axilla. Ultrasound-guided core needle biopsy was performed. Final diagnosis: granular cell tumour

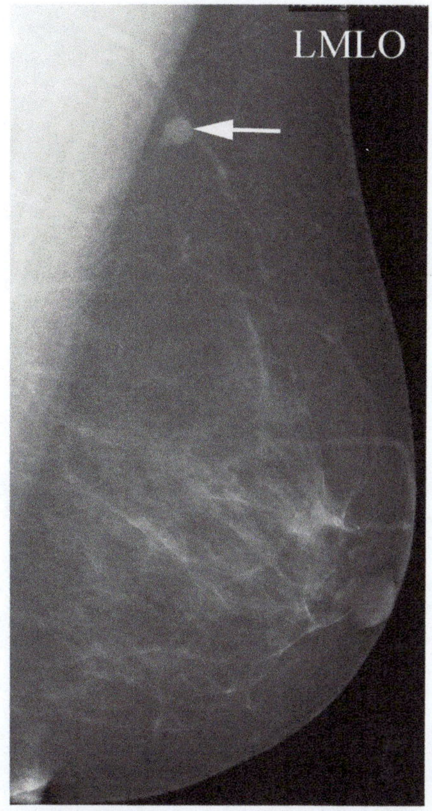

Fig. 14 A 64-year-old asymptomatic female presented for a screening mammogram. MLO view of the left breast shows an 8-mm well-defined ovoid mass in the left upper outer quadrant (*arrow*). Final diagnosis: schwannoma

distinction from other spindle cell lesions such as metaplastic carcinomas, fibroepithelial lesions with minor epithelial components, fibromatosis and myofibroblastoma, among others, is challenging and most result in surgical excision [31, 32].

Extra-axillary lesions

The axilla also includes muscles and bones of the shoulder and upper rib cage. Therefore, recognising that an axillary mass is within or beneath the muscle is essential in forming an appropriate differential diagnosis. Although extra-axillary lesions are rare, benign and malignant muscular neoplasms may be encountered (Fig. 15). Intramuscular myxoma is a benign neoplasm arising from fibroblasts, which produce excessive mucopolysaccharide, accounting for their complex appearance on US and heterogeneous signal on MR imaging. Most commonly involving the heart, they can occur at other sites including subcutaneous tissue, aponeurotic tissue, bone, the genitourinary system and skin. They can be associated with fibrous dysplasia (Mazabraud's syndrome). On imaging, intramuscular myxoma typically presents as a slowly enlarging mass that is often complex on US and most often demonstrates T1 hypointensity, T2 hyperintensity, a T1 perilesional fat rind, and rim and internal enhancement on MR. As these lesions may be indistinguishable from myxoid liposarcoma on imaging; biopsy is essential for diagnosis [33].

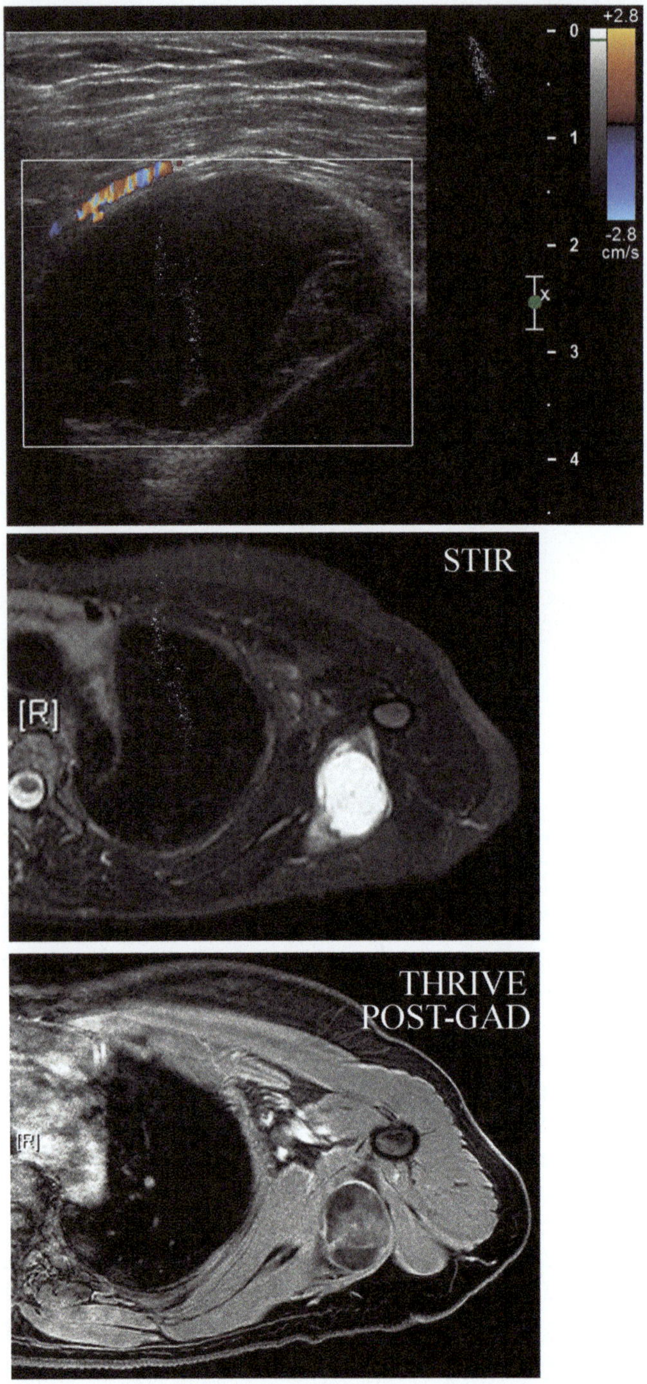

Fig. 15 A 43-year-old female presents with a stable left axillary mass for 3–4 years, which the patient reports to fluctuate with her menstrual cycle. MLO and CC views reveal no focal mammographic abnormality (not shown here). **b** Ultrasound demonstrated a complex oval mass with cystic and solid components lying within the muscle. Colour Doppler analysis demonstrates some peripheral blood flow. **c** Axial STIR and **d** axial post-gadolinium sequences demonstrate an ovoid lesion within the latissmus dorsi muscle at the level of the axilla, which was hypointense to muscle on T1-weighted images (not shown here) and shows increased signal intensity on the fluid-sensitive STIR sequence shown here. Post-gadolinium imaging shows some internal enhancement. CT-guided needle biopsy was performed. Final diagnosis: intramuscular myxoma of the latissimus dorsi

Conclusions

Knowledge of the normal axillary anatomy aids in determining the underlying aetiology of an axillary mass. The differential diagnosis of an axillary mass is broad, including skin lesions, infections, haematoma, lymphadenopathy (hyperplastic, inflammatory, neoplastic or metastatic), accessory breast tissue, fibroadenoma, fibrocystic change, post-operative fluid collections, primary breast cancer and intramuscular neoplasms. For most cases, imaging evaluation entails diagnostic mammography and targeted ultrasound. If intervention is warranted, FNA or core needle biopsies are safe and accurate methods for diagnosis and for guiding the management of an axillary mass.

References

1. Ecanow JS et al (2013) Axillary staging of breast cancer: what the radiologist should know. Radiographics 33(6):1589–1612
2. Mainiero MB et al (2010) Axillary ultrasound and fine-needle aspiration in the preoperative evaluation of the breast cancer patient: an algorithm based on tumor size and lymph node appearance. AJR Am J Roentgenol 195(5):1261–1267
3. Krishnamurthy S et al (2002) Role of ultrasound-guided fine-needle aspiration of indeterminate and suspicious axillary lymph nodes in the initial staging of breast carcinoma. Cancer 95(5):982–988
4. Damera A et al (2003) Diagnosis of axillary nodal metastases by ultrasound-guided core biopsy in primary operable breast cancer. Br J Cancer 89(7):1310–1313
5. Abdsaleh S, Azavedo E, Lindgren PG (2004) Ultrasound-guided large needle core biopsy of the axilla. Acta Radiol 45(2):193–196
6. Nori J et al (2005) Role of axillary lymph node ultrasound and large core biopsy in the preoperative assessment of patients selected for sentinel node biopsy. Radiol Med 109(4):330–344
7. Kim KH et al (2008) The safety and efficiency of the ultrasound-guided large needle core biopsy of axilla lymph nodes. Yonsei Med J 49(2):249–254
8. Topal U et al (2005) Role of ultrasound-guided core needle biopsy of axillary lymph nodes in the initial staging of breast carcinoma. Eur J Radiol 56(3):382–385
9. Bancroft LW et al., A.-.
10. Bedi DG et al (2008) Cortical morphologic features of axillary lymph nodes as a predictor of metastasis in breast cancer: in vitro sonographic study. AJR Am J Roentgenol 191(3): 646–652
11. Shetty MK, Carpenter WS (2004) Sonographic evaluation of isolated abnormal axillary lymph nodes identified on mammograms. J Ultrasound Med 23(1):63–71
12. Choi YJ et al (2009) High-resolution ultrasonographic features of axillary lymph node metastasis in patients with breast cancer. Breast 18(2):119–122

13. Deurloo EE et al (2003) Reduction in the number of sentinel lymph node procedures by preoperative ultrasonography of the axilla in breast cancer. Eur J Cancer 39(8):1068–1073
14. Gogas J et al (2002) Granular cell tumor of the breast: a rare lesion resembling breast cancer. Eur J Gynaecol Oncol 23(4):333–334
15. Kopans, D.B.I.L.-R., Philadelphia and New York.
16. Laor T et al (2004) MRI appearance of accessory breast tissue: a diagnostic consideration for an axillary mass in a peripubertal or pubertal girl. AJR Am J Roentgenol 183(6): 1779–1781
17. Sever AR et al (2012) Preoperative needle biopsy of sentinel lymph nodes using intradermal microbubbles and contrast-enhanced ultrasound in patients with breast cancer. AJR Am J Roentgenol 199(2):465–470
18. Garcia-Ortega MJ et al (2011) Pretreatment axillary ultrasonography and core biopsy in patients with suspected breast cancer: diagnostic accuracy and impact on management. Eur J Radiol 79(1):64–72
19. Alvarez S et al (2006) Role of sonography in the diagnosis of axillary lymph node metastases in breast cancer: a systematic review. AJR Am J Roentgenol 186(5):1342–1348
20. Houssami N et al (2011) Preoperative ultrasound-guided needle biopsy of axillary nodes in invasive breast cancer: meta-analysis of its accuracy and utility in staging the axilla. Ann Surg 254(2):243–251
21. Houssami N et al (2014) Clinical utility of ultrasound-needle biopsy for preoperative staging of the axilla in invasive breast cancer. Anticancer Res 34(3):1087–1097
22. Giuliano AE et al (2011) Axillary dissection vs no axillary dissection in women with invasive breast cancer and sentinel node metastasis: a randomized clinical trial. JAMA 305(6):569–575
23. Cools-Lartigue J, Meterissian S (2012) Accuracy of axillary ultrasound in the diagnosis of nodal metastasis in invasive breast cancer: a review. World J Surg 36(1):46–54
24. Cools-Lartigue J et al (2013) Preoperative axillary ultrasound and fine-needle aspiration biopsy in the diagnosis of axillary metastases in patients with breast cancer: predictors of accuracy and future implications. Ann Surg Oncol 20(3):819–827
25. Adeniran A et al (2004) Granular cell tumor of the breast: a series of 17 cases and review of the literature. Breast J 10(6): 528–531
26. DeMay RM, Kay S (1984) Granular cell tumor of the breast. Pathol Annu 19(Pt 2):121–148
27. Yang WT et al (2006) Sonographic and mammographic appearances of granular cell tumors of the breast with pathological correlation. J Clin Ultrasound 34(4):153–160
28. Nasser H et al (2010) Malignant granular cell tumor: case report with a novel karyotype and review of the literature. Ann Diagn Pathol 14(4):273–278
29. Dialani V et al (2011) Breast schwannoma. Case Rep Med 2011: 930841
30. Uchida N, Yokoo H, Kuwano H (2005) Schwannoma of the breast: report of a case. Surg Today 35(3):238–242
31. C. Fletcher, D.H.o.T., Churchill Livingstone, New York, NY, USA, 3rd edition, 2007.
32. Gultekin SH, Cody HS 3rd, Hoda SA (1996) Schwannoma of the breast. South Med J 89(2):238–239
33. Murphey MD et al (2002) Imaging of soft-tissue myxoma with emphasis on CT and MR and comparison of radiologic and pathologic findings. Radiology 225(1):215–224

17

Fibromuscular dysplasia: what the radiologist should know: a pictorial review

L. Varennes · F. Tahon · A. Kastler · S. Grand · F. Thony · J. P. Baguet · O. Detante · E. Touzé · A. Krainik

Abstract
Fibromuscular dysplasia (FMD) is an idiopathic, segmentary, non-inflammatory and non-atherosclerotic disease that can affect all layers of both small- and medium-calibre arteries. The prevalence of FMD is estimated between 4 and 6 % in the renal arteries and between 0.3 and 3 % in the cervico-encephalic arteries. FMD most frequently affects the renal, carotid and vertebral arteries, but it can theoretically affect any artery. Radiologists play an important role in the diagnosis of FMD, and good knowledge of FMD's signs will certainly help reduce the delay between the first symptoms and diagnosis. The common string-of-beads aspect is well known, but less common presentations also have to be considered. These less common imaging findings include vascular loops, fusiform vascular ectasia, arterial dissection, aneurysm and subarachnoid haemorrhage. These radiologic presentations should be known by radiologists in order to diagnose possible FMD, particularly when present in young females or when associated with personal or familial hypertension, to reduce the delay between the onset of the first symptom and the final diagnosis. The patients have to be referred to specialised FMD centres for dedicated management.

Teaching Points

- *Fibromuscular dysplasia is not a rare disease.*
- *Radiologists should recognise less common presentations to orient specific management.*
- *Vascular loops, fusiform vascular ectasia and a "string-of-beads" aspect are typical presentations.*
- *Arterial dissection, aneurysm and subarachnoid haemorrhage are less typical radiologic presentations.*

Keywords Fibromuscular dysplasia · Radiology · Arteries · Aneurysm

L. Varennes · F. Tahon · A. Kastler · S. Grand · A. Krainik (✉)
Department of Neuroradiology and MRI, University Hospital of Grenoble, CS 10217-38043, Grenoble Cedex 09, France
e-mail: akrainik@chu-grenoble.fr

L. Varennes · F. Thony
Department of Radiology, University Hospital of Grenoble, CS 10217-38043, Grenoble Cedex 09, France

J. P. Baguet
Department of Cardiology, Mutualist Hospital Group of Grenoble, 38028 Grenoble cedex 1, France

O. Detante
Department of Neurology, University Hospital of Grenoble, CS 10217-38043, Grenoble Cedex 09, France

E. Touzé
Department of Neurology, University Caen Basse Normandie, Inserm U919, CHU Côte de Nacre, Caen, France

Introduction

Fibromuscular dysplasia (FMD) is an idiopathic, segmentary, non-inflammatory and non-atherosclerotic disease that can affect all layers of both small- and medium-calibre arteries. Although not known, the FMD prevalence in the general population is considered to be low by several authors [1]. The cause and pathophysiology of FMD are still unknown [2, 3]. Clinical manifestations of FMD are primarily dependent on the vessels that are involved. FMD most frequently affects the renal, carotid and vertebral arteries, but can be found in all territories [3]. It is a potentially serious disease, especially in the cervico-encephalic location, where it can lead to severe stenosis, hypoperfusion, aneurysm, subarachnoid haemorrhage, dissection or arterial occlusion [3–5].

FMD is often not considered in the differential diagnosis because radiological aspects can be difficult to diagnose and the symptoms reported are not specific. Therefore, the mean delay from symptoms to diagnosis has been reported to be up to 4.1 years [6].

Radiologists play an important role in the diagnosis of FMD, and a good knowledge of FMD's presentations should help to reduce the delay between the first symptoms and final diagnosis. The objective of this review is therefore to raise radiologists' awareness of FMD's epidemiology, pathophysiology, clinical presentation, typical and atypical radiological aspects and possible complications.

Epidemiology

The prevalence of FMD is estimated between 4 and 6 % in the renal arteries and between 0.3 and 3 % in the cervico-encephalic arteries [2, 7–9]. However, most data stem from series of consecutive angiograms performed in symptomatic patients and therefore cannot be considered representative. Several authors believe that these prevalence values are underestimated because FMD is frequently asymptomatic [10–12]. In a review combining the results of 4 studies including 3,181 asymptomatic patients who had undergone a renal angiography before kidney transplant donation, 4.4 % (139 subjects) presented FMD lesions [1]. In another study among 20,244 consecutive autopsies performed at the Mayo Clinic over a 25-year period, only 4 subjects had cervical FMD (0.02 %) [13].

FMD is most frequently revealed in the kidneys in young patients with resistant hypertension secondary to fibrodysplastic renal artery stenosis (RAS). FMD is found in about 1 % of hypertensive patients and represents the second leading cause of renovascular hypertension after atherosclerotic disease. As for cervico-encephalic FMD, the symptoms are not specific.

In 2012, Olin et al. [6] included 447 cases from the FMD registry from nine states in the USA, the largest number of patients included in any study to date. The most frequently described symptoms or conditions were hypertension (63.8 %), headaches (52.4 %), pulsatile tinnitus (27.5 %), dizziness (26 %) and neck pain (22 %). This study showed a clear female prevalence (91 %), and the mean age at diagnosis was 51.9 years. In 6 % of cases, FMD was discovered randomly. Affected arteries were mainly renal arteries (79.7 %), extracranial carotid (74.4 %) and vertebral (36.6 %) arteries, mesenteric arteries (26 %) and intracranial carotid arteries (17 %). Sixty-five per cent of patients with renal FMD lesions also had cervico-encephalic artery lesions, and vice versa.

Several studies have reported a lower frequency of FMD lesions in the carotid arteries compared with renal arteries [1, 3, 14–16]. In 1982, Mettinger et al. found 58 % renal artery involvement versus 32 % carotid artery involvement based on a systematic review of 36 studies, including 1,197 patients with FMD [9]. This difference can be explained as FMD is more frequently symptomatic in renal arteries through the onset of hypertension [3], which also tends to increase its prevalence. Moreover, at the time of this study, multi-detector computed tomography (CT) was not as available a diagnostic tool as it is today. Indeed, easy access to computed tomographic angiography (CTA) and better knowledge of cervico-encephalic FMD, which is now looked for systematically in patients with renal artery lesions, may explain the differences in cervico-encephalic FMD lesion prevalence found in more recent studies [6].

Pathophysiology

FMD's pathophysiology remains unclear. Some authors suggest a role played by estrogenic impregnation given the female predominance. The predominance of right renal artery lesions suggests a mechanical component because the right kidney is more mobile than the left one; the mechanism may involve compression of the vasa vasorum leading to ischaemia. The vasa vasorum are small blood vessels that wind along arteries whose calibres are larger than 1 mm. They feed the adventitia and the external two-thirds of the media. There are relatively few in the carotid and renal arteries, possibly a feature of FMD [13]. Smoking could also be a risk factor. Autosomal dominant transmission with incomplete penetrance and variable expressivity is suggested in 6–10 % familial types; no specific gene has been identified, though [17]. Moreover, a study performed over 9 years in 106 patients who had repeated angiograms showed either a progression or a stabilisation of FMD lesions but no lesion regression was seen [9].

Typical and variant aspects

Typical aspects

Classifications

The first case of histologically proven carotid FMD was published by Connett and Lansche in 1965 [18]. Later, a classification of FMD based on renal artery lesions was described in 1971 by Harrison and MacCormack [19], then revised by Stanley in 1996 [20]. This classification is based on the most affected arterial layer: the intimal type, medial type or subadventitial type. The authors report that several forms can co-exist in the same patient. These lesions were later described in carotid arteries in autopsies [3].

(1) The intimal type corresponds to fibrous circumferential intimal thickening with proliferation of subendothelial connective tissue. The internal elastic lamina is always preserved, and the media and adventitia are normal. This

form is mainly found in children, rarely in adults (5 %). It appears as focal truncal stenosis (Fig. 1).

(2) The medial type is the most frequent (60–70 %) and corresponds to a rarefaction of smooth media muscle cells replaced by fibrosis. The intima, internal elastic lamina and adventitia are normal. It appears as a succession of dilatations and multifocal stenoses with a characteristic string-of-beads aspect. It is mainly discovered in females aged 30–50 years (Fig. 2).

(3) The perimedial or subadventitial type (10–20 % of cases) corresponds to excessive elastic tissue in the external area of the media. Its aspect is close to the medial type with fewer dilatations that do not exceed the diameter of the normal artery. Stenosis often appears tubular (Fig. 3).

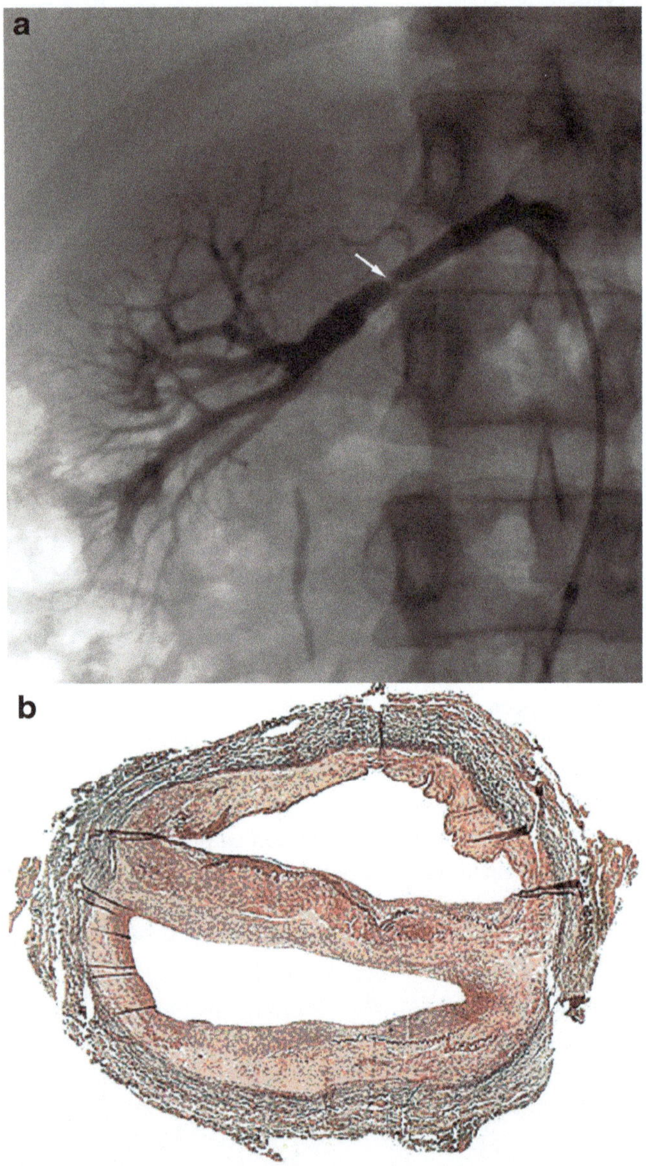

Fig. 1 Example of intimal FMD lesions. **a** Renal angiogram showing short focal stenosis (*white arrow*) of the right renal artery, in favour of intimal FMD. **b** Colour histological slide of intimal FMD showing circumferential focal thickening. Media and adventitia are normal

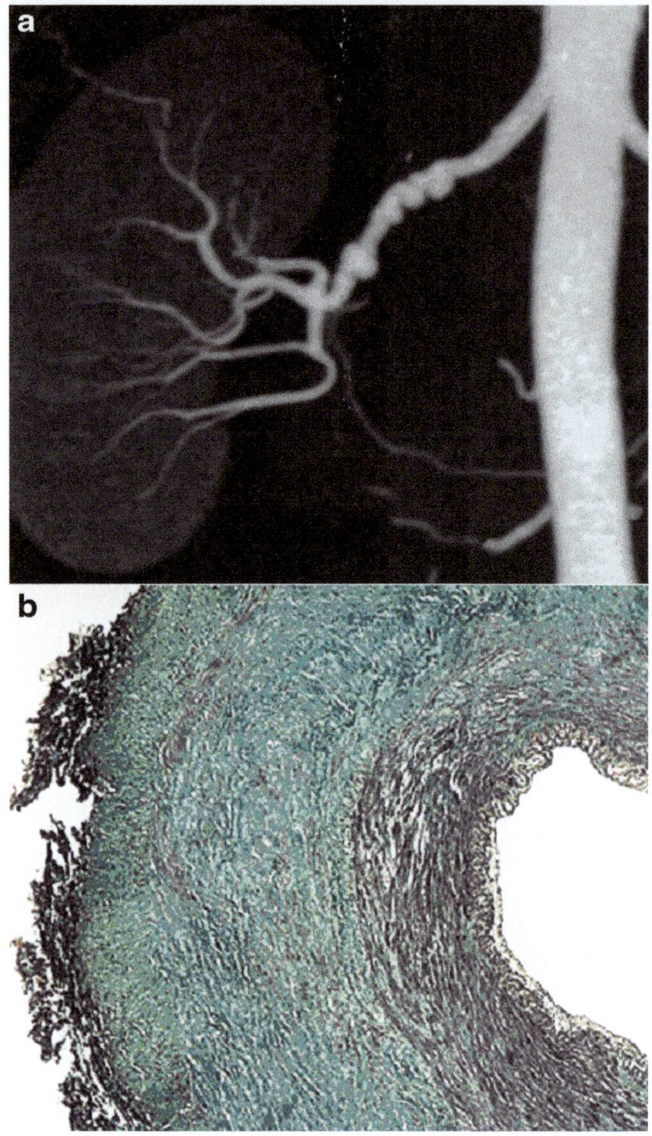

Fig. 2 Example of medial FMD lesions. **a** Renal CTA with coronal plane MIP reconstruction, showing the typical "string-of-beads" aspect of the right renal artery, in favour of medial FMD. **b** Colour histological slide of medial FMD showing extensive medial fibrosis. Intima and adventitia are normal

This classification is not frequently used in daily practice because several types may co-exist in the same patient and/or the same artery. Today, pathological samples are analysed in exceptional circumstances. Kincaid et al.'s angiographic classification based on a series of 125 patients [21] is more commonly used. The purpose of Kincaid's classification is to distinguish the multifocal (multiple stenosis or string-of-beads aspect), unifocal (short stenosis less than 1 cm long), tubular (stenosis more than 1 cm long) and mixed types. The string-of-beads aspect is the most characteristic aspect of FMD and indicates the presence of

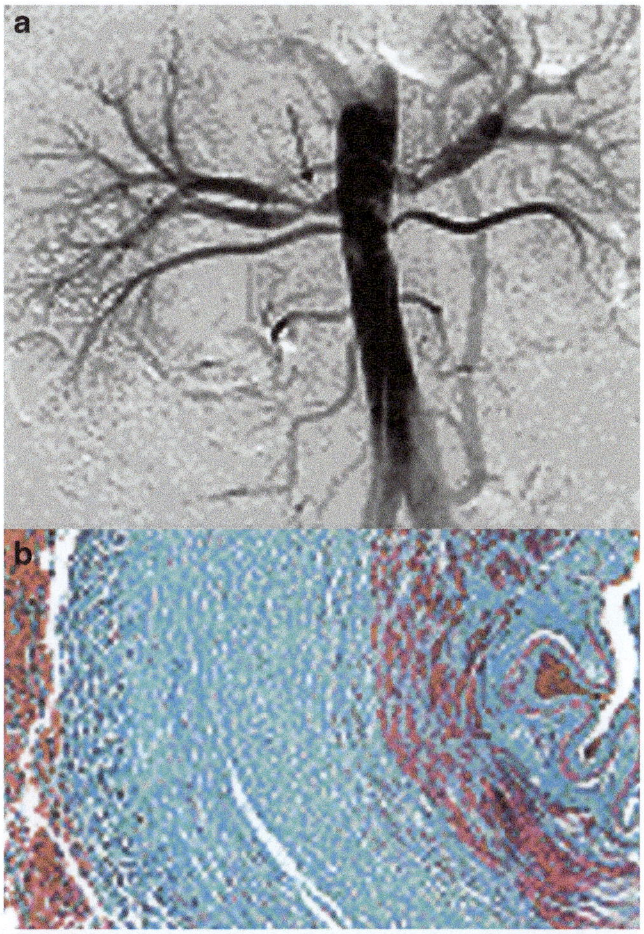

Fig. 3 Example of perimedial FMD lesions. **a** Aorta angiogram showing a long stenosis (*black arrow*) of the right renal artery, in favour of perimedial FMD. **b** Colour histological slide of perimedial FMD showing extensive perimedial fibrosis

medial lesions [1]. The other angiographic aspects are less specific to a histological type.

In 2012, Savard et al. [22] proposed a simplified classification based only on two angiographic cervico-encephalic subtypes of FMD: the multifocal (presence of ≥2 stenoses on a given vessel segment with or without the typical string-of-beads appearance) and unifocal (presence of a single focal or tubular stenosis) types. Interestingly, Savard et al. showed significant clinical differences depending on the subtype such as median age at diagnosis of FMD, hypertension, sex distribution, initial blood pressure and current smoking.

Diagnostic tools

Figure 4 shows the diagnostic strategies, advantages and drawbacks of different imaging techniques.

In case of renal impairment, Doppler ultrasound shows an accelerated blood flow in renal arteries with stenoses. It also allows studying the size of the kidneys, which is a good evaluation criterion for disease severity and follow-up [17].

Magnetic resonance angiography (MRA) and CTA present high specifities for detecting renal artery stenosis due to FMD (92 and 84 % respectively), but have relatively low sensitivities (64 and 62 % respectively) [1]. Although, MRA has a poorer spatial resolution (1–2 mm) compared with CTA, its main advantage is still the non-ionising technique. Finally, although gadolinium-based contrast material is still safer than iodine-based contrast media, gadolinium-based contrast agents should not to be used in patients with an estimated glomerular filtration rate<30 ml/min/1.73 m^2 because of concerns about nephrogenic systemic fibrosis [6]. In these patients, non-contrast MR angiography techniques with time-of-flight sequences can be used especially in ultra-high field MRI equipment. Nonetheless, to date, no published studies have validated the use of time-of-flight sequences for the diagnosis of FMD compared with angiography or other non-invasive imaging modalities [23]. A recent study comparing contrast-enhanced MRA with conventional angiography showed a sensitivity of 97 % and specificity of 93 % for FMD diagnosis. MRA was more sensitive for detecting the string-of-beads appearance (97 %) than detecting a >50 % stenosis (68 %) [24].

CTA has the best sensitivity/specificity ratio (1) and allows reconstruction of the renal arterial vasculature [23] but requires contrast media injection. High spatial resolution and short acquisition time are the major advantages of the current CTA studies. This technology allows visualisation of a greater volume per unit time, resulting in reduced pulsation and stair-step artefacts. CTA has the ability to generate three-dimensional multiplanar and volume-rendered images. Assessment of the renal arteries should be performed using vascular windows on a dedicated three-dimensional workstation. It is imperative to review the data sets using multiple reconstruction formats, including multiplanar reformatted images, shaded surface display and maximum-intensity projections. The use of all these reformats in addition to the axial "raw data" has been shown to improve the sensitivity and specificity of this imaging modality [25].

Although the diagnosis of cervico-encephalic FMD can be suspected with Doppler ultrasound in case of vascular loops, ectasia, intimal flap or aliasing, it is most frequently established with cross-sectional imaging, using CTA of the supra-aortic trunks (SAT), MRA or in some cases conventional angiography. These imaging techniques present better sensitivity in detecting lesions of the middle and distal portions of the internal carotid and vertebral arteries at the level of the C1 and C2 vertebrae [1], which are the most frequently affected segments [3].

Multi-row detector CTA allows a detailed evaluation of the extracranial and intracranial cerebrovasculature with the ability to identify FMD, dissections, cerebral aneurysms and atherosclerosis. Moreover, the images can be reconstructed in

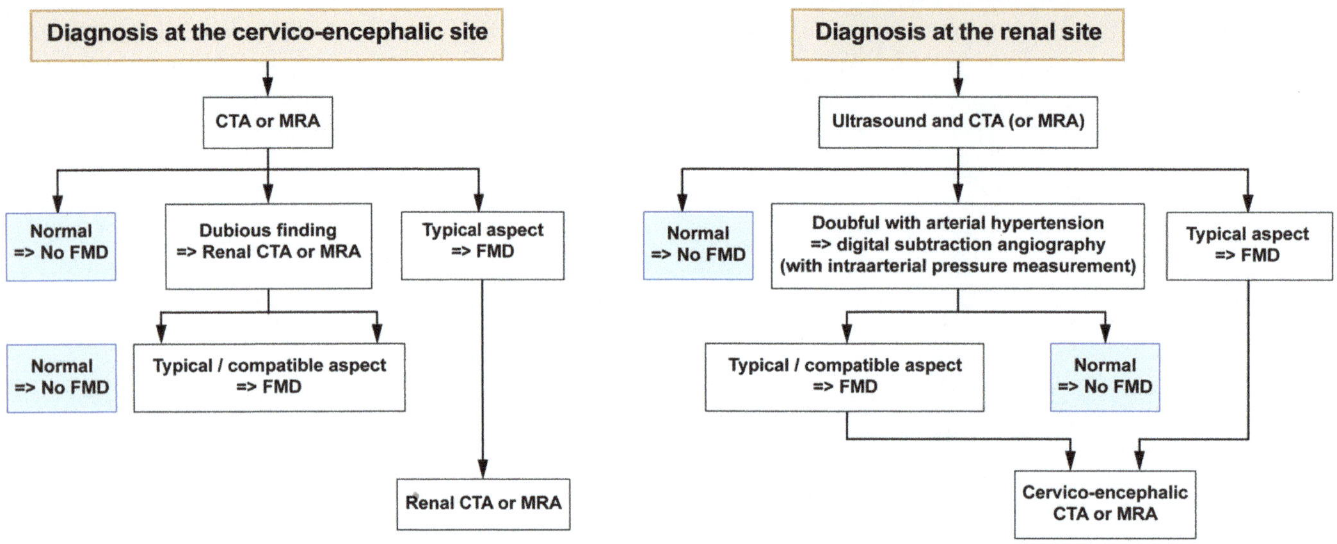

	Advantages	Drawbacks
Ultrasound	Easy access, cheap, safety, hemodynamic exploration, high sensitivity for detection of significant stenoses	Operator-dependent, poor specificity
CTA	High sensitivity, high specificity, high spatial resolution, short acquisition time	Iodine injection (risk of allergia or renal failure), X-irradiation, no hemodynamic explorartion
MRA	Safety, moderate sensitivity, moderate specificity	Specific contraindications, moderate spatial resolution, no hemodynamic exploration
Digital subtraction angiography	High spatial resolution, short acquisition time	Iodine injection (risk of allergia or renal failure), X-irradiation, invasive procedure

Fig. 4 Flow chart illustrating imaging algorithms in case of suspected DFM for both the renal or cervico-encephalic level. The table shows the advantages and drawbacks of the different diagnostic tests

maximal intensity and three-dimensional projections, allowing detailed anatomic visualisation.

No clinical studies have validated the use of MRA compared with catheter-based angiography for the diagnosis of cerebrovascular FMD. Consequently, the specificity and sensitivity of MRA in the diagnosis of FMD are not known. Nevertheless, MRA may have the benefit of detecting FMD-associated SAT dissections when T1 fat-saturation images are acquired simultaneously with time-of-flight or gadolinium-enhanced images [26].

Despite the improvements in non-invasive screening techniques, negative results do not exclude the diagnosis of FMD. In case of high clinical suspicion, use of diagnostic arteriography [1, 9] or endovascular ultrasound can be discussed if therapeutically relevant. Indeed, catheter-based angiography remains the gold standard imaging modality for renovascular FMD because of its unsurpassed spatial resolution (<0.1 mm) [1, 3].

Imaging acquisition protocols To date there are no existing imaging protocol recommendations specific to FMD diagnosis. In our institution, the following protocols are currently used for both the initial diagnosis and follow-up:

- Renal

– CTA

An ROI is placed in the abdominal aorta; density tracking is used with a threshold set at 180 HU and 3-s delay. Seventy ml of Omnipaque 350 is used. ANgioCT is performed from the diaphragm to pubis. The slice thickness is 1 mm, with the following settings: 120 kV, 300 mAs.

– MRA

This protocol can be randomly used in both 1.5- and 3-T scanners: Coronal 3D FFE angioMR after injection of 0.2 ml/kg of Dotarem at 2 ml/s. Slice thickness is set at 0.8 mm (total slices 65), TR: 5 ms, TE: 1,79 ms.

- SAT

– CTA

An ROI is set in the aortic arch with a 75-DH threshold with no delay. Acquisition is set from the tracheal bifurcation to 4 cm above the dorsum salae. Injection of 60 ml of Omnipaque 350 is at 5 cc/s. Slice thickness is 0.9 mm with 240 mAs, 120 kV.

– MRA

Coronal 3D FFE angioMR is carried out after injection of 0.2 ml/kg of Dotarem at 1.2 ml/s. Slice thickness is set at 0.7 mm (total slices 105) with the following settings: TR: 4 ms, TE: 1.57 ms.

Preferential locations, clinical manifestation and radiological diagnostic criteria

1. Renal arteries The renal arteries are the most frequently affected location of FMD lesions. In 1997, in a series of 104 hypertensive patients with renal artery FMD, 80 % were middle-aged females with preserved renal function. In 54 % of the cases, the lesions were bilateral, and they involved the branches in 42 % of the cases. Multifocal string-of-beads lesions were found in 84 % of the cases. The unifocal type most often affected young males, with tighter stenosis and more frequent downstream lesions [27].

FMD renal involvement does not necessarily lead to arterial hypertension, and progression toward kidney failure is rare, even in cases of bilateral lesions [1, 12]. In case of stenosis in a patient with hypertension and renal FMD, the severity of stenosis and its relation to hypertension can only be asserted in case of asymmetrical kidney size. Measuring intrarenal arterial pressure compared to intra-aortic pressure can also assess the severity of stenosis. Thus, in case of a significant difference (>20 mmHg), hypertension can be attributed to the FMD lesions and therefore lead to renal angioplasty.

Even in cases of non-significant renal artery stenosis, the progression of the lesions ought to be monitored. In nearly one-third of cases, occurrence of a new lesion, worsening stenosis or an extending aneurysm can be visualised in these patients [21].

2. Cervico-encephalic arteries The advent of multi-detector CT and the increase in awareness among physicians about the cervico-encephalic location of FMD have certainly participated in increasing the its prevalence. In 1982, Mettinger and Ericson, from an analysis of the literature about FMD, reported a prevalence of cervico-encephalic FMD lesions of 32 % (in about 1,100 patients) [9]. In 2012, Olin et al. [6] reported a much higher prevalence of 74 % (in 447 cases from the FMD registry from nine states in the USA).

Although the most frequent symptoms of FMD are non-specific (headache, dizziness, neck pain) [6], some clinical manifestations of cervico-encephalic FMD are more serious, such as transient ischaemic attack (TIA), stroke, subarachnoid haemorrhage and arterial dissection. FMD mainly affects the internal carotid artery in its extracranial part, but all territories can be affected [17].

TIA and ischaemic stroke can be due to either arterial stenosis, leading to hypoperfusion and clot emboli, or to spontaneous extracranial arterial dissection. In case of intracranial dissection, haemorrhage most often occurs. FMD can also lead to subarachnoid haemorrhage (SAH) because of the occurrence of an intracranial dissection or a rupture of intracranial aneurysms (mainly due to the rupture of the internal elastic lamina in the medial types of FMD) [17].

3. Radiological diagnostic criteria There are no formal radiological diagnostic criteria, but it is well established that the string-of-beads aspect found in renal or cervico-encephalic locations on arteriography, CTA or MRA is highly suggestive of FMD. Focal or tubular lesions on angiography allow determining the diagnosis when they are typical [28]. Another frequent finding suggestive of an FMD diagnosis is the presence of a "web-like" defect at the origin of the internal carotid artery [3, 29].

In such situations, lesions may be discrete at the cervical level and typical at the renal level. Thus, imaging of the renal arteries will help to establish the diagnosis. The opposite situation is also true, and performing imaging of the renal arteries is recommended in a patient presenting discrete but suggestive lesions in the cervico-encephalic arteries so as to confirm the diagnosis, and vice versa (Figs. 5 and 6) [30].

Intracranial FMD with a typical string-of-beads aspect (basilar artery, carotid, middle cerebral artery) is usually an intracranial extension of extracranial lesions [29].

Less typical presentations (Fig. 12)

Less typical locations

FMD can occur in almost any artery, including those that supply the intestines (mesenteric arteries) and the upper (brachial arteries) and lower limbs (iliac arteries). In many patients, FMD is found in more than one artery, which argues for a systemic disease. In 2012, Olin et al. [6] reported that FMD affects mesenteric arteries in 26.3 %, upper extremity arteries in 15.9 % and lower extremity arteries in 6 %. No aortic location was reported in this study. To date, it is not possible to determine whether the coronary artery involvement is due to atherosclerosis or fibromuscular dysplasia.

Arterial dissection

According to Olin et al., out of 447 cases of FMD, 19.7 % had an arterial dissection [6]. In 75 % of cases, the dissection was located in the carotid artery, 22 % in the renal artery and 17 % in a vertebral artery.

Renal artery dissection may occur in 5–10 %, especially in case of renal artery tubular stenosis [31]. It may be responsible of renal infarct by total occlusion or distal emboli, leading to

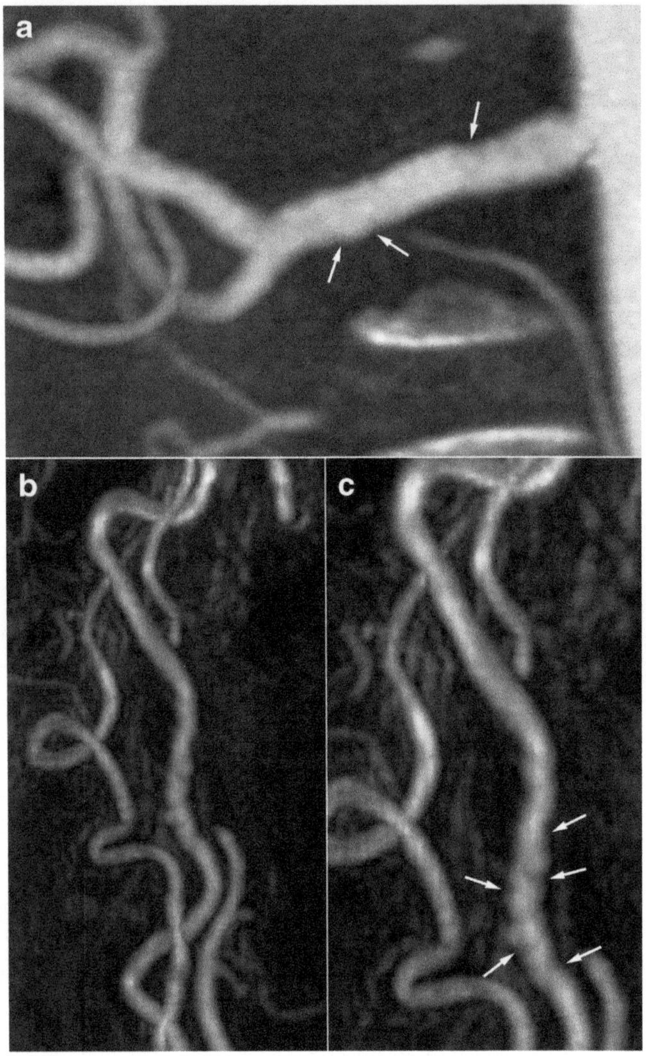

Fig. 5 Radiologic findings in a 68-year-old female patient who suffered from an inferior myocardial infarct secondary to spontaneous dissection of the right coronary artery. **a** Renal coronal CTA MIP reconstruction showing moderate involvement of the right renal artery (*white arrows*). **b** and **c** Three-dimensional gadolinium-enhanced MRA reconstructions in the same patient showing the typical string-of-beads aspect (*white arrows*) of the internal carotid artery, highly suggestive of FMD

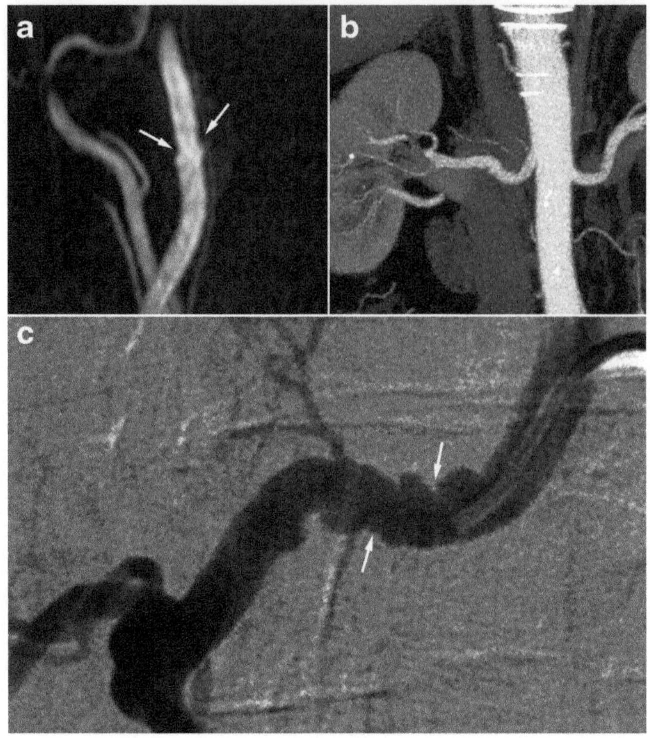

Fig. 6 Radiologic findings in a 62-year-old male patient with arterial hypertension. **a** Gadolinium-enhanced MRA with MIP reconstruction showing typical but discrete involvement of the internal carotid artery (*white arrows*). **b** Renal CTA, coronal MIP reconstruction in the same patient showing a typical aspect of a medial string-of-beads dysplasia of the right renal artery. **c** Right renal angiogram confirming the typical aspect of the right renal artery, in favour of FMD

sudden pain in the flank, haematuria and/or rapidly progressive hypertension [1].

Extracranial dissection of the neck arteries, symptomatic or not, may occur as a complication of FMD lesions [4, 32]. However, it is not sufficient to establish a final diagnosis of FMD. In our experience, out of 64 patients with FMD, more than half of the cervico-encephalic artery dissections were discovered unexpectedly (unpublished data). Spontaneous dissection of a cervical artery is a frequent cause of stroke in young adults and may be associated with FMD in 15–20 % of cases [33, 34]. For this reason, physicians should consider FMD in patients with cervico-encephalic artery dissection, particularly if it is spontaneous, multifocal or in an atypical location. This situation should lead to further exploration of the renal arteries. The same approach could be proposed in case of a pseudoaneurysm that might correspond to the aftermath of a dissection.

Aneurysms/vascular ectasia

Single or multiple aneurysms are frequent in FMD patients [5, 35]. Their prevalence reached 17 % in Olin et al.'s series [6]. Their preferential locations are the renal arteries (33 %) where large aneurysms may develop, notably in medial FMD. Their rupture remains a rare complication. They may also be responsible for distal emboli or even arteriovenous fistula when rupturing in the renal vein [36]. The most frequent locations are the following: carotid (21 %), aortic (19.7 %) and coeliac (15.8 %). A strong association also exists between FMD and intracranial aneurysm, accounting for 11.8 % of the aneurysms in the series reported by Olin et al. Several authors report a 22–51 % prevalence of intracranial aneurysms in patients with FMD in the carotid and/or vertebral arteries [9, 29, 37, 38]. Nonetheless, these results come from a series of cerebral angiograms for the most part undertaken for hypertension. In 1998, in a meta-analysis of 18 studies including 615 FMD patients, Cloft et al. found a 24 % prevalence of intracranial aneurysms [39]. However, in the 212 patients without SAH, the prevalence was 7.3 %, which remains higher than the prevalence expected in the general population, around 2.3 % [40]. One may here suggest the diagnosis of FMD in patients with intracranial aneurysm and/or carotid ectasia, particularly in young females, especially in cases of an associated personal or familial history of hypertension.

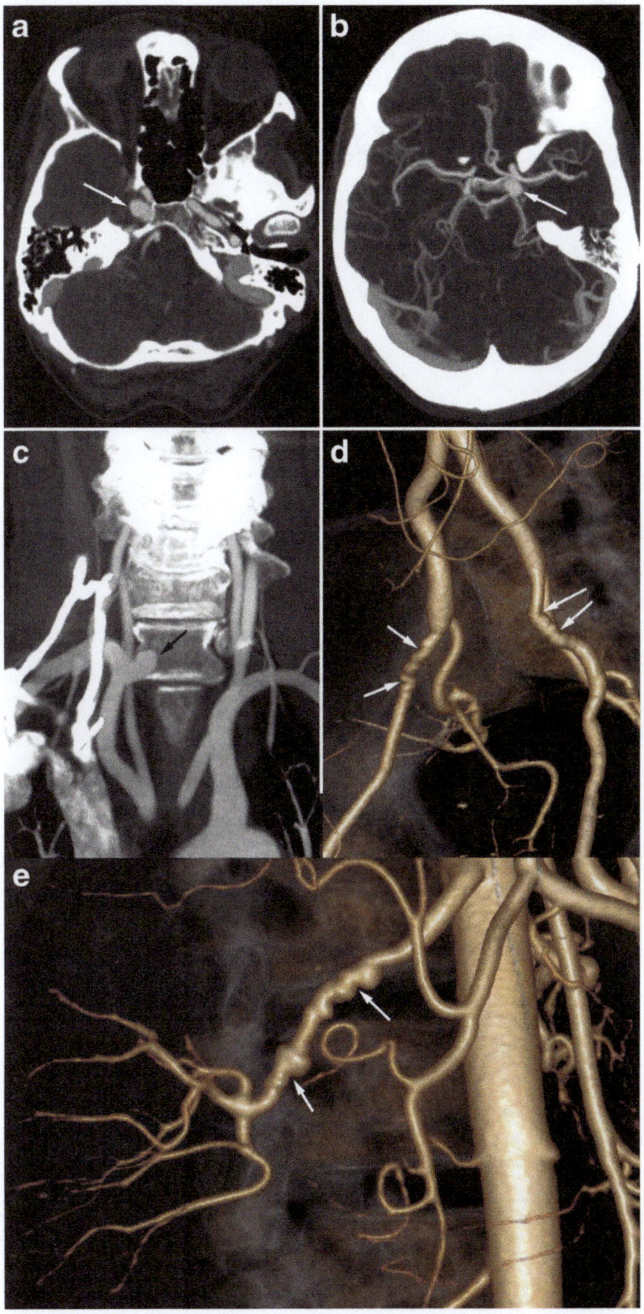

Fig. 7 Radiologic findings in a 56-year-old female patient presenting with non-specific headaches. **a** and **b** Cerebral CTA showing bilateral carotid aneurysms with intracavernous development (*white arrows*). **c** Coronal CTA MIP reconstruction of the supra-aortic trunks, showing a right subclavicular aneurysm (*black arrow*). **d** and **e** Three-dimensional volume-rendered abdominal CTA showing typical medial FMD affecting the external iliac arteries (*white arrows*, **d**) and the right renal artery (*white arrows*, **e**)

In some cases, these aneurysms have an intracavernous development and may be bilateral (Fig. 7). They therefore do lead to SAH but can be responsible for cavernous sinus syndrome. An exceptional case of a carotid-cavernous fistula has even been described [35]. Loops and/or fusiform vascular ectasia in the subpetrous segment of the internal carotid arteries is also frequently found in FMD patients [30].

Unexplained SAH

SAH found in FMD patients is usually a consequence of subarachnoid intracranial aneurysm rupture (Figs. 8 and 9) [3]. SAH has also been described in patients with no visible aneurysm on angiography but with ruptured of microaneurysms of the basilar artery at autopsy (Fig. 10) [41]. These SAHs can also stem from intracranial dissection [30, 42]. The diagnosis is suggested on arteriography (Figs. 4, 11 and 12). For intracranial dissection with SAH re-bleeds, usually endovascular or neurosurgical treatment can be proposed. In the case the arteriography at 3 months showed an ad integrum restitution of the artery.

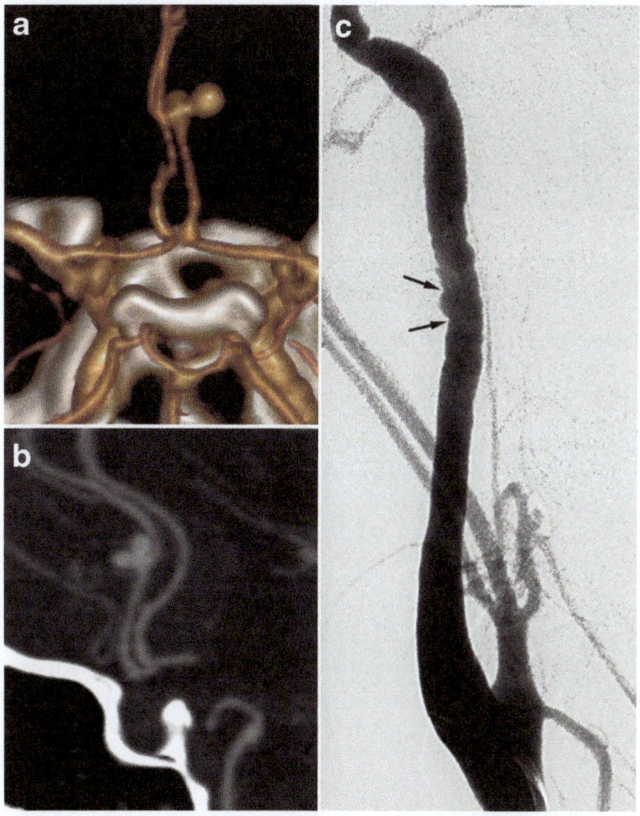

Fig. 8 Radiologic findings in a 38-year-old female patient presenting with non-traumatic spontaneous subarachnoid haemorrhage. **a** Three-dimensional volume-rendered cerebral CTA showing a right pericallosal artery aneurysm. **b** Cerebral CTA sagittal MIP reconstruction of the same aneurysm. **c** Therapeutic arteriography revealed typical right carotid artery medial FMD lesions (*black arrows*)

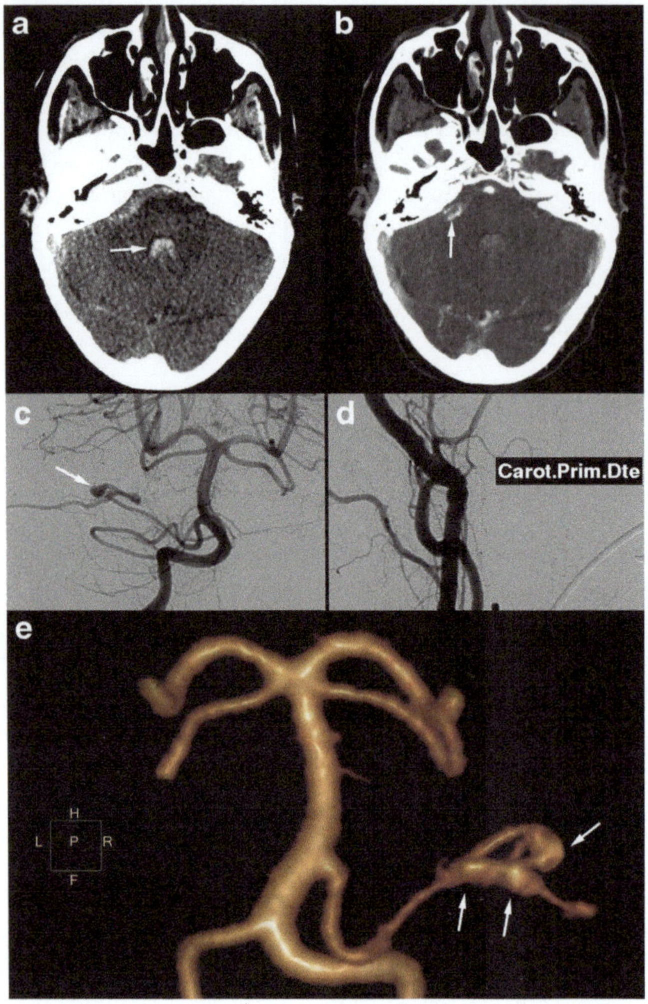

Fig. 9 Radiologic findings in a 70-year-old female patient presenting a right-hemisphere non-traumatic SAH with tetraventricular inundation. **a** Cerebral non-enhanced CT showing SAH and intraventricular haemorrhage. **b** Cerebral CTA showing a dissecting aneurysm of the right antero-inferior cerebellar artery. **c** Angiogram of the right vertebral artery in arterial phase confirming the dissecting aneurysm of the right antero-inferior cerebellar artery (*white arrow*). **d** Right common carotid angiogram showing the typical string-of-beads aspect, in favour of FMD. **e** Cerebral 3D volume-rendered CTA of the dissecting aneurysm of the right antero-inferior cerebellar artery (*white arrows*)

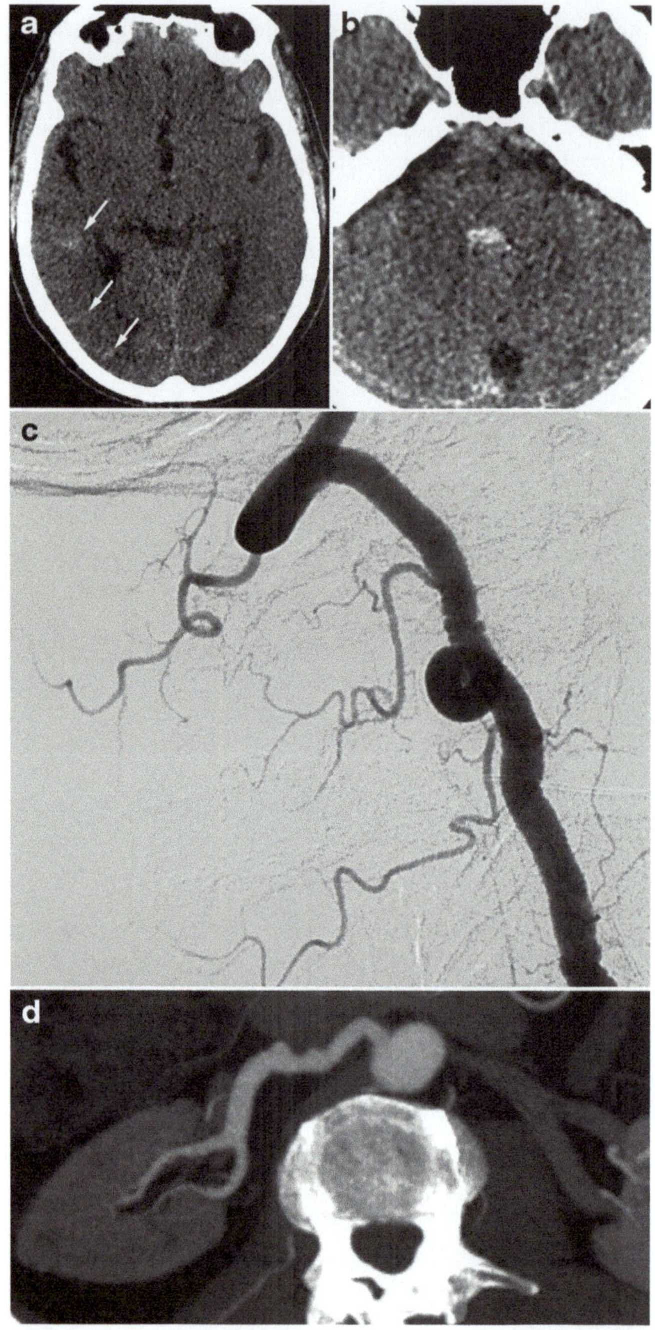

Fig. 10 Radiologic findings in a 65-year-old male patient with SAH of the posterior fossa. The CTA shows no particular signs. The arteriography found typical FMD lesions in the right vertebral artery. The renal CT shows ectasia of the right renal artery termination. **a** and **b** Cerebral non-enhanced CT showing right temporo-occipital SAH (*white arrows*) associated with intraventricular haemorrhage (V4). **c** Right vertebral angiogram showing the typical string-of-beads aspect. **d** Renal CTA, curved reconstructions of the right renal artery showing ectasia of the distal part of the right renal artery

Thus, the presence of non-traumatic SAH, especially in a young female patient, wherever it may be located and whatever its size, should bring up the diagnosis and discussion of a cervico-encephalic artery and renal artery examination during the diagnostic work-up [30].

Differential diagnoses (Fig. 13)

First of all, one must ensure that the images do not stem from vasospasm or stationary waves related to catheter use and/or the injection of a contrast agent. This is manifested by regular undulations with no significant stenosis, which are reversible after injection of a vasodilator and/or removal of the catheter [43].

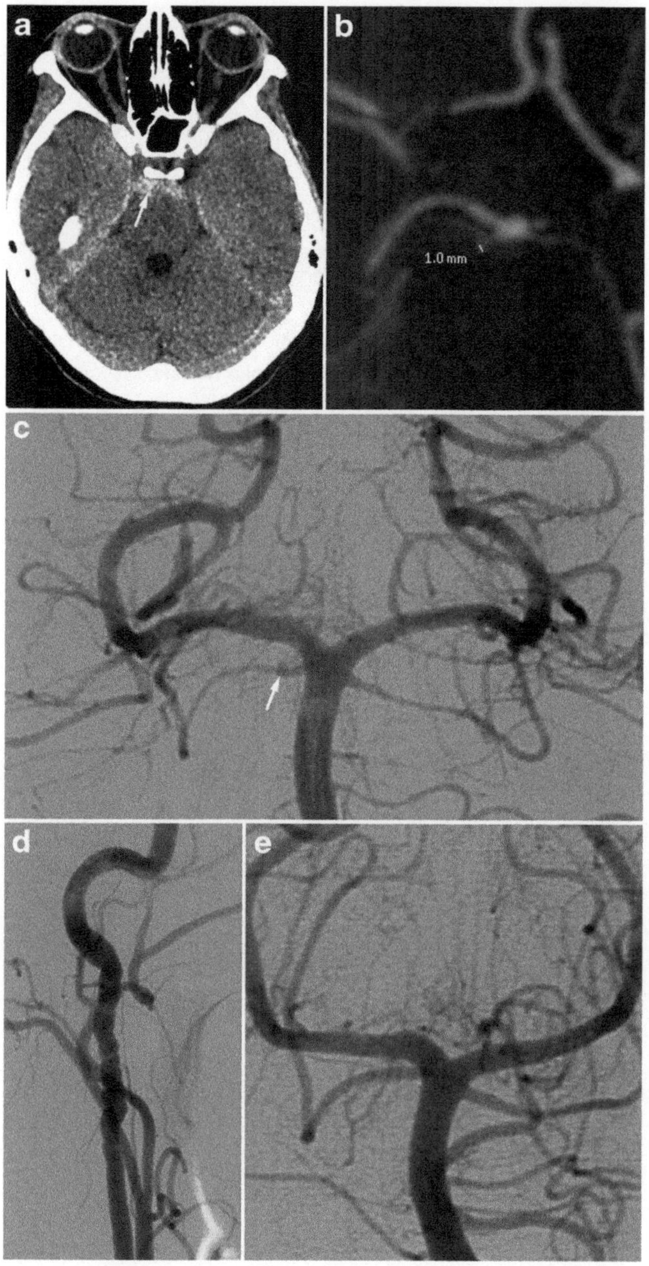

Fig. 11 Radiologic findings in a 48-year-old female presenting with posterior headaches. The initial CT shows SAH of the posterior fossa. The angiography found dissection of the right superior cerebellar artery. Study of the supra-aortic arteries shows typical FMD images. Ad integrum restitution at 3 months. **a** Cerebral non-enhanced CT showing prepontine SAH (*white arrow*). **b** and **c** Cerebral CTA and angiogram showing a dissection of the right superior cerebellar artery. **d** Right carotid angiogram showing showing classical FMD imaging findings. **e** The 3-month follow-up angiography showing ad integrum restitution of the artery, in favour of arterial dissection

Marfan or vascular Ehlers-Danlos syndrome should be discussed when presented with aneurysmal lesions and/or multiple dissections, particularly with a compatible morphotype or in a suggestive family context [1]. These diagnoses rely on associated phenotypic traits and genetic tests: acrogeric dysmorhy, distal joint laxity and tiny skin elasticity (confirmed by detection of the COL3A1 gene mutation) [44].

Vasculitis may mimic FMD lesions, but in most cases the presence of systemic inflammation provides the diagnosis [1].

Atherosclerotic lesions usually occur in a different setting. Most focal lesions are preferentially located at the ostium of the arteries or at a bifurcation. Most FMD patients are young and have few or no cardiovascular risk factors or aortic atheromatous plaques [1].

Finally, segmental arterial mediolysis (SAM) should be suggested in cases of an association of digestive tract artery lesions, notably the gastroduodenal artery. The similarity between the chronic vacular lesions of SAM and FMD lesions raises the question of a common pathophysiological stem of these lesions, one perhaps being a progressive form of the other [45, 46].

With typical string-of-beads lesions involving the renal and/or carotid arteries, possible differential diagnoses are limited.

Treatment/management

Treatment for patients with FMD may include medical therapy and surveillance; endovascular therapy for stenosis (angioplasty with or without stenting), dissection (stents) or aneurysms (coils, stents); or surgery. Therapeutic decisions depend on the nature and location of vascular lesions (stenosis versus dissection versus aneurysm), the presence and severity of symptoms, prior to vascular events related to FMD, the presence and size of aneurysms, and comorbid conditions.

The lack of knowledge about the natural history of FMD and the insufficient number of randomised studies comparing different therapeutic approaches does not allow adequate evaluation of the effectiveness of different therapeutic options. In patients who had an ischaemic stroke antiplatelet therapy is generally introduced, although its efficacy has never been demonstrated specifically for symptomatic patients with FMD.

Patients with symptomatic FMD lesions that are accessible to surgery and with low perioperative risk can be good candidates for surgery because the long-term anatomical results are good and most surgical techniques are well known.

However, because of recent advances in interventional radiology techniques, including angioplasty with or without stenting showed, patients treated percutaneously have fewer complications. This is why patients who present recurring symptoms resulting from haemodynamic instability, despite medical treatment, may be offered percutaneous angioplasty as it is considered the most reasonable treatment option. However, the results of long-term percutaneous angioplasty are still poorly understood [3].

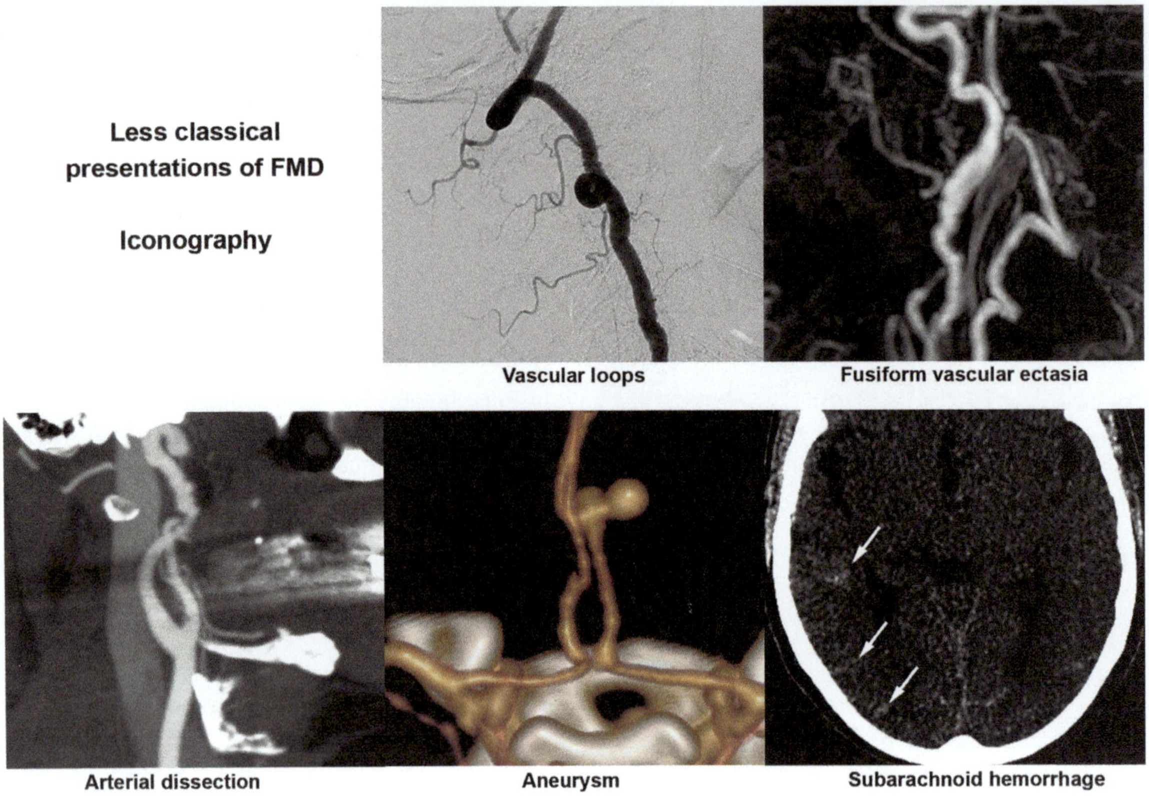

Fig. 12 Summary of less typical imaging findings in FMD

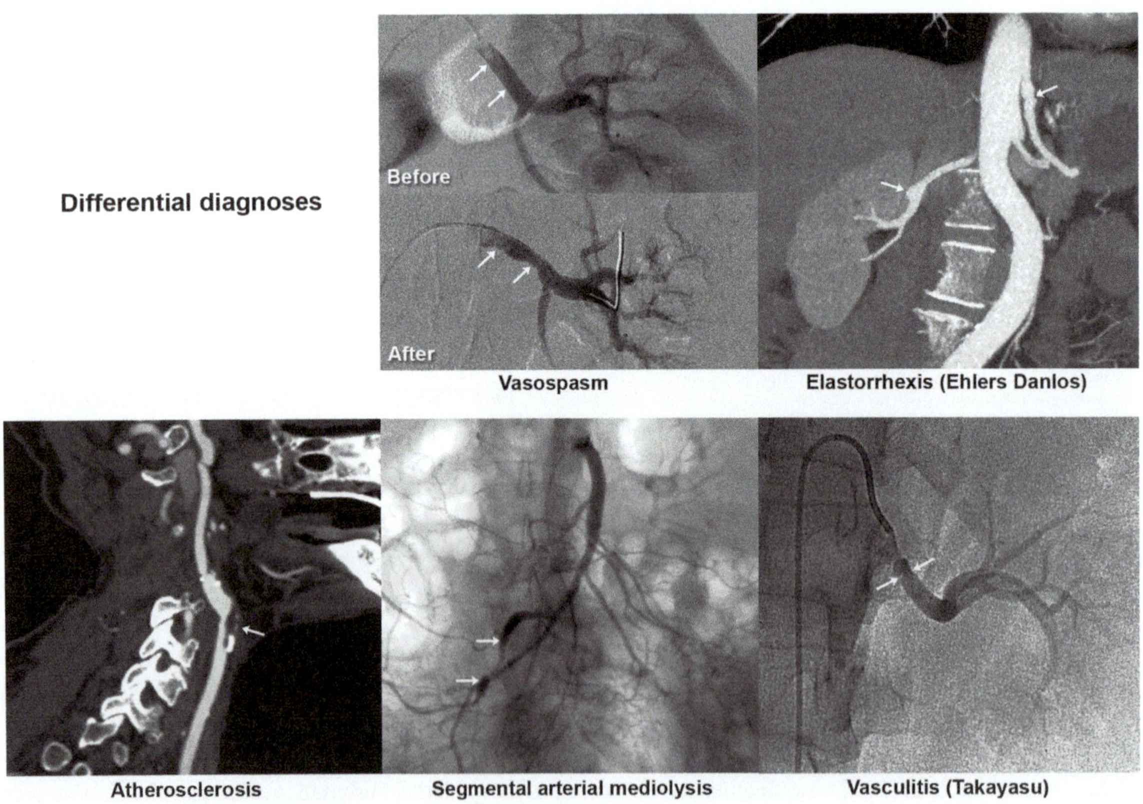

Fig. 13 Summary of classical differential diagnoses

Conclusion

FMD is a systemic non-atheromatous, non-inflammatory disease that affects females more than males. Renal and cervicoencephalic arteries are the most frequently affected sites. However, FMD may affect any artery. Radiologists play an important role in the diagnosis of FMD. A better knowledge of this disease is critical to shorten the delay between the first symptoms and final diagnosis. Common imaging findings of FMD, mainly the usual string-of-beads aspect, are well known. However, it is important to recognise less common presentations of FMD, such as vascular loops, fusiform vascular ectasia, arterial dissection, aneurysm and subarachnoid haemorrhage, to suggest the diagnosis and to conduct further investigations.

References

1. Plouin PF, Perdu J, La Batide-Alanore A, Boutouyrie P, Gimenez-Roqueplo AP, Jeunemaitre X (2007) Fibromuscular dysplasia. Orphanet J Rare Dis 2:28
2. Pasquini M, Trystram D, Oppenheim C, Ploin P, Touzé E (2011) Dysplasie fibromusculaire cervicale et intracrânienne. Press Med 40:713–719
3. Touze E, Oppenheim C, Trystram D et al (2010) Fibromuscular dysplasia of cervical and intracranial arteries. Int J Stroke 5(4):296–305
4. Hugenholtz H, Pokrupa R, Montpetit VJ, Nelson R, Richard MT (1982) Spontaneous dissecting aneurysm of the extracranial vertebral artery. Neurosurgery 10(1):96–100
5. Zimmerman R, Leeds NE, Naidich TP (1977) Carotid-cavernous fistula associated with intracranial fibromuscular dysplasia. Radiology 122(3):725–726
6. Olin JW, Froehlich J, Gu X et al (2012) The United States Registry for Fibromuscular Dysplasia: results in the first 447 patients. Circulation 125(25):3182–3190
7. Houser OW, Baker HL Jr (1968) Fibromuscular dysplasia and other uncommon diseases of the cervical carotid artery: angiographic aspects. Am J Roentgenol Radium Ther Nucl Med 104(1):201–212
8. Manelfe C, Clarisse J, Fredy D, André J, Crouzet G (1974) Dysplasies fibromusculaires des artères cervico-céphaliques. J Neuroradiol 1:149–231
9. Mettinger KL (1982) Fibromuscular dysplasia and the brain. II. Current concept of the disease. Stroke 13(1):53–58
10. Blondin D, Lanzman R, Schellhammer F et al (2010) Fibromuscular dysplasia in living renal donors: still a challenge to computed tomographic angiography. Eur J Radiol 75(1):67–71
11. Neymark E, LaBerge JM, Hirose R et al (2000) Arteriographic detection of renovascular disease in potential renal donors: incidence and effect on donor surgery. Radiology 214(3):755–760
12. Cragg AH, Smith TP, Thompson BH et al (1989) Incidental fibromuscular dysplasia in potential renal donors: long-term clinical follow-up. Radiology 172(1):145–147
13. Schievink WI, Bjornsson J (1996) Fibromuscular dysplasia of the internal carotid artery: a clinicopathological study. Clin Neuropathol 15(1):2–6
14. Mettinger KL, Ericson K (1982) Fibromuscular dysplasia and the brain. I. Observations on angiographic, clinical and genetic characteristics. Stroke 13(1):46–52
15. Begelman SM, Olin JW (2000) Fibromuscular dysplasia. Curr Opin Rheumatol 12(1):41–47
16. Stanley JC, Fry WJ, Seeger JF, Hoffman GL, Gabrielsen TO (1974) Extracranial internal carotid and vertebral artery fibrodysplasia. Arch Surg 109(2):215–222
17. La Batide A, Perdu J, Ploin P (2007) Dysplasie fibromusculaire artérielle. Press Med 36:1016–1023
18. Connett MC, Lansche JM (1965) Fibromuscular hyperplasia of the internal carotid artery: report of a case. Ann Surg 162:59–62
19. Harrison EG Jr, McCormack LJ (1971) Pathologic classification of renal arterial disease in renovascular hypertension. Mayo Clin Proc 46(3):161–167
20. Stanley J (1996) Renal artery fibrodysplasia. In: Renal Vascular Disease, Novick A, Scoble J, Hamilton G (eds). WB Saunders, London, 21–23
21. Kincaid OW, Davis GD, Hallermann FJ, Hunt JC (1968) Fibromuscular dysplasia of the renal arteries. Arteriographic features, classification, and observations on natural history of the disease. Am J Roentgenol Radium Ther Nucl Med 104(2):271–282
22. Savard S, Steichen O, Azarine A, Azizi M, Jeunemaitre X, Plouin PF (2012) Association between 2 angiographic subtypes of renal artery fibromuscular dysplasia and clinical characteristics. Circulation 126(25):3062–3069
23. Vasbinder GB, Nelemans PJ, Kessels AG et al (2004) Accuracy of computed tomographic angiography and magnetic resonance angiography for diagnosing renal artery stenosis. Ann Intern Med 141(9): 674–682, discussion 682
24. Willoteaux S, Faivre-Pierret M, Moranne O et al (2006) Fibromuscular dysplasia of the main renal arteries: comparison of contrast-enhanced MR angiography with digital subtraction angiography. Radiology 241(3):922–929
25. Sabharwal R, Vladica P, Coleman P (2007) Multidetector spiral CT renal angiography in the diagnosis of renal artery fibromuscular dysplasia. Eur J Radiol 61(3):520–527
26. Furie DM, Tien RD (1994) Fibromuscular dysplasia of arteries of the head and neck: imaging findings. AJR Am J Roentgenol 162(5): 1205–1209
27. Pannier-Moreau I, Grimbert P, Fiquet-Kempf B et al (1997) Possible familial origin of multifocal renal artery fibromuscular dysplasia. J Hypertens 15(12 Pt 2):1797–1801
28. Haute Autorité de Santé (2010) Protocole national de diagnostic et de soins : dysplasie fibromusculaire syptomatologique chez l'adulte. HAS, Paris.Available via http://www.hassante.fr/portail/upload/docs/application/pdf/2011-06/synthese_medecin_traitant_sur_la_dysplasie_fibromusculaire_chez_ladulte.pdf. Accessed November 2010
29. Osborn AG, Anderson RE (1977) Angiographic spectrum of cervical and intracranial fibromuscular dysplasia. Stroke 8(5):617–626
30. Varennes L, Tahon F, Grand S, et al. (2012) Aspect typique et variantes de la dysplasie fibro-musculaire des artères à destinée encéphalique. French Journeys of Radiology, Paris. Available via http://pe.sfrnet.org/ModuleConsultationPoster/consultationPoster.aspx?intIdPoster=5465. Accessed October 2012
31. Lacombe M (2001) Isolated spontaneous dissection of the renal artery. J Vasc Surg 33(2):385–391
32. Ringel SP, Harrison SH, Norenberg MD, Austin JH (1977) Fibromuscular dysplasia: multiple "spontaneous" dissecting aneurysms of the major cervical arteries. Ann Neurol 1(3):301–304
33. Schievink WI (2001) Spontaneous dissection of the carotid and vertebral arteries. N Engl J Med 344(12):898–906

34. Debette S, Leys D (2009) Cervical-artery dissections: predisposing factors, diagnosis, and outcome. Lancet Neurol 8(7): 668–678
35. Bellot J, Gherardi R, Poirier J, Lacour P, Debrun G, Barbizet J (1985) Fibromuscular dysplasia of cervico-cephalic arteries with multiple dissections and a carotid-cavernous fistula. A pathological study. Stroke 16(2):255–261
36. Goncharenko V, Gerlock AJ Jr, Shaff MI, Hollifield JW (1981) Progression of renal artery fibromuscular dysplasia in 42 patients as seen on angiography. Radiology 139(1):45–51
37. Stanley JC, Gewertz BL, Bove EL, Sottiurai V, Fry WJ (1975) Arterial fibrodysplasia. Histopathologic character and current etiologic concepts. Arch Surg 110(5):561–566
38. Mettinger KL, Soderstrom CE (1978) Pathogenetic profile of TIA before 55. A three-year investigation. J Neurol Sci 36(3):341–348
39. Cloft HJ, Kallmes DF, Kallmes MH, Goldstein JH, Jensen ME, Dion JE (1998) Prevalence of cerebral aneurysms in patients with fibromuscular dysplasia: a reassessment. J Neurosurg 88(3):436–440
40. Rinkel GJ, Djibuti M, Algra A, van Gijn J (1998) Prevalence and risk of rupture of intracranial aneurysms: a systematic review. Stroke 29(1):251–256
41. van de Nes JA, Bajanowski T, Trubner K (2007) Fibromuscular dysplasia of the basilar artery: an unusual case with medico-legal implications. Forensic Sci Int 173(2–3):188–192
42. Andersen CA, Collins GJ Jr, Rich NM, McDonald PT (1980) Spontaneous dissection of the internal carotid artery associated with fibromuscular dysplasia. Am Surg 46(4):263–266
43. Lehrer H (1967) The physiology of angiographic arterial waves. Radiology 89(1):11–19
44. Poloskey SL, Kim E, Sanghani R et al (2012) Low yield of genetic testing for known vascular connective tissue disorders in patients with fibromuscular dysplasia. Vasc Med 17(6):371–378
45. Gaud S, Cridlig J, Claudon M, Diarrassouba A, Kessler M, Frimat L (2010) Segmental arterial mediolysis and renovascular hypertension. Nephrol Ther 6(7):597–601
46. Chao CP (2009) Segmental arterial mediolysis. Semin Interv Radiol 26(3):224–232

18

Indications and selection of MR enterography vs. MR enteroclysis with emphasis on patients who need small bowel MRI and general anaesthesia: results of a survey

Michael R. Torkzad · Gabriele Masselli · Steve Halligan · Aytek Oto · Henning Neubauer · Stuart Taylor · Arun Gupta · Jens Brøndum Frøkjær · Ian C. Lawrance · Christopher J. Welman · Anne Negård · Olle Ekberg · Michael Patak · Thomas Lauenstein

Abstract

Aims To survey the perceived indications for magnetic resonance imaging of the small bowel (MRE) by experts, when MR enteroclysis (MREc) or MR enterography (MREg) may be chosen, and to determine how the approach to MRE is modified when general anaesthesia (GA) is required.

Materials and methods Selected opinion leaders in MRE completed a questionnaire that included clinical indications (MREg or MREc), specifics regarding administration of enteral contrast, and how the technique is altered to accommodate GA.

Results Fourteen responded. Only the diagnosis and follow-up of Crohn's disease were considered by over 80 % as a valid MRE indication. The remaining indications ranged between 35.7 % for diagnosis of caeliac disease and unknown sources of gastrointestinal bleeding to 78.6 % for motility disorders. The majority chose MREg over MREc for all indications (from 100 % for follow-up of caeliac disease to 57.7 % for tumour diagnosis). Fifty per cent of responders had needed to consider MRE under GA. The most commonly recommended procedural change was MRI without enteral distention. Three had experience with intubation under GA (MREc modification).

M. R. Torkzad (✉)
Department of Radiology, Oncology, Radiation Sciences, Uppsala University, Uppsala, Sweden
e-mail: michael.torkzad@gmail.com

G. Masselli
Umberto I Hospital, Radiology Department, Sapienza University, Rome, Italy

S. Halligan
Center for Medical Imaging, University College London, London, UK

A. Oto
Department of Radiology, University of Chicago, Chicago, IL, USA

H. Neubauer
Department of Paediatric Radiology, University Hospital Wuerzburg, Wuerzburg, Germany

S. Taylor
Center for Medical Imaging, University College London, London, UK

A. Gupta
Intestinal Imaging, St Mark's Hospital, Harrow, UK

J. B. Frøkjær
Department of Radiology, Aalborg University Hospital, Aalborg, Denmark

I. C. Lawrance
School of Medicine and Pharmacology, University of Western Australia and Centre for Inflammatory Bowel Disease, Fremantle Hospital, Fremantle, Australia

C. J. Welman
Department of Radiology, Fremantle Hospital, Fremantle, Australia

A. Negård
Abdominal and Children's Radiology, Department of Radiology, Akershus University Hospital, Lørenskog, Norway

O. Ekberg
Department of Clinical Sciences/Medical Radiology, Lund University; Diagnostic Centre of Imaging and Functional Medicine Lund University Skåne University Hospital, Malmö, Sweden

M. Patak
Klinik Hirslanden, Witellikerstrasse 40, Zürich, Austria

T. Lauenstein
Department of Diagnostic and Interventional Radiology and Neuroradiology, University Hospital Essen, Essen, Germany

Conclusion Views were variable. Requests for MRE under GA are not uncommon. Presently most opinion leaders suggest standard abdominal MRI when GA is required.
Main messages
- *Experts are using MRE for various indications.*
- *Requests for MRE under general anaesthesia are not uncommon.*
- *Some radiologists employ MREc under general anaesthesia; others do not distend the small bowel.*

Keywords Small bowel · MRI · Crohn's disease · General anaesthesia

Abbreviations

CT	Computerised tomography
ECCO	European Crohn's and Colitis Organisation
EL	Evidence level
ESGAR	European Society of Gastrointestinal and Abdominal Radiology
GA	General anaesthesia
MRE	Magnetic resonance imaging of small bowel
MREc	Magnetic resonance imaging performed by means of enteroclysis
MREg	Magnetic resonance imaging performed by means of oral intake (or nasogastric tube), also called enterography follow-through or hydro-MRI
MRI	Magnetic resonance imaging
NG	Nasogastric
SB	Small bowel

Introduction

In a recent evidence-based consensus for assessment of small bowel (SB) inflammatory disease [1] jointly from the European Crohn's and Colitis Organisation (ECCO) and European Society of Gastrointestinal and Abdominal Radiology (ESGAR), it was stated that (abbreviation added to suit our article): "Magnetic resonance imaging (MRI) of the small bowel (MRE) and colon requires fast imaging techniques and luminal distension [Evidence Level (EL) 2]. MRE has similar diagnostic accuracy and similar indications to CT, but with the major advantage of not imparting ionising radiation [EL 1]".

While most radiologists recommend distention for adequate SB assessment, methods to achieve this vary. Some use enterography (oral administration) or enteroclysis (nasojejunal intubation with the tube tip in close proximity to the ligament of Treitz). Improved capability of MRI to diagnose SB pathology has generated increasing requests to perform these examinations in patients who require general anaesthesia (GA). Demand is particularly increasing in the paediatric age group, not least in an attempt to limit exposure to ionising radiation. SB distension with large volumes of orally administered fluids, however, is generally considered a contraindication in GA, or heavy sedation, given the risk of aspiration [2–5]. To deliberately distend the SB with fluids would, therefore, be contradictory to this general rule.

To date there are no published data on the safety or otherwise of performing MRE under GA, nor is there any guidance on any required protocol modifications.

The purposes of this study were to:

1. Survey key opinion leaders regarding their current indications and protocols for undertaking MRE.
2. To document their attitudes and experience of performing MRE under GA in order to issue guidance for this specific clinical scenario.

Materials and methods

Two radiologists (MRT and TL) devised the questionnaire, which covered four broad topic areas addressed by a series of multiple choice questions, together with space for free comments.

The questionnaire was sent to recognised opinion leaders, chosen via a history of prior indexed publications, supplemented by the chief investigators personal knowledge of their work and contributions in the field. Twenty-four radiologists were identified initially and each contacted on up to three occasions for an initial response with a goal to recruit at least ten completed responses. If responses were incomplete, participants were again contacted. The topic areas addressed were as follows:

Part I (questions 1–12): The first topic covered the number of examinations performed annually and the imaging modality of choice for named different pathologies with an emphasis on magnetic resonance enterography (MREg) vs. magnetic resonance enteroclysis (MREc).

Part II (questions 13–20): The preference(s) of opinion leaders for SB distension including type of contrast agent, desired signal characteristics, and mode and rate of administration.

Part III (questions 21–25): Experience with MRI under GA was canvassed including any changes in indications in comparison to routine MRE. Specifically experts were asked if they favored MRI without SB distension, instead of MRE when GA was required, and whether they would rather choose an alternative modality (e.g. CT).

Part IV (questions 26–39): These related to protocol modifications made by experts if they performed SB MRI under GA.

The results were entered in Excel file sheets and expressed as percentages of the responses.

Results

Fourteen experts completed the questionnaire. Two of the invitees were not radiologists and chose not to participate, and two others mentioned that they were working at the same institution as the responding 14 and wanted to avoid duplication. The other six invitees did not respond. Among the responders, all interpreted between 100 and 500 small bowel MRIs annually, averaging 222.

Part I

All experts (14 out of 14 or 100 %) advocate MRI for follow-up of SB Crohn's disease with most advocating MREg (13 out of 14, 93 %) as opposed to MREc (1 out of 14, Fig. 1). The majority used MRI to confirm/refute an initial diagnosis of SB Crohn's disease with 93 % (13 out of 14) choosing MRE (of whom 11 or 79 % chose MREg).

For studying SB motility disorders 79 % (11 out of 14) chose MRE (10 out of 14 or 71 % MREg).

The most frequent indications where MRE (MREg or MREc) was ***not chosen*** by the majority of experts as the imaging modality of choice were (followed by the proportion who preferred other radiologic and non-radiologic methods of valuation): the evaluation of serosal tumour implants (10 out of 14 or 71 %), diagnosis of caeliac disease (9 out of 14 or 64 %), unknown source of gastrointestinal bleeding after negative colonoscopy and gastroduodenoscopy (9 out of 14 or 64 %), and follow-up (8 out of 14 or 57 %) and diagnosis (7 out of 14 or 50 %) of SB tumours (Fig. 1). In all the other conditions, as mentioned in Fig. 1, MRE was preferred.

Interestingly, MREg was always more frequently favoured than MREc, between 0 % (follow-up of caeliac disease with MREc and MREg favoured by none and 8 experts, respectively) to 43 % (diagnosis of small bowel tumours with MREc and MREg favoured by 3 and 4 experts, respectively).

Part II

Position of the patient

The prone position was clearly favoured (12 experts out of 14 or 86 %), with supine positioning as second (2 experts out of 14 or 14 %).

Type of oral contrast agent

Among the contrast agents specified, mannitol was the most common among the experts (4 experts out of 14 or 29 %), followed by VoLumen (3 experts out of 14 or 21 %), sorbitol (2 experts out of 14 or 14 %) and tap water by one expert (1 out of 14 or 7 %). Four experts chose other contrast agents [locust bean gum (LBG) by two researchers and polyethylene glycol solution (PEG) and Glycoprep-C at one centre each]. The most common feature among all experts was their choice of contrast agents that had the signal characteristics of water, i.e. double phasic being high signal on T2 weighting and low signal on T1 weighting.

Fig. 1 The choice of examinations by different experts for different diseases. *Blue bars*: MREc or MR enterlocysis; *red bar*: MREg or MR enterography; *yellow bar*: other free choices of both radiological imaging methods or any other possible means

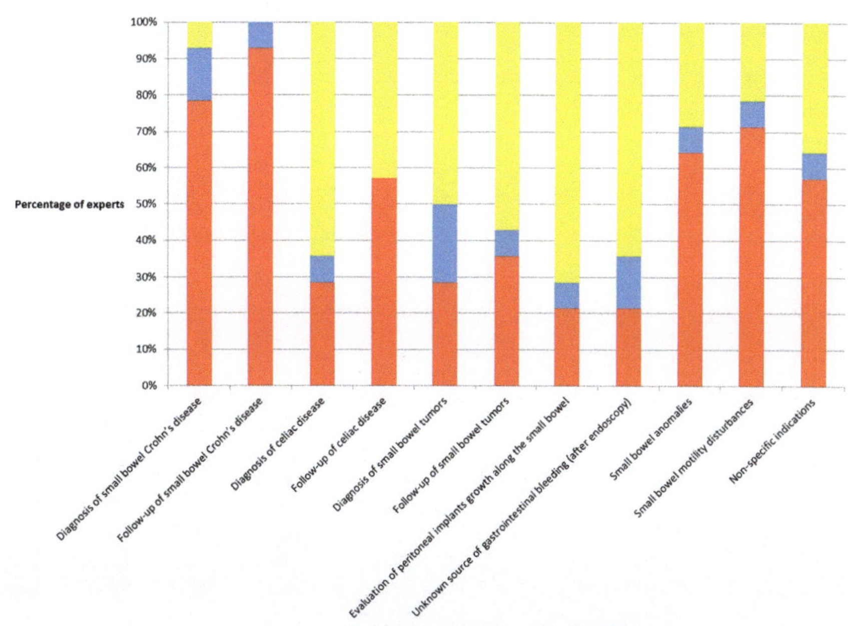

Factors influencing the rate and volume of the administered contrast agent

The volume of oral agent ingested during MREg was influenced primarily by patient compliance, even though a fixed volume was planned to be given at the start of the procedure. The time allowed for ingestion was always fixed and thus it was the rate of administration that resulted in the differences in administered oral agent volumes. For MREc, monitoring progression of the contrast agent with a fixed rate seemed to be most influential in the determination of the administration rate (Figs. 2 and 3).

Part III

MRI under GA was performed only at 8 out of 14 (57 %) of the centres. In half of the centres with (4 out of 14) and half of those without (3 out of 14), the possibility of MRI under GA had led to the request to perform MRE under GA.

When asked to do MRE under GA 3 out of 14 (21 %) experts did not recommend MRI (Fig. 4). Eight experts out of 14 (57 %), however, would perform standard abdominal MRI (4 out of 14 or 29 %), e.g. with no SB distension or choosing some form of intubation (4 out of 14 or 29 %). Intubation would be done either as an MREc alone or an MREc with the addition of a stomach tube to drain excessive stomach fluid. Three experts perform MRE under GA.

Part IV

This section dealt with modifications employed if there was a question of combining MRE with a GA. Most cases where GA is requested are young children who cannot comply with the examination. However there are some patients who require GA because of impaired cognitive function or mental retardation. Patient age has an important role. The number of experts employing prone positioning decreased to 6 out of 14 (41 %), 3 choosing supine, 3 choosing whatever position was easiest for the anaesthesiologist and one choosing right decubitus. It should be considered that a supine patient is in the most convenient position for the anaesthesiologist unless specific issues warrant other positions.

An almost equal number of experts, 4 out of 14 (27 %) and 3 out of 14 (36 %), employed endoscopic methods and/or fluoroscopy for nasojejunal tube insertion if enteroclysis would be employed under these circumstances, respectively.

Of the experts questioned only three had first-hand experience with MRE under GA (initials blinded). Most of the differences in their protocols are related to differences in MREc in general. The major differences among the authors that are related to MREc being done under GA is the use of one tube (n= 2 participants) or two tubes (n=1 participant) method. The latter participant tries to combine upper gastrointestinal endoscopy under GA (which patients usually need for various reasons) with MREc under GA. The endoscopist inserts both tubes with the tip in the stomach, and the radiologist then advances one tube to its position at the level of the Treitz ligament. He or she uses two nasogastric tubes for drainage of any regurgitated fluids from the intestines into the stomach during MRE.

Discussion

This survey illustrates a degree of discrepancy among experts performing MRE. Considering the proportion agreeing on a valid indication for MRE, only two indications exceeded

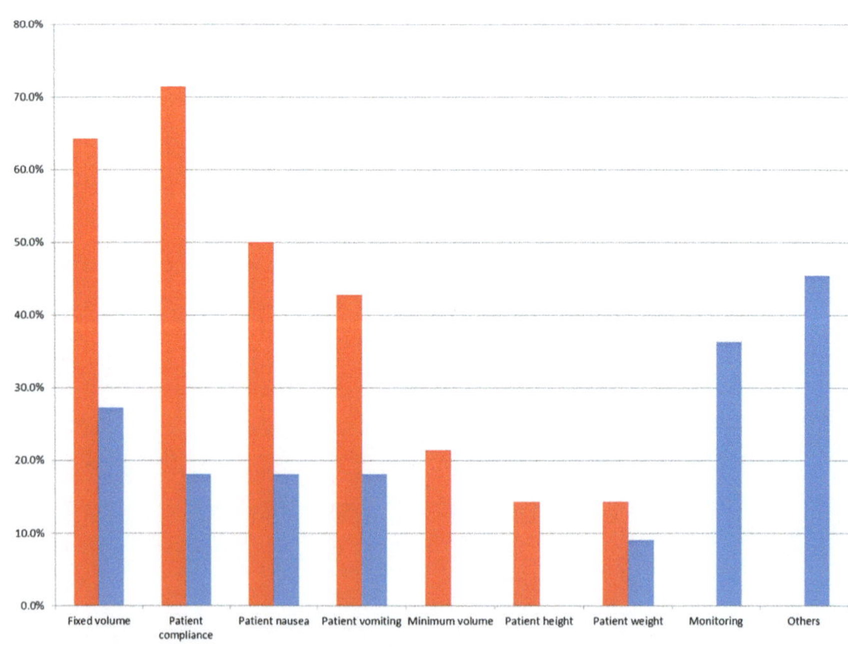

Fig. 2 Factors influencing the volume of enteral contrast agents. *Blue bars*: MREc or MR enterlocysis; *red bar*: MREg or MR enterography

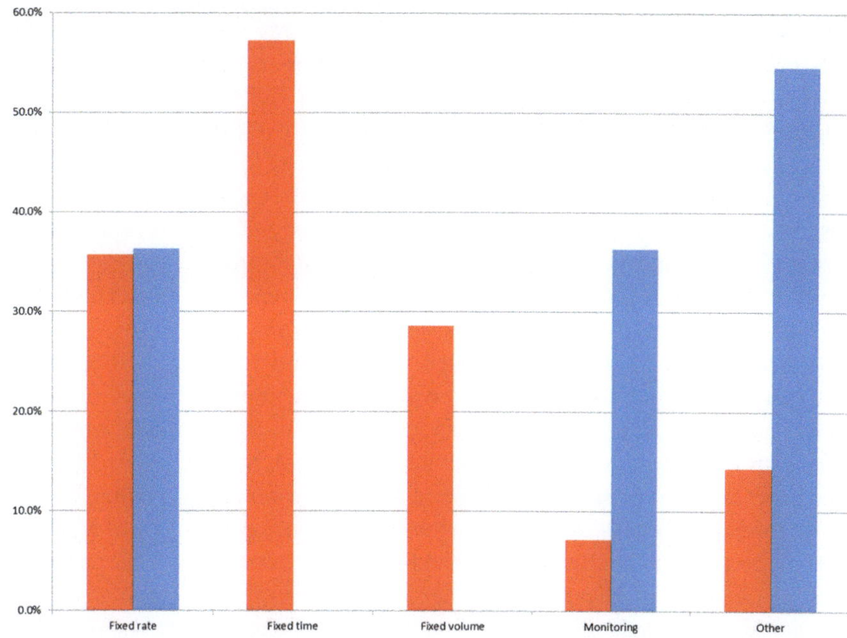

Fig. 3 Factors influencing the rate of administration of enteral agent. *Blue bars*: MREc or MR enterlocysis; *red bar*: MREg or MR enterography

80 %: the initial diagnosis and follow-up of Crohn's disease [6–18]. Otherwise, we observed a wide variation among our experts regarding other indications for MRE. These ranged from 29 % suggesting MRE for evaluation of serosal carcinomatosis (oral presentation at the European Congress of Radiology 2014 by MRT) and ischaemia [19] to 79 % for motility studies [20–29].

Such variation in opinion and perceived indications may depend on the wide experimental potential for MRE as well as the academic orientation of our experts. These experts are more known for their research and inclined to test new applications. Experience may also contribute to variation in the responses we observed [30, 31]. Small bowel diseases are varied, many are relatively uncommon, and it is time-consuming for each research group to accrue sufficient numbers of cases and report them, and for other researchers to confirm the initial observations. Only Crohn's disease has been studied in large numbers and by many individuals and

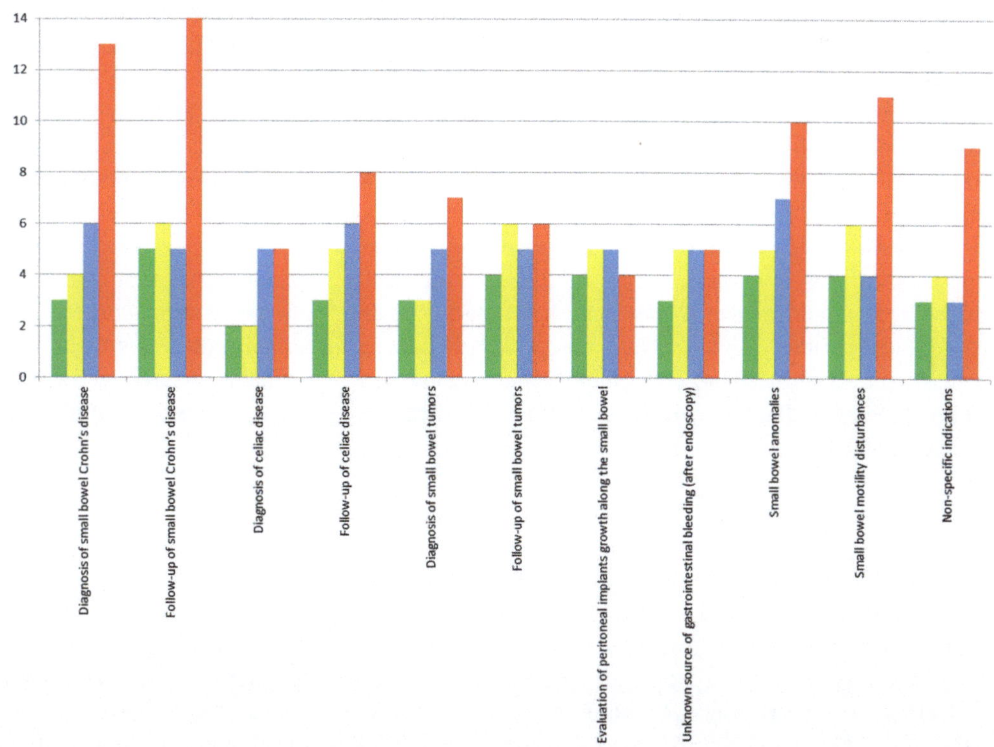

Fig. 4 Change in methodology in the number of experts when confronted with the dilemma of doing MRI under general anaesthesia. *Green bar*: MRE is not the best alternative (among those with access to MRI under general anaesthesia). *Yellow bar*: MRE is not the best alternative (among those with or without access to MRI under GA). *Blue bar*: distention is not essential and therefore MRI of the abdomen is sufficient. *Red bar*: how participant answered to indications for MRE in part I

groups. Oftentimes CT of the small intestine is preferred to MRE because of the availability and lower cost. MRE, however, offers diagnostic advantages in addition to a lack of ionising radiation, and MRE can also be performed without intravenous contrast agents if there is renal insufficiency [32].

We did not focus on the technique and imaging sequences required for MRE, which deserves a separate study. The amount of enteral agent [33], its timing [34], osmolarity [35], type of agent [36, 37], its concentration [38], type of antiperistaltic agent [39, 40], additives such as erythromycin and enema [41], MRI sequences used [42, 43] and field strength [44] are just some possible modifications. Unfortunately most if not all protocol modifications have been undertaken on healthy volunteers. Some areas have not been touched. One area specifically not covered was administration of intravenous contrast agents as this was not expected to change because of GA. The authors had been asked to mention what parts of the protocol they would change if performing MRE under GA. Colon distention, though shown to improve small bowel distention, is rarely used. Furthermore, employing an enema in an unconscious patient inside an MR machine is probably never used. Nonetheless no one reported enema administration when asked about protocol modifications due to patients undergoing GA. Among the questions we posed, there was no single factor that was considered by at least 80 % of our experts as important for determining the volume and/or rate of the agent administered. The factors that the experts agreed upon were that the signal characteristic of the agent was biphasic, behaving like water, and that the patient was examined prone.

We, however, focused more on the choice between MREc and MREg as this has been more controversial and more studied, albeit only in patients with Crohn's disease [45, 46]. In brief patients prefer MREg [46], while radiologists prefer MREc images [46–50]. MREc probably demonstrates more superficial ulcerations than MREg [18]. The joint position statement from ECCO and ESGAR also considered enteroclysis as likely better for the diagnosis of partial small bowel obstruction in Crohn's disease [2], though no statistically significant advantage was evident in the studies referenced [50]. For other patients, such as those with malignancies or gastrointestinal bleeding, every tumour site is important. This is probably reflected in higher proportions of our experts choosing MREc than any other indication, though still less than MREg. Studies such as that from Gupta et al. [51] with MREg have shown such good results that one can understand why experts prefer MREg. In this particular study, recruiting patients with Peutz-Jeghers syndrome, patients preferred capsule endoscopy over MREg and one might speculate that this preference would be more exaggerated if MREc had been offered.

Half of our experts had been exposed to the scenario of MRE under GA, an observation regardless of whether MRI under GA was available at their own centre. Most experts when confronted with this dilemma still opted for MRI, but used a standard approach. This choice suggests that MRI is such a powerful method that most experts still consider it advantageous to do MRI as opposed to choosing another modality.

The change in methods due to GA can be based on two aspects. One is that MRI may not be much better than other available methods (e.g. CT) that could easily replace MRI. The other is that SB distention is not important and the risk of SB distention outweighs any potential benefits. In some cases such as unknown GI bleeding no one would risk MRI with, or without, SB distention as the first choice. For diagnosis and follow-up of SB Crohn's disease and motility disturbances, however, there are some who consider that the benefits of MRI outweigh its risk. Our study demonstrates that the widespread use of MRE has led to requests for it in patients who otherwise require GA under anaesthesia. Considering the risks associated with GA, therefore, it seems prudent to employ other available modalities such as CT if the benefit from MRI does not justify the risk of GA. If the benefit of MRI seems to outweigh the risk of GA, then a decision must be made on how valuable the distention is. Finally, if distention is required and MRE is employed, then based on the experience of radiologists in this study, MREc is the preferred method, avoiding major filling of the stomach and having more control over gastric filling (perhaps via a separate gastric tube).

Our study has several shortcomings. First, the selection process of the experts could be questioned, i.e. who qualifies as an expert. Most of our researchers are from the Western hemisphere and Australia. Clearly they have more experience with Crohn's disease than certain other diseases, e.g. small bowel tuberculosis. Despite this, the variation in responses was so striking that we expect that with the inclusion of more international experts with more heterogeneous backgrounds this variation would only become even more prominent. Second, it has become common practice to use the Delphi process, or similar approaches, for examining agreement among experts. Our main concern was centred on MRE under GA and other areas were touched on only briefly. For many potential indications there are no existing publications in the available literature and so the Delphi process (or its modifications) and/or systematic review and meta-analysis are impossible.

Conclusion

Most experts clearly prefer MREg over MREc. There are many emerging indications for MRE. When confronted by the prospects of performing MRE under GA many experts would still do MRI with or without small bowel distention rather than choosing another modality. This article, however, demonstrates that more work is needed to address the fundamental issues concerning MRE. MRE is usually performed by a few enthusiastic individuals working at separate centres and there is a need for more collaborative work putting the ideas and experiences of these individuals together.

References

1. Panes J, Bouhnik Y, Reinisch W, Stoker J, Taylor SA, Baumgart DC et al (2013) Imaging techniques for assessment of inflammatory bowel disease: joint ECCO and ESGAR evidence-based consensus guidelines. J Crohn's Colitis 7:556–585
2. Arlachov Y, Ganatra RH (2012) Sedation/anaesthesia in paediatric radiology. Br J Radiol 85(1019):e1018–e1031
3. Shankar VR (2008) Sedating children for radiological procedures: an intensivist's perspective. Pediatr Radiol 38(Suppl 2):S213–S217
4. Dalal PG, Murray D, Cox T, McAllister J, Snider R (2006) Sedation and anesthesia protocols used for magnetic resonance imaging studies in infants: provider and pharmacologic considerations. Anesth Analg 103(4):863–868
5. Schulte-Uentrop L, Goepfert MS (2010) Anaesthesia or sedation for MRI in children. Curr Opin Anaesthesiol 23(4):513–517
6. Hafeez R, Punwani S, Boulos P, Bloom S, McCartney S, Halligan S et al (2011) Diagnostic and therapeutic impact of MR enterography in Crohn's disease. Clin Radiol 66(12):1148–1158
7. Steward MJ, Punwani S, Proctor I, Adjei-Gyamfi Y, Chatterjee F, Bloom S et al (2012) Non-perforating small bowel Crohn's disease assessed by MRI enterography: derivation and histopathological validation of an MR-based activity index. Eur J Radiol 81(9):2080–2088
8. Hafeez R, Greenhalgh R, Rajan J, Bloom S, McCartney S, Halligan S et al (2011) Use of small bowel imaging for the diagnosis and staging of Crohn's disease—a survey of current UK practice. Br J Radiol 84(1002):508–517
9. Tolan DJ, Greenhalgh R, Zealley IA, Halligan S, Taylor SA (2010) MR enterographic manifestations of small bowel Crohn disease. Radiographics 30(2):367–384
10. Punwani S, Rodriguez-Justo M, Bainbridge A, Greenhalgh R, De Vita E, Bloom S et al (2009) Mural inflammation in Crohn disease: location-matched histologic validation of MR imaging features. Radiology 252(3):712–720
11. Casciani E, Masselli G, Di Nardo G, Polettini E, Bertini L, Oliva S et al (2011) MR enterography versus capsule endoscopy in paediatric patients with suspected Crohn's disease. Eur Radiol 21(4):823–831
12. Masselli G, Casciani E, Polettini E, Lanciotti S, Bertini L, Gualdi G (2006) Assessment of Crohn's disease in the small bowel: prospective comparison of magnetic resonance enteroclysis with conventional enteroclysis. Eur Radiol 16(12):2817–2827
13. Masselli G, Brizi MG, Menchini L, Minordi L, Vecchioli SA (2005) Magnetic Resonance Enteroclysis imaging of Crohn's. Radiol Med 110(3):221–233
14. Frøkjaer JB, Larsen E, Steffensen E, Nielsen AH, Drewes AM (2005) Magnetic resonance imaging of the small bowel in Crohn's disease. Scand J Gastroenterol 40(7):832–842
15. Lawrance IC, Welman CJ, Shipman P, Murray K (2009) Correlation of MRI-determined small bowel Crohn's disease categories with medical response and surgical pathology. World J Gastroenterol 15(27):3367–3375
16. Ziech ML, Bossuyt PM, Laghi A, Lauenstein TC, Taylor SA, Stoker J (2012) Grading luminal Crohn's disease: which MRI features are considered as important? Eur J Radiol 81(4):e467–e472
17. Bickelhaupt S, Froehlich JM, Cattin R, Patuto N, Tutuian R, Wentz KU et al (2013) Differentiation between active and chronic Crohn's disease using MRI small-bowel motility examinations—initial experience. Clin Radiol 68(12):1247–1253
18. Torkzad MR, Ullberg U, Nyström N, Blomqvist L, Hellström P, Fagerberg UL (2012) Manifestations of small bowel disease in pediatric Crohn's disease on magnetic resonance enterography. Inflamm Bowel Dis 18(3):520–528
19. Lauenstein TC, Ajaj W, Narin B, Göhde SC, Kröger K, Debatin JF et al (2005) MR imaging of apparent small-bowel perfusion for diagnosing mesenteric ischemia: feasibility study. Radiology 234(2): 569–575
20. Froehlich JM, Patak MA, von Weymarn C, Juli CF, Zollikofer CL, Wentz KU (2005) Small bowel motility assessment with magnetic resonance imaging. J Magn Reson Imaging 21(4):370–375
21. Bickelhaupt S, Pazahr S, Chuck N, Blume I, Froehlich JM, Cattin R et al (2013) Crohn's disease: small bowel motility impairment correlates with inflammatory-related markers C-reactive protein and calprotectin. Neurogastroenterol Motil 25(6):467–473
22. Bickelhaupt S, Froehlich JM, Cattin R, Raible S, Bouquet H, Bill U et al (2014) Software-assisted small bowel motility analysis using free-breathing MRI: feasibility study. J Magn Reson Imaging 39(1): 17–23
23. Cullmann JL, Bickelhaupt S, Froehlich JM, Szucs-Farkas Z, Tutuian R, Patuto N et al (2013) MR imaging in Crohn's disease: correlation of MR motility measurement with histopathology in the terminal ileum. Neurogastroenterol Motil 25(9):749–e577
24. Menys A, Atkinson D, Odille F, Ahmed A, Novelli M, Rodriguez-Justo M et al (2012) Quantified terminal ileal motility during MR enterography as a potential biomarker of Crohn's disease activity: a preliminary study. Eur Radiol 22(11):2494–2501
25. Menys A, Taylor SA, Emmanuel A, Ahmed A, Plumb AA, Odille F et al (2013) Global small bowel motility: assessment with dynamic MR imaging. Radiology 269(2):443–450
26. Menys A, Helbren E, Makanyanga J, Emmanuel A, Forbes A, Windsor A et al (2013) Small bowel strictures in Crohn's disease: a quantitative investigation of intestinal motility using MR enterography. Neurogastroenterol Motil 25(12):967–e775
27. Torkzad MR, Vargas R, Tanaka C, Blomqvist L (2007) Value of cine MRI for better visualization of the proximal small bowel in normal individuals. Eur Radiol 17(11):2964–2968
28. Yacoub JH, Oto A (2014) New magnetic resonance imaging modalities for Crohn disease. Magn Reson Imaging Clin N Am 22(1):35–50
29. Yacoub JH, Obara P, Oto A (2013) Evolving role of MRI in Crohn's disease. J Magn Reson Imaging 37(6):1277–1289
30. Negaard A, Mulahasanovic A, Reisaeter LA, Aasekjaer K, Sandvik L, Klow NE (2008) Crohn's disease evaluated with magnetic resonance enteroclysis: diagnostic performance of experienced and inexperienced readers before and after training. Acta Radiol 49(9):967–974
31. Negaard A, Sandvik L, Mulahasanovic A, Berstad AE, Klöw NE (2006) Magnetic resonance enteroclysis in the diagnosis of small-intestinal Crohn's disease: diagnostic accuracy and inter- and intra-observer agreement. Acta Radiol 47(10):1008–1016
32. Masselli G, Gualdi G (2013) CT and MR enterography in evaluating small bowel diseases: when to use which modality? Abdom Imaging 38(2):249–259
33. Kinner S, Kuehle CA, Herbig S, Haag S, Ladd SC, Barkhausen J et al (2008) MRI of the small bowel: can sufficient bowel distension be

achieved with small volumes of oral contrast? Eur Radiol 18(11): 2542–2548
34. Kuehle CA, Ajaj W, Ladd SC, Massing S, Barkhausen J, Lauenstein TC (2006) Hydro-MRI of the small bowel: effect of contrast volume, timing of contrast administration, and data acquisition on bowel distention. AJR Am J Roentgenol 187(4):W375–W385
35. Ajaj W, Goyen M, Schneemann H, Kuehle C, Nuefer M, Ruehm SG et al (2005) Oral contrast agents for small bowel distension in MRI: influence of the osmolarity for small bowel distention. Eur Radiol 15(7):1400–1406
36. Ajaj W, Goehde SC, Schneemann H, Ruehm SG, Debatin JF, Lauenstein TC (2004) Oral contrast agents for small bowel MRI: comparison of different additives to optimize bowel distension. Eur Radiol 14(3):458–464
37. Ajaj W, Goehde SC, Schneemann H, Ruehm SG, Debatin JF, Lauenstein TC (2004) Dose optimization of mannitol solution for small bowel distension in MRI. J Magn Reson Imaging 20(4):648–653
38. Lauenstein TC, Schneemann H, Vogt FM, Herborn CU, Ruhm SG, Debatin JF (2003) Optimization of oral contrast agents for MR imaging of the small bowel. Radiology 228(1):279–283
39. Gutzeit A, Binkert CA, Koh DM, Hergan K, von Weymarn C, Graf N et al (2012) Evaluation of the anti-peristaltic effect of glucagon and hyoscine on the small bowel: comparison of intravenous and intramuscular drug administration. Eur Radiol 22(6):1186–1194
40. Froehlich JM, Daenzer M, von Weymarn C, Erturk SM, Zollikofer CL, Patak MA (2009) Aperistaltic effect of hyoscine N-butylbromide versus glucagon on the small bowel assessed by magnetic resonance imaging. Eur Radiol 19(6):1387–1393
41. Lauenstein TC, Vogt FM, Herborn CU, DeGreiff A, Debatin JF, Holtmann G (2003) Time-resolved three-dimensional MR imaging of gastric emptying modified by IV administration of erythromycin. AJR Am J Roentgenol 180(5):1305–1310
42. Neubauer H, Pabst T, Dick A, Machann W, Evangelista L, Wirth C et al (2013) Small-bowel MRI in children and young adults with Crohn disease: retrospective head-to-head comparison of contrast-enhanced and diffusion-weighted MRI. Pediatr Radiol 43(1):103–114
43. Maccioni F, Patak MA, Signore A, Laghi A (2012) New frontiers of MRI in Crohn's disease: motility imaging, diffusion-weighted imaging, perfusion MRI, MR spectroscopy, molecular imaging, and hybrid imaging (PET/MRI). Abdom Imaging 37(6):974–982
44. Patak MA, von Weymarn C, Froehlich JM (2007) Small bowel MR imaging: 1.5T versus 3T. Magn Reson Imaging Clin N Am 15(3): 383–393, vii
45. Torkzad MR, Lauenstein TC (2009) Enterclysis versus enterography: the unsettled issue. Eur Radiol 19(1):90–91
46. Lawrance IC, Welman CJ, Shipman P, Murray K (2009) Small bowel MRI enteroclysis or follow through: which is optimal? World J Gastroenterol 15(42):5300–5306
47. Negaard A, Sandvik L, Berstad AE, Paulsen V, Lygren I, Borthne A et al (2008) MRI of the small bowel with oral contrast or nasojejunal intubation in Crohn's disease: randomized comparison of patient acceptance. Scand J Gastroenterol 43(1):44–51
48. Masselli G, Casciani E, Polettini E, Gualdi G (2008) Comparison of MR enteroclysis with MR enterography and conventional enteroclysis in patients with Crohn's disease. Eur Radiol 18(3): 438–447
49. Masselli G, Vecchioli A, Gualdi GF (2006) Crohn disease of the small bowel:MR enteroclysis versus conventional enteroclysis. Abdom Imaging 31(4):400–409
50. Negaard A, Paulsen V, Sandvik L, Berstad AE, Borthne A, Try K et al (2007) A prospective randomized comparison between two MRI studies of the small bowel in Crohn's disease, the oral contrast method and MR enteroclysis. Eur Radiol 17(9):2294–2301
51. Gupta A, Postgate AJ, Burling D, Ilangovan R, Marshall M, Phillips RK et al (2010) A prospective study of MR enterography versus capsule endoscopy for the surveillance of adult patients with Peutz-Jeghers syndrome. AJR Am J Roentgenol 195(1):108–116

19

Research education in Europe: an opinion paper by the European Society of Radiology

European Society of Radiology (ESR)

Abstract Research is a major positive driver for radiology. Therefore, research education needs to be a major topic for the radiology leadership, including the research committee of the ESR. Professional (radiological and non-radiological) and scientific publications as well as Research Committee questionnaires provide the basis for this opinion paper. Although radiology is well-positioned to deal with current and future challenges, there are still some gaps, such as the presence of radiology in basic research, radiology-specific research versus research services for other disciplines, need of adaptation to new research topics, general attitude towards research, issues of career planning, lack of incentives for researchers, gender issues with loss of women from the researcher pipeline, limited financing of research education and variability between countries and institutions. There is no easy answer to such challenges. However, all stakeholders, from the ESR to subspecialty societies, university departments, general radiology departments and the individual radiologist must recognise and promote research within their competencies. Many means and structures are already available but need to be used more extensively and systematically. Additional means need to be developed, scientific and professional trends must be actively followed, and minimal standards in research education should be maintained throughout Europe.

Main Messages

- *Radiology research includes a broad spectrum, from basic to health services research.*
- *Research education needs to be widely available and systematically promoted.*
- *Existing means such as the European Institute for Biomedical Imaging Research (EIBIR) need to be advanced.*
- *New developments in research topics and professional life must be continuously monitored and evaluated.*

European Society of Radiology (ESR) (✉)
Neutorgasse 9/2, 1010 Vienna, Austria
e-mail: communications@myesr.org

Introduction

Radiology is a research-driven discipline. It needs to remain so and will expand into new research areas. Radiology covers basic scientific research, technical developments, applied clinical research and health services research in order to contribute to patient wellbeing, referring physicians, healthcare organisations and society. Evidence-based medicine has not yet played a very important role in radiology, but is here to stay [1] and will be applied by policy makers in most countries. Currently, the evidence for radiology practice is largely unsupported by high-level evidence and pays little heed to patient outcome.

To limit ourselves to clinical applications will not be sufficient. Disciplines contributing to basic research will have the best opportunity to apply and evaluate new knowledge early. Such knowledge promotes teaching. Those who teach will be recognised as the intellectual owners of procedures and diagnostic tools and are likely to be asked to advise on protocols, guidelines and in remuneration schemes. All this could be taken over by professionals from other disciplines, many of whom already have well-funded research activities, strategic plans and substantial expertise.

Research is a positive driver for radiology for other reasons, too, as it attracts the best staff, is the basis for third party financing and opens new business opportunities. This does not mean that the hard working, well-trained, clinical radiologist should be sidelined. He or she fulfils a very important role for patients, clinical departments, hospitals and the healthcare system. Their work may support at least part of research infrastructure and equipment and provides clinical data essential for many types of research. However, to recruit, motivate and provide consistent career planning for researchers is especially demanding and requires special attention from radiology leaders.

This White Paper is not a general statement regarding research but rather concentrates on research education. We have more than enough reason to plan research education, which is an important prerequisite when recruiting and maintaining research-oriented staff, allowing them to perform high-quality research and in order to be credible partners for clinical colleagues and other stakeholders in medical research.

After the initial training phase, there is a brain drain into non-academic settings where payment is often better and work is more compatible with family life or dual careers. Gender issues are commonly perceived as an additional burden to department leaderships but also represent a strength considering the input of diverse opinions and attitudes.

This paper analyses gaps in current research education. The analysis is based on two questionnaires sent to national and specialty societies throughout Europe, one of which has been published in *Insights into Imaging* [2]. Current educational activities include several means to promote research in radiology, many of which have already been applied successfully in single institutions, individual countries or even throughout Europe, but probably not in a systematic fashion. For future solutions, many of the existing programmes may be further developed, expanded or concentrated, broadened or focused, be combined with other activities, be better promoted, or become better accessible, for instance by using teleconferencing. However, many institutions and individuals will contribute to research and research education, including the individual European states and their institutions and societies, European regulations, societies, their committees, individual universities, university hospitals, research groups and individual radiology leaders.

Gaps in radiological research and research education, current activities and future solutions

Presence of radiology in basic research

Radiologists are often involved in the application and clinical assessment of technical innovation rather than performing their own laboratory-based research or epidemiological studies. Innovation-related research is important and should be continued. However, in order to have an impact on funding agencies and major university programmes, radiologists must be involved in basic research with an emphasis on both biological and physical topics.

Education relating to basic research is primarily the responsibility of universities. There are a number of M.D./Ph.D. programmes related to radiological topics throughout Europe [3], but also shorter programmes such as summer schools (http://www.excite.ethz.ch/). Radiological societies probably cannot (and should not) influence university programmes directly. However, radiology chairpersons should actively and systematically be involved in research activities by the scientific societies. There may be a need for an association of university radiologists or a research-oriented academy in order to increase participation of university hospitals in research education. Such an entity may best work under the umbrella of the ESR to avoid duplication of effort. The US-based Association of University Radiologists (AUR) and its affiliated groups such as the Radiology Research Alliance (RRA) (http://aur.org/AffinityGroups/http://aur.org/AffinityGroups/) may represent an interesting example.

The ESR is already very active in basic research, mainly through its EIBIR (European Institute for Biomedical Imaging Research, www.eibir.org) organisation. The ESR could further contribute to basic and clinical research activities through further activities driven by its research committee in the fields of imaging biomarkers, standardisation, imaging biobanks and personalised medicine. Studies resulting from this strategic planning should be operated by EIBIR. On the practical side, the European Congress of Radiology (ECR), European School of Radiology (ESOR) and the European subspecialty societies may contribute by systematically including basic research in their programmes and activities, adapted to the educational levels of their main audiences. The authors are aware that sessions and courses including basic research are not mainstream and would have to be tailored carefully to the needs of the general radiology audience in order to fulfil its goals; for example, by providing interactive courses including both basic researchers and clinical radiologists, similar to courses provided by other societies, including the International Society for Magnetic Resonance in Medicine (ISMRM).

The training in radiology through a medical residency system has proved to provide an adequate formation to the future specialists in clinical radiology. However, residency programmes tend to be tilted towards an almost purely clinical approach, which can lead to a deficit in research education.

It is mandatory to include an adequate training in the basic principles of research and evidence-based medicine in a thorough and comprehensive radiology curriculum in order to train a complete radiologist. This research education includes a satisfactory formation in the elements of the scientific methods, understanding the basic statistical knowledge in order to critically read and assess scientific publications, and an introduction to the design of research studies and scientific publishing (scientific posters and communications, articles). Training should be carried out under the supervision of the pertinent experienced trainers, and with an adequate degree of supervision appropriate to the status and training year of the trainee [4–6]. In that sense, the European Training Curriculum for Radiology developed by the ESR provides a valuable template to assure a basic education.

The radiology residency's final goal is to develop a complete specialist in general radiology and all trainees should be completely trained in all fields and disciplines in order to achieve this target. However, radiology training can also be a starting point to those trainees who would rather focus on a research-oriented career than on a more clinically-oriented practice. Mentors and tutors of the radiology departments in charge of radiology trainees can help in orienting and guiding those trainees without losing the principle of an adequate and general formation.

Research is a discipline that benefits from scientific exchange and, furthermore, taking into consideration the increasingly global society we live in, where international interchange is a usual practice. As a global and international society, the ESR and its associated institutions could take a leading role in providing a frame for scientific and research exchange programmes for radiology trainees.

Radiology-specific research versus research services

Radiology is important for the research undertaken by other disciplines; for example, as a service by acquiring, evaluating, communicating and storing imaging biomarker data. Such activities contribute to research in radiology as they connect radiologists to a research network and transfer knowledge from statistical methods, quality control, good manufacturing practice (GMP), industry-based research and university-based research into radiology. However, it does not directly give the radiologists a substantial role in basic research. Research education needs to take this important source of knowledge into account and needs to provide basic knowledge in the relevant topics.

Equally important, radiological research activities should not remain limited to a service to clinical partners, but original questions should arise from radiology itself, and the respective research methodology must be taught to radiologists. Radiology needs to broaden its research activities, from animal studies to randomised clinical trials and thus obtain an autonomous role in basic and clinical research. Radiology is also well suited to epidemiological research; for example, through the management of image databases and by providing and developing biomarkers. In order to survive in the current and future healthcare environment, radiology may not be sufficiently active in providing its own data on patient outcomes related to radiological diagnoses and therapeutic interventions. Various training opportunities by the ESR and EIBIR represent the basic framework for future development.

New research topics

New research topics develop continuously, and radiology as well as radiological education must follow such developments. New radiological research topics may originate from clinical questions. Examples include new surgical techniques requiring preoperative imaging for proper indication, surgical planning, early detection of complications and follow-up. Similar questions arise in non-surgical disciplines; for instance, after the introduction of new medication. There are also more general trends requiring imaging support, such as the increased interest in obesity, lifestyle issues and ageing. Imaging biomarkers are important in many disciplines, such as oncology, cardiology, rheumatology, liver surgery and orthopaedic surgery. Personalised medicine is another area of potential growth where radiology will have an important role.

There may also be research opportunities at the intersection with other disciplines, sometimes unexpectedly. Behavioural research may involve radiology; for example, in the assessment of the role of training, of fatigue or of incentive drivers. Imaging of new materials provided by material science is another example of where radiologists are commonly involved; for instance, in the assessment of new orthopaedic or cardiac implants.

Radiology needs to monitor such new opportunities and draw its own conclusions in a systematic fashion. First of all, radiologists, particularly those associated with academic institutions, need knowledge of current basic research as well as clinical research and what topics are becoming active. We should not rely simply on the interest of a few individuals but we need professional background as well as organisational representation. Professional background can be obtained by dual education, such as M.D./Ph.D. programs, or dual appointments, such as physicists, biologists or clinicians employed in radiology departments. Radiological societies, above all the ESR, should firmly anchor basic research topics in their programme. Individual radiology leaders should lobby their universities to provide educational and research programs, such as M.D./Ph.D. programs, basic research summer schools and joint series of lectures. Those associated with journals should try to attract and support publication of basic research papers. Although such work may be of less interest to many readers, it may foster important discussions. All academically active radiologists can contribute to this process, from serving as a reviewer for journals up to the editors. Societies also have the power to promote basic research through prizes and through the construction of their meeting programs.

Attitude

The commonly cited “Generation Y”, those born between 1980 and 2000, may have a reputation which is worse than it actually deserves. However, limited working hours, predictable careers and meaningful work contents may not favour research activities alongside a busy clinical schedule [7]. At the same time, some senior radiologists may not see research and research education as important as the ESR Working Group on Research Educations might hope. When time and other resources are limited, research competes with clinical work and clinical training and may easily lose.

In turn, the many positive facets of Generation Y should be addressed. Empathy and true interest in meaningful work are typical for this generation and may lead to an extra effort in research. To convince Generation Y of the importance of research and research education for the future of their discipline is crucial. Most important in this process are radiology leaders and other role models, such as basic researchers, who should promote the concept of radiology as a research-oriented discipline.

The even younger "Generation Z" (digital natives, born after 2000) will soon start to enter medical school and will expect systematic use of digital technologies for teaching and research. Similar to Generation Y, Generation Z is eager to learn and to achieve a meaningful goal. This general motivation should be reinforced by radiology training programs that need to focus on the science aspects of the specialty.

Meaningful work, application of computer sciences, and adaptation of time schedules are in the hands of radiology leaders, universities and research societies. The ESR should emphasise the importance of research and research education, whilst recognising academic leaders within society.

Career planning

The previously mentioned questionnaires indicate that career planning is an important topic and that relevant gaps are perceived. Training currently does not sufficiently emphasise grant applications, research ethics or required basic science. To promote and teach such activities may be too demanding for some teaching institutions, especially in a non-academic setting, but even for some university institutions. Family-friendly working models may not be sufficiently available in many countries and institutions, further impinging on motivation to perform research.

In Europe, residency programs and other curricula tend to be less formalised than, for example, in the USA. Within the research education working group there was no consensus regarding the effect of such lack of formalisation: does this lead to a waste of time and loss of focus, or is this academic freedom or avoidance of unnecessary bureaucracy? Generation Y may give the answer, as they like predictable career paths and select residency programs according to factors such as reliability and predictability.

Admittedly, the lower European formalisation is not proven to be inferior to the USA system; for instance, when looking at research productivity [8]. However, formal systems are better able to detect and correct underperforming individuals and institutions.

The risky business of research projects can be made more predictable by several measures; training in methodology, providing statistical and other scientific counselling, sharing the risk by working in research groups with more than one project, regular meetings and reporting, in order to identify deviation from the planned track. Day-to-day management of research careers will help young researchers in their longer education to attain promotion to staff positions. One possibility is to offer clinical fast track for those committed to research with strictly organised access to topics with limited training positions; for example, interventional radiology training. This is the task of radiology chairs but may be facilitated by carefully adapting the European and national training charters in order to better accommodate such career tracks.

Another important topic is the "pipeline leakage", with capable researchers leaving the scientific track before reaching senior staff positions. Systematic career planning by radiology chairs is probably the best way to avoid preventable loss of careers. This includes scouting for open positions for the younger, not yet connected radiologists, as well as preparation for applications to leading positions.

Such promotion of research is not an easy task. Clinical routine work remains the basis of all radiology. To find a way to promote researchers without frustrating clinical radiologists remains an art of leadership.

Incentives

There must be intrinsic motivation to perform research and to participate in research education in order to enjoy working as a researcher. The willingness to contribute to human knowledge, to develop the discipline of radiology and to foster patient wellbeing are strong intrinsic motivations [9]. To identify such individuals is another important task for radiology leaders, possibly supported by the hospitals' human resources departments. However, even highly motivated residents need some incentive not to lag behind purely clinical colleagues of the same age. Clinicians may be promoted to clinical staff physician earlier than researchers with their longer education path. In the long run, trainees may also look at salaries in the academic versus private practice system. The impact of lower salaries in the academic system must be offset not only by intrinsic motivation but also by extrinsic factors such as academic rewards. The responsibilities are with the chairpersons of the departments of radiology who should ensure that salaries are similar to clinical salaries in their own institutions and not too low in comparison to other institutions competing for the same radiologists. They cannot do this without the help of programmes for financing of protected time or support personnel. In addition, universities (and faculties of medicine) as well as scientific societies have means to compensate active research by academic promotion and by invitations to speak at prestigious meetings. When chairpersons make decisions regarding congress participation, research activities should be a top criterion.

Gender issues

The proportion of women in medical school, in residency and more recently in staff positions is increasing. Childbearing at least for a certain period of time does not allow to work full time, may lead to reduced research in favour of clinical activity and may reduce the status of women who wish to remain in the competitive research environment. Women may be less inclined than men to choose a research career, and the brain drain from the academic system is more pronounced for women than men (http://www.gleichstellung.uzh.ch/politik/gleichstellungsmonitoring/GLM_Datentabellen_2013.pdf). At the University of Zurich, 1991–1993, 46.8 % of newly registered students were women. However, in 2013, the percentage of female full professors was 19.5 % instead of the expected half of all positions at University of Zurich. Another reason to formally address women in radiology relates to the fact that a mixed leadership has been shown to be more successful than single-gender groups. When reviewed from an economical point of view, net income growth for companies with women board members has averaged 14 % over the past 6 years compared with 10 % for those with no female board representation [10].

To keep the increasingly female radiology workforce in academic institutions is a standard task for radiology chairs, hospitals and universities. Quota may not be the best way to reach this but may be taken into consideration if voluntary programmes are not successful. However, the efforts of each individual staff member are as important. They provide role models, may actively recruit female candidates for research career tracks, and ensure that females are adequately represented in search committees. A discussion of this topic is provided in the bestselling book "Lean in" by Facebook's COO, Sheryl Sandberg [11], and in the multi-editor book, "The Glass Ceiling in the 21st Century: Understand Barriers to Gender Equality" [12].

Financing of research education

Funding constraints have occasionally been noted in the ESR research committee questionnaires. Indeed, training in general and research education specifically must compete with tighter budgets and stricter resource allocation models such as diagnosis-related groups, leaving no or little room for cross-subsidising research and teaching by healthcare funds.

Even under economic pressure, chairpersons have means to promote research. Workload is not always evenly distributed during the day, during the week or during all seasons. There tend to be low activity periods in clinical radiology; for instance, in the mornings before patients seen in outpatient clinics appear in the radiology department, or in summer when elective hospitalisations may be slower. Also, there are university programmes and private foundations willing to finance protected time. There is also a leadership aspect: such resources may be attributed in a competitive fashion. Radiology leaders are responsible for insisting on such efforts especially during periods of frustrations after rejected applications. Universities, societies such as the ESR, the European Union and industry may assist in efforts to finance research and research education. They may provide grants for protected time, research fellowships, summer schools, courses and other activities promoting research and research education.

Variability

The position and the organisation of research education varies between countries but also between institutions within the same country. For students and level 1 residents (years 1–3 of the European curriculum) (www.myesr.org/html/img/pool/ESR_2014_ESR-EuropeanTrainingCurriculum_web_Dec.pdf), there is minimal compulsory research education specific to radiology. However, voluntary courses are often available even at these early levels. Many countries and individual universities provide M.D./Ph.D. programmes as well as shorter courses for topics such as good clinical practice courses (GCP). Training on the job and participation at society meetings such as the ECR are also often used as a means to promote research education. Variability between institutions is not necessarily a bad thing but also the expression of the freedom of research. However, it means that some of the potential to recruit future researchers is not fully realised. Nevertheless, research education is too important not to use the potential of all capable individuals. Institutions with less active programmes and countries with a less formalised research programmes and research education should agree to minimal activities. European societies play an important role through strategic statements, rules and regulations such as the European Training Charter, as well as their educational activities. Teach the teachers programmes may assist in reducing variability between programmes and countries, and are probably underused in radiology.

Conclusions

Research education is the pacemaker for research-driven radiology of the future. This paper investigates how current gaps can be filled in research education and training. There are no easy solutions, but to advance is well within the remit and capacity of the various players in the field, from the ESR and its committees to the individual radiologist. Many means are already available but may need to be more systematically applied, existing structures such as EIBIR need to be strengthened, and leaders need to consistently and unequivocally emphasise the role of research for radiology.

Acknowledgments This article was kindly prepared by the ESR Research Committee (Chairman: H.-U. Kauczor), Working Group on Research Education and Training (Members: Juerg Hodler, Hans Ulrich Kauczor, Birgit Ertl-Wagner, David Wilson, Anders Persson, Siarhei Kharuzhyk, Ervin László Berenyi, Marc Dewey, Pablo Rodriguez-Carnero) on behalf of the European Society of Radiology (ESR). It was approved by the ESR Executive Council on January 2015.

References

1. Sardanelli F, Hunink MG, Gilbert FJ, Di Leo G, Krestin GP (2010) Evidence-based radiology: why and how? Eur Radiol 20(1):1–15
2. European Society of Radiology (ESR) (2012) Education in research: results of a survey commissioned by the research committee of the European Society of Radiology. Insights Imaging 3:535–542
3. European Society of Radiology (ESR) (2013) MD PhD programmes with relevance to imaging. Results from a European survey. Insights Imaging 4:409–415
4. Barker CF (2013) Making imaging research a part of radiology resident training. Acad Radiol 20(2):135–136
5. Costello JR, Mullins ME, Votaw JR, Karolyi DR, Kalb B, Gonzales P et al (2013) Establishing a new radiology residency research track. Acad Radiol 20(2):243–248
6. Sundgren PC (2012) Mentoring radiology residents in clinical and translational research. Acad Radiol 19(9):1110–1113
7. The Economist (2013) Generations in the workplace. Winning the generation game. The Economist Newspaper Limited, London
8. Spitzmueller D, Hodler J, Seifert B, Zanetti M (2010) Radiological research activity 1998–2007: relationship to gross domestic product, health expenditure and public expenditure on education. Insights Imaging 2010(1):269–280
9. Buddeberg-Fischer B, Christen S, Weishaupt D, Hoffmann A, Kubik-Huch RA (2011) Professional satisfaction of radiologists in Switzerland. Swiss Med Wkly 141:w13271
10. Credit Suisse Research Institute, Mary Curtis Christine Schmid, Marion Struber. Editorial deadline, 13 July 2012, https://www.credit-suisse.com/newsletter/doc/gender_diversity.pdf
11. Sandberg S (2013) Lean in: women, work, and the will to lead. Alfred A. Knopf, New York
12. Barreto M, Ryan MK, Schmitt MT (2009) The glass ceiling in the 21st century: understanding barriers to gender equality. American Psychological Association, Washington

20

Imaging of haemodialysis: renal and extrarenal findings

Ferruccio Degrassi · Emilio Quaia · Paola Martingano · Marco Cavallaro · Maria Assunta Cova

Abstract Electrolyte alterations and extra-renal disorders are quite frequent in patients undergoing haemodialysis or peritoneal dialysis. The native kidneys may be the site of important pathologies in patients undergoing dialysis, especially in the form of acquired renal cystic disease with frequent malignant transformation. Renal neoplasms represents an important complication of haemodialysis-associated acquired cystic kidney disease and imaging surveillance is suggested. Extra-renal complications include renal osteodistrophy, brown tumours, and thoracic and cardiovascular complications. Other important fields in which imaging techniques may provide important informations are arteriovenous fistula and graft complications.

Teaching points

- *Renal neoplasms represent a dreaded complication of haemodialysis.*
- *In renal osteodystrophy bone resorption typically manifests along the middle phalanges.*
- *Brown tumours are well-defined lytic lesions radiographically, possibly causing bone expansion.*
- *Vascular calcifications are very common in patients undergoing haemodialysis.*
- *Principal complications of the AV fistula consist of thrombosis, aneurysms and pseudoaneurysms.*

Keywords Haemodialysis · Acquired cystic kidney disease · Renal neoplasm · Renal osteodystrophy · Dialysis access complications

F. Degrassi (✉) · E. Quaia · P. Martingano · M. Cavallaro · M. A. Cova
Department of Radiology, Cattinara Hospital, University of Trieste, Strada di Fiume 447, 34149 Trieste, Italy
e-mail: ferruccio.degrassi@alice.it

Introduction

End-stage renal disease occurs when chronic renal failure progresses to the point that the kidneys are permanently functioning at less than 10 % of their capacity, namely the glomerular filtration rate (GFR) is permanently lower than 15 ml/min/1.73 m^2. End-stage renal disease used to be a lethal condition until the advent of long-term haemodialysis and renal transplantation. In the USA, diabetic nephropathy, hypertension and glomerulonephritis cause approximately 75 % of end-stage renal disease in patients undergoing haemodialysis.

The dialysis is the exchange of solutes and waste products via either an extracorporeal membrane (haemodialysis) or a peritoneal membrane (continuous ambulatory or cycling peritoneal dialysis). As far as haemodialysis is concerned, the solute removal primarily depends on passive diffusion across a semipermeable membrane. Blood and dialysate flow rates are adjusted to replenish the supply of incoming solute available for diffusion [1]. The efficiency of ultrafiltration depends on the water permeability of the device and the surface area [1]. Haemodialysis has a higher clearance rate for low-molecular-weight substances such as urea [1]. Peritoneal dialysis should be performed in infants and patients with relative contraindications to haemodialysis such as severe vascular disease, active bleeding, haemorrhagic diathesis or cardiovascular instability.

The clinical constellation of signs and symptoms of end-stage renal disease is known as uraemic syndrome. Various problems related to the vascular access in patients on haemodialysis [2] are also common since the peritoneal dialysis catheter leads to the risk of peritonitis and local infections. Patients with end-stage renal failure are susceptible to all the complications of any underlying condition such as diabetes and hypertension as well as other metabolic and physiologic derangements. In addition, chronic immunosuppression makes patients with end-stage renal disease prone to infections, tuberculosis included [3].

Imaging plays an essential role in the assessment of the possible renal and extra-renal complications in patients undergoing long-term haemodialysis.

Chronic renal failure

Chronic renal failure can result from numerous renal parenchymal diseases, the most common being glomerulonephritis, diabetes, hypertension and the polycystic kidney disease. Diabetes and hypertension are now recognised as the leading causes of chronic renal failure in the USA [4]. Often, patients only seek medical attention when the renal disease has progressed to the uraemic stage since adult patients are usually unaware of their advancing renal failure until the GFR has decreased to less than 15 ml per minute, namely end-stage renal disease [4].

Ultrasound (US) with Doppler US examination of intrarenal vessels is the imaging modality of choice to be employed in patients with renal failure and is commonly performed early in the clinical course [5]. Chronic renal failure manifests with a reduction of renal dimensions that develops over months or years. US reveals a reduced renal length and reduced renal cortical thickness with an increased renal cortical echogenicity often associated with poor visibility of the renal pyramids and the renal sinus, marginal irregularities, parenchymal cysts and also papillary calcifications (Fig. 1a–b). Colour Doppler US reveals a reduced renal vascularity and increased RI values measured at the level of the segmental and interlobular arteries [6, 7] according to the stage of chronic renal failure. The capability of renal RI to aid in the prediction of renal dysfunction progression has been demonstrated. US follow-up of native scarred kidneys is indicated in patients with chronic renal failure treated with dialysis or renal transplantation because they develop the acquired cystic kidney disease (ACKD) with a significantly increased risk of solid and cystic renal malignancies. CT confirms the US findings by revealing reduced renal length and cortical thickness (Fig. 2).

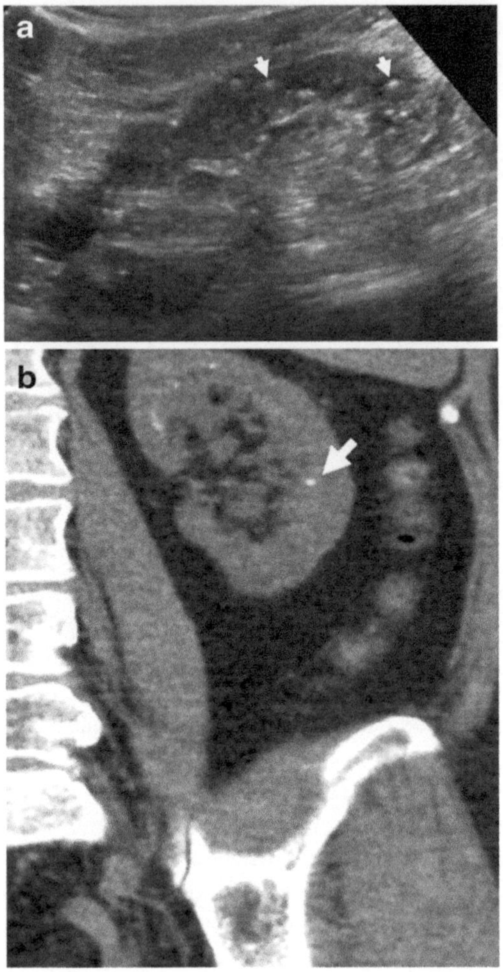

Fig. 1 a–b: **a** Grey-scale US and (**b**) unenhanced CT, coronal reformations. Papillary calcifications in a patient undergoing long-term dialysis, appearing as hyperchoic spots on renal pyramids. Papillary calcifications may also be observed in analgesic nephropathy, in sarcoidosis, primary hyperparathyroidism, diabetes mellitus and medullary sponge kidney

Renal abnormalities in long-term haemodialysis

Acquired cystic kidney disease

ACKD was first described by Dunnil et al. (1977) and is characterised by the development of numerous fluid-filled cysts in patients with end-stage renal disease who have undergone prolonged dialysis but without a history of hereditary cystic disease (Fig. 3a, b). After 1–3 years of haemodialysis, 10–20 % of patients have ACKD, 40–60 % after 3–5 years of haemodyalisis and more than 90 % after 5–10 years of haemodialysis. The cysts measure 0.5 to 2 cm in diameter, contain clear fluid, are lined by either a hyperplastic or a flattened tubular epithelium, and often contain calcium oxalate crystals. They probably form as a result of obstruction of tubules by interstitial fibrosis or oxalate crystals. Frequently, some cysts may develop a haemorrhagic pattern causing

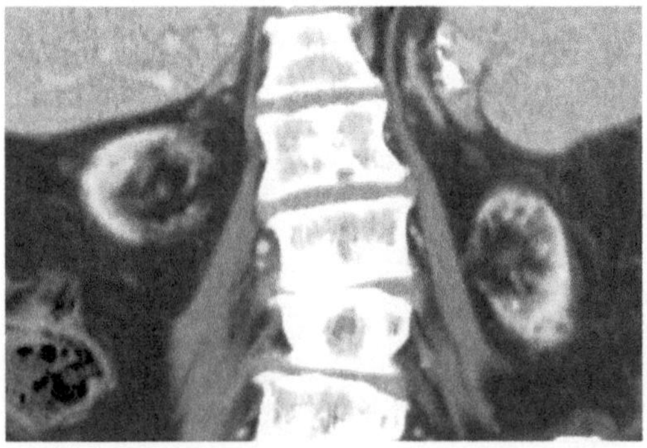

Fig. 2 Chronic renal failure in a 76-year-old female. CT image of kidneys reveals a short length and diffuse reduction of renal cortical thickness

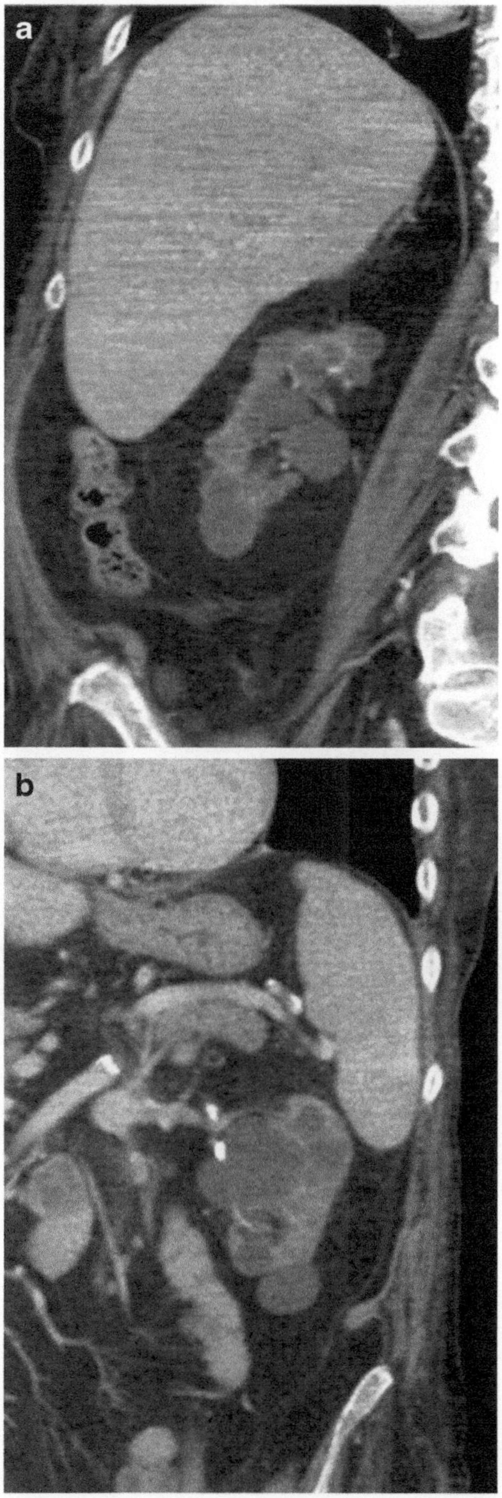

Fig. 3 **a**, **b**: Unenhanced (**a**) and contrast-enhanced CT (**b**). Acquired cystic kidney disease in a patient undergoing long-term haemodialysis

haematuria (Fig. 4a, b). The likelihood of the development of ACKD increases with the duration of haemodialysis, and it is higher in male and older patients. Other factors such as the underlying renal insufficiency and serum creatinine level have no significant influence on the development of ACKD. The development of renal cell carcinoma in the wall of the cysts is the most serious complication of ACKD. The prevalence of renal cell carcinoma in patients with dialysis-associated ACKD undergoing long-term haemodialysis is increased, being in the range of 3–6 %. The prevalence is similar in patients with ACKD undergoing renal transplantation.

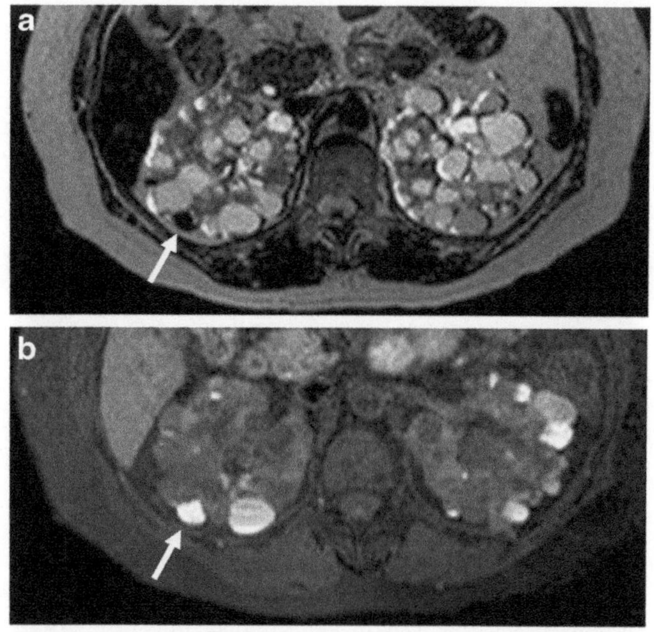

Fig. 4 **a**, **b**: Haemorrhagic renal cyst (*arrow*) in the right kidney in a patient undergoing long-term haemodialysis. The cyst appears hypointense on T2-weighted MR sequences (**a**) and hyperintense on T1-weighted MR sequences (**b**)

Renal neoplasms

An increased incidence of renal tumours has been reported in patients with end-stage renal disease [8]. Renal cell carcinoma (RCC) presents with a frequency three to six times higher in patients receiving haemodialysis than in the general population [8]. Observations provide histological evidence that renal cell neoplasms are prone to develop in relatively young patients with renal failure when their uraemia is treated by long-term dialysis. The incidence of renal carcinoma increases with the duration of dialysis [8].

Other studies indicate that the stimulus for neoplastic growth comes with a cystic transformation of the kidneys. A very strong association with ACKD and an increased incidence of papillary renal tumours have been observed in many studies [9]. More than 80 % of all patients with end-stage renal disease developing a renal tumour actually have underlying ACKD [8]. Since these tumours are multiple and very often small in size, the ratio of histological RCC subtypes is shifted toward papillary renal carcinoma and papillary renal cell adenoma [8].

Renal tumours developing in patients undergoing haemodialysis present at an earlier age compared to the general population, with a higher incidence in males, [8, 10–12], and they frequently are bilateral (9 %) and multi-centric (50 %) [5]. The papillary hyperplasia in the cyst is thought to be a precursor of the papillary carcinoma. Papillary-cell renal cell carcinoma accounts for about half the cases identified in patients undergoing haemodialysis, while it does not exceed 10 % in the general population (Fig. 5a–c) [13–16].

CT seems to provide better diagnostic accuracy than US or MR imaging in the detection of renal tumours in patients undergoing haemodialysis (Fig. 6a–c) [17, 18].

The leading sign of the tumour is the space occupied by the lesion localised in the atrophic renal parenchyma; the size of the distinguishable tumour is about 5 mm in diameter when causing the bulging of the renal surface [9]. Smaller lesions under the kidney surface may remain undetected, especially when ultrasound or plain CT is used [19]. Renal parenchymal atrophy in the end stage of glomerulonephritis or interstitial nephritis is the main limitation of ultrasound in imaging the kidneys in dialysis patients [9], while the enhancement of small nodular foci could help identify smaller tumours inside the renal parenchyma if multi-detector row computed tomography with isotropic resolution is used [9].

It is generally agreed that there is a need for regular surveillance of patients with ACKD for the early detection of renal cell carcinoma [17, 18].

Although regular follow-up trans-abdominal ultrasound or conventional helical CT is able to detect larger masses, Ferda et al. have shown that the capabilities of multi-detector row computed tomography offer more accurate imaging of multiple renal tumours in ESRD patients [9]. However, some authors maintain that the performance of periodic ultrasound controls allows achieving the early diagnosis and treatment of tumours of the kidney in patients in dialysis [20].

There is no clear consensus about screening in the long-term dialysis population. The current literature indicates that most patients will develop acquired renal cysts after 3–7 years on dialysis, the latter associated with a 1.6–7.0 % incidence of

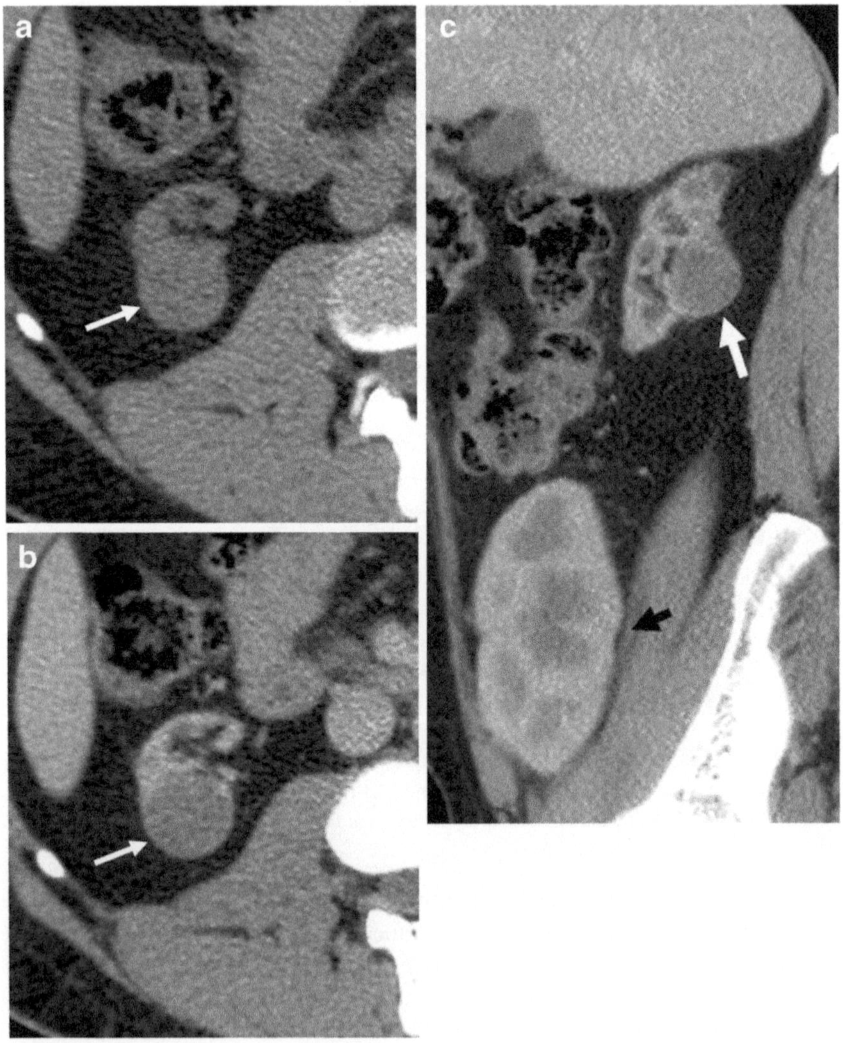

Fig. 5 a–c: Unenhanced (**a**) and contrast-enhanced CT, transverse plane (**b**) and sagittal reformation (**c**). Rounded lesion (white arrow) of the right kidney in a patient after renal allograft transplantation (*black arrow*). The lesion shows indeterminate enhancement (an increase of 10 HU after contrast injection). The dissected specimen proved to be a papillary renal cell carcinoma. There was no sign of acquired cystic renal disease

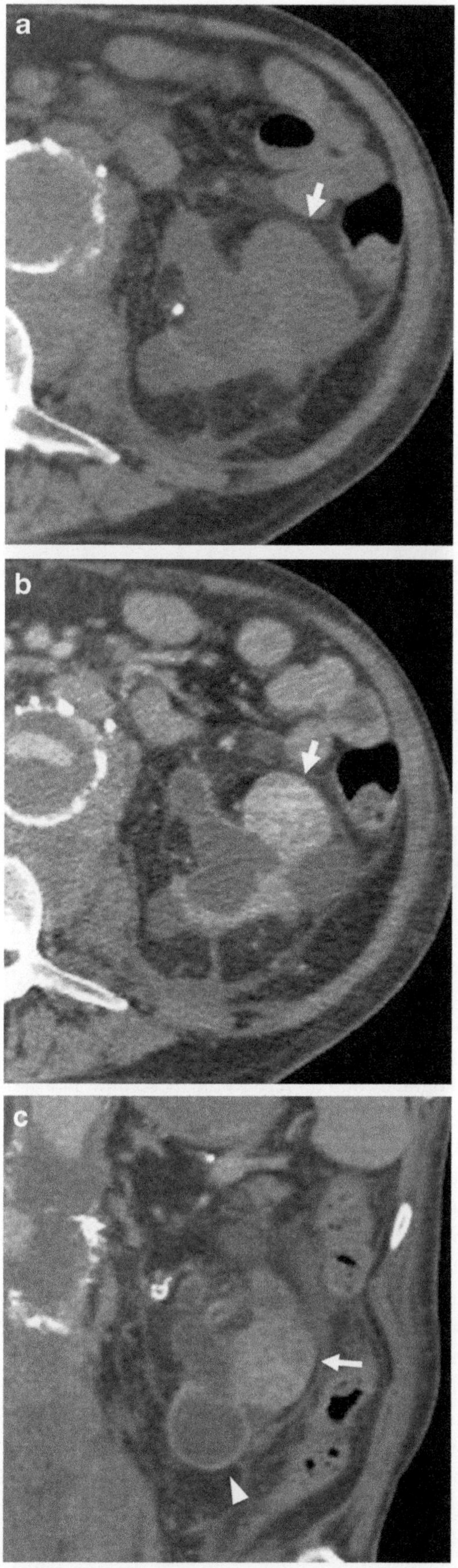

◀ **Fig. 6 a–c**: ACKD in a patient who has been undergoing haemodialysis for 10 years. **a** Unenhanced and contrast-enhanced CT, transverse plane (**b**) and coronal reformation (**c**). Both kidneys present multiple cysts; one of these at the inferior pole of the left kidney presents uniform thickening of the wall (Bosniak IIF) (*arrowhead*). Moreover a solid enhancing lesion, about 3 cm in size, is evident on the left kidney (*arrow*) corresponding to a clear-cell renal cell carcinoma

RCC. This has led some authors to recommend routine screening for RCC in patients who have been on dialysis for longer than 3 years, including subsequent transplant recipients [21]. Some authors have found that screening with computed tomography or ultrasound increases life expectancy by about 1.6 years among 20-year-old patients with a life expectancy of 25 years [22].

Extra-renal complications in patients undergoing long-term haemodialysis

Musculoskeletal system

Patients with chronic renal disease and on haemodialysis may develop many different musculoskeletal abnormalities, including secondary hyperparathyroidism, osteomalacia, osteosclerosis, osteoporosis, amyloidosis and a variety of crystal deposition diseases [23].

Other abnormalities related to the biochemical disturbance of chronic renal failure include soft tissue/vascular calcifications and crystalline arthropathies.

Musculoskeletal sequelae predominantly related to dialysis include an aluminium toxicity manifesting as osteomalacia from ingestion of aluminium salts in phosphate-binding antiacids used to control hyperphosphataemia, amyloidosis and destructive spondyloarthropathy.

Dialysis-related amyloidosis is a frequent and major complication in long-term dialysis patients, and it presents with carpal tunnel syndrome, cystic bone lesions, destructive spondylarthropathy, arthritis, periarthritis and systemic organ involvement [24].

Destructive spondyloarthropathy is characterised by rapidly progressive radiographic abnormalities, including the loss of intervertebral disc space, erosion of the subchondral bone in the adjacent vertebral bodies and new bone formation (Fig. 7). In some patients, destructive changes may be severe, simulating infective spondylitis: the persistence of low signal intensity on T2-weighted images generally permits excluding infections [23].

Avascular necrosis, osteomyelitis (Fig. 8a, b), septic arthritis, tendinosis/tendon rupture and bursitis/synovitis are caused by a combination of chronic renal failure, steroid/ immunosuppressants and dialysis [25].

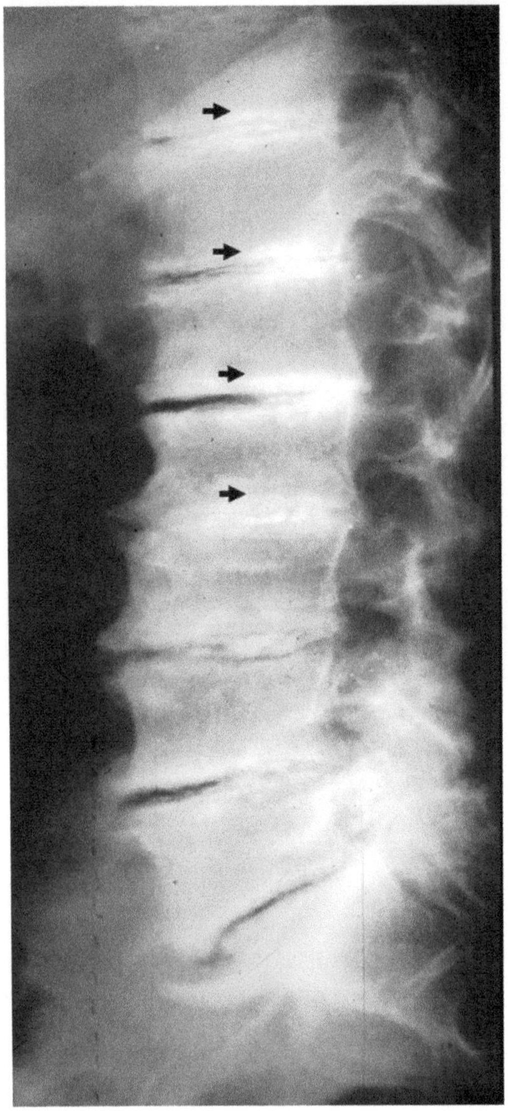

Fig. 7 Plain x-ray film of the spine. Diffuse osteosclerosis of the spine in a patient undergoing chronic haemodialysis. Diffuse sub-endplate densities at multiple contiguous levels (*arrows*), a pattern known as "rugger-jersey spine"

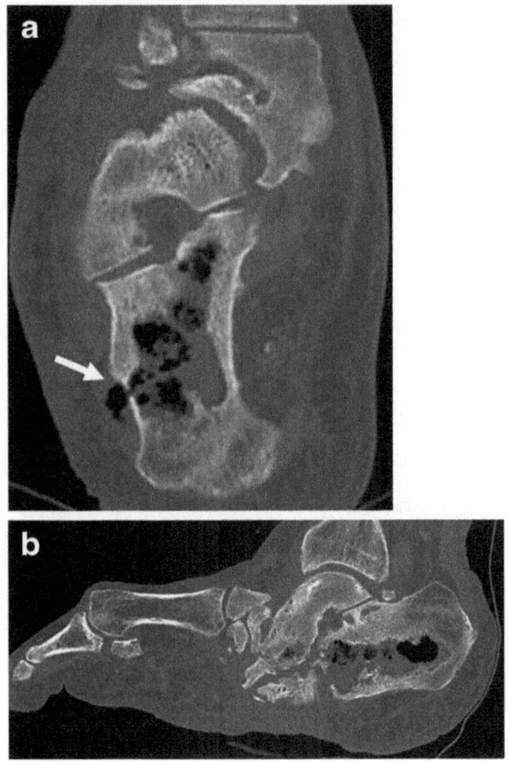

Fig. 8 **a**, **b**: Unhenanced CT axial (**a**), sagittal plane. Osteomyelitis of the tarsus in a 72-year-old male with chronic renal failure under dialysis. Extensive bone alterations involving all the tarsal bones with important areas of ostelysis associated with areas of osteosclerosis. The infection extensively involves the calcaneus with intraosseous fluid and gas components. A fistula with subcutaneous soft tissue is visible on the lateral side of the calcaneus (*arrow*)

Renal osteodystrophy

Abnormalities involving the musculoskeletal system are numerous and frequent in patients with chronic renal insufficiency. Chronic renal insufficiency, haemodialysis, peritoneal dialysis, renal transplantation and administration of different medications provoke complex biochemical disturbances of the calcium-phosphate metabolism with a wide spectrum of bone and soft tissue abnormalities named renal osteodystrophy [26]. Renal osteodystrophy is a global term applied to all pathological features of bone in patients with chronic renal failure and it includes osteomalacia or rickets according to the age of the patient, secondary hyperparathyroidism with bone resorption, periosteal reaction, brown tumours, osteosclerosis, osteoporosis, soft tissue and vascular calcifications.

Multiple factors play a role in creating renal osteodystrophy including a deficiency in the active form of vitamin D due to impaired renal metabolism and an increase in the parathormone secretion due to hyperphosphataemia causing hypocalcaemia by precipitating calcium [5].

Radiography still represents the most important and widely performed technique [27] to identify the alterations of renal osteodystrophy. Radionuclide imaging, computed tomography and magnetic resonance imaging are less frequently indicated and are mainly used for more sensitive and precise identifications (aseptic bone necrosis, infection, Looser's zones), morphological presentations (spinal infection with neural compromise) and the differential diagnosis of complications (destructive spondyloarthropathy versus spinal infection).

The osteoclastic bone resorption affects the surfaces of the bone and may be subperiosteal, intracortical, endosteal, trabecular, subchondral, subligamentous and subtendinous. Early radiographic changes of subperiosteal bone resorption may be demonstrated at the phalangeal tufts and the radial aspects of the middle phalanges of the second and the third hand fingers (Fig. 9a, b) [26]. Early subperiosteal resorption produces the loss of definition of the cortical bone with a characteristic lace-like appearance, which later on progresses to

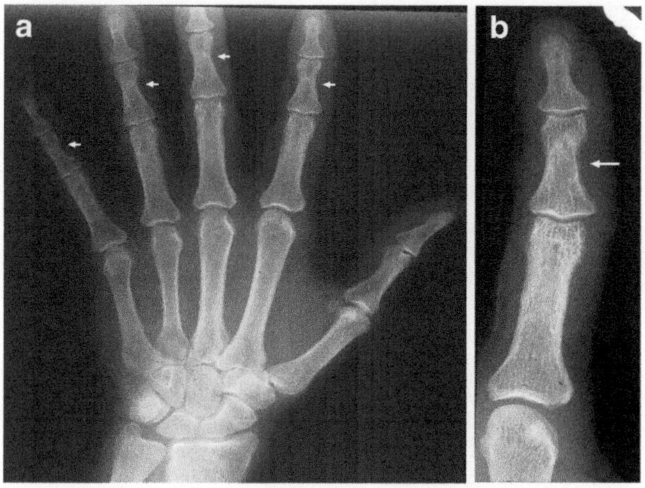

Fig. 9 **a**, **b**: **a** Radiographic image of the left hand in a patient undergoing chronic haemodialysis. **b** Magnification. Secondary hyperparathyroidism with bone resorption along the radial aspects of the middle phalanges of the fingers (*arrows*)

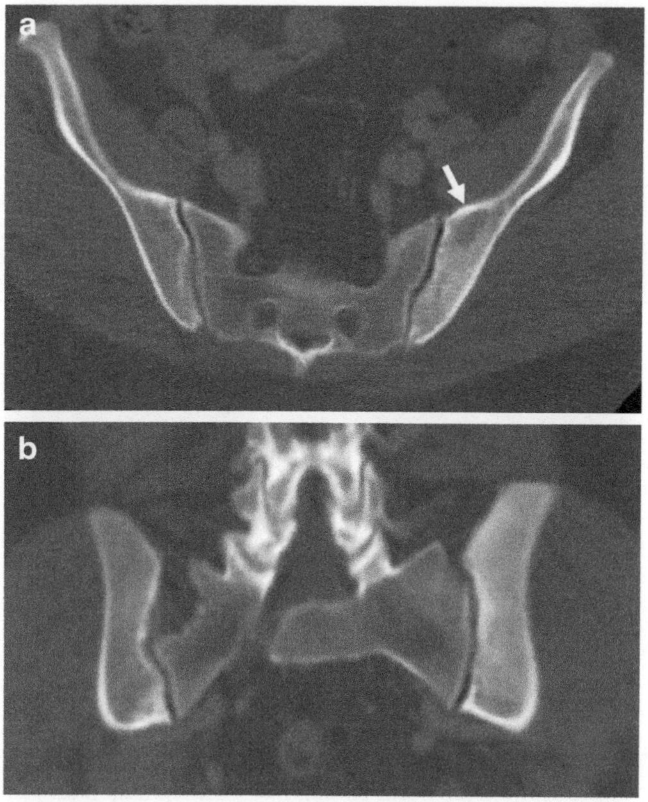

Fig. 10 **a**, **b**: Unenhanced CT. Sacral region, axial plane (**a**) and coronal reformation (**b**). Renal osteodystrophy of the left iliac wing with diffuse bone sclerosis and some areas of resorption (*arrows*) due to secondary hyperparathyroidism in a patient undergoing chronic haemodialysis

complete cortical disappearance. The advanced bone resorption of the terminal phalanges may result in acro-osteolysis with separation of the tuft and the base of the phalanx. Subperiosteal resorption is frequently combined with intracortical tunnelling and endosteal resorption, which causes scalloped defects of the inner cortical contour. In advanced disease, the widespread trabecular resorption within the medullary bone may be seen with a loss of definition and the disappearance of trabeculae. The most typical manifestation of trabecular bone resorption appears at the cranial vault and is named the 'salt and pepper' skull [26].

Subchondral bone resorption may affect different articulations, most commonly the sacroiliac, sternoclavicular and acromioclavicular joints, intervertebral discs and the symphysis pubis. Radiographic changes at the sacroiliac joints are similar to those seen in ankylosing spondylitis and include the widening of the joint space and subchondral bone erosions surrounded by osteosclerosis [26].

Subligamentous and subtendinous bone resorption occurs at numerous sites, especially at the ischial tuberosities, femoral trochanters and the insertions of the coracoclavicular ligaments.

Periosteal new bone production may be seen in patients with advanced hyperparathyroidism affecting the metatarsals, femur, pelvis, humerus, radius, ulna, metacarpals and phalanges.

Osteosclerosis is frequently found in patients with renal osteodystrophy and secondary hyperparathyroidism (Fig. 10a, b). Bone sclerosis in renal osteodystrophy may affect different skeletal elements but it usually predominates in the axial skeleton. One of the typical findings includes broad osteosclerosis localised below the endplates of the vertebral bodies with normal density of the middle parts ('rugger jersey' appearance) [26].

Radiographic signs of osteomalacia are a bone density decrease with a loss of definition of the cortical bone and coarsening of the trabecular pattern. Looser's zones (i.e. Milkman's fractures, pseudofractures) are rare but pathognomic features, which are most common in the medial part of the femoral neck, pubic rami, ilii, scapulae, ribs and acromion. Looser's zones represent unmineralised osteoid and are seen as lucent lines perpendicular to the cortex, frequently symmetric in location.

Rickets-like changes may occur in the immature skeleton and reflect an abnormal endochondral ossification. Radiographic features include osteopenia with softening and bending of bones, widening of the growth plate as well as the cupping, expansion, demineralisation and disorganisation of the metaphysis [26].

The osteoporotic bone is characterised by the thinning of cortices and trabeculae. These features are most evident in skeletal elements rich in cancellous bone (spine, proximal femur and forearm). In advanced osteoporosis the loss of trabeculae with pathological fractures may occur. In the vertebral column the disappearance of transverse trabeculae with preservation of the vertical compression trabeculae results in characteristic vertical striations. The final results are pathological fractures with wedge-shaped, biconcave (fish vertebrae) or flattened vertebral bodies and vertebral column deformities. Vertebral fractures can be evaluated subjectively or using quantitative methods. In general, the sensitivity of radiography is poor; 30 % to 50 % of bone tissue has to be lost before osteoporosis can be detected on routine radiographs [26].

Brown tumours

Brown tumours are a form of cystic fibrous osteitis, the end stage of bone remodelling in primary or secondary hyperparathyroidism [28]. In patients with chronic renal failure brown tumours represent an extreme and serious complication of renal osteodystrophy [28–31]. Brown tumours are caused by the localised replacement of bone by vascularised fibrous tissue (osteitis fibrosa cystica) resulting from parathyroid hormone-stimulated osteoclastic activity [5]. Patients with renal osteodystrophy who have brown tumours actually have autonomously functioning parathyroid glands or tertiary hyperparathyroidism [5]. The fibrous tissue contains giant cells, and the lesions may become cystic, following necrosis and liquefaction [5]. These lesions represent a reparative cellular process rather than a neoplastic process and are located in areas of intense bone resorption (Fig. 11a, b) [5, 32].

Brown tumours occur as single or multiple radiolucent lesions and can be found both within bone and in the adjacent soft tissues. When left untreated, they can undergo central necrosis and cyst formation [5]. Radiographically, brown tumours are well-defined lytic lesions, often eccentric or cortical, that may cause endosteal scalloping and bone expansion.

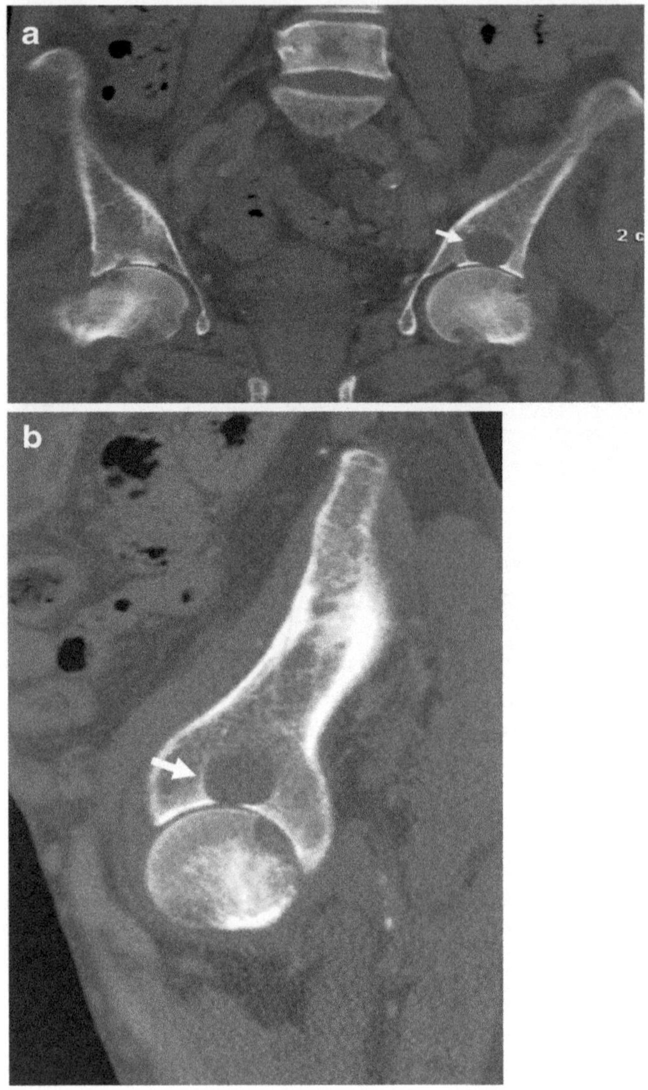

Fig. 11 **a**, **b**: Unenhanced CT, coronal (**a**) and sagittal (**b**) reformations. Brown tumour in a patient undergoing chronic haemodialysis with tertiary hyperparathyroidism. The brown tumour appears as a lytic lesion of the ilium (*arrow*)

Soft tissue and vascular metastatic calcification

Biochemical disturbance of chronic renal failure includes vascular and soft tissue metastatic calcifications and crystalline arthropathies. Vascular calcifications manifest as both medial and intimal calcifications of the arteries and are a hallmark of the accelerated atherosclerosis observed in uraemia [33].

Calcific uraemic arteriolopathy is a rare but life-threatening complication estimated to occur in 1 % of patients with chronic renal disease and in 4.1 % of patients undergoing maintenance haemodialysis [34]. Articular calcinosis is characterised by the deposition of a large amount of calcium around the periarticular regions, and it is commonly noticed over the shoulder, elbow and hip joints [35]. Even visceral (myocardial and pericardial) calcifications may occur in patients undergoing haemodialysis.

Vascular calcifications are very common in end-stage renal disease, especially in patients undergoing haemodialysis (Fig. 12a, b) [36, 37]. The mechanisms of vascular calcification are hyperphosphataemia and elevated calcium (Ca) and phosphate (P) products [38, 39].

Vascular calcification induces the stiffening of the vessel wall and reduces the vascular compliance [40]. Iwasa et al. showed a much higher rate of intracranial artery calcification in haemodialysis patients than in the general population, and this finding has been reported to be an independent risk factor for ischaemic stroke. The most frequently involved sites of calcification in haemodialysis patients were the internal carotid artery and the vertebral arteries [41].

Cardiovascular complications

Cardiovascular complications are common in patients with chronic renal failure and are related to atherosclerosis and hyperlipidaemia, hypertension due to sodium retention and alterations in the renin-angiotensin axis, myocardial dysfunction and pericarditis. More than 50 % of end-stage renal disease patients treated with chronic haemodialysis die from cardiovascular diseases, including congestive heart failure due to the increase of the left ventricular afterload: volume overload between dialyses,

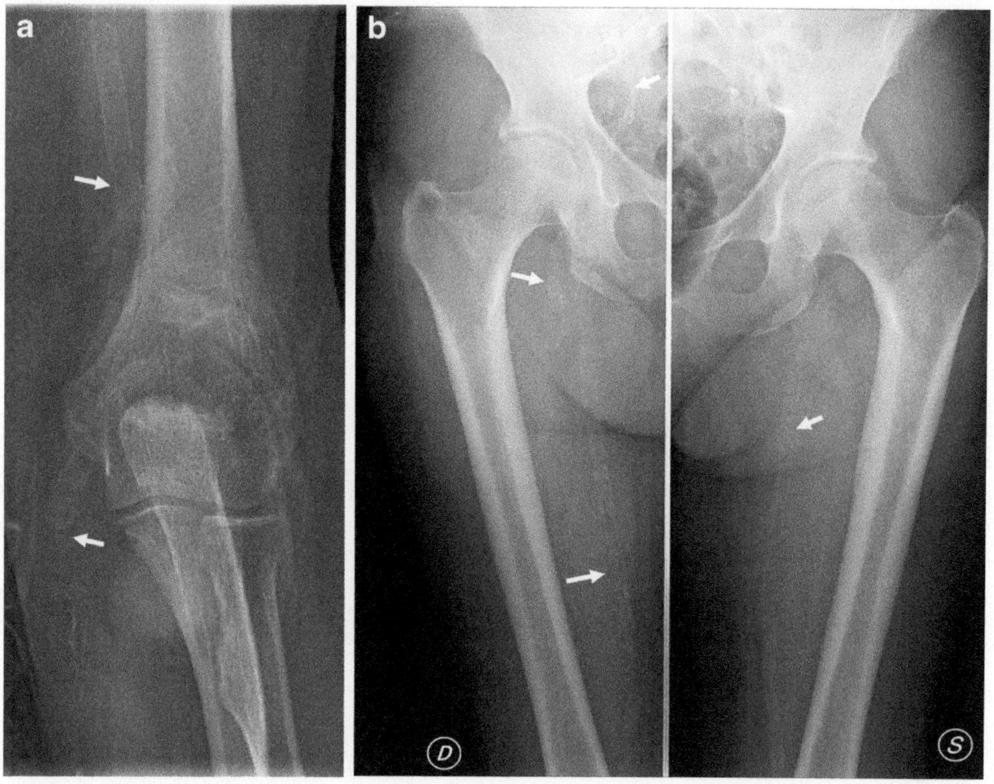

Fig. 12 **a**, **b**: Radiographic images of several skeletal segments of different patients (all undergoing long-term haemodialysis) show diffuse calcifications of the peripheral arteries (*arrows*). Vascular calcifications appear as both medial and intimal calcifications of arteries

hypertension, increased arterial stiffness, anaemia, vascular access flow (arteriovenous fistula) and sympathetic activation. Patients undergoing dialysis present a higher risk of atherosclerosis, also for underlying diabetes mellitus and/or hypertension as causes of end-stage renal disease [4]. Atherosclerosis involves the main and all the peripheral arteries including the intrarenal arteries. Calcifications of the myocardium, coronary arteries and cardiac valves are frequently observed in patients with end-stage renal disease [40, 42].

Cardiovascular calcification lesions can lead to the development of a number of clinically significant complications, including myocardial ischaemia, myocardial infarction, impaired myocardial function, congestive heart failure, cardiac valve insufficiency and cardiac arrhythmias [43, 44]. It has been demonstrated that B2-microglobulin amyloid deposits are extensively localised in the hearts of long-term haemodyalisis patients [45], in particular at the level of the endocardium, myocardium and wall of the small vessels [24].

Thoracic complications

Patients with chronic renal failure may present several abnormal findings visible on chest radiography due to changes in the phosphorus and calcium metabolism, changes in haemostasis, arterial hypertension, fluid retention or due to dialysis.

The thoracic complications of haemodialysis may be classified into two main topics: cardiovascular and pulmonary [46].

Cardiovascular findings include aortic calcification, cardiomegaly, calcifications of the coronary arteries, pericardial effusion, pulmonary thromboembolism and intra-atrial thrombus [46].

The most frequent pulmonary abnormalities include interstitial and alveolar oedema due to congestive heart failure, pleural effusion, lung atelectasis, metastatic pulmonary calcifications and calcifications of the bronchial walls, pleura and chest wall vessels. Lung parenchymal abnormalities visible on CT include areas of ground-glass opacity, interlobular septal thickening, parenchymal fibrosis scars, emphysema bullae, peribronchovascular interstitial thickening, increased vascular calibre, bronchiectasis, and thickening of the pleura and fissures [46].

The frequency of pulmonary infections in uraemic patients is higher compared to the general population, with evidence of parenchymal consolidation and/or pleural effusion [46].

Staphylococcus aureus continues to be the most common (20.8 %) cause of bacterial infection among patients on long-term haemodialysis [46]. Patients on haemodialysis are at increased risk of developing active tuberculosis after primary infection, activation of quiescent disease or reactivation of pre-existing tuberculosis infection [46].

Neurologic complications

Patients with end-stage renal disease frequently have central nervous system abnormalities, some of them related to end-stage renal disease itself and others related to problems secondary to haemodialysis [47].

The most common neurologic complications in this patient group include focal white matter lesions, cerebral atrophy, dialysis encephalopathy, hypertensive encephalopathy, cerebral infarction, intracerebral haemorrhage, posterior reversible encephalopathy syndrome, osmotic demyelination syndrome, cerebral infection, sinus vein thrombosis and dialysis disequilibrium syndrome. Peripheral neuropathy is also common in patients with chronic renal failure [5].

Acute cerebrovascular disease is one of the most frequent causes of morbidity and mortality in patients on long-term haemodialysis treatment. Cerebral ischaemia and infarction are important risk factors for stroke and are caused by the occlusion of the small, deeply penetrating cerebral arteries. Haemodialysis patients are at greater risk of cerebral haemorrhage because of anticoagulant therapies (e.g., heparin and low-molecular-weight heparins), defects of platelet adhesion, anaemia and inadequate control of hypertension. Cerebral haemorrhage may be intraparenchymal, subdural, epidural or subarachnoid. Patients with end-stage renal disease also have predisposing factors that lead to sinus vein thrombosis.

Haematologic abnormalities

Haematologic abnormalities are among the most consistent manifestations of uraemia [4]. These abnormalities include anaemia, bleeding and granulocyte and platelet dysfunction. The primary causes of anaemia in chronic renal failure are deficiency of erythropoietin, which is a glycoprotein normally produced by the kidney, and iron deficiency due to a reduced iron intake and frequent blood sampling. Erythropoietin therapy has improved the general status of patients with chronic renal failure. In patients with uraemic syndrome the fat bone marrow is progressively replaced by haematopoietic marrow content with a hypointense appearance on T1-weighted MR images in various anatomical regions (especially the spine and upper and lower limb bones). A haemorrhagic diathesis is common in patients with chronic renal failure. Spontaneous non-traumatic bleeding may affect the perinephric and subcapsular spaces, renal parenchyma or collecting system. Gastrointenstinal bleeding is also common in uraemic patients [5].

Encapsulating peritoneal sclerosis

Although medical considerations may dictate the choice of continuous ambulatory peritoneal dialysis (CAPD) or haemodialysis for some patients, most cases of renal failure are treatable with either method.

Therefore, it is important to recognise some potentially fatal complications of CAPD that must be detected at an early stage in order to allow a prompt interruption of CAPD and direct the patient toward the haemodialysis treatment only.

Encapsulating peritoneal sclerosis is an uncommon serious complication of CAPD [48] associated with significant morbidity and mortality.

In a large study by Rigby and Hawley [49], the overall prevalence of encapsulating peritoneal sclerosis is 0.7 %; however, the prevalence increases to 19.4 % in patients who have been on CAPD [49] for more than 8 years.

Encapsulating peritoneal sclerosis is a condition characterised by fibrotic thickening of the peritoneum, which can progress to the encasement or encapsulation of the small-bowel loops with a resultant bowel obstruction. The peritoneal thickening can be smooth or irregular and nodular, and mild peritoneal thickening typically progresses to diffuse, severe peritoneal thickening and eventually peritoneal calcification.

Peritoneal thickening progresses to peritoneal encapsulation of the involved small-bowel loops, a process that has been described as the "cocooning" of the small bowel, by a sheath of fibrous, sclerosed peritoneum.

The small-bowel loops are often centrally collected by encapsulating the fibrotic peritoneum. The fibrotic process may appear as a mass of small bowel loops tethered together. Ultimately, small-bowel necrosis with perforation may occur.

In encapsulating peritoneal sclerosis, the fibrotic, thickened peritoneal membranes can result in loculated ascites. Since the small bowel becomes involved, tethered and mass-like, the tethered small bowel may also produce loculated fluid collections.

Numerous other complications related to peritoneal dialysis have been described, including catheter dysfunction, haematoma, dialysate leak and hydrothorax [50].

Dialysis access complications

Repeated access to the circulation is essential to perform an adequate maintenance haemodialysis. End-stage renal failure patients requiring long-term haemodialysis need a durable vascular access, and the maintenance of an acceptable vascular access is an important issue for patients with renal failure. Haemodialysis is usually performed with an internal arteriovenous fistula (AVF) or polytetrafluoroethylene (PTFE, Teflon) graft, also known as a prosthetic bridge graft (PBG). Surgically constructed arteriovenous (AV) fistulas (radio- or brachiocephalic), synthetic AV grafts or a venous catheter positioned in a central vein are common means of establishing a vascular access for long-term haemodialysis.

Vascular stenosis is the major cause of access failure. The treatment of stenosis with percutaneous interventions, angioplasty, endoluminal vascular stents or thombolysis as an alternative to surgery has been shown to increase the chance of survival for patients with AVF and PBG dialysis [51]. Several surveillance techniques can be used for the prompt detection of access stenosis development. Colour Doppler US [52] and digital subtraction angiography [53] are most commonly used for the detection of access stenosis, while contrast-enhanced multi-detector CT [54] and MR angiography of shunts [55] have recently been introduced. Angiographic evaluation via puncture of the brachial artery is indicated when an interventional procedure is planned.

Arteriovenous fistulas

The AV fistula is considered the best long-term vascular access for haemodialysis because it provides adequate blood flow, is long-lasting and has a lower complication rate than other types of access. A nephrologist or surgeon creates an AV fistula. As a result, the vein grows larger and stronger, making repeated needle insertions for haemodialysis treatments easier. AV fistulas also present some disvantages, including the incomplete maturation of the vein, and a 1–4-month period may be required before the AV fistula can be used. Fistula dysfunction is the most common reason for a second intervention and recurrent hospitalisation. The rate of AVF complications increases with age and the erythropoietin dose as well as among patients with a history of a previous failed shunt [56]. The clinical symptoms include poor flow with loss of thrill in the graft, enlarging pseudoaneurysm or ipsilateral limb swelling.

The main complications of AV fistula include thrombosis with occlusion or stenosis of the venous outflow (Fig. 13a, c) as well as aneurysm or pseudoaneurysm of the venous tract (Fig. 14a, c) close or distal to the anastomosis with the radial artery [57]. In particular, the venous outflow obstruction is the most common cause of AVF thrombosis and poor dialysis.

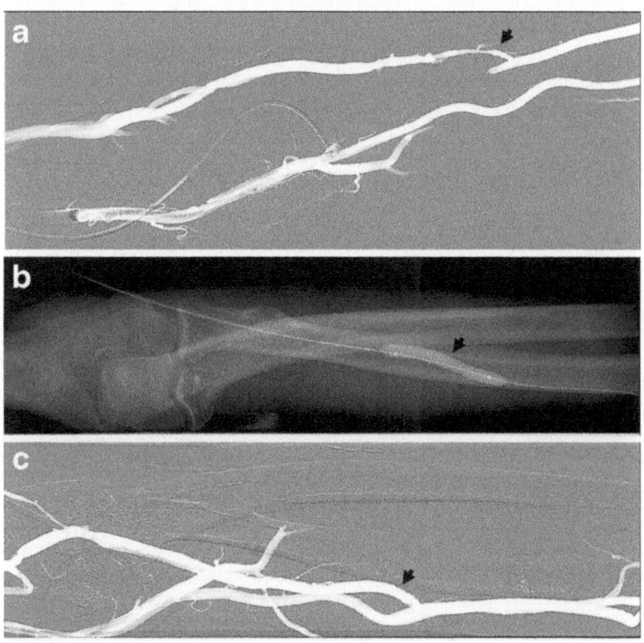

Fig. 13 a–c: An 80-year-old male patient with chronic renal failure undergoing haemodialysis. Stenosis (about 5 cm in length) of outflow of AVF of the arm (*arrow*) (**a**), treated by angioplasty (**b**) with recovery of the normal patency (**c**)

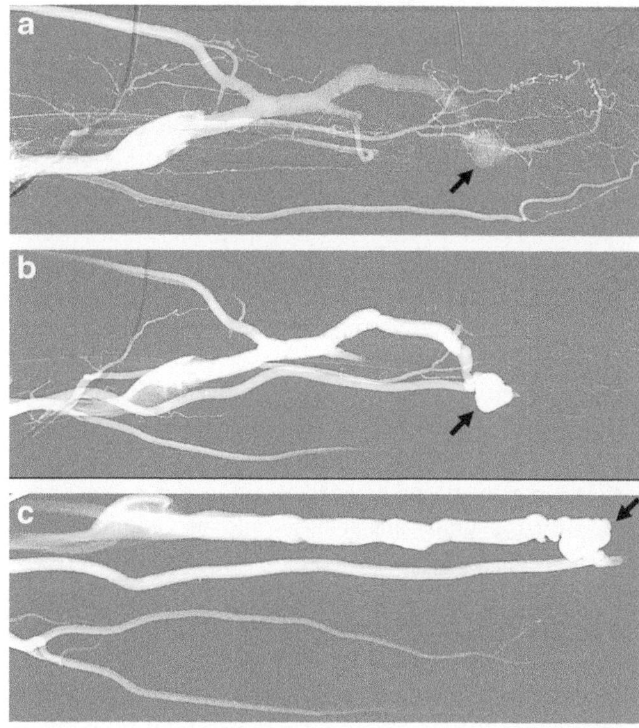

Fig. 14 a–c: AVF of the forearm at the level of the metaphysis of the radius in a 70-year-old patient with chronic renal failure under dialysis. Outflow perianastomotic pseudoaneurysms (*arrows*). Vein aneurysms or pseudoaneurysms are located in the puncture site

Most typically, pseudoaneurysms are found in areas of repeated puncture or surgical anastomosis.

Complications of the arterial tract of AVFs are rare. Proximal arterial disease, the occlusion or arterial anastomotic stenosis are readily shown by digital subtraction angiography. The arterial stenosis appears as a narrowed area adjacent to or between areas of graft ectasia. The laceration of the radial artery may determine a haematoma with compression of the nervous structures in the carpal tunnel.

Arteriovenous grafts

The AV fistula with its long patency rate and low complication profile is usually the first choice for vascular access creation. However, when superficial veins are not suitable for the AV fistula creation, or they have all been exhausted as a result of repeated AV fistula procedures, arteriovenous grafts using expanded polytetrafluoroethylene (PTFE) are an alternative [58]. The PTFE graft—prosthetic bridge graft (PBG)—consists of a synthetic catheter inserted and sutured into an artery, usually the radial artery, and a vein, usually the cephalic or the basilic vein.

Unlike the arteriovenous fistula used for chronic haemodialysis, the AV graft can be used immediately. Just as in natural AVF, the non-dominant arm should be used first [58]. Compared to properly formed fistulas, grafts tend to have more problems with clotting and infections and require earlier replacement. However, a well-cared-for graft can last several years.

The overall complication rate for AV grafts is twice as that of AV fistulas. The most common complication associated with the AV graft is venous outflow obstruction with graft thrombosis, which accounts for 85 to 90 % of problems with haemodialysis. PBGs have a shorter mean patency than native AVFs. The most common causes of failure include the surgical twisting or kinking of the graft during implantation, arterial plugs, stenosis of the venous anastomosis or an unsuspected venous stenosis. Venous stenosis results in problems that have the net effect of causing inadequate dialysis. Stenosis most frequently involves the venous anastomosis, but it may occur anywhere within the system composed by the graft, anastomosis and its draining veins. Complete thrombosis is easily identified when it involves the graft or the entire venous limb. Moreover, AV grafts may produce complications related to arterial inflow stenosis, arterial anastomotic stenosis, intragraft stenosis, graft pseudoaneurysm and graft degeneration. Treatment options are either a surgical revision or endovascular stent graft placement.

Dialysis access catheters

The high thrombosis rate of AVF and PBGs and the high recurrence rates after thrombolysis and angioplasty have led to consideration of performing haemodialysis with percutaneously inserted venous catheters. Nowadays, venous catheters are often taken into consideration as a long-term solution for haemodialysis because of the improvement in biomaterials available for catheters. Percutaneous venous catheters present the advantage of being placed on an outpatient basis; moreover, they do not require any maturation period, and they prevent repeated punctures of the AVF. The disavantages are represented by the fact that venous catheters are cosmetically less acceptable, and the achievable peak of flow rates are lower than with AVFs and PBGs.

A venous catheter positioned in a central vein (usually the right internal jugular vein or, less frequently, the femoral or subclavian veins) through the subclavian vein for a temporary access has two chambers to allow a two-way flow of blood. Once a catheter has been placed, the needle insertion is not necessary. Catheters are not ideal for permanent access, and their patency is maintained via a heparin-saline infusion by flushing the catheter with 2 or 3 ml of heparin (2,000–3,000 units) twice daily (every 12 h). They can clog, become infected, and cause stenosis or complete thrombosis of the central vein in which they are placed. However, if there is a need to starting haemodialysis immediately, a catheter will work for several weeks or months while the permanent access is gradually developing.

References

1. Cohen AJ, AH ed (MP1991) *Use of dialytic procedures in the intensive care units*. Intensive care medicine, ed. I.R. Rippe JM, Alpert JS, Fink, Little, Brown and Company: Boston. 742–764
2. Stuart S et al (2009) Complications of continuous ambulatory peritoneal dialysis. Radiographics Rev Public Radiol Soc North Am Inc 29(2):441–460
3. Richardson RM (2012) The diagnosis of tuberculosis in dialysis patients. Semin Dial 25(4):419–422
4. DG W (ed) (1992) Chronic renal failure. Cecil textbook of medicine, ed. S.L. Wyngaarden JB, Bennett JC, Saunders: Philadelphia. 533–541
5. Quaia E, SS (ed) (2011) Imaging of Dialysis Radiological Imaging of the Kidney, ed. Q. Springer. 793–810
6. Petersen LJ et al (1995) The pulsatility index and the resistive index in renal arteries in patients with hypertension and chronic renal failure. Nephrol Dial Transplant Off Public Eur Dial Transplant Assoc Eur Ren Assoc 10(11):2060–2064
7. Petersen LJ et al (1997) The pulsatility index and the resistive index in renal arteries. Associations with long-term progression in chronic renal failure. Nephrol dial Transplant Off Public Eur Dial Transplant Assoc Eur Ren Assoc 12(7):1376–1380
8. Denton MD et al (2002) Prevalence of renal cell carcinoma in patients with ESRD pre-transplantation: a pathologic analysis. Kidney Int 61(6):2201–2209
9. Ferda J et al (2007) Computed tomography of renal cell carcinoma in patients with terminal renal impairment. Eur J Radiol 63(2):295–301
10. Doublet JD et al (1997) Renal cell carcinoma of native kidneys: prospective study of 129 renal transplant patients. J Urol 158(1): 42–44
11. Pope JC, Koch MO, Bluth RF (1994) Renal cell carcinoma in patients with end-stage renal disease: a comparison of clinical significance in patients receiving hemodialysis and those with renal transplants. Urology 44(4):497–501
12. Kliem V et al (1997) Risk of renal cell carcinoma after kidney transplantation. Clin Transplant 11(4):255–258
13. Hoshida Y et al (1999) Renal neoplasias in patients receiving dialysis and renal transplantation: clinico-pathological features and p53 gene mutations. Transplantation 68(3):385–390
14. Ishikawa I, Kovacs G (1993) High incidence of papillary renal cell tumours in patients on chronic haemodialysis. Histopathology 22(2): 135–139
15. Takebayashi S et al (2000) Renal cell carcinoma in acquired cystic kidney disease: volume growth rate determined by helical computed tomography. Am J Kidney Dis the off J National Kidney Found 36(4):759–766
16. Roy C et al (2005) Papillary renal cell carcinoma in allograft kidney. Eur Radiol 15(4):661–665
17. Scandling JD (2007) Acquired cystic kidney disease and renal cell cancer after transplantation: Time to rethink screening? Clin J Am Soc Nephrol 2(4):621–622

18. Schwarz A et al (2007) Renal cell carcinoma in transplant recipients with acquired cystic kidney disease. Clin J Am Soc Nephrol 2(4): 750–756
19. Fleischmann D (2003) Multiple detector-row CT angiography of the renal and mesenteric vessels. Eur J Radiol 45(Suppl 1):S79–S87
20. Bellido JA et al (2007) [Early ultrasound detection of renal tumors in patients with end stage renal disease in dialysis]. Arch Esp Urol 60(9):1 079–83
21. Filocamo MT et al (2009) Renal cell carcinoma of native kidney after renal transplantation: clinical relevance of early detection. Transplant Proc 41(10):4197–4201
22. Hurst FP et al (2011) Incidence, predictors and associated outcomes of renal cell carcinoma in long-term dialysis patients. Urology 77(6): 1271–1276
23. Theodorou DJ, Theodorou SJ, Resnick D (2002) Imaging in dialysis spondyloarthropathy. Semin Dial 15(4):290–296
24. Niwa T (2001) Dialysis-related amyloidosis: pathogenesis focusing on AGE modification. Semin Dial 14(2):123–126
25. Katz R, ML (2007) Carmichael J, et al., Musculoskeletal manifestations of chronic renal failure and dialysis, in Radiological Society of North America scientific assembly and annual meeting program, Chicago
26. Jevtic V (2003) Imaging of renal osteodystrophy. Eur J Radiol 46(2): 85–95
27. States LJ (2001) Imaging of metabolic bone disease and marrow disorders in children. Radiol Clin North Am 39(4):749–772
28. Bereket A et al (2000) Brown tumour as a complication of secondary hyperparathyroidism in severe long-lasting vitamin D deficiency rickets. Eur J Pediatr 159(1–2):70–73
29. Cicconetti A, Matteini C, Piro FR (1999) [Differential diagnosis in a case of brown tumor caused by primary hyperparathyroidism]. Minerva stomatol 48(11):553–558
30. Jeren-Strujic B et al (2001) Secondary hyperparathyroidism and brown tumor in dialyzed patients. Ren Fail 23(2):279–286
31. Fatma LB et al (2010) Brown tumors in patients with chronic renal failure and secondary hyperparathyroidism: report of 12 cases. Saudi J Kidney Dis Transpl an Off Publ Saudi Cent Organ Transpl Saudi Arabia 21(4):772–777
32. Lessa MM et al (2005) Brown tumor of the facial bones: case report and literature review. Ear Nose Throat J 84(7):432–434
33. Ketteler M et al (2005) Pathogenesis of vascular calcification in dialysis patients. Clin Exp Nephrol 9(4):265–270
34. Trent JT, Kirsner RS (2001) Calciphylaxis: diagnosis and treatment. Adv Skin Wound Care 14(6):309–312
35. Datta C et al (2005) Tumoral calcinosis. Indian J Dermatol Venereol Leprol 71(4):293–294
36. Raggi P et al (2002) Cardiac calcification in adult hemodialysis patients. A link between end-stage renal disease and cardiovascular disease? J Am Coll Cardiol 39(4):695–701
37. Jono S et al (2000) Phosphate regulation of vascular smooth muscle cell calcification. Circ Res 87(7):E10–E17
38. Gelev S et al (2008) Vascular calcification and atherosclerosis in hemodialysis patients: what can we learn from the routine clinical practice? Int Urol Nephrol 40(3):763–770
39. Giachelli CM et al (2001) Vascular calcification and inorganic phosphate. Am J Kidney Dis Off J National Kidney Found 38(4 Suppl 1): S34–S37
40. Guerin AP et al (2000) Arterial stiffening and vascular calcifications in end-stage renal disease. Nephrol Dial Transplant off Publ Eur Dial Trans Assoc Eur Ren Assoc 15(7):1014–1021
41. Iwasa Y et al (2012) Prevalence of intracranial artery calcification in hemodialysis patients–a case-control study. Int Urol Nephrol 44(4): 1223–1228
42. Braun J et al (1996) Electron beam computed tomography in the evaluation of cardiac calcification in chronic dialysis patients. Am J kidney dis Off J National Kidney Found 27(3):394–401
43. London GM et al (2000) Calcification of the aortic valve in the dialyzed patient. J Am Soc Nephrol JASN 11(4):778–783
44. Ribeiro S et al (1998) Cardiac valve calcification in haemodialysis patients: role of calcium-phosphate metabolism. Nephrol Dial Transplant Off Public Eur Dial Transplant Assoc Eur Ren Assoc 13(8):2037–2040
45. Takayama F et al (2001) Dialysis-related amyloidosis of the heart in long-term hemodialysis patients. Kidney Int Suppl 78:S172–S176
46. Lakadamyali H, Ergun T (2008) Thorax CT findings in symptomatic hemodialysis patients. Transplant Proc 40(1):71–76
47. Brouns R, De Deyn PP (2004) Neurological complications in renal failure: a review. Clin Neurol Neurosurg 107(1):1–16
48. Kawaguchi Y et al (2005) Recommendations on the management of encapsulating peritoneal sclerosis in Japan, 2005: diagnosis, predictive markers, treatment, and preventive measures. Perit Dial Int J Int Soc Perit Dial 25(Suppl 4):S83–S95
49. Rigby RJ, Hawley CM (1998) Sclerosing peritonitis: the experience in Australia. Nephrol Dial Transplant Off Publ Eur Dial Transplant Assoc Eur Ren Assoc 13(1):154–159
50. Zandieh S et al (2014) Radiological diagnosis of dialysis-associated complications. Insights Imaging 5(5):603–617
51. van der Linden J et al (2002) Short- and long-term functional effects of percutaneous transluminal angioplasty in hemodialysis vascular access. J Am Soc Nephrol JASN 13(3):715–720
52. Doelman C et al (2005) Stenosis detection in failing hemodialysis access fistulas and grafts: comparison of color Doppler ultrasonography, contrast-enhanced magnetic resonance angiography, and digital subtraction angiography. J Vasc Surg 42(4):739–746
53. Froger CL et al (2005) Stenosis detection with MR angiography and digital subtraction angiography in dysfunctional hemodialysis access fistulas and grafts. Radiology 234(1):284–291
54. Rooijens PP et al (2008) Multi-slice computed tomographic angiography for stenosis detection in forearm hemodialysis arteriovenous fistulas. J Vasc Access 9(4):278–284
55. Pinto C et al (2006) Time-resolved MR angiography with generalized autocalibrating partially parallel acquisition and time-resolved echo-sharing angiographic technique for hemodialysis arteriovenous fistulas and grafts. J Vasc Interv Radiol JVIR 17(6):1003–1009
56. Salahi H et al (2006) Complications of arteriovenous fistula in dialysis patients. Transplant Proc 38(5):1261–1264
57. Rodriguez HE et al (2005) Arteriovenous access: managing common problems. Perspect Vasc Surg Endovasc Ther 17(2):155–166
58. Nikeghbalian S, Bananzadeh A, Yarmohammadi H (2006) Difficult vascular access in patients with end-stage renal failure. Transplant Proc 38(5):1265–1266

21

Dual-energy CT after radiofrequency ablation of liver, kidney, and lung lesions: a review of features

Frederik Vandenbroucke[1] · Steven Van Hedent[1] · Gert Van Gompel[1] · Nico Buls[1] · Gordon Craggs[1] · Jef Vandemeulebroucke[2,3] · Pablo R. Ros[4] · Johan de Mey[1]

Abstract Early detection of residual tumour and local tumour progression (LTP) after radiofrequency (RF) ablation is crucial in the decision whether or not to re-ablate. In general, standard contrast-enhanced computed tomography (CT) is used to evaluate the technique effectiveness; however, it is difficult to differentiate post-treatment changes from residual tumour. Dual-energy CT (DECT) is a relatively new technique that enables more specific tissue characterisation of iodine-enhanced structures because of the isolation of iodine in the imaging data. Necrotic post-ablation zones can be depicted as avascular regions by DECT on greyscale- and colour-coded iodine images. Synthesised monochromatic images from dual-energy CT with spectral analysis can be used to select the optimal keV to achieve the highest contrast-to-noise ratio between tissues. This facilitates outlining the interface between the ablation zone and surrounding tissue. Post-processing of DECT data can lead to an improved characterisation and delineation of benign post-ablation changes from LTP. Radiologists need to be familiar with typical post-ablation image interpretations when using DECT techniques. Here, we review the spectrum of changes after RF ablation of liver, kidney, and lung lesions using single-source DECT imaging, with the emphasis on the additional information obtained and pitfalls encountered with this relatively new technique.

Teaching Points

- *Technical success of RF ablation means complete destruction of the tumour.*
- *Assessment of residual tumour on contrast-enhanced CT is hindered by post-ablative changes.*
- *DECT improves material differentiation and may improve focal lesion characterisation.*
- *Iodine maps delineate the treated area from the surrounding parenchyma well.*

Keywords Dual-energy CT · Radiofrequency ablation · Liver · Lung · Kidney

✉ Frederik Vandenbroucke
spovef@uzbrussel.be

1 Department of Radiology, UZ Brussel (VUB), Laarbeeklaan 101, Brussels, Belgium

2 Department of Electronics and Informatics, Vrije Universiteit Brussel, Brussels, Belgium

3 Department of Medical IT, iMinds, Ghent, Belgium

4 Department of Radiology, University Hospitals Case Medical Center/Case Western Reserve University, Cleveland, OH, USA

RF Ablation

Minimally invasive therapies are increasingly used in patients with malignant tumours, who are not suitable candidates for surgical resection. The aim of local ablative therapy is to induce cell death. Radio-frequency (RF) ablation has attracted much attention in the last decade because of its technological improvements and has become a well-established technique to treat primary and secondary hepatic malignancies, as well as kidney and lung tumours.

Technical success following RF ablation is due to the complete destruction of the tumour. In case of incomplete necrosis of the tumoral volume, re-ablation of residual tumour can be pursued in order to improve technique effectiveness. For this reason, it is crucial to evaluate the results of the procedure early after ablation. The ideal imaging technique should show the degree of necrosis of the malignant mass and detect residual tumour.

Imaging immediately after ablation also allows for the detection of post-procedural complications and provides a baseline for future follow-up comparisons. Unfortunately, the assessment of residual tumour, usually by means of contrast-enhanced computed tomography (CT), is hindered by post-ablative changes, particularly at the periphery of a treated lesion where blood flow is greatest [1, 2].

On pathology this represents a haemorrhagic rim corresponding to an early inflammatory reaction to the necrotic tissue [3, 4]. Today, contrast-enhanced CT is the standard approach to image early post-ablative changes in the liver [5, 6], kidney [7], and lung [8]. However, some investigators have reported that although complete necrosis may appear clearly on contrast-enhanced CT, these findings do not always correlate with histopathological conclusions, which suggests that there is limited diagnostic accuracy in the detection of residual tumours [9–12].

Dual-energy CT

A well-known drawback of standard CT is that a number of different materials or tissues may show similar attenuation behaviour at single radiation energy levels and, with that, similar corresponding Hounsfield numbers. This poor attenuation difference can be partially resolved by using dual-energy CT (DECT) technology with material decomposition [13]. DECT is able to achieve tissue attenuation sampling at two different energy spectra, which results in more specific information beyond the typical Hounsfield units.

For already several years, three main technical approaches have been developed by various vendors for the acquisition of dual-energy data: a single-source rapid kilovolt peak-switching technique, a dual-source technique with an angular offset, and finally use of a dual-layer detector that discriminates between high- and low-energy photons [13]. The first two techniques obtain dual-energy data simultaneously at two different energy levels at typically 80 and 140 kVp, although dual-source systems can also operate at 100 and 140 kVp (with an additional tin filter) in case of larger patient sizes. The third technique uses the detected high- and low-energy signal components in one CT acquisition. More recently, a non-simultaneous, single-source technique has been reported that applies a sequential data acquisition and a coregistration motion correction algorithm [14]. It has been shown that DECT improves material differentiation and works especially well in materials with large atomic numbers, such as iodine and calcium, because their strong photoelectric effect causes high attenuation at lower photon energies [15]. The material decomposition technique assumes that for any tissue an equivalent mixture of

Table 1 Early and long-term findings after RF ablation of liver lesions in successful and unsuccessful results, with the added value of the DECT technique

		Early findings	Long-term findings
Successful	General findings	Non-enhancing area on contrast-enhanced CT Regular hypervascular peripheral rim Central hyperattenuation is indecisive for success	Regular borders of the ablation zone Reduction in size
	Added value of DECT	Iodine void area Improved contrast on the 40-keV images Excellent conspicuity of the ablation zone on iodine-coded images	Sharp depiction of the ablation zone's edge on iodine images
Unsuccessful	General findings	Irregular rim Focal nodular thickening at the border	Focal hypervascular nodule (HCC) Nodular attenuation differences around the ablation zone (hypovascular metastasis)
	Added value of DECT	Higher residual tumour-to-liver contrast on iodine images Increased attenuation of iodine on the low-keV images for detection of subtle residual tumour	Better contrast between LTP and liver parenchyma on iodine images

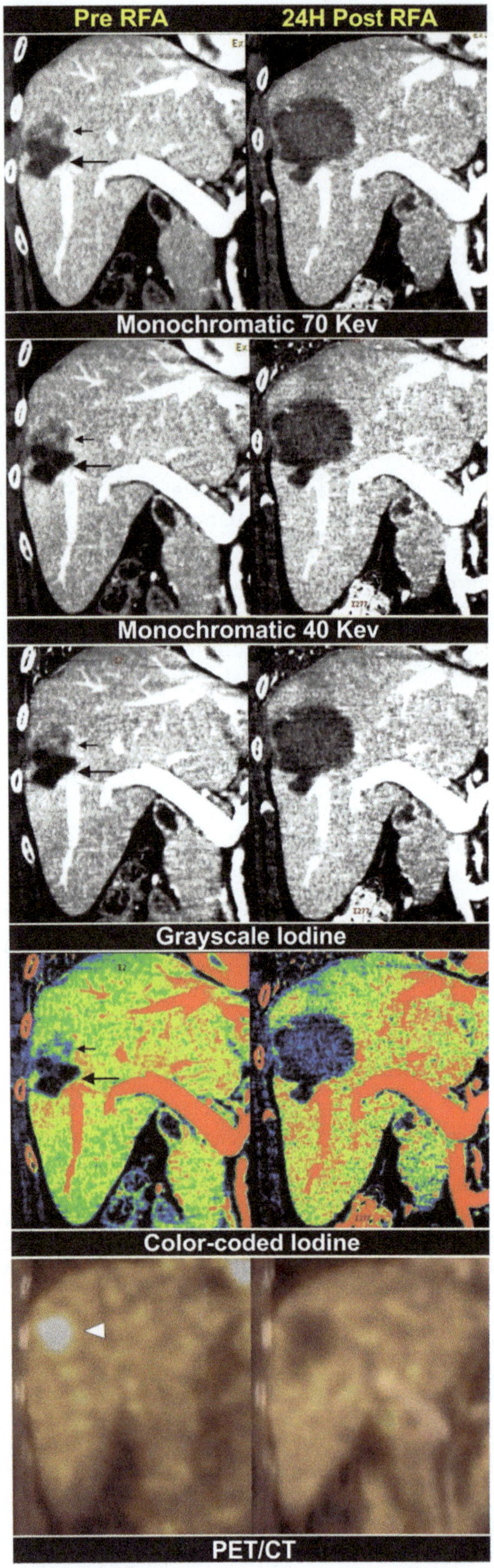

Fig. 1 Hypovascular liver metastasis. A 53-year-old female undergoes surgery for rectal carcinoma and then receives RF ablation in a focal liver lesion. Eight months later, a local tumour progression (first column) at the cranial side of the ablation zone (*large arrow*) can be seen as an intermediate density (*small arrow*). In this straightforward case, the tumoral tissue is equally well depicted on the 40- and 70-keV images as on the greyscale iodine images. Noise is more prominent on the 40-keV image however. Iodine maps are encoded using a rainbow template with a colour coding from high to low iodine concentration, being from red (through yellow) to blue respectively. The intermediate colour represents a tumour (*small arrow*). On PET/CT a vivid FDG uptake is seen (*arrowhead*). Twenty-four hours after a second RF ablation (second column), a sharp delineated ablation zone is found. On all reconstructions, the avascular nature of the ablation zone is well demonstrated. The contrast with the surrounding liver parenchyma appears highest on the colour-coded iodine map. No FDG uptake is seen on the PET/CT image. The PET/CT 3 months later (not shown) does not show signs of tumoral activity

water and iodine exists with similar spectral attenuation properties. Consequently, after a material decomposition calculation process, two base material maps can be displayed, representing the concentrations of water and iodine in each voxel. In contrast studies, these concentrations correspond to real water/iodine concentrations in blood. All other materials (e.g. bone, fat) are described as a mixture of both of these base materials and will appear as hyper- or hypodensity in the base pair maps. Iodine concentrations can be accurately quantified. A recent study showed a 0.55 mg/cc mean error when comparing calculated and true iodine concentrations in renal masses [16]. These calculated iodine concentrations (mg/cc) can be displayed for any region of interest (ROI) as either a greyscale- or colour-coded iodine image. Such iodine maps obtained from DECT images are not a surrogate for dynamic perfusion CT, as they merely provide a visualisation of the iodine distribution in the tissues at one point in time.

In addition to calculating base material maps, synthesised or synthesised monochromatic images from dual-energy CT, representing CT values (HU) over a range of 40 to 140 keV, can also be obtained. Compared to high-keV, low-keV images (closer to the k-edge of iodine) typically provide improved contrast between different structures, e.g. between a tumour and surrounding normal parenchyma after injection of iodinated contrast material. On the other hand, noise is more prominent in these lower keV images [17]. Synthesised monochromatic images at 77 keV correspond best to the effective energy of a single-energy

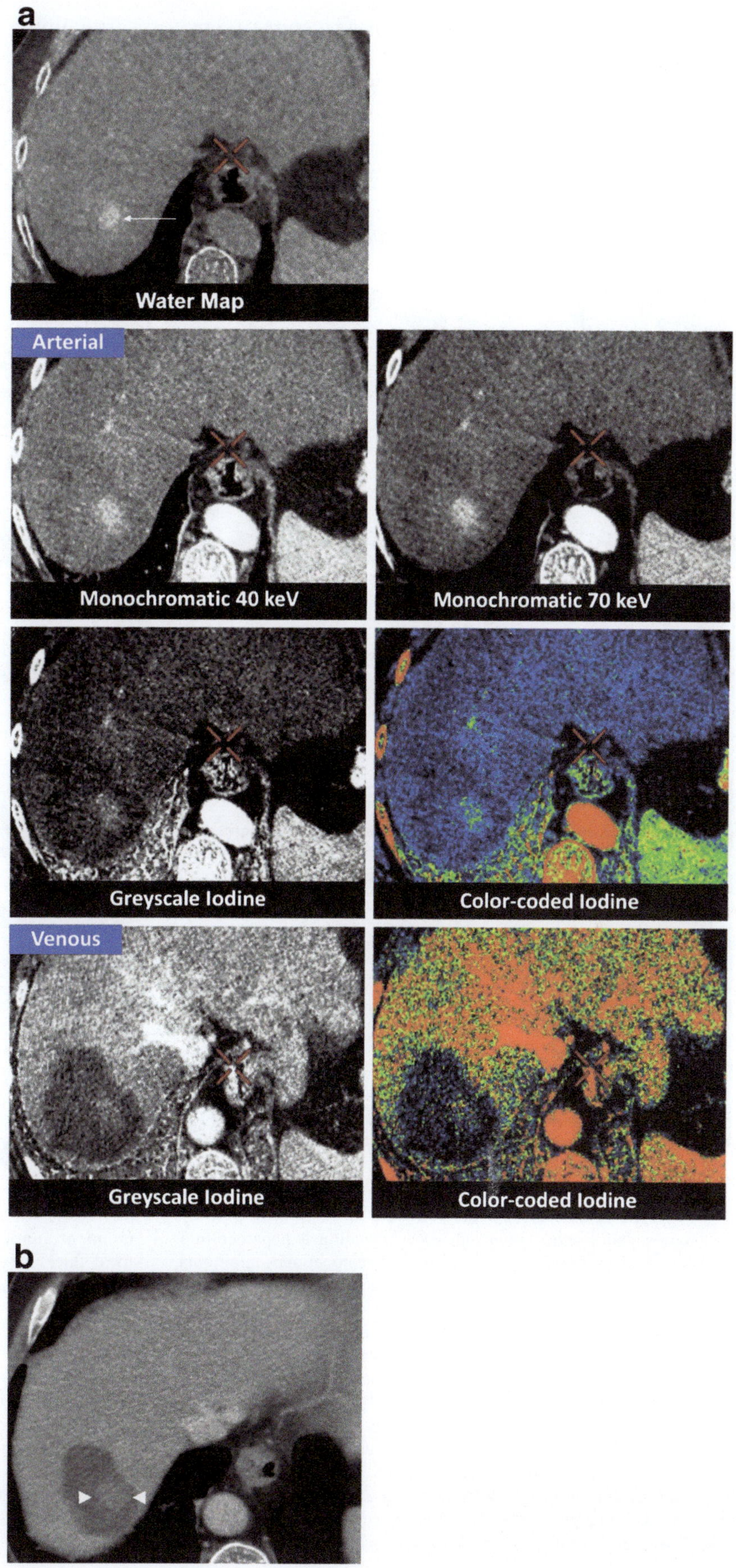

Fig. 2 Hypervascular metastasis. A 63-year-old male undergoes follow-up CECT in the arterial phase 4 years after ablation of a renal cell carcinoma. This reveals a 26-mm hypervascular lesion in segment VII of the liver, which is histopathologically proven to be a metastasis of the RCC. RF ablation is performed. **a** Twenty-four hours after the ablation, a DECT is performed. The water map image shows a centrally located hyperdensity in the ablation zone (*arrow*), corresponding to intense charring and desiccation of the treated lesion. Note that this hyperdensity is less visible on the iodine maps. The arterial phase image does not demonstrate any focal hypervascularity at the border of the ablation zone. No rim enhancement can be seen. The delineation of the total ablation zone is better depicted on the portal-venous phase greyscale- and colour-coded iodine images, because the amount of iodine in the liver parenchyma is higher. **b** On the 1-year follow-up CECT, a smooth delineation of the ablation zone is noticed, which serves as proof of the technical success of the ablation. The central hyperdensity however is still noticeable (*arrowheads*)

120-kV scan [18], such that the image contrast simulates a traditional single-energy CT scan. By assessing the DECT images, an optimised keV window based on the contrast-to-noise ratio between tissues can be calculated. In RF ablation, an improved contrast is typically obtained between the ablation zone and surrounding normal liver parenchyma. A scatterplot analysis, which estimates the material concentration in each voxel, can also help to differentiate different structures in the ROIs. Research is currently ongoing with regard to adequate quantification of the acquired DECT data. Several potential candidate parameters are

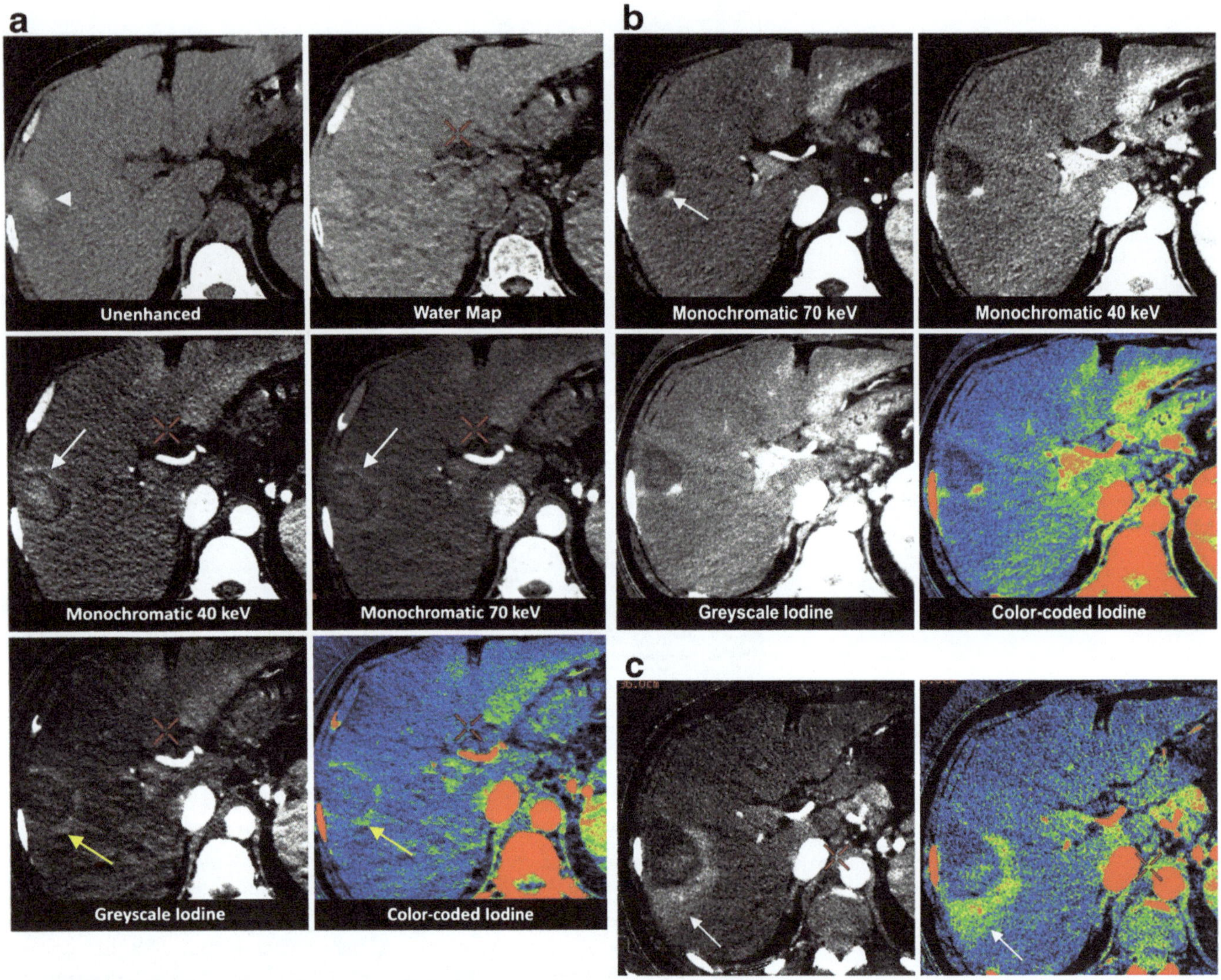

Fig. 3 Hepatocellular carcinoma. A 43-year-old male with cirrhosis undergoes gadolinium enhanced MRI, revealing a hepatocellular carcinoma in segment VII, typical for a hepatocellular carcinoma, which is confirmed through biopsy. **a** Twenty-four hours after RF ablation, the patient undergoes a standard unenhanced CT scan and a contrast-enhanced DECT. The unenhanced CT shows a central area of high attenuation (*arrowhead*) within the ablation zone, which has a lower visibility on the water map reconstruction. The central hyperdensity is well noticeable on the synthesised monochromatic 40-keV but less so on the 70-keV images, and it is hardly visible on the iodine images. On the 40- and 70-keV synthesised monochromatic images, the ablation zone can be depicted as a lesion with a hypervascular peripheral rim (*white arrows*). On the greyscale- and colour-coded iodine images, we can better appreciate the focal hypervascular thickening at the posterior border (*yellow arrows*) than with the synthesised monochromatic images. **b** Due to the suspicious nature of the focal thickening seen in **a**, a shorter follow-up period is adhered to and a DECT is performed 5 weeks post-RF ablation. A focal hypervascular nodule is well depicted on the 70-keV (*white arrow*) images, although more clearly observable on the 40-keV ones; however again it is more evident on the greyscale- and colour-coded iodine images. Biopsy of this region confirms residual HCC. **c** Twenty-four hours after the second ablation, the greyscale- and colour-coded iodine images show significant iodine rim uptake around the ablation zone in the arterial phase (*arrows*). Therefore, a focal hypervascular remnant cannot be appreciated. This rim disappears on the venous phase (not shown). MRI after 10 weeks reveals no signs of reactivation

Table 2 Early and long-term findings after RF ablation of kidney lesions in successful and unsuccessful results, with the added value of the DECT technique

		Early findings	Long-term findings
Successful	General findings	Non-enhancing area on the contrast-enhanced CT Often wedge shaped because of peripheral infarctions Streaky soft tissue attenuations in the perirenal fat	Regular borders of the ablation zone Slow reduction in size Fat between the ablation zone and normal kidney parenchyma
	Added value of DECT	Improved contrast on the 40-keV images Clear differentiation between avascular and viable tissues on iodine images	Sharp depiction of the ablation zone's edge on the iodine images
Unsuccessful	General findings	Persistent enhancement at the border of the ablation zone	Nodular attenuation difference around the ablation zone
	Added value of DECT	Iodine concentrations that are similar to the original tumour, with quantitative assessment Higher lesion-to-liver contrast on the iodine images	Intermediate iodine concentration between the ablation zone and normal kidney parenchyma at the level of the tumour

being screened for usefulness within the RFA context, such as CT numbers (i.e. Hounsfield unit curves) [19, 20], contrast-to-noise ratios [20, 21] or iodine concentrations [22]. Compared to standard CT, DECT may have the potential to improve focal lesion characterisation, and it is a promising tool to supply quantitative data in addition to traditional morphological information. The associated radiation dose with DECT will depend on the applied technology. Although specific clinical studies comparing the dose efficiency of different technologies are still lacking, current data suggest that DECT imaging with dual-source systems does not necessarily cause additional radiation exposure for the patient compared to standard CT [17, 23, 24]. Radiation dose data on the rapid kilovolt peak–switching technique to date are still inconclusive and reports from other approaches are scarce or nonexistent [25]. However, the increased informational content and post-processing flexibility of DECT data create additional opportunities for dose saving, such as the creation of virtual unenhanced images from a contrast-enhanced scan [25].

The purpose of this pictorial essay is to display post-ablative changes on contrast-enhanced CT with a single-source rapid kilovolt peak-switching technique in order to identify the additional information provided by DECT imaging and to describe the pitfalls of this relatively new technique in the evaluation of RF ablation's technical success.

DECT imaging protocol

Fast kilovoltage switching CT was performed on a 64-slice CT (Discovery CT750 HD, GE Healthcare, Milwaukee, WI, USA) after IV administration of 120 cc contrast at 2.5 cc/s. Scan data were acquired at 40-mm collimation using predefined GSI protocols at $CTDI_{vol}$ values between 15.02 and 25.53 mGy. Fixed tube currents (between 375 and 600 mA) were used as our DECT scanning mode is not compatible with the automated tube current modulation system of the scanner. Images were processed on a workstation (AW4.4; GE Healthcare) using the Gemstone Spectral imaging application. Three types of images were reconstructed for analysis: synthesised monochromatic images from 40 to 140 keV, greyscale- and colour-coded iodine images (with 'rainbow' colour map).

Liver ablation

Necrosis caused by thermal damage is characterised by an absence of blood perfusion, resulting in a non-

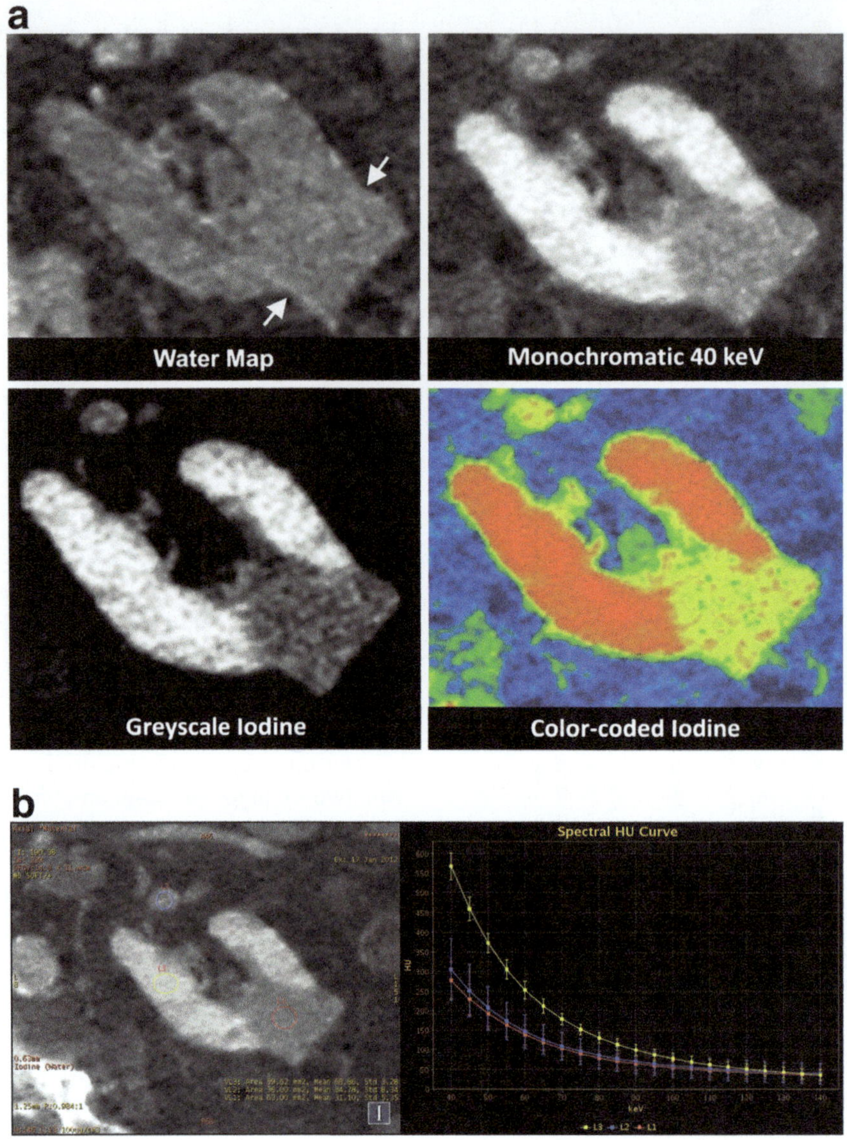

Fig. 4 Renal cell carcinoma. An ultrasound reveals a renal mass in a 72-year-old male. **a** Venous phase DECT confirms a lesion in the left kidney. On the water map images, the lesion is exophytic and isodense compared to the kidney parenchyma (*arrows*). The synthesised monochromatic 40-keV greyscale-coded and colour-coded iodine images show a hypovascular lesion compared to the kidney parenchyma. A biopsy demonstrates a renal clear cell carcinoma. **b** On the iodine-coded image (left), three ROIs are selected: L1 (red) in the RCC; L2 (blue) in the renal vein; L3 (yellow) in the unaffected kidney parenchyma. The estimated amounts of iodine in the ROIs are presented in the right lower corner (mean value and standard deviation in 100 $\mu g/cm^3$). On the spectral HU curve (right), the renal vein (L2) and RCC (L1) represent overlapping curves, suggesting similar iodine content. The normal kidney parenchyma (L3) has a markedly higher curve in the lower keV range, confirming a higher iodine uptake. **c** Axial (left column) and coronal (right column) reconstructions from a contrast-enhanced venous phase DECT, 24 h post-RF ablation. The water map images show very poor hyperattenuation in the ablated zone (*arrowheads*). The contrast difference between the ablation zone and the kidney parenchyma is well demonstrated on the synthesised monochromatic 40- and 70-keV images. The colour-coded iodine images show well-depicted areas of intermediate density on the axial reconstructions (*black arrows*) surrounding the ablation zone. The axial images of the synthesised monochromatic reconstructions less clearly visualise these regions. The multiplicity suggests a benign post-ablative finding, probably corresponding to transient thermal damage to the bordering kidney parenchyma. No definitive conclusion can be made concerning residual tumour solely relying on these images. However, compared to the pre-ablation imaging, we can assume that the tissue in question is a normal kidney parenchyma. At the outer margin of the ablation zone, a region of intermediate density is depicted. The coronal reconstructions are essential to prove the continuity with regard to the kidney parenchyma (*white arrows*). **d** On the follow-up CECT 15 months later, the focally enhanced tissue at the lateral side shows no signs of growth (*arrow*), thus confirming the absence of residual tumour

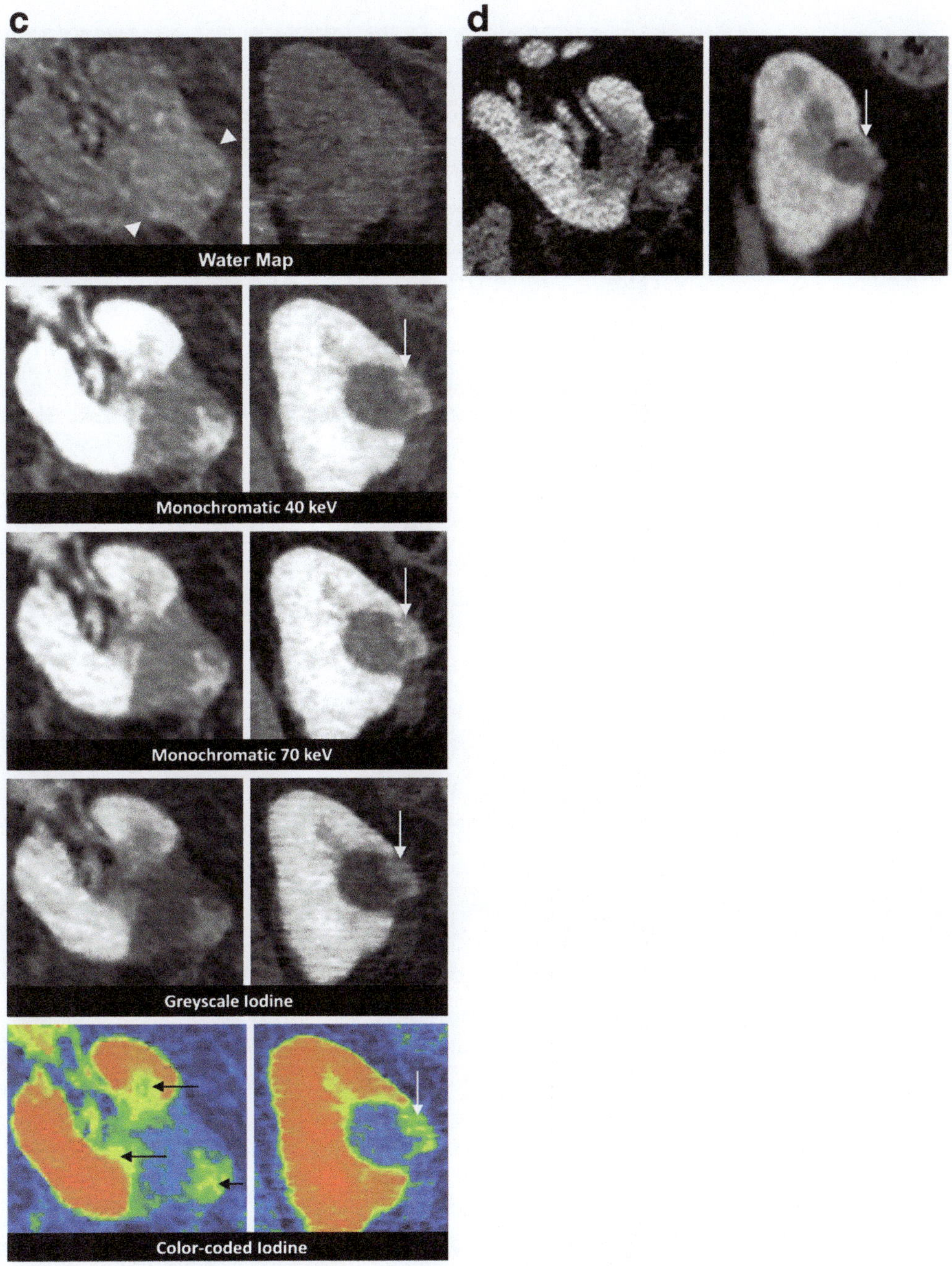

Fig. 4 (continued)

enhancing area on contrast-enhanced CT (Table 1). Due to this lack of internal vascularity, iodine maps are well suited for delineating the treated area from the liver parenchyma (Figs. 1 and 2a). Dual-energy CT has the possibility to extract iodine from the enhanced images to create water map images and thus potentially skip true unenhanced images, as shown in Fig. 3a. This undoubtedly offers a considerable advantage in limiting radiation dose exposure [23]. However, a drawback is that current DECT techniques do not produce water map images with the same contrast-to-noise ratio as true unenhanced images [26].

Frequently, a hyperattenuation centrally within the ablation zone can be seen on unenhanced images [27]. It is thought that this area of high density correlates to a region of greater cellular disruption in the centre of the ablation zone [3], reportedly caused by the intense charring of the severely desiccated coagulated lesion [28]. It has usually disappeared by the time the next follow-up CT examination takes place, but can

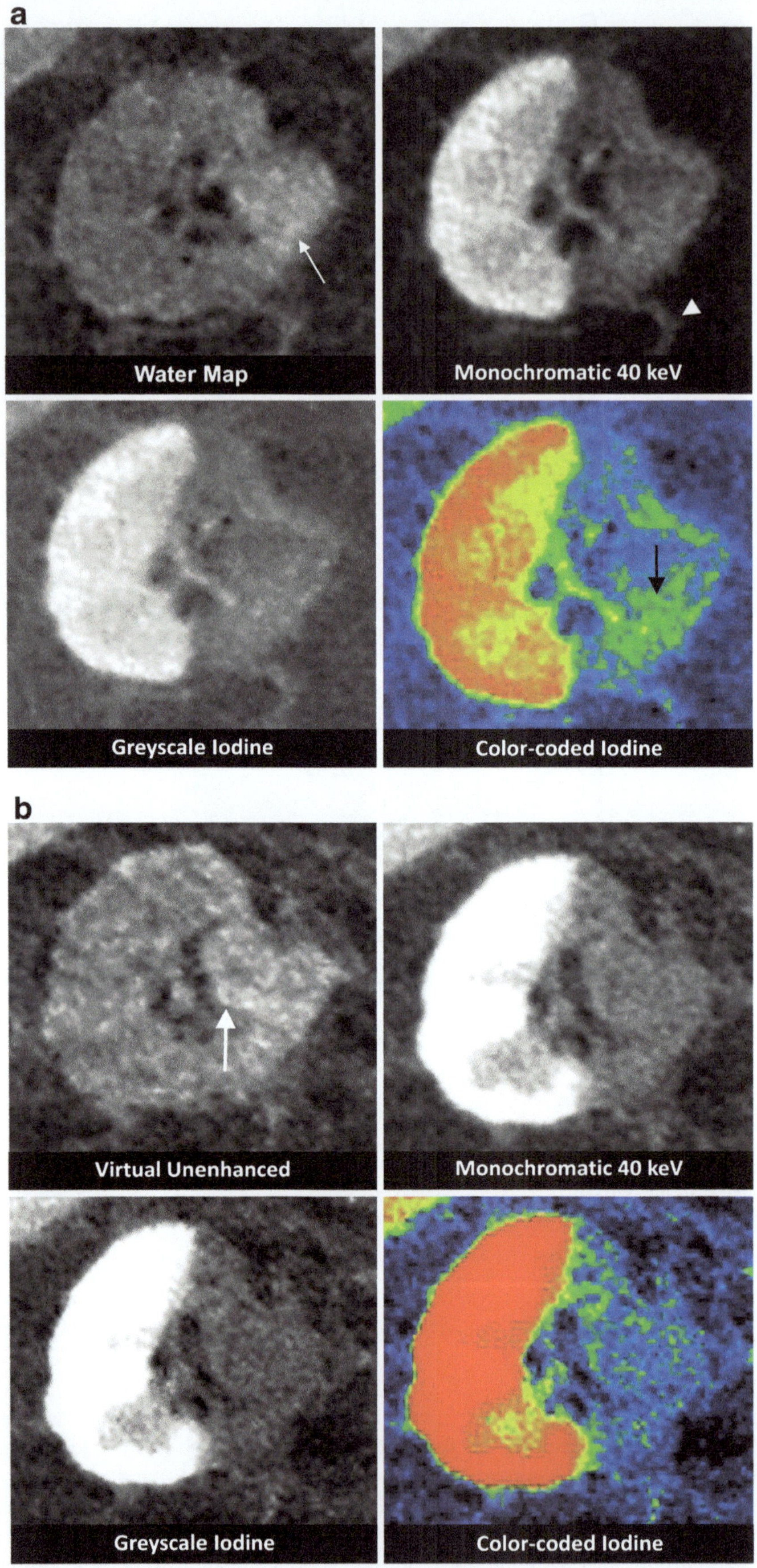

Fig. 5 Renal cell carcinoma. A lesion in the right kidney of a 73-year-old male is confirmed as being a hypernephroma through biopsy. The patient is treated with RF ablation, while cooling the pyelum with a double j-stent. **a** The DECT obtained 24 h post ablation shows a hyperdense region in the ablation zone on the water map images (*white arrow*). On the synthesised monochromatic 40-keV images, a sharp delineation of the ablation border is assessed, without the presence of any internal hyperdensity in the ablation zone. A post-procedural, streaky, soft-tissue attenuation can be seen in the surrounding perirenal fat (*arrowheads*). The avascular zone is well depicted on the greyscale- and colour-coded iodine images. In this window level, some yellowish coloured pixels are seen in the centre of the ablation zone on the colour-coded iodine images (*black arrow*), lying in the extension of a branch of the renal artery, explainable as being spilled iodine due to arterial perfusion. **b** DECT reconstructions at a 3-month follow-up stage show an overall stability in the size of the ablation zone. The ablated zone is still slightly hyperdense on the water map image (*arrow*). There is no uptake of iodinated contrast on the greyscale- and colour-coded iodine images, which proves that this area is completely avascular and confirms that the colour pixels seen in **a** were not a sign of tumour activity

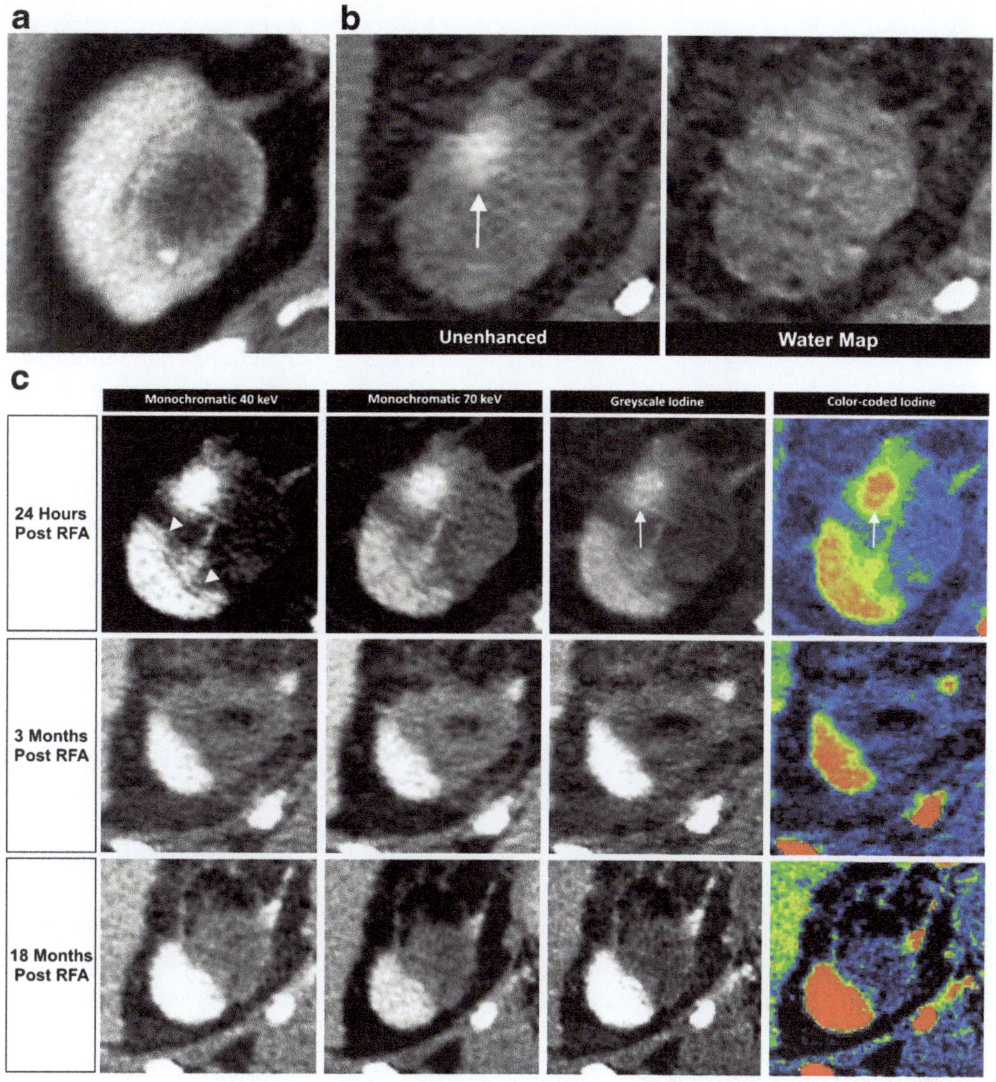

Fig. 6 Renal cell carcinoma. A 40-year-old female is diagnosed with a suspicious lesion in the right kidney on ultrasound. After consulting her urologist, the patient opts for RF ablation. **a** CECT shows a thick-walled cystic lesion in the right upper pole, graded as a Bosniak 4 cyst. **b** The true unenhanced polychromatic CT image (left), 24 h post ablation, shows a hyperdense change in the ablation zone (*arrow*). This finding cannot be confirmed on the water map reconstructions. **c** The imaging appearance of the ablation zone 24 h (*first row*), 3 months (*second row*), and 18 months (*third row*) after RF ablation. On the 24-h post-ablation series, the delineation of the ablation zone is clearly observable on all reconstructed images; however, the 40 keV image is of superior quality when compared to the 70-keV image (*arrowheads*). On the iodine-coded images, the internal high attenuation is unexpectedly (no iodine content) still visible within the avascular zone (*arrows*). No suspicious nodular enhancement is observed at the border of the ablation zone. DECT from 3- and 18-month follow-up depicts an involution of the avascular zone. There is a loss of the internal high-attenuation changes. There is no evidence of local tumour progression

persist for a longer time [29] (Fig. 2b). This hyperattenuation is observable on both the water map and true unenhanced images. Despite the absence of iodine, this can also be seen on the iodine-coded images, since the hyperattentuated area is represented as a combination of both water and iodine after material decomposition (Fig. 2a). Meticulous comparison of water and iodine-coded images allows for differentiation of this central hyperattenuation after RF ablation and structures enhancing after IV contrast administration. The reader should however be aware of the lower image quality of water images with respect to true unenhanced images (Fig. 3a), as also reported on dual-source DECT [20]. Similar to the study of Lee et al. [20], we observed sharp depiction of the edge of the ablation zone of the iodine images. Contrary to their findings obtained using a dual-source DECT system, our experience with single-source DECT images did not prove an internal homogeneity of the ablation zone on the iodine images.

Immediately after ablation, it is common to find a hyper-attenuating halo surrounding the ablation zone on CECT, correlated to an increase in arterial perfusion due to capillary leakage from thermal damage [30]. The circumferential enhancement is predominantly visible on the arterial phase and can be very prominent in some cases (Fig. 3c), obscuring the interpretation of residual tumour. An irregular or nodular rim can indicate the presence of residual tumour, although benign variations do occur [30–32]. When focal thickening at the border of the ablation zone is unclear, a shorter follow-up period is recommended [32]. Previous studies have shown that a hypervascular rim remains visible in 89 % of cases after 1 month, in 56 % of cases between 1 and 3 months, and in 22 % of cases between 3 and 6 months [33]. Ideally, the volume of

Table 3 Early and long-term findings after RF ablation of lung lesions in successful and unsuccessful results, with the added value of the DECT technique

		Early findings	Long-term findings
Successful	General findings	Partial or circumferential ground-glass opacification surrounding the treated tumour	Reduction in size
	Added value of DECT	Vanishing of the iodine uptake in the treated tumour, with a clear delineation of the avascular zone on the iodine-coded images	Shrinkage of the avascular zone
Unsuccessful	General findings	Lack of ground-glass opacification around a part of the tumour is not decisive of success	Centrally located enhancements - Enhancement not already present immediately after the RF ablation Growth of the ablation zone Change from ground-glass to solid opacity
	Added value of DECT	Improved contrast of iodine in the lesion on the 40-keV and iodine-coded images 'Enhancing' of a part of the tumour on the 40-keV compared to the water map image	Internal iodine uptake in the ablation zone

thermal necrosis exceeds the limits of the metastasis by 1 cm in all dimensions [34]. Residual tumour will persist as a focal nodular enhancement in the periphery of the ablation zone (Fig. 3b). For dual-energy CT, the increased attenuation of iodine on the low-keV (e.g. around 40 keV) images is better suited for detecting any subtle density differences around the ablation zone (Fig. 3b). Adding colour-coding enhances the visibility of the contrast in the image.

The water-iodine material decomposition can highlight areas containing iodinated contrast. Iodine maps are superior to synthesised monochromatic images for the qualification of contrast uptake. Consequently, a hypervascular nodule with a higher inflow of iodine is better depicted on the iodine maps when compared to synthesised monochromatic images (Fig. 2b).

Kidney ablation

Ablation zones in the kidneys lack iodine content and are often wedge shaped because of peripheral infarctions [35] (Table 2). Determining a tumour's iodine concentration before RF ablation can provide a baseline for future follow-up assessments (Fig. 4a, b). Iodine concentrations that are similar to the original tumour post ablation can be a sign of local tumour progression. The iodine content can be assessed qualitatively as well as quantitatively in the investigated ROI (Fig. 4b).

When evaluating the contrast uptake in a lesion, it is imperative to compare the lesion's density on the water map images to that on the synthesised monochromatic images in order to be able to appraise possible 'enhancement'. The iodine content can be assessed qualitatively based on the iodine-coded images as well as quantitatively when expressed in iodine concentrations (mg/ml) (Fig. 4b) in the investigated ROI. Enhancement can also be demonstrated by comparing the iodine concentration in the lesion to a surrounding vascular structure after an IV contrast injection. When evaluating colour-coded iodine maps, it is important to compare iodine concentrations in the ROI to those in adjacent structures, because windowing (as a diagnostic tool) causes variability in the colour spectrum.

As with liver lesions, the extent of necrosis in the ablation zone can be assessed more accurately on 40-keV rather than on 70-keV synthesised monochromatic images. Also, the iodine maps show clear differentiation between avascular and viable tissues. Adjacent to the avascular zone, regions of intermediate vascularity can be seen that appear most pronounced on colour-coded iodine images (Fig. 4c). This may correspond to

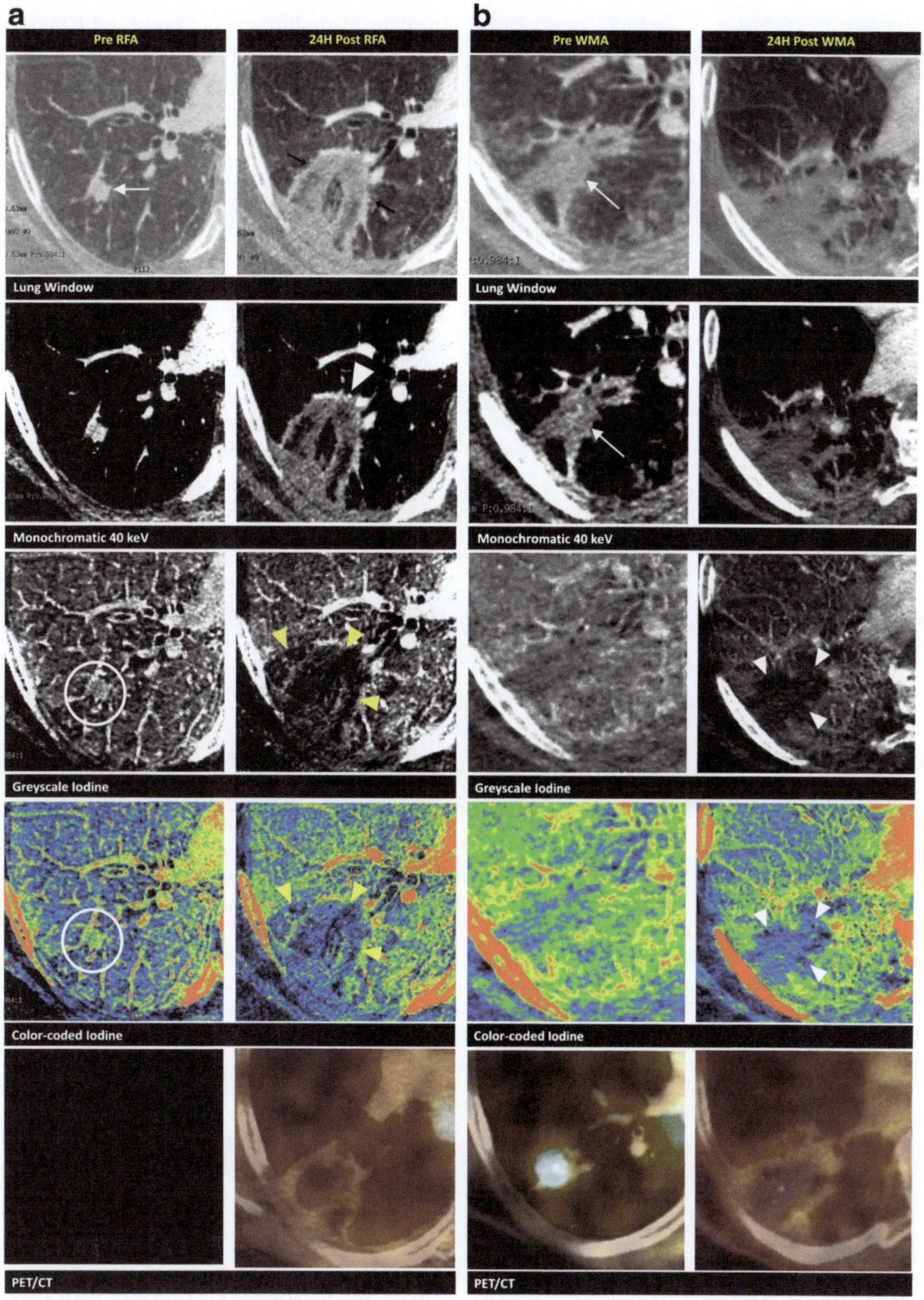

transient thermal damage to the adjacent kidney parenchyma, causing a temporary blood flow decrease in this area. Multi-planar reconstructions are vital in the assessment of questionable regions after the RF

◀ **Fig. 7** Pulmonary metastases. A 77-year-old female, with a known melanoma, undergoes a PET/CT that shows a hypermetabolic nodule in the right upper lobe (not in our possession). The biopsy is non-conclusive. The therapeutic option is RF ablation. **a** Imaging is performed before (first column) and 24 h after (second column) RF ablation. The 70-keV lung window shows a focal nodule of 11 mm (*white arrow*) in proximity of a blood vessel. This nodule is hyperdense on the synthesised monochromatic 40-keV images and shows iodine content on the greyscale- and colour-coded iodine maps (*circles*). Destructive lung parenchyma is seen after the ablation as an irregular hyperdensity on the lung window (*black arrows*). The synthesised monochromatic 40-keV reconstructions show very heterogeneous densities in this region. The vessel on the anterior side is still intact (*white arrowhead*). On the iodine maps, we clearly observe the absence of iodine uptake (*yellow arrowheads*). PET/CT shows no activity in this region. **b** Imaging is performed before (first column) and 24 h after (second column) microwave ablation (MWA). After 6 months, a well-circumscribed consolidation is seen on the 70-keV lung window and synthesised monochromatic 40-keV image (*arrows*). The greyscale- and colour-coded iodine maps show no focal iodine uptake. This consolidation is hypermetabolic on PET/CT. As a result of the discrepancy between the morphologic and metabolic imaging methods, and the proximity of the blood vessel, which could lead to a heat-sink effect, the patient opts for further focal thermal treatment through microwave ablation. Twenty-four hours after ablation, a large heterogeneously shaped density is recognised on the lung window. The greyscale- and colour-coded iodine maps very clearly show the zone without internal contrast uptake (*arrowheads*) when compared to the 40-keV images. Again, a photopenic area is seen on the PET/CT image

ablation procedure (Fig. 4c). Although avascularity is by definition a sign of successful ablation, the ablation zone can show remnants of iodine concentration, possibly due to the extravasation of iodine which itself is caused by vascular damage (Fig. 5a).

The majority of ablation zones are hypodense in nature; however, it is not uncommon to have a variable degree of haemorrhagic necrosis in the necrotic area. This degree of attenuation is not predictive of technique effectiveness (Fig. 6c). Since the quality of the water maps is less compared to the true unenhanced images, spontaneous hyperdensity may be missed by this reconstruction technique (Fig. 6b).

In the contrast to rim enhancement that is commonly found in liver ablations, this phenomenon has only been observed occasionally in ablated renal parenchyma [25]. If present, it resolves quickly and is only marginally visible after 3 months [36]. Post-ablative changes in the perirenal fat are predominantly seen as streaky soft tissue attenuations (Fig. 5a), which resolve to a dominant band or halo over time (Fig. 4d). Long-term follow-up findings include the development of fat between the ablation zone and normal kidney parenchyma [37, 38] (Fig. 4d). The majority of kidney ablations show little to no reduction in size within the first 6 to 12 months [39, 40]; however, earlier shrinkage is not uncommon (Fig. 6c).

Lung ablation

When performing RF ablation of lung lesions, the goal is to achieve an avascular region, void of any iodine enhancement (Table 3). Dual-energy CT in the lungs can depict an abnormal blood flow distribution, improving the detection of acute pulmonary embolism [41]. In addition, we believe that the complete avascular ablative area post ablation is well depicted on the iodine-coded images as an iodine-void area. Therefore, iodine mapping may be an excellent method to evaluate the technique effectiveness and also delineates a more realistic assessment of the necrotic zone after ablation (Fig. 7a). On CECT imaging, the absence of iodine uptake in an ablated lung lesion is hard to identify since the boundary between the ablated and non-ablated tissue cannot be clearly defined (Fig. 8).

The typical finding on lung window CT during and after RF ablation is ground-glass opacification surrounding the treated tumour, which is fully circumferential (Fig. 8) in the majority of cases, but can also be partial (Fig. 9a). It is less common to find ground-glass opacification along the electrode tract. These ground-glass changes typically lead to an overestimation of the necrosis zone by 2–4 mm [42]. The distinction between the inner necrotic zone and the outer haemorrhagic viable zone is not clear on CT imaging; thus, the effective necrotic zone is easily overestimated [8]. As a result, the boundary between the ablated and non-ablated zones cannot be clearly defined using traditional morphologic imaging (Fig. 7b).

It is unclear how the iodine images provide a more realistic view of the necrotic zone after ablation. Kawai et al. [43] evaluated the feasibility of distinguishing ground-glass opacification in adenocarcinomas from that in a haemorrhage or inflammation. They found that there was an increased iodine-related attenuation in adenocarcinomas, but not in a pulmonary haemorrhage or in inflammatory changes. These findings led us to investigate the possible benefits of using iodine maps to distinguish residual tumours (Fig. 9) from the common post-ablative changes found in lung ablation. On follow-up CECT, centrally located enhancements or enhancements that were not present immediately after the RF ablation are indicative of malignancy [44]. Even without enhancement, growth of the ablation zone (after 8 to 10 weeks) or any peripheral nodule is a cause for concern. A change from ground-glass opacity to solid opacity also requires further investigation [43]. Positron

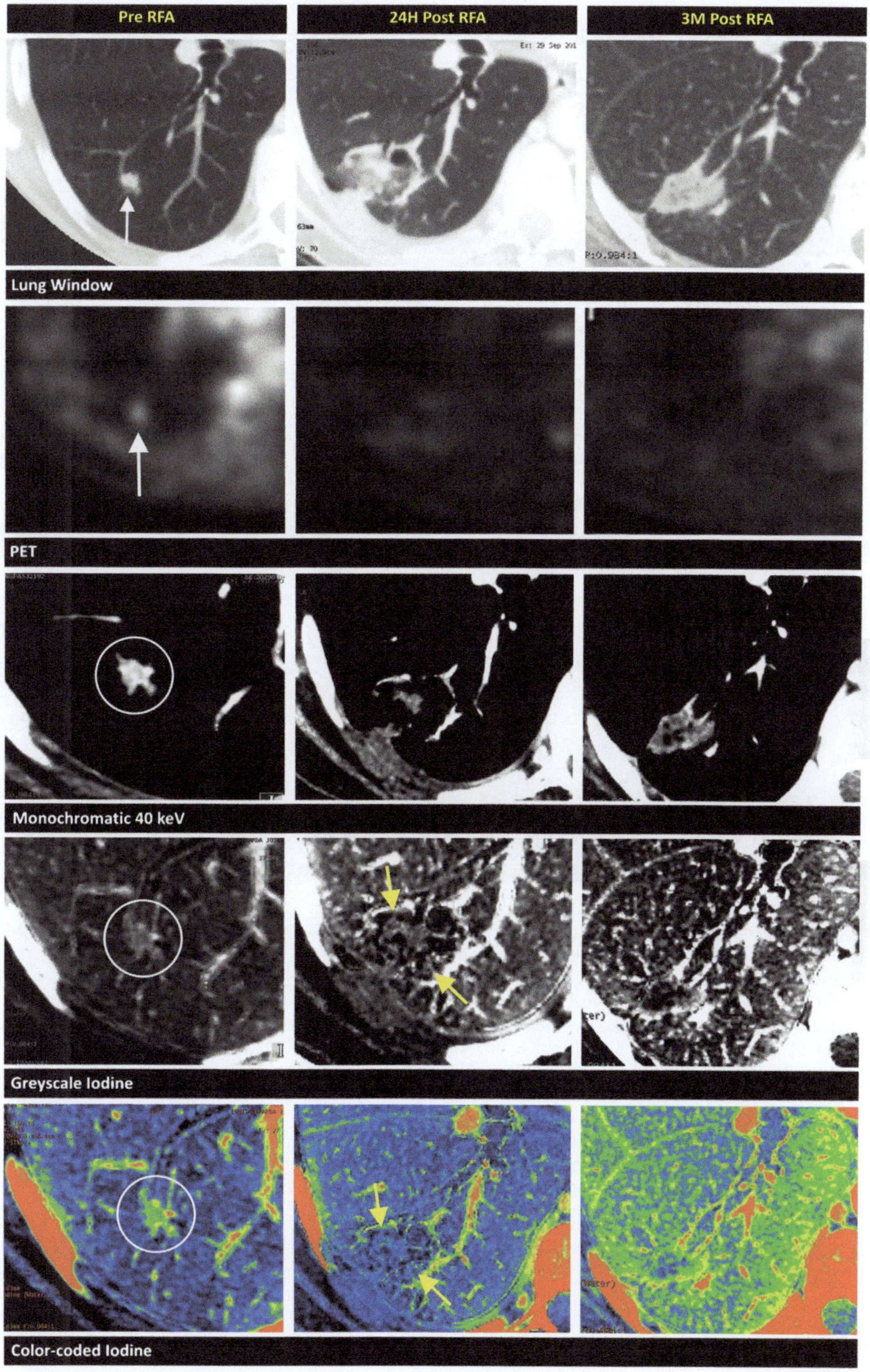

Fig. 8 Pulmonary metastases. A 69-year-old female, with a history of breast cancer diagnosed 9 years prior, shows a hypermetabolic nodule in the inferior lobe of the right lung on PET/CT. A biopsy reveals a metastasis of a ductal mammary carcinoma. An RF ablation is performed. Imaging of the lesion 1 day before (first column), **24 h** after (second column), and 3 months after (third column) complete RF ablation is performed. Before ablation, an 8-mm well-circumscribed nodule is depicted on the synthesised monochromatic 70-keV lung window, FDG-avid on the PET scan (*white arrows*). Internal vascularisation is clearly observable on the contrast-enhanced, synthesised monochromatic 40-keV, greyscale- and colour-coded iodine images (*circles*). The changes found 24 h post ablation are a ground-glass appearance (*yellow arrowheads*) around the lesion and the vanishing of the previously seen iodine uptake in the lesion. The post-ablative avascular zone surrounding the necrotic lesion can be delineated on the iodine images as darker areas (*yellow arrows*). On the lung window images after 3 months, the treated area has transformed into a homogeneous, well-delineated area of high attenuation. PET/CT images reveal no activity after the RF ablation. The greyscale- and colour-coded iodine images show a reduction in size of the avascular region

emission tomography/CT is considered the optimal follow-up tool after focal ablation in the lung. Residual disease can be detected through tracer uptake, most likely at the periphery of the ablation zone (Fig. 9b). On follow-up, increased or new metabolic activity located centrally (Fig. 7b) or at the outer rim

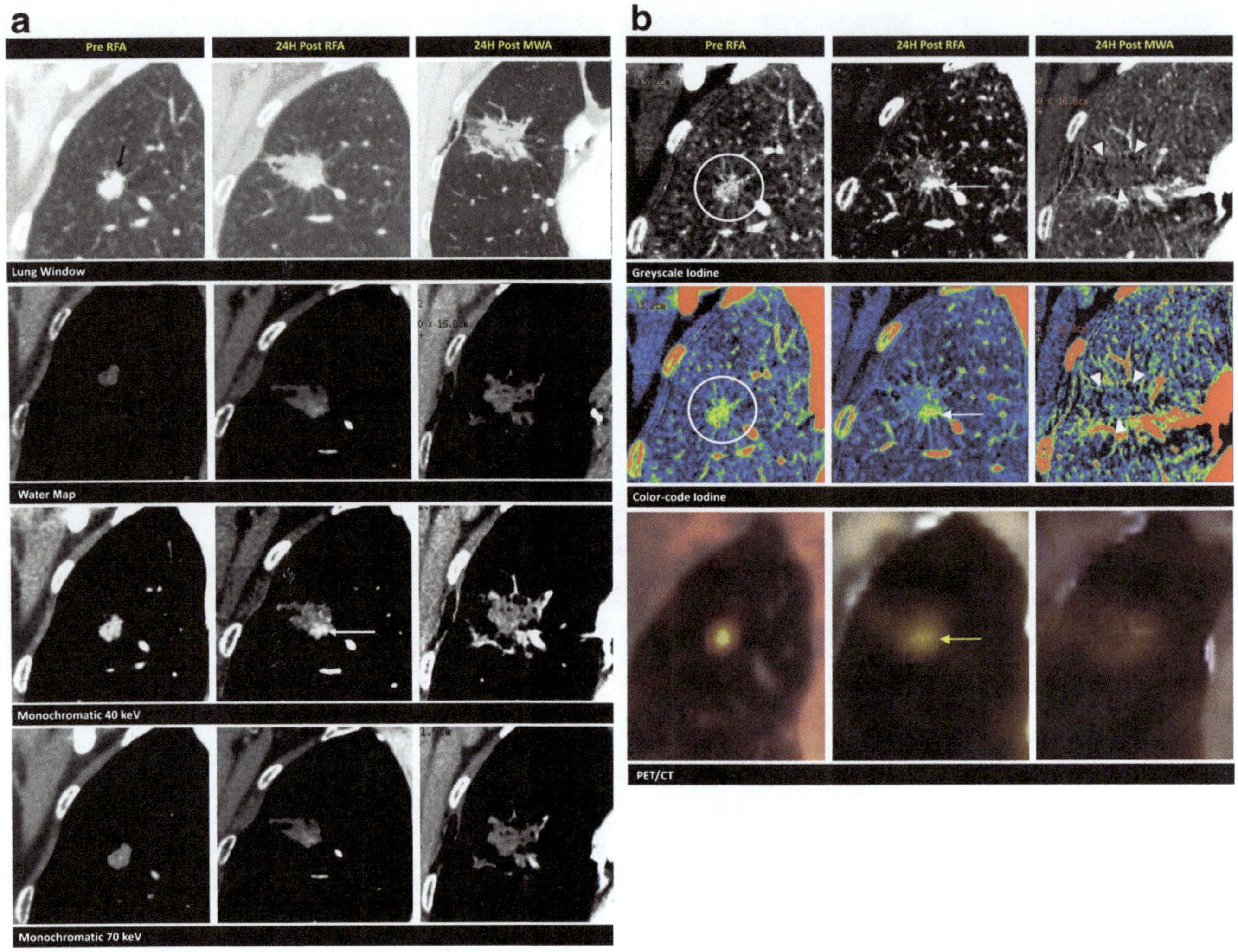

Fig. 9 Pulmonary metastases. A focal lung nodule is found in a 65-year-old female diagnosed with ovarian carcinoma. A biopsy reveals a non-small-cell carcinoma. A multidisciplinary team meeting leads to the choice for RF ablation treatment. Coronal reconstructions of the lesion in the right upper lobe before (first column), 24 h after the first RF ablation (second column), and 24 h after microwave ablation (third column) are demonstrated. **a** A focal nodule of 9 mm in the upper lobe is seen on the 70-keV lung window (*black arrow*) prior to the ablation. This nodule is "enhanced" on the synthesised monochromatic images compared to the water map image. This "increase in density" is better appreciated on the 40-keV rather than on the 70-keV images. Twenty-four hours after the first ablation, the spicular nodule appears enlarged on the lung windows. On the 40-keV image, a focal enhancement (*arrow*) is noted at the inferior border of the ablation zone, again more clearly visible compared to the 70-keV image. After re-ablation with microwave technique, we notice more important changes on the lung window than after the first ablation. **b** The iodine content of the hypermetabolic lesion before the RF ablation is most observable on the greyscale- and colour-coded iodine images (*circles*). The nodule is hypermetabolic on PET/CT. Twenty-four hours after the first ablation, the greyscale- and colour-coded iodine maps clearly show the focal area of iodine uptake (*white arrows*) on the inferior border. PET/CT confirms hypermetabolic remnants (*yellow arrow*). After re-ablation, the larger area of thermal damage has lost its internal focal iodine uptake, which is most appreciable on the iodine-coded images (*arrowheads*). Images after the re-ablation lack FDG uptake on PET/CT

of the ablation zone is a sign of progressive tumour activity [44].

Conclusion

Post-ablative changes can hamper the evaluation of post-ablation zones. Our pictorial review illustrates the potential improvements that DECT provides in the differentiation of tissues. We believe that DECT can be a valuable asset in the differentiation of residual tumours from benign inflammatory changes, commonly found after the ablation of liver, kidney, and lung tumours. Further investigation is required because of the limited clinical experience with this relatively new technique.

References

1. Vogt FM, Antoch G, Veit P et al (2007) Morphologic and functional changes in nontumorous liver tissue after radiofrequency ablation in an in vivo model: comparison of 18 F-FDG PET/CT, MRI, ultrasound, and CT. J Nucl Med 48:1836–1844
2. Lee JM, Jin GY, Goldberg SN et al (2004) Percutaneous radiofrequency ablation for inoperable non-small cell lung cancer and metastases: preliminary report. Radiology 230:125–134
3. Goldberg SN, Gazelle GS, Compton CC, Mueller PR, Tanabe KK (2000) Treatment of intrahepatic malignancy with radiofrequency ablation: radiologic-pathologic correlation. Cancer 88:2452–2463
4. Miao Y, Ni Y, Bosmans H et al (2001) Radiofrequency ablation for eradication of renal tumor in a rabbit model by using a cooled-tip electrode technique. Ann Surg Oncol 8:651–657
5. 5 Choi H, Loyer EM, DuBrow RA et al. (2001) Radio-frequency ablation of liver tumors: assessment of therapeutic response and complications. Radiographics 21 Spec No:S41-54
6. Schraml C, Clasen S, Schwenzer NF et al (2008) Diagnostic performance of contrast-enhanced computed tomography in the immediate assessment of radiofrequency ablation success in colorectal liver metastases. Abdom Imaging 33:643–651
7. Atwell TD, Schmit GD, Boorjian SA et al (2013) Percutaneous ablation of renal masses measuring 3.0 cm and smaller: comparative local control and complications after radiofrequency ablation and cryoablation. AJR Am J Roentgenol 200:461–466
8. Yamamoto A, Nakamura K, Matsuoka T et al (2005) Radiofrequency ablation in a porcine lung model: correlation between CT and histopathologic findings. AJR Am J Roentgenol 185:1299–1306
9. Lu DS, Yu NC, Raman SS et al (2005) Radiofrequency ablation of hepatocellular carcinoma: treatment success as defined by histologic examination of the explanted liver. Radiology 234:954–960
10. Kim YS, Rhim H, Lim HK et al (2006) Completeness of treatment in hepatocellular carcinomas treated with image-guided tumor therapies: Evaluation of positive predictive value of contrast-enhanced CT with histopathologic correlation in the explanted liver specimen. J Comput Assist Tomogr 30:578–582
11. Rendon RA, Kachura JR, Sweet JM et al (2002) The uncertainty of radio frequency treatment of renal cell carcinoma: findings at immediate and delayed nephrectomy. J Urol 167:1587–1592
12. Hataji O, Yamakado K, Nakatsuka A et al (2005) Radiological and pathological correlation of lung malignant tumors treated with percutaneous radiofrequency ablation. Intern Med 44:865–869
13. Johnson TR, Fink C, Schönberg SO, Reiser MF (2011) Dual energy CT in clinical practice. Springer
14. Morsbach F, Wurnig MC, Muller D, Krauss B, Korporaal JG, Alkadhi H (2014) Feasibility of single-source dual-energy computed tomography for urinary stone characterization and value of iterative reconstructions. Investig Radiol 49:125–130
15. Johnson TR, Krauss B, Sedlmair M et al (2007) Material differentiation by dual energy CT: initial experience. Eur Radiol 17:1510–1517
16. Chandarana H, Megibow AJ, Cohen BA et al (2011) Iodine quantification with dual-energy CT: phantom study and preliminary experience with renal masses. AJR Am J Roentgenol 196:W693–700
17. Coursey CA, Nelson RC, Boll DT et al (2010) Dual-energy multidetector CT: how does it work, what can it tell us, and when can we use it in abdominopelvic imaging? Radiographics 30:1037–1055
18. Yagi M, Ueguchi T, Koizumi M et al (2013) Gemstone spectral imaging: determination of CT to ED conversion curves for radiotherapy treatment planning. J Appl Clin Med Phys 14:173–186
19. Wang Q, Shi G, Qi X, Fan X, Wang L (2014) Quantitative analysis of the dual-energy CT virtual spectral curve for focal liver lesions characterization. Eur J Radiol 83:1759–1764
20. Lee SH, Lee JM, Kim KW et al (2011) Dual-energy computed tomography to assess tumor response to hepatic radiofrequency ablation: potential diagnostic value of virtual noncontrast images and iodine maps. Investig Radiol 46:77–84
21. Lv P, Lin XZ, Chen K, Gao J (2012) Spectral CT in patients with small HCC: investigation of image quality and diagnostic accuracy. Eur Radiol 22:2117–2124
22. Li Y, Shi G, Wang S, Wang S, Wu R (2013) Iodine quantification with dual-energy CT: phantom study and preliminary experience with VX2 residual tumour in rabbits after radiofrequency ablation. Br J Radiol 86:20130143
23. Henzler T, Fink C, Schoenberg SO, Schoepf UJ (2012) Dual-energy CT: radiation dose aspects. AJR Am J Roentgenol 199: S16–25
24. Song KD, Kim CK, Park BK, Kim B (2011) Utility of iodine overlay technique and virtual unenhanced images for the characterization of renal masses by dual-energy CT. AJR Am J Roentgenol 197: W1076–1082
25. Ganguli S, Brennan DD, Faintuch S, Rayan ME, Goldberg SN (2008) Immediate renal tumor involution after radiofrequency thermal ablation. J Vasc Interv Radiol 19:412–418
26. Sahni VA, Shinagare AB, Silverman SG (2013) Virtual unenhanced CT images acquired from dual-energy CT urography: accuracy of attenuation values and variation with contrast material phase. Clin Radiol 68:264–271
27. Kim YN, Rhim H, Choi D et al (2011) The effect of radiofrequency ablation on different organs: ex vivo and in vivo comparative studies. Eur J Radiol 80:526–532
28. Morimoto M, Sugimori K, Shirato K et al (2002) Treatment of hepatocellular carcinoma with radiofrequency ablation: radiologic-histologic correlation during follow-up periods. Hepatology 35:1467–1475
29. Park MH, Rhim H, Kim YS, Choi D, Lim HK, Lee WJ (2008) Spectrum of CT findings after radiofrequency ablation of hepatic tumors. Radiographics 28:379–390, discussion 390–372
30. Gillams AR, Lees WR (2005) Radiofrequency ablation of colorectal liver metastases. Abdom Imaging 30:419–426
31. Nghiem HV, Francis IR, Fontana R et al (2002) Computed tomography appearances of hypervascular hepatic tumors after percutaneous radiofrequency ablation therapy. Curr Probl Diagn Radiol 31: 105–111
32. Vandenbroucke F, Vandemeulebroucke J, Ilsen B et al. (2014) Predictive value of pattern classification 24 hours after radiofrequency ablation of Liver metastases on CT and positron emission tomography/CT. J Vasc Interv Radiol 25:1240–9. 10.1016/j.jvir.2014.04.020
33. Marcovich R, Aldana JP, Morgenstern N, Jacobson AI, Smith AD, Lee BR (2003) Optimal lesion assessment following acute radio frequency ablation of porcine kidney: cellular viability or histopathology? J Urol 170:1370–1374
34. Lencioni R, Cioni D, Bartolozzi C (2001) Percutaneous radiofrequency thermal ablation of liver malignancies: techniques, indications, imaging findings, and clinical results. Abdom Imaging 26: 345–360
35. Tan BJ, El-Hakim A, Morgenstern N, Semerdzhiev Y, Smith A, Lee BR (2004) Comparison of laparoscopic saline infused to dry radio frequency ablation of renal tissue: evolution of histological infarct in the porcine model. J Urol 172:2007–2012
36. Merkle EM, Nour SG, Lewin JS (2005) MR imaging follow-up after percutaneous radiofrequency ablation of renal cell carcinoma: findings in 18 patients during first 6 months. Radiology 235:1065–1071

37. Kawamoto S, Permpongkosol S, Bluemke DA, Fishman EK, Solomon SB (2007) Sequential changes after radiofrequency ablation and cryoablation of renal neoplasms: role of CT and MR imaging. Radiographics 27:343–355
38. Smith S, Gillams A (2008) Imaging appearances following thermal ablation. Clin Radiol 63:1–11
39. Gervais DA, McGovern FJ, Arellano RS, McDougal WS, Mueller PR (2003) Renal cell carcinoma: clinical experience and technical success with radio-frequency ablation of 42 tumors. Radiology 226: 417–424
40. Svatek RS, Sims R, Anderson JK, Abdel-Aziz K, Cadeddu JA (2006) Magnetic resonance imaging characteristics of renal tumors after radiofrequency ablation. Urology 67:508–512
41. Zhang LJ, Zhao YE, Wu SY et al (2009) Pulmonary embolism detection with dual-energy CT: experimental study of dual-source CT in rabbits. Radiology 252:61–70
42. Bojarski JD, Dupuy DE, Mayo-Smith WW (2005) CT imaging findings of pulmonary neoplasms after treatment with radiofrequency ablation: results in 32 tumors. AJR Am J Roentgenol 185: 466–471
43. Kawai T, Shibamoto Y, Hara M, Arakawa T, Nagai K, Ohashi K (2011) Can dual-energy CT evaluate contrast enhancement of ground-glass attenuation? Phantom and preliminary clinical studies. Acad Radiol 18:682–689
44. Abtin FG, Eradat J, Gutierrez AJ, Lee C, Fishbein MC, Suh RD (2012) Radiofrequency ablation of lung tumors: imaging features of the postablation zone. Radiographics 32:947–969

22

Beyond PET/CT in Hodgkin lymphoma: a comprehensive review of the role of imaging at initial presentation, during follow-up and for assessment of treatment-related complications

Abhishek R. Keraliya [1,2] · **Sree Harsha Tirumani** [1,2] · **Atul B. Shinagare** [1,2] · **Nikhil H. Ramaiya** [1,2]

Abstract
Objective The purpose of this article is to provide a comprehensive review of the role of imaging modalities other than PET/CT in the management of Hodgkin lymphoma (HL). PET/CT is the imaging modality of choice in the management of Hodgkin's lymphoma (HL). However, imaging modalities other than PET/CT such as plain radiographs, ultrasound, CT, MRI and nuclear imaging can help in various stages of clinical management of HL, including the initial workup and post-treatment surveillance. Both CT and MRI help in detecting recurrences, treatment-related pulmonary, cardiovascular and abdominal complications as well as second malignancies. Familiarity with expected post-treatment changes and complications on surveillance images can help radiologists guide patient management. The purpose of this article is to provide a comprehensive review of the role of imaging modalities other than PET/CT in the management of Hodgkin lymphoma (HL).
Main Messages
- *Surveillance of HL patients is usually performed with plain radiographs and CT.*
- *Follow-up imaging can depict normal post-treatment changes or treatment-related complications.*
- *Imaging is important for the timely detection of second malignancies in HL patients.*

✉ Abhishek R. Keraliya
akeraliya@partners.org

1 Department of Radiology, Harvard Medical School, Brigham and Women's Hospital, 75 Francis Street, Boston, MA 02115, USA

2 Department of Imaging, Harvard Medical School, Dana Farber Cancer Institute, 450 Brookline Avenue, Boston, MA 02215, USA

Keywords Hodgkin lymphoma · PET/CT · Computed tomography · MRI ultrasound

Introduction

Hodgkin lymphoma (HL) accounts for approximately 10 % of all lymphomas diagnosed in the developed world annually [1]. The WHO classification divides HL into two main types: classical HL (CHL) and nodular lymphocyte predominance HL (NLPHL). CHL is further subdivided into four histological subtypes: nodular sclerosis CHL (NSCHL), mixed cellularity CHL (MCCHL), lymphocyte-rich CHL (LRCHL) and lymphocyte-depleted CHL (LDCHL) [2]. HL has bimodal age distribution with most patients diagnosed between 15 and 30 years of age, followed by another peak in adults over the age of 50. HL is usually confined to the lymph nodes. Cervical and mediastinal lymph nodes are the most common site of lymph nodal involvement in HL. In mediastinal lymph nodes, prevascular and paratracheal subsets are most commonly affected. Isolated infradiaphragmatic lymphadenopathy occurs in less than 10 % of patients at diagnosis [3]. Extranodal involvement is less common in HL than in NHL and seen in only 10–15 % of patients. The most frequent sites of extranodal involvement are bone, bone marrow, lung and liver [4].

HL is now curable in more than 80 % of cases owing to significant therapeutic advances in the form of newer chemotherapeutic drugs, advances in radiotherapy and stem cell transplantation [5]. Treatment for HL usually depends on the stage at diagnosis, histological subtype and prognostic factors. According to National Comprehensive Cancer Network (NCCN) guidelines, the initial evaluation of patients with HL includes detailed history and physical examination, evaluation of performance status, laboratory investigations (blood counts, ESR, LDH, liver and renal function tests) and radiological investigations (chest radiograph, PET/CT, contrast-enhanced CT). Staging for HL is based on the Cotswolds modification of the Ann Arbor staging system.

Patients with HL are usually classified into four groups: early-stage favourable (stage I–II with no unfavourable factors), early-stage unfavourable (grade I–II with any of the unfavourable factors), advanced favourable (clinical stage III or IV with zero to three adverse risk factors listed below) and advanced unfavourable (clinical stage III or IV with four or more adverse risk factors listed below). Large mediastinal adenopathy (>33 % of the thoracic width on the chest x-ray, ≥10 cm on CT), presence of B symptoms, more than 2 or 3 nodal sites of disease or an ESR of 50 or more are unfavourable prognostic factors for patients with stage I and II disease. Assessment of prognosis is important for formulating management strategies.

For patients with advanced-stage HL, the International Prognostic Factors Project has developed an International Prognostic Index with a prognostic score that is based on the following seven adverse factors: age more than 45 years, male gender, stage IV disease, albumin level below 4.0 g/dl, haemoglobin level below 10.5 g/dl, white blood cell count more than 15,000/mm^3, absolute lymphocytic count less than 600/mm^3 or a lymphocyte count less than 8 % of the total WBC count [6].

Chemotherapy or combination chemotherapy plus low dose involved field radiation therapy (LD-IFRT) is the standard treatment option in HL. The most common chemotherapeutic regimes used for HL are ABVD (doxorubicin, bleomycin, vinblastine, dacarbazine), Stanford V (doxorubicin, vinblastine, mechlorethamine, vincristine, bleomycin, etoposide and prednisone) and BEACOPP (bleomycin, etoposide, doxorubicin, cyclophosphamide, vincristine, procarbazine and prednisone). Patients with nonbulky stage IA or IIA disease are considered to have clinical early-stage disease. These patients are candidates for chemotherapy, combined modality therapy or radiation therapy alone [7]. The number of cycles is determined by the pre-treatment prognostic factors (favourable or unfavourable disease) and the rate of response to treatment. The treatment for HL also depends on the patient's performance state and the response to treatment. ABVD, Stanford V or escalated BEACOPP is the preferred therapy for patients with advanced HL. For patients with refractory HL or who relapse after chemotherapy and involved-field radiation therapy, second-line chemotherapeutic agents, biological therapy (such as rituximab) and autologus stem cell transplant are treatment options. The role of consolidation radiotherapy after chemotherapy in patients with advanced HL is controversial; however involved-field radiotherapy (IF-RT) is beneficial for patients with partial response after chemotherapy according to a prospective randomised trial of 739 patients with advanced HL [8].

Due to improved long-term survival, treatment-related complications have emerged as an important cause of morbidity and mortality in patients with HL. Early and accurate diagnosis of treatment-related cardiovascular and pulmonary complications and second malignancies are of paramount importance to continue the survival benefit in these patients, especially in those treated with mantle field radiation.

Imaging, especially PET/CT, plays a key role in the diagnosis, staging, response assessment, prognostication and surveillance of patients with HL. Though FDG-PET/CT is the imaging modality of choice in HL, other modalities such as conventional radiographs, ultrasound (US), CT and magnetic resonance imaging (MRI) are often used in the evaluation of lymphoma at various stages of management. In this article, we review the role of various imaging modalities beyond FDG-PET/CT in the management of HL with emphasis on imaging features of treatment-related complications.

PET/CT in Hodgkin's Lymphoma

According to NCCN, 18 F-Fluoro-DeoxyGlucose (FDG) positron emission tomography (PET)/computed tomography (CT) is the corner stone for initial staging and evaluation of treatment response in HL. Response to treatment with chemotherapy or combined modality therapy is assessed by restaging with FDG-PET/CT at midcycle (interim PET/CT) or completion of treatment. FDG-PET positivity at the treatment completion is an adverse prognostic factor for disease-free survival [9]. Metabolic imaging with PET often leads to either upstaging or downstaging in approximately 15–40 % of patients with Hodgkin lymphoma with impact on management in about 5–15 % [10, 11]. Several studies have established the role of interim FDG-PET in the prognosis of HL during chemotherapy. PET is particularly useful in the evaluation of a post-treatment residual mass in patients after the completion of therapy, with positive FDG-PET associated with a significantly poorer progression-free survival [12]. Negative interim FDG-PET/CT is highly predictive of progression-free survival, even more than the International Prognostic Score (IPS) [13, 14]. According to a prospective study, the sensitivity and specificity of FDG PET to predict relapse are 79 % and 97 %, respectively, with a negative predictive value more than 90 % in HL patients after the completion of chemotherapy [15]. Negative PET study reliably rules out disease relapse. However, the positive predictive value of PET is variable, which is an important limitation of PET, and a biopsy is necessary to confirm the diagnosis of a relapse [16]. FDG-PET/CT is also useful in radiation treatment planning and helps in better delineation of the radiation field without increasing radiation volumes [17]. There are some important limitations of FDG-PET/CT. FDG uptake can also be seen in post-treatment inflammation, infection, brown fat and normal physiologic metabolic activity, which can lead to false-positive results. Similarly, low-grade histological subtypes and minimal residual disease can give false-negative results.

Imaging beyond PET at initial staging

The most typical presentation of HL is painless, enlarged superficial lymphadenopathy with systemic symptoms such as fever, night sweats, fatigue and weight loss. Patients with intrathoracic lymphadenopathy may present with respiratory symptoms such as cough, dyspnoea and chest pain. Chest radiography can be performed as the initial investigation in these patients. Chest X-ray provides preliminary information about involvement of the mediastinum and lungs. Bulky mediastinal lymphadenopathy at diagnosis is an unfavourable prognostic factor in patients with HL and can be quantified by measuring using the mediastinal mass ratio. Cotswolds modification of the Ann Arbor staging system defines bulky disease as a mediastinal mass exceeding one third of the internal transverse diameter of the thorax at the T5/6 intervertebral disc level on a posteroanterior chest radiograph (Fig. 1) [18]. US is often helpful in confirming enlarged nodes and guiding biopsy, particularly cervical lymph nodes, the most common nodal group affected in patients with HL. US can be useful for evaluation of extranodal sites of involvement in the abdomen (e.g., gallbladder, kidney) and image-guided biopsy of focal lesions in solid organs such as the liver and spleen [19].

CT can be performed for further evaluation of abnormalities detected on chest x ray. CT can help in depicting other areas of lymph node enlargement that are not obvious on chest radiographs. On CT, HL is characterised by the presence of a discrete anterior mediastinal mass with a lobulated contour with homogeneous soft-tissue attenuation. Large lymph nodal masses can have a heterogeneous appearance with low attenuation areas representing necrosis, haemorrhage or cystic degeneration (Fig. 1). CT is particularly useful for exact anatomical delineation of lymph nodal involvement and in formulating treatment plans and radiation fields.

Although PET/CT remains the corner stone for initial staging and response assessment at the completion of treatment in patients with HL, MRI plays an important part in management of patients with HL. The role of MRI is particularly important in paediatric and younger patients because of exposure to ionising radiation in diagnostic modalities such as CT and PET/CT. In recent years, diffusion-weighted imaging (DWI) has been emerging as a radiation-free alternative to PET/CT for staging of various malignancies including lymphoma [20]. DWI is a functional MRI technique that depicts differences in the mobility of water in tissues. Hypercellular tumours exhibit more restricted water diffusion than normal tissues, which is reflected as high signal intensity on DWI with low apparent diffusion coefficient (ADC) values. DWI-MRI has sensitivity up to 97 % and is a feasible alternative to PET/CT for follow-up and treatment response assessment in patients with FDG-avid lymphoma [21, 22]. The whole body-DWI technique does not need specific equipment and is well tolerated by patients thanks to the relatively shorter acquisition time, which is longer than the acquisition time for CT but shorter than for PET/CT. The use of higher magnetic field strength (3 T) has a higher signal-to-noise ratio (SNR), which improves the ability of lesion detection. The cost of a WB-MRI is roughly equal to the cost for an 18F-FDG PET/CT examination. MRI is also useful in evaluation of intracranial disease and spinal cord involvement because of better soft tissue resolution. In the thorax, MRI is beneficial for assessment of chest wall, vascular, cardiac and pleural and brachial plexus involvement [23].

Central venous thrombosis and compression: Superior vena cava (SVC), brachiocephalic or internal jugular veins can be directly compressed by the mediastinal adenopathy with development of SVC syndrome. Lymphoma is responsible for about 10 % of malignant SVC obstruction cases [24]. SVC and brachiocephalic venous thrombosis can also complicate chemotherapy catheter placement in patients with HL. Contrast-enhanced chest CT is the modality of choice for evaluation of SVC obstruction and to differentiate between venous thrombosis and extrinsic compression. Chest wall venous collaterals and characteristic focal hyperenhancement of liver ("hot-spot sign") is seen with SVC or brachiocephalic vein obstruction due to opening of caval-mammary-phrenic–hepatic capsule-portal pathways (Fig. 1). In this pathway, blood flows from the internal mammary vein to the inferior phrenic vein. The inferior phrenic vein then communicates with hepatic capsular veins, which in turn drain into the intrahepatic portal tributaries. Focal non-mass-like contrast enhancement is seen along the superior aspect of the liver with dilated inferior phrenic veins and hepatic capsular veins [25, 26].

Central nervous system (CNS) involvement in HL is rare with an overall reported incidence of 0.2–0.5 % [27]. Intracranial HL is usually seen in patients with relapsed and progressive disease as a part of widespread systemic involvement. The most common histological subtypes of CHL associated with CNS involvement are MCHL and NSHL. Evaluation of CNS involvement in HL on FDG-PET is limited by the intense physiologic FDG uptake in the brain. CT with intravenous contrast and MRI are useful in such instances. Spinal cord compression is a rare complication of HL, occurring usually in the setting of progressive and advanced disease. As the initial symptom of HL, it is extremely rare, with only a few cases reported in the literature [28]. Prompt diagnosis is crucial as early surgical decompression, radiation therapy and chemotherapy are imperative to prevent irreversible neurological deficits. MR imaging of the spine, without and with the use of gadolinium-based contrast material, is

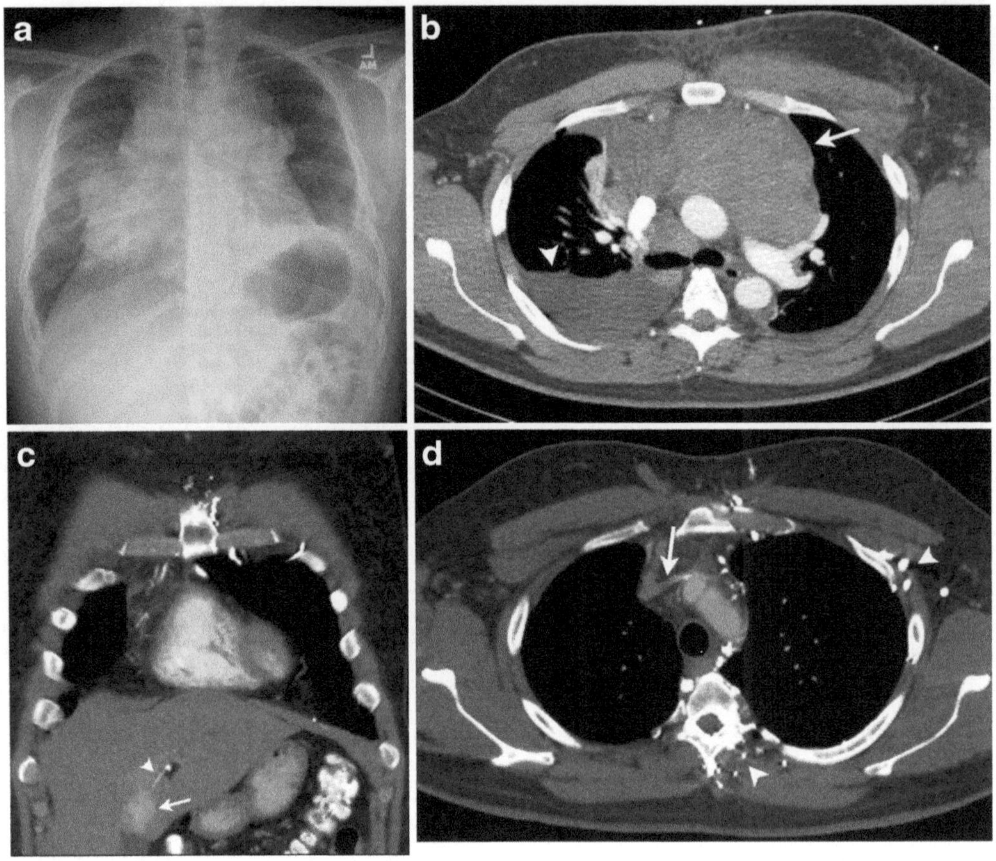

Fig. 1 A 39-year-old male with increasing cough, night sweats and weight loss since 2 months. **a** Frontal chest radiograph demonstrates bulky mediastinal lymphadenopathy exceeding one third of the internal transverse diameter of the thorax. **b** Axial contrast-enhanced CT image reveals large conglomerate anterior mediastinal lymph nodal mass (*arrow*) and right-sided pleural effusion (*arrowhead*). Biopsy of lymph nodal mass was suggestive of nodular sclerosing HL. Follow-up CT study after treatment with chemotherapy and mediastinal radiation complicated by chronic venous thrombosis. **c** Coronal contrast-enhanced CT image shows focal hyperenhancement (*arrow*) in segment IV of the liver due to reflux in a capsular vein (*arrowhead*) communicating with the inferior phrenic vein (not shown). **d** Axial contrast-enhanced CT image demonstrates chronic occlusion of the left brachiocephalic vein (*arrow*) with multiple chest wall and paravertebral venous collaterals on the left side (*arrowheads*)

the standard for the diagnosis of malignant spinal cord compression (Fig. 2) [29].

Imaging beyond PET during follow-up

Due to the long-term risks and complications of the therapies of HL, regular follow-up of treated patients with HL is important. The follow-up schedule depends on the age of patients, staging at the time of diagnosis and type of treatment given. Physical examinations and blood tests are performed every 3 to 6 months for the first 2 years, then every 6 to 12 months for the next 3 years and then annually [30]. The NCCN guidelines recommend imaging techniques such as chest radiographs or chest CT and abdomen and pelvis CT to be performed every 6 months for the first 2 years and then annually for the next 3 years. If the neck is involved in the radiation treatment field, thyroid function tests are performed annually. The overall 5-year survival rate for early-stage HL in children and adolescent population is more than 90 % [31]. However, up to 10 % of patients with early-stage and up to 25 % patients with advanced-stage HL relapse after first-line therapy [32]. In addition to detecting long-term treatment-related complications, the goal of the surveillance scans is to detect local and distant recurrences of lymphoma. Recurrent lymphoma has the same appearance as primary HL; however pulmonary parenchymal involvement is more common in recurrent HL. The various patterns of parenchymal involvement include a pulmonary nodule or mass, lobar or segmental consolidation with an air bronchogram and a reticular pattern with peribronchovascular and interlobular septal thickening [33]. Findings suggestive of recurrent disease in the radiation field include an alteration in the contour of the radiation fibrosis with an increase in size, convex borders, appearance of homogeneous opacity with obliteration of the air bronchogram and filling of the bronchi (Fig. 3) [34].

Restaging CT examinations often demonstrate findings that represent expected post-treatment changes. Dystrophic lymph

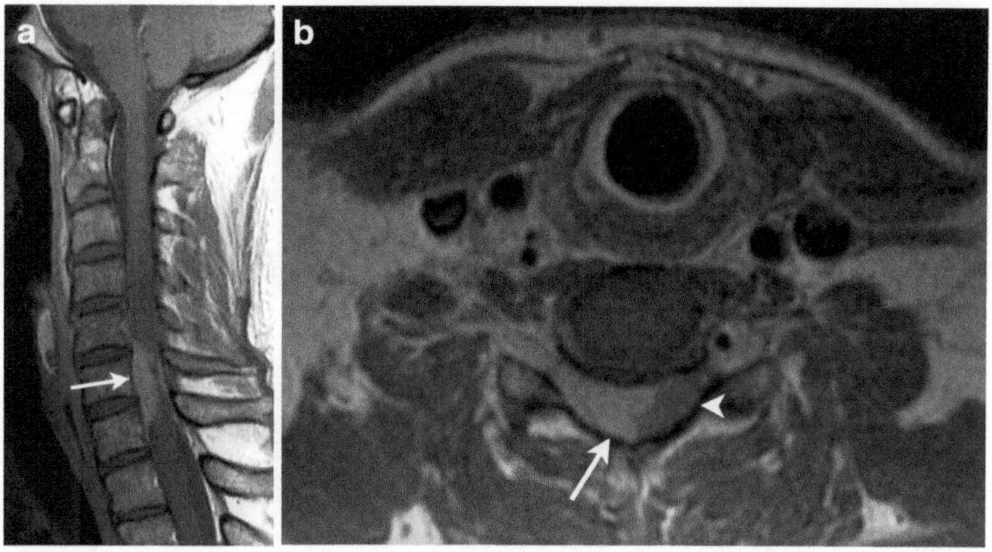

Fig. 2 A 36-year-old male with newly diagnosed nodular sclerosing HL presenting with numbness in his right hand. **a** Sagittal contrast-enhanced T1-weighted image of the cervical spine demonstrates enhancing epidural soft tissue (*arrow*) at the C4 to C6 vertebral levels. **b** Axial contrast-enhanced T1-weighted image demonstrates epidural enhancing soft tissue (*arrow*) with significant compression and mass effect on the cervical spinal cord (*arrowhead*)

nodal calcification is seen in approximately 2–8 % of treated patients with HL following radiation or chemotherapy (Fig. 4). Lymph nodal calcification in untreated patients is seen in less than 1 % of patients with aggressive histological subtypes of HL [35]. In treated patients, dystrophic calcification represents treatment-induced necrosis and is associated with good prognosis and long-term survival [36]. Absence of spleen is another finding on imaging that can be encountered in patients with HL. Before effective chemotherapy and radiotherapy were available and staging was crucial to differentiate limited-stage disease from extensive-stage disease, splenectomy was often performed in patients with HL as 20–35 % with clinically limited disease confined to above the diaphragm will have occult splenic involvement [37].

Rebound hyperplasia of the thymus occurs in 10 to 25 % of patients treated with chemotherapy [38]. Thymic rebound usually occurs 1 to 11 months after completion of chemotherapy because of reactive lymphoid hyperplasia in response to withdrawal of chemotherapy and is usually self-limiting and reversible [39]. It is important to differentiate thymic rebound from recurrent mediastinal disease. CT features that favour thymic regrowth over lymphomatous thymic involvement or thymic tumour are a diffusely enlarged thymus that maintains the normal thymic morphology with a smooth contour, uniform density without invasion of adjacent tissues and absence of pericardial or pleural effusion (Fig. 5).

Until the 1990s in the prechemotherapy era, radiation therapy was often used as a single modality in the treatment of HL with more extended fields and higher doses than in current radiotherapy techniques [40]. In patients who have received infradiaphragmatic radiotherapy, various abdominal organs could be affected by side effects of radiation. Radiation-induced liver disease (radiation hepatitis) has a threshold of 30–35 Gy for the whole liver. Radiation-induced liver injury demonstrates an acute phase occurring within 3 months of exposure characterised by hyperaemia, venous congestion

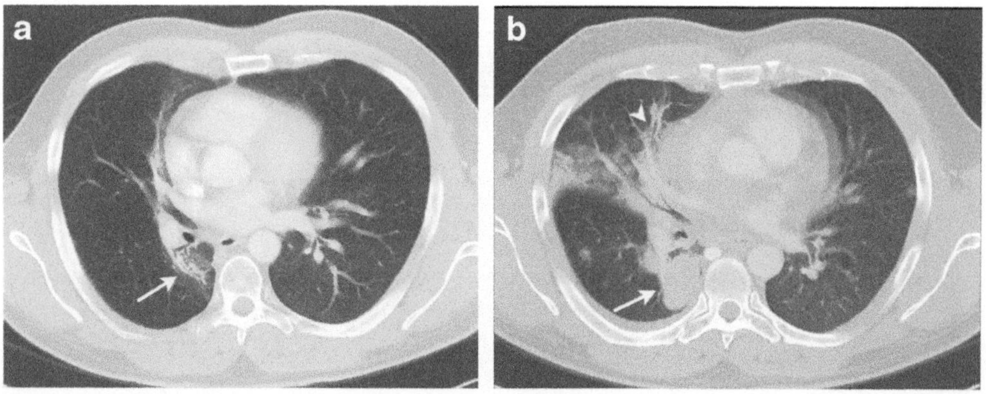

Fig. 3 A 35-year-old male with a history of HL treated 3 years ago with chemotherapy and mediastinal radiation presenting with relapsed HL in the radiation field. **a** Axial CT image in lung window settings shows well-demarcated area of parenchymal distortion and traction bronchiectasis in a paramediastinal location in the right lower lobe (*arrow*) suggestive of post-radiation changes. **b** Axial CT image in lung window settings after 3 years shows the appearance of a lobulated mass within the radiation field with obliteration of the previously visualised air bronchogram (*arrow*). New appearance of ground-glass opacities with consolidation (*arrowhead*) is seen in the right middle lobe

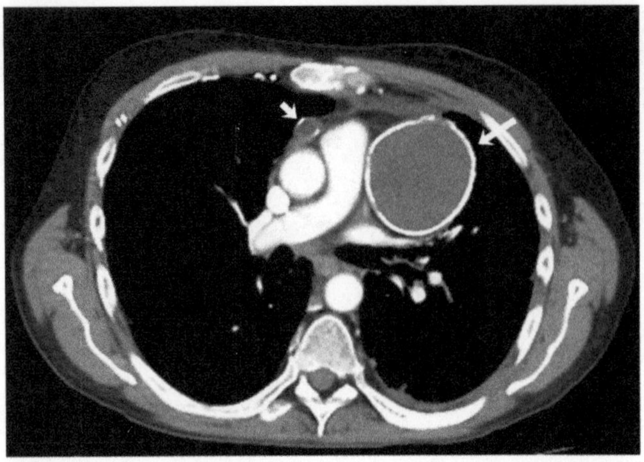

Fig. 4 A 37-year-old male with a history of HL treated with chemotherapy and mediastinal radiation 5 years ago. Axial contrast-enhanced CT image reveals anterior mediastinal lymphadenopathy with peripheral calcification (*arrows*)

and fatty infiltration and a chronic phase with development of fibrosis and architectural distortion. On CT it appears as a sharply demarcated area of hypodensity corresponding to the radiation ports; however, in case of background fatty infiltration of liver, the irradiated area appears hyperdense compared to adjacent liver parenchyma. Radiation-induced pancreatic injury is characterised by parenchymal atrophy and fibrosis. The spleen is also radiosensitive and splenic atrophy occurs at doses of 35–40 Gy [41]. The upper poles of the kidneys (more commonly the left kidney because of its higher anatomical position than the right) can be affected by radiation. Radiation-induced cortical thinning and atrophy of the upper poles of the kidneys are well demarcated from the rest of the renal parenchyma and frequently seen on follow-up studies in patients with HL (Fig. 6) [42]. Uncommonly, lymphomatous involvement in the abdomen and pelvis can fistulise with the gastroitestinal tract resulting in tumour-bowel fistula (TBF). TBF can occur either spontaneously or following treatment with radiotherapy or chemotherapy. Gastrosplenic fistula can occur in association with gastric or splenic lymphoma and clinically manifests with epigastric pain and upper gastrointestinal bleeding [43, 44]. CT is the investigation of choice for the diagnosis of TBF with demonstration of a tract following oral contrast administration (Fig. 7).

Radiation therapy causes destruction of haematopoietic marrow elements and their replacement by fatty marrow elements usually occurring 3 to 6 weeks following radiotherapy; this is characterised by fatty replacement of marrow and manifests on MRI as T1 hyperintensity with a sharp demarcation corresponding to the radiation port [45]. Bone marrow recovery after radiation therapy can be reversible or irreversible depending on the amount of radiation given. Partial or complete recovery usually occurs at low doses (less than 30 Gy). Permanent fatty marrow replacement is usually seen above the dose of 36 Gy with very little chance of complete recovery [46].

Complications of treatment

The main cause of increased mortality and morbidity among long-term survivors of HL are treatment-related development of secondary cancers, drug-related toxicities, radiation-induced pulmonary, cardiovascular and abdominal complications, thyroid disorders and myelosuppresion.

Cardiovascular toxicity Cardiovascular toxicity in treated patients with HL can be due to doxorubicin and/or radiation. The cause-specific mortality for cardiovascular disease is approximately 10 % [47]. The cumulative incidence of adverse cardiac events in patients treated for HL is more than 20 % 25 years after radiotherapy and prior mediastinal radiation is a long-term risk factor for increased cardiovascular mortality and morbidity in HL patients, especially with doses above 30 Gy [48, 49]. Radiation produces dose-dependent cardiac damage through several different mechanisms. Radiation-induced cardiovascular complications can be acute, such as acute pericarditis, or chronic, such as coronary artery disease, valvular heart disease, decreased ventricular function, arrhythmia and chronic pericarditis. Initial evaluation of coronary artery disease is done with stress echocardiography or nuclear scintigraphy to look for inducible ischaemia. Patients with a

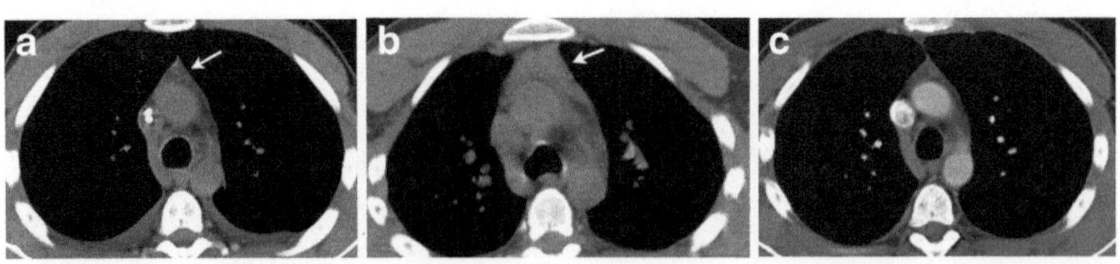

Fig. 5 A 22-year-old male with relapsed HL shows thymic rebound after second-line chemotherapy. **a** Axial non-contrast CT image shows triangular low-attenuation anterior mediastinal soft tissue (*arrow*) suggestive of normal thymus. **b** Axial non-contrast CT image after 3 months of chemotherapy shows diffusely enlarged thymus (*arrow*). The thymic contour is maintained with smooth margins and absence of surrounding vascular invasion. **c** Axial non-contrast CT image 4 months after completion of chemotherapy shows resolution of thymic enlargement with similar appearance of thymus compared to pretreatment study

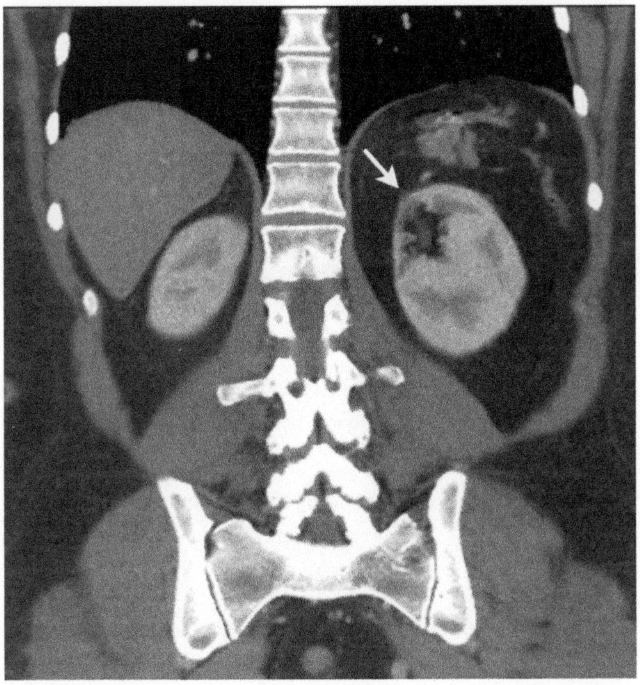

Fig. 6 A 49-year-old female with a history of nodular sclerosing HL treated 23 years ago with mantle and paraaortic radiation to a total dose of 36 Gy. Coronal reformatted image of contrast-enhanced CT shows cortical thinning of the upper pole of the left kidney (*arrow*). Note the absence of spleen from the prior splenectomy

positive stress test can be further evaluated with coronary CT angiography. Coronary calcifications are frequently visualised at follow-up chest CT in patients with treated HL (Fig. 8). Patients treated with radiation therapy are also at higher risk for development of noncoronary arteriosclerotic vascular disease including subclavian and carotid artery stenosis (Fig. 8). In a retrospective study of 414 patients treated with radiation therapy, Hull et al. found the incidence of noncoronary atherosclerotic disease was 2 % at 5, 3 % at 10 and 7 % at 20 years [50]. Radiation-induced pericardial disease can manifest in the form of pericarditis or pericardial effusion and is seen in 20 to 40 % of patients treated with mantle field radiation [51]. Echocardiography and MRI are useful modalities for the evaluation of pericardial disease. Radiation-induced valvular disease can manifest as both stenosis and insufficiency.

Anthracyclines cause dose-dependent cardiac toxicity that can produce irreversible cardiomyopathy. Left ventricular dysfunction has been reported to occur in 5 % of patients at cumulative doses as low as 240 mg/m^2 [52]. Monitoring of left ventricular function with echocardiography, radionuclide angiography or less commonly cardiac MRI is recommended in patients who have received anthracycline-based chemotherapy. A multiple-gated acquisition (MUGA) scan is particularly useful for determination of the ejection fraction in HL patients before and after they undergo chemotherapy. A 10 % decline of the left ventricular ejection fraction (LVEF) below the lower limit of normal or an absolute decline of 45 % or decline of 20 % at any level is indicative of cardiac function deterioration. The risk of cardiac toxicity increases with combined treatment (doxorubicin and radiation) compared to either treatment given alone [48, 53, 54].

Pulmonary toxicity Like cardiovascular toxicity, pulmonary toxicity in HL patients can be due to radiotherapy or cytotoxic chemotherapy.

Radiation-induced pulmonary toxicity Newer radiotherapy techniques such as involved-site radiation therapy (ISRT) and intensity-modulated radiation therapy (IMRT) deliver less radiation to uninvolved normal organs compared to conventional involved-field or extended-field radiation therapy and reduce the long-term pulmonary and cardiovascular toxicity [55]. The degree of radiation damage depends on multiple factors such as the total radiation dose, fractionation, dose rate, volume of the lungs receiving a specified dose and beam arrangement [56].

Radiologic manifestations are usually confined to the lung tissue within the radiation port and are dependent on the

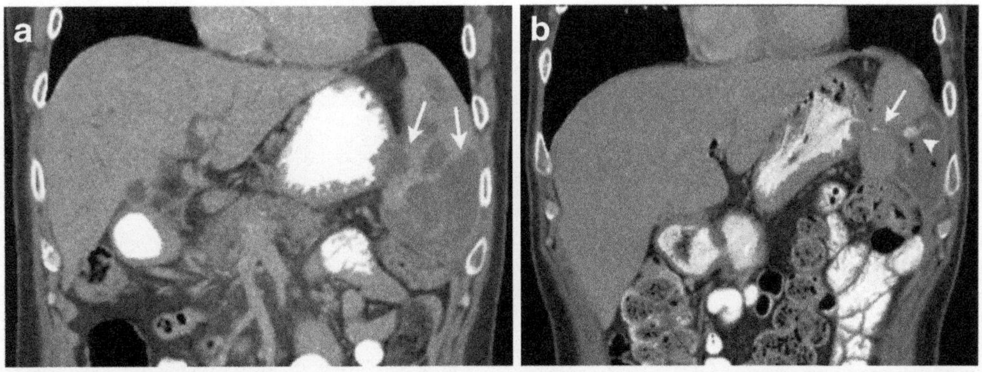

Fig. 7 A 49-year-old male with relapsed HL with splenic lesions treated with second-line chemotherapy. **a** Coronal contrast-enhanced CT image shows splenomegaly with multiple low-attenuation splenic lesions (*arrows*). **b** Coronal contrast-enhanced CT image 4 months after treatment with second-line chemotherapy demonstrates communication between the stomach and spleen (*arrow*) with the presence of hyperdense oral contrast material (*arrowhead*) and air specs in a low-attenuation splenic lesion suggestive of gastrosplenic fistula

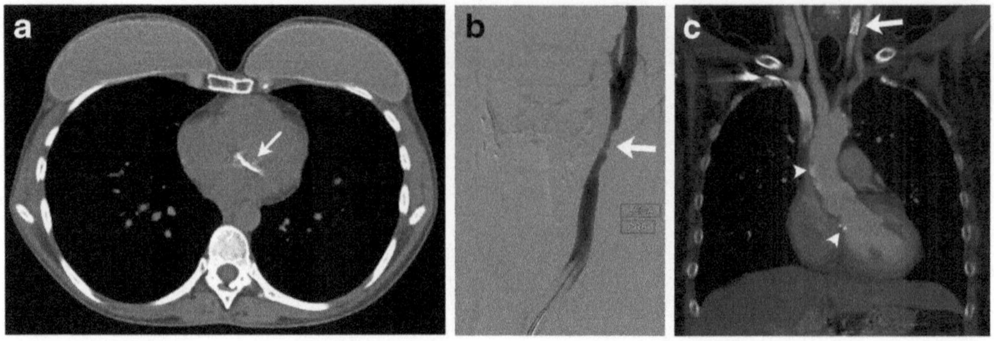

Fig. 8 Cardiovascular complications. **a** A 38-year-old female with a history of nodular sclerosing HL at the age of 12 treated with chemotherapy and upper mantle radiation. Axial non-enhanced CT image shows mitral valve calcification (*arrow*). Note the bilateral mastectomies with a breast prosthesis from prior breast cancer. **b** A 40-year-old female with a history of nodular sclerosing HL at the age of 15 treated with chemotherapy and upper mantle radiation. Digital subtraction angiogram of the left carotid artery shows moderate to severe narrowing of the left distal common carotid artery (*arrow*). **c** Coronal reformatted image of contrast-enhanced CT during follow-up shows the presence of a stent in the left common carotid artery (*arrow*). Note the presence of aortic arch and right coronary artery calcifications (*arrowheads*). Also note the absence of spleen from the prior splenectomy

interval after completion of treatment. Radiation-induced lung injury is divided into two clinical stages: the early stage characterised by radiation pneumonitis and late stage characterised by chronic radiation fibrosis. Early radiation pneumonitis usually occurs about 4–12 weeks after completion of radiation therapy and is characterised by ground-glass opacification, consolidation and atelectasis within the radiation portals. Radiation fibrosis usually develops within 6–12 months after completion of radiation therapy. Typical features of radiation fibrosis include a well-demarked area of volume loss, linear scarring or consolidation, parenchymal distortion and traction bronchiectasis, ipsilateral mediastinal shift and adjacent pleural thickening [34, 57].

Bleomycin- and cyclophosphamide-induced pulmonary toxicity Bleomycin is commonly used in chemotherapy regimens of HL. Bleomycin-induced lung injury usually occurs in 3 %–20 % of treated patients [58]. HRCT is more sensitive than chest radiographs in identifying bleomycin-induced lung abnormalities. Common manifestations of bleomycin-induced lung disease are diffuse alveolar damage, nonspecific interstitial pneumonia (NSIP) and bronchiolitis obliterans organising pneumonia (BOOP) (Fig. 9). Cyclophosphamide can cause pulmonary haemorrhage and diffuse alveolar damage. CT manifestations of NSIP include patchy ground-glass opacities combined with reticular opacities in peripheral subpleural distribution. BOOP is characterised by bilateral asymmetrical ground-glass opacities or airspace consolidation in a peripheral or peribronchial distribution [59, 60].

Second malignancies Second malignancies are the leading cause of death in long-term survivors of HL. Risk factors depend on the type of second malignancy and include the radiation dose and field, chemotherapy agents and doses administered, history of smoking and sex and age of the patient [61]. The maximum risk of a second cancer is at 5 to 9 years after chemotherapy alone, but after combined modalities the risk remains for 25 years or longer [62]. Solid tumours account for more than 50 % of second malignancies developing after 15 or more years of follow-up in patients treated for HL [63]. Lung and breast cancers are the most common secondary cancers in patients with HL due to their proximity to the radiation portal (Fig. 10a) [64]. Other solid tumours that have an increased incidence among HL survivors include gastrointestinal cancers, bone and soft tissue tumours, thyroid cancers, malignant melanoma, bladder cancer and malignant mesothelioma. The risk of developing secondary cancer is lower with combined modality treatment than with radiotherapy alone as the initial treatment [61, 63, 65, 66].

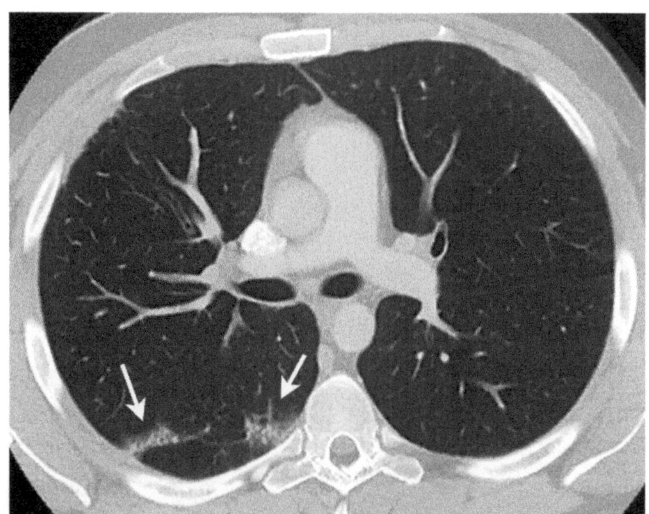

Fig. 9 A 22-year-old male with nodular sclerosing HL on treatment with an ABVD regimen and complaining of new onset cough without fever. Axial contrast-enhanced lung window CT image shows patchy ground-glass opacities in the right lower lobe with peripheral subpleural distribution suggestive of drug toxicity

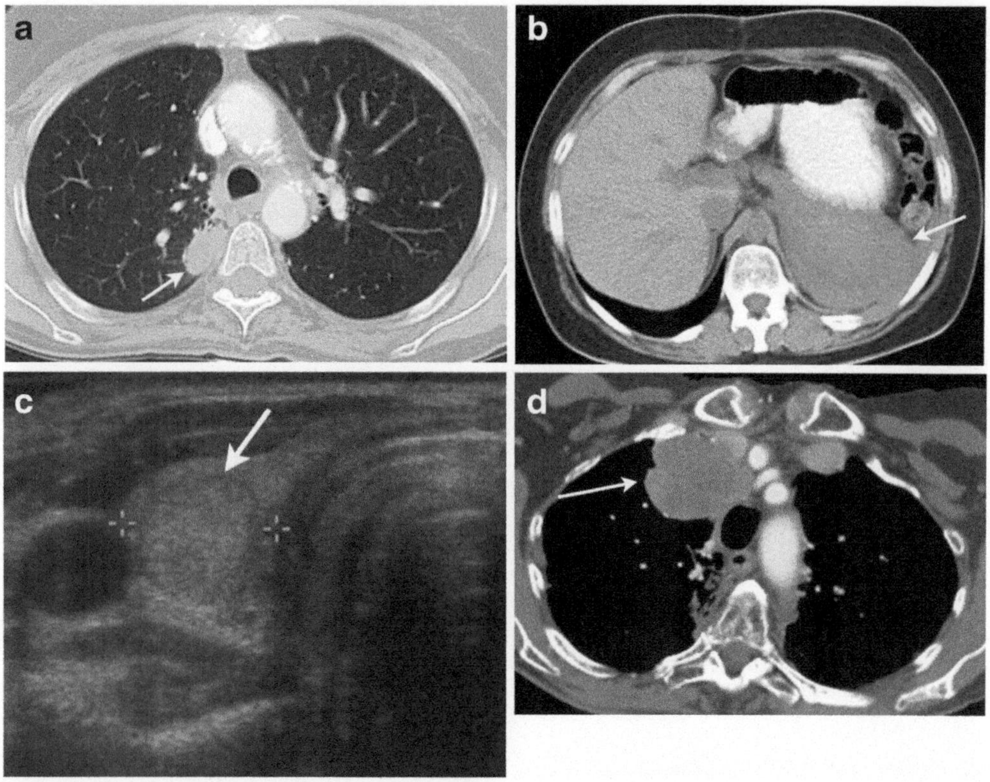

Fig. 10 Second malignancies in patients with HL. **a** A 40-year-old female with a history of nodular sclerosing HL at the age of 15 treated with chemotherapy and upper mantle radiation. Axial contrast-enhanced lung window CT image shows a soft tissue mass within the right paramediastinal radiation field. Pathology was suggestive of adenocarcinoma of the lung. **b** A 24-year-old female presenting with upper abdominal pain and fullness with a prior history of HL at the age of 13 treated with splenectomy and radiation. Axial non-enhanced CT image of the upper abdomen shows a soft tissue mass lesion in the left upper abdomen (*arrow*). Pathology was suggestive of mesothelioma. **c** A 48-year-old female with a history of nodular sclerosing HL at the age of 15 treated with chemotherapy, mantle and pelvic radiation. Transverse greyscale ultrasound image shows a solid nodule in the right lobe of the thyroid (*arrow*). Fine-needle aspiration cytology from the nodule was suggestive of papillary thyroid carcinoma. **d** A 56-year-old female presenting with shortness of breath, intermittent cough and weight loss with a prior history of HL treated with radiation 40 years ago. Axial contrast-enhanced CT image shows a large heterogeneously enhancing anterior mediastinal mass (*arrow*). Pathology was suggestive of radiation-induced sarcoma

The risk of lung cancer is substantially increased in patients with HL treated with radiotherapy or chemotherapy, especially among smokers. The overall survival of non-small-cell lung cancer (NSCLC) in the setting of treated HL is inferior compared to patients with de novo lung cancer [67]. Breast cancers after HL typically occur after a long latency of 10–15 years and are associated with young age at irradiation. Annual breast screening (mammography or MRI) beginning no later than 8 to 10 years after treatment completion or at age 40 (whichever occurs earlier) is recommended for woman who have received chest or axillary radiation [68].

Patients with HL have a 20-fold increased risk of mesothelioma after radiotherapy. Mesothelioma arises from the mesothelial cells forming the serosal membranes of body cavities. Pleural and peritoneal cavities are frequent sites of involvement. Patients with lymphoma-associated malignant mesothelioma have younger age at diagnosis and longer overall survival compared with those with asbestos-associated mesothelioma [69]. CT is the primary imaging modality used for the evaluation of malignant pleural mesothelioma. Pleural mesothelioma presents as pleural thickening, pleural-based nodules, pleural effusion, thickening of interlobular fissures and pleural calcifications. The tumour frequently causes invasion of the chest wall, pericardium, heart and diaphragm. MRI is particularly helpful in detecting chest wall and mediastinal involvement because of the improved soft tissue contrast resolution [70, 71]. The CT features of malignant peritoneal mesothelioma are peritoneal- or omental-based masses as well as irregular or nodular peritoneal thickening with or without ascites (Fig. 10b) [72].

Radiotherapy is the main cause of thyroid cancers after HL, since the thyroid gland is a highly radiosensitive organ and is frequently exposed to radiation because of its location in neck (Fig. 10c). The risk of developing various thyroid abnormalities such as thyroid cancer, Grave's disease, thyroiditis, hypothyroidism, nodular thyroid disease and thyroid atrophy is more than 50 % in patients with HL [40, 73, 74].

Patients with HL who received subdiaphragmatic radiotherapy have a dose-dependent increased risk of gastric cancer. The risk is further increased in patients who also received chemotherapy with MOPP (mechlorethamine, vincristine, procarbazine and prednisone) or BEACOPP regimes containing procarbazine. The stomach cancer risk is also increased in patients who are treated with dacarbazine, a component of the ABVD regimen, frequently used in patients with HL [75].

Radiation-induced sarcoma (RIS) is rare and associated with higher doses of radiation and with the use of concurrent chemotherapy (Fig. 10d). The mean latency period for post-radiation bone and soft tissue sarcomas ranges from 4 to 17 years [76]. Post-radiation sarcoma usually arises in or near the radiation field [77].

Imaging plays an important role in the timely detection of second malignancies in patients with HL. Knowledge of the history and site of prior radiotherapy can help the radiologists to increase the index of suspicion of second malignancies.

Conclusion

In conclusion, although PET/CT remains the cornerstone for initial staging and response assessment at the completion of treatment in patients with HL, imaging modalities other than PET/CT often help in the initial workup of patients with HL. Treatment for HL usually depends upon the stage at diagnosis, histological subtype and prognostic factors, and chemotherapy or combination chemotherapy plus low-dose involved-field radiation therapy (LD-IFRT) is the standard treatment option in HL. Treatment response is assessed by restaging PET/CT using the Deauville criteria. Surveillance of HL patients after treatment is performed with plain radiographs and CT. Follow-up imaging can depict normal post-treatment changes or complications including second malignancies. Familiarity with expected post-treatment changes and complications on surveillance scans can help radiologists to guide patient management.

Disclosures A.B. Shinagare was awarded an RSNA research grant starting in July 2014. No disclosures are reported for the remaining authors.

References

1. Jemal A, Siegel R, Ward E, Hao Y, Xu J, Thun MJ (2009) Cancer statistics, 2009. CA Cancer J Clin 59:225–249
2. Campo E, Swerdlow SH, Harris NL, Pileri S, Stein H, Jaffe ES (2011) The 2008 WHO classification of lymphoid neoplasms and beyond: evolving concepts and practical applications. Blood 117: 5019–5032
3. Vassilakopoulos TP, Angelopoulou MK, Siakantaris MP et al (2006) Pure infradiaphragmatic Hodgkin's lymphoma. Clinical features, prognostic factor and comparison with supradiaphragmatic disease. Haematologica 91:32–39
4. Guermazi A, Brice P, de Kerviler EE et al (2001) Extranodal Hodgkin disease: spectrum of disease. Rad Rev Pub Radiol Soc North America, Inc 21:161–179
5. Siegel R, Naishadham D, Jemal A (2013) Cancer statistics, 2013. CA Cancer J Clin 63:11–30
6. Hasenclever D, Diehl V (1998) A prognostic score for advanced Hodgkin's disease. International prognostic factors project on advanced Hodgkin's disease. N Engl J Med 339:1506–1514
7. Armitage JO (2010) Early-stage Hodgkin's lymphoma. N Engl J Med 363:653–662
8. Aleman BM, Raemaekers JM, Tomisic R et al (2007) Involved-field radiotherapy for patients in partial remission after chemotherapy for advanced Hodgkin's lymphoma. Int J Radiat Oncol Biol Phys 67:19–30
9. de Wit M, Bohuslavizki KH, Buchert R, Bumann D, Clausen M, Hossfeld DK (2001) 18FDG-PET following treatment as valid predictor for disease-free survival in Hodgkin's lymphoma. Ann Oncol Off J Euro Soc Med Oncol/ESMO 12:29–37
10. Bednaruk-Mlynski E, Pienkowska J, Skorzak A et al (2015) Comparison of positron emission tomography/computed tomography with classical contrast-enhanced computed tomography in the initial staging of Hodgkin lymphoma. Leuk lymphoma 56:377–382
11. Juweid ME (2006) Utility of positron emission tomography (PET) scanning in managing patients with Hodgkin lymphoma. Hematol Edu Prog Am Soc Hematol Am Soc Hematol Educ Prog 259–265: 510–251
12. Naumann R, Vaic A, Beuthien-Baumann B et al (2001) Prognostic value of positron emission tomography in the evaluation of post-treatment residual mass in patients with Hodgkin's disease and non-Hodgkin's lymphoma. Br J Haematol 115:793–800
13. Gallamini A, Rigacci L, Merli F et al (2006) The predictive value of positron emission tomography scanning performed after two courses of standard therapy on treatment outcome in advanced stage Hodgkin's disease. Haematologica 91:475–481
14. Gallamini A, Hutchings M, Rigacci L et al (2007) Early interim 2-[18 F]fluoro-2-deoxy-D-glucose positron emission tomography is prognostically superior to international prognostic score in advanced-stage Hodgkin's lymphoma: a report from a joint Italian-Danish study. J Clin Oncol Off J Am So Clin Oncol 25: 3746–3752
15. Guay C, Lepine M, Verreault J, Benard F (2003) Prognostic value of PET using 18 F-FDG in Hodgkin's disease for posttreatment evaluation. J Nuc Med Off Pub Soc Nuc Med 44:1225–1231
16. El-Galaly TC, Mylam KJ, Brown P et al (2012) Positron emission tomography/computed tomography surveillance in patients with Hodgkin lymphoma in first remission has a low positive predictive value and high costs. Haematologica 97:931–936
17. Girinsky T, Auperin A, Ribrag V et al (2014) Role of FDG-PET in the implementation of involved-node radiation therapy for Hodgkin lymphoma patients. Int J Radiat Oncol Biol Phys 89:1047–1052
18. Bradley AJ, Carrington BM, Lawrance JA, Ryder WD, Radford JA (1999) Assessment and significance of mediastinal bulk in Hodgkin's disease: comparison between computed tomography and chest radiography. J Clin Oncol Off J Am Soc Clin Oncol 17: 2493–2498
19. McInnes MD, Kielar AZ, Macdonald DB (2011) Percutaneous image-guided biopsy of the spleen: systematic review and meta-analysis of the complication rate and diagnostic accuracy. Radiology 260:699–708

20. Mayerhoefer ME, Karanikas G, Kletter K et al (2014) Evaluation of diffusion-weighted MRI for pretherapeutic assessment and staging of lymphoma: results of a prospective study in 140 patients. Clinical Cancer Res Off J Am Assoc Cancer Res 20:2984–2993
21. Stephane V, Samuel B, Vincent D et al (2013) Comparison of PET-CT and magnetic resonance diffusion weighted imaging with body suppression (DWIBS) for initial staging of malignant lymphomas. Eur J Radiol 82:2011–2017
22. Mayerhoefer ME, Karanikas G, Kletter K, et al. Evaluation of diffusion-weighted magnetic resonance imaging for follow-up and treatment response assessment of lymphoma: results of an 18 F-FDG-PET/CT-controlled prospective study in 64 patients. Clinical cancer research: an official journal of the American Association for Cancer Research 2015
23. Carter BW, Wu CC, Khorashadi L et al (2014) Multimodality imaging of cardiothoracic lymphoma. Eur J Radiol 83:1470–1482
24. Wilson LD, Detterbeck FC, Yahalom J (2007) Clinical practice. Superior vena cava syndrome with malignant causes. N Engl J Med 356:1862–1869
25. Dahan H, Arrive L, Monnier-Cholley L, Le Hir P, Zins M, Tubiana JM (1998) Cavoportal collateral pathways in vena cava obstruction: imaging features. AJR Am J Roentgenol 171:1405–1411
26. Kapur S, Paik E, Rezaei A, Vu DN (2010) Where there is blood, there is a way: unusual collateral vessels in superior and inferior vena cava obstruction. Radiog Rev Pub Radiol Soc North Am Inc 30:67–78
27. Hirmiz K, Foyle A, Wilke D et al (2004) Intracranial presentation of systemic Hodgkin's disease. Leuk lymphoma 45:1667–1671
28. Rabhi M, Ennibi K, Chaari J (2007) Toloune F [Hodgkin's disease presenting with spinal cord compression]. Rev Neurol 163:1109–1112
29. Katabathina VS, Restrepo CS, Betancourt Cuellar SL, Riascos RF, Menias CO (2013) Imaging of oncologic emergencies: what every radiologist should know. Radiog Rev Pub Radio Soc North Am Inc 33:1533–1553
30. Engert A, Eichenauer DA, Dreyling M, Group EGW (2009) Hodgkin's lymphoma: ESMO clinical recommendations for diagnosis, treatment and follow-up. Ann Onco Off J Euro Soc Med Oncol/ESMO 20(Suppl 4):108–109
31. Smith MA, Seibel NL, Altekruse SF et al (2010) Outcomes for children and adolescents with cancer: challenges for the twenty-first century. J Clin Oncol Off J Am Soc Clin Oncol 28:2625–2634
32. Daw S, Wynn R, Wallace H (2011) Management of relapsed and refractory classical Hodgkin lymphoma in children and adolescents. Br J Haematol 152:249–260
33. Vargas HA, Hampson FA, Babar JL, Shaw AS (2009) Imaging the lungs in patients treated for lymphoma. Clin Radiol 64:1048–1055
34. Choi YW, Munden RF, Erasmus JJ et al (2004) Effects of radiation therapy on the lung: radiologic appearances and differential diagnosis. Radiog Rev Pub Radiol Soc North Am Inc 24:985–997, discussion 998
35. Apter S, Avigdor A, Gayer G, Portnoy O, Zissin R, Hertz M (2002) Calcification in lymphoma occurring before therapy: CT features and clinical correlation. AJR Am J Roentgenol 178:935–938
36. Strijk SP (1985) Lymph node calcification in malignant lymphoma. Presentation of nine cases and a review of the literature. Acta Radiol Diagn 26:427–431
37. Castellino RA (1992) Diagnostic imaging studies in patients with newly diagnosed Hodgkin's disease. Ann Oncol Off J Euro Soc Med Oncol/ESMO 3(Suppl 4):45–47
38. Nasseri F, Eftekhari F (2010) Clinical and radiologic review of the normal and abnormal thymus: pearls and pitfalls. Radiog Rev Pub Radiol Soc North Am Inc 30:413–428
39. Zhen Z, Sun X, Xia Y et al (2010) Clinical analysis of thymic regrowth following chemotherapy in children and adolescents with malignant lymphoma. Jpn J Clin Oncol 40:1128–1134
40. Brennan S, Hann LE, Yahalom J, Oeffinger KC, Rademaker J (2008) Imaging of late complications from mantle field radiation in lymphoma patients. Radiol Clin N Am 46:419–430
41. Kwek JW, Iyer RB, Dunnington J, Faria S, Silverman PM (2006) Spectrum of imaging findings in the abdomen after radiotherapy. AJR Am J Roentgenol 187:1204–1211
42. Izzedine H, Cluzel P, Deray G (2007) Renal radiation-induced arterial stenosis. Kidney Int 71:1188
43. Tirumani SH, Baez JC, Jagannathan JP, Shinagare AB, Ramaiya NH (2013) Tumor-bowel fistula: what radiologists should know. Abdom Imaging 38:1014–1023
44. Dellaportas D, Vezakis A, Fragulidis G, Tasoulis M, Karamitopoulou E, Polydorou A. Gastrosplenic fistula secondary to lymphoma, manifesting as upper gastrointestinal bleeding. Endoscopy 2011; 43 Suppl 2 UCTN:E395
45. Daldrup-Link HE, Henning T, Link TM (2007) MR imaging of therapy-induced changes of bone marrow. Eur Radiol 17:743–761
46. Casamassima F, Ruggiero C, Caramella D, Tinacci E, Villari N, Ruggiero M (1989) Hematopoietic bone marrow recovery after radiation therapy: MRI evaluation. Blood 73:1677–1681
47. Aleman BM, van den Belt-Dusebout AW, Klokman WJ, Van't Veer MB, Bartelink H, van Leeuwen FE (2003) Long-term cause-specific mortality of patients treated for Hodgkin's disease. J Clin Onco Off J Am Soc Clin Oncol 21:3431–3439
48. Galper SL, Yu JB, Mauch PM et al (2011) Clinically significant cardiac disease in patients with Hodgkin lymphoma treated with mediastinal irradiation. Blood 117:412–418
49. Hancock SL, Tucker MA, Hoppe RT (1993) Factors affecting late mortality from heart disease after treatment of Hodgkin's disease. JAMA J Am Med Assoc 270:1949–1955
50. Hull MC, Morris CG, Pepine CJ, Mendenhall NP (2003) Valvular dysfunction and carotid, subclavian, and coronary artery disease in survivors of hodgkin lymphoma treated with radiation therapy. JAMA J Am Med Assoc 290:2831–2837
51. Adams MJ, Hardenbergh PH, Constine LS, Lipshultz SE (2003) Radiation-associated cardiovascular disease. Crit Rev Oncol/Hematol 45:55–75
52. Swain SM, Whaley FS, Ewer MS (2003) Congestive heart failure in patients treated with doxorubicin: a retrospective analysis of three trials. Cancer 97:2869–2879
53. Hodgson DC (2011) Late effects in the era of modern therapy for Hodgkin lymphoma. Hematol/Ed Prog Am Soc Hematol Am Soc Hematol Ed Prog 2011:323–329
54. Busia A, Laffranchi A, Viviani S, Bonfante V, Villani F (2010) Cardiopulmonary toxicity of different chemoradiotherapy combined regimens for Hodgkin's disease. Anticancer Res 30:4381–4387
55. Specht L, Yahalom J, Illidge T et al (2014) Modern radiation therapy for Hodgkin lymphoma: field and dose guidelines from the international lymphoma radiation oncology group (ILROG). Int J Radiat Oncol Biol Phys 89:854–862
56. Graves PR, Siddiqui F, Anscher MS, Movsas B (2010) Radiation pulmonary toxicity: from mechanisms to management. Semin Radiat Oncol 20:201–207
57. Park KJ, Chung JY, Chun MS, Suh JH (2000) Radiation-induced lung disease and the impact of radiation methods on imaging features. Radiograp Rev Pub Radiol Soc North Am Inc 20:83–98
58. Froudarakis M, Hatzimichael E, Kyriazopoulou L et al (2013) Revisiting bleomycin from pathophysiology to safe clinical use. Critical Rev Onco/Hematol 87:90–100
59. Rossi SE, Erasmus JJ, McAdams HP, Sporn TA, Goodman PC (2000) Pulmonary drug toxicity: radiologic and pathologic manifestations. Radiograp Rev Pub Radiol Soc North Am Inc 20:1245–1259
60. Cella L, Liuzzi R, D'Avino V et al (2014) Pulmonary damage in Hodgkin's lymphoma patients treated with sequential chemo-

radiotherapy: predictors of radiation-induced lung injury. Acta Oncol 53:613–619
61. Hodgson DC, Gilbert ES, Dores GM et al (2007) Long-term solid cancer risk among 5-year survivors of Hodgkin's lymphoma. J Clin Oncol Off J Am Soc Clin Oncol 25:1489–1497
62. Swerdlow AJ, Higgins CD, Smith P et al (2011) Second cancer risk after chemotherapy for Hodgkin's lymphoma: a collaborative British cohort study. J Clin Oncol Off J Am Soc Clin Oncol 29: 4096–4104
63. Ng AK, Bernardo MV, Weller E et al (2002) Second malignancy after Hodgkin disease treated with radiation therapy with or without chemotherapy: long-term risks and risk factors. Blood 100:1989–1996
64. Nyandoto P, Muhonen T, Joensuu H (1998) Second cancer among long-term survivors from Hodgkin's disease. Int J Radiat Oncol Biol Phys 42:373–378
65. Dores GM, Metayer C, Curtis RE et al (2002) Second malignant neoplasms among long-term survivors of Hodgkin's disease: a population-based evaluation over 25 years. J Clin Oncol Off J Am Soc Clin Oncol 20:3484–3494
66. Franklin J, Pluetschow A, Paus M et al (2006) Second malignancy risk associated with treatment of Hodgkin's lymphoma: meta-analysis of the randomised trials. Ann Oncol Off J Eur Soc Med Oncol/ESMO 17:1749–1760
67. Milano MT, Li H, Constine LS, Travis LB (2012) Variables affecting survival after second primary lung cancer: a population-based study of 187 Hodgkin's lymphoma patients. J Thor Dis 4:22–29
68. Ng A, Constine LS, Advani R et al (2010) ACR appropriateness criteria: follow-up of Hodgkin's lymphoma. Curr Probl Cancer 34: 211–227
69. Chirieac LR, Barletta JA, Yeap BY et al (2013) Clinicopathologic characteristics of malignant mesotheliomas arising in patients with a history of radiation for Hodgkin and non-Hodgkin lymphoma. J Clin Oncol Off J Am Soc Clin Oncol 31:4544–4549
70. Wang ZJ, Reddy GP, Gotway MB et al (2004) Malignant pleural mesothelioma: evaluation with CT, MR imaging, and PET. Radiograp Rev Pub Radiol Soc North Am Inc 24:105–119
71. Yamamuro M, Gerbaudo VH, Gill RR, Jacobson FL, Sugarbaker DJ, Hatabu H (2007) Morphologic and functional imaging of malignant pleural mesothelioma. Eur J Radiol 64:356–366
72. Park JY, Kim KW, Kwon HJ et al (2008) Peritoneal mesotheliomas: clinicopathologic features, CT findings, and differential diagnosis. AJR Am J Roentgenol 191:814–825
73. Hancock SL, Cox RS, McDougall IR (1991) Thyroid diseases after treatment of Hodgkin's disease. N Engl J Med 325:599–605
74. Shafford EA, Kingston JE, Healy JC, Webb JA, Plowman PN, Reznek RH (1999) Thyroid nodular disease after radiotherapy to the neck for childhood Hodgkin's disease. Br J Cancer 80:808–814
75. Morton LM, Dores GM, Curtis RE et al (2013) Stomach cancer risk after treatment for Hodgkin lymphoma. J Clin Oncol Off J Am Soc Clin Oncol 31:3369–3377
76. Sheppard DG, Libshitz HI (2001) Post-radiation sarcomas: a review of the clinical and imaging features in 63 cases. Clin Radiol 56:22–29
77. O'Regan K, Hall M, Jagannathan J et al (2011) Imaging of radiation-associated sarcoma. AJR Am J Roentgenol 197:W30–36

23

Current updates on the molecular genetics and magnetic resonance imaging of focal nodular hyperplasia and hepatocellular adenoma

Maneesh Khanna · Subramaniyan Ramanathan · Najla Fasih · Nicola Schieda · Vivek Virmani · Matthew D. F. McInnes

Abstract

Focal nodular hyperplasia (FNH) and hepatocellular adenomas (HCAs) constitute benign hepatic neoplasms in adults. HCAs are monoclonal neoplasms characterised by an increased predilection to haemorrhage and also malignant transformation. On the other hand, FNH is a polyclonal tumour-like lesion that occurs in response to increased perfusion and has an uneventful clinical course. Recent advances in molecular genetics and genotype-phenotype correlation in these hepatocellular neoplasms have enabled a new classification system. FNHs are classified into the typical and atypical types based on histomorphological and imaging features. HCAs have been categorised into four subtypes: (1) HCAs with HNF-1α mutations are diffusely steatotic, do not undergo malignant transformation, and are associated with familial diabetes or adenomatosis. (2) Inflammatory HCAs are hypervascular with marked peliosis and a tendency to bleed. They are associated with obesity, alcohol and hepatic steatosis. (3) HCAs with β-catenin mutations are associated with male hormone administration and glycogen storage disease, frequently undergo malignant transformation and may simulate hepatocellular carcinoma on imaging. (4) The final type is unclassified HCAs. Each of these except the unclassified subtype has a few distinct imaging features, often enabling reasonably accurate diagnosis. Biopsy with immunohistochemical analysis is helpful in difficult cases and has strong implications for patient management.

Teaching points

- *FNHs are benign polyclonal neoplasms with no risk of haemorrhage or malignancy.*
- *HCAs are benign monoclonal neoplasms classified into four subtypes based on immunohistochemistry.*
- *Inflammatory HCAs show an atoll sign with a risk of bleeding and malignant transformation.*
- *HNF-1α HCAs are steatotic HCAs with minimal complications and the best prognosis.*
- *β-Catenin HCA shows variable MRI features and a high risk of malignancy.*

Keywords Focal nodular hyperplasia · Hepatocellular adenoma · MRI · Molecular genetics · Immunohistochemistry

M. Khanna · S. Ramanathan · N. Fasih · N. Schieda · V. Virmani · M. D. F. McInnes
Department of Diagnostic Imaging, The Ottawa Hospital, University of Ottawa, Ontario, Canada

M. Khanna
Department of Radiology, Hamad General Hospital, Hamad Medical Corporation, Doha, Qatar

S. Ramanathan
Department of Radiology, Al-Wakra Hospital, Hamad Medical Corporation, Doha, Qatar

S. Ramanathan (✉)
Al-Wakra Hospital, Hamad Medical Corporation, PO Box 82228, Doha, Qatar
e-mail: subbu2000@yahoo.com

Introduction

Benign hepatocellular lesions in adults can be divided into two main categories according to their pathogenesis: regenerative lesions, composed mainly of focal nodular hyperplasia

(FNH), and neoplastic lesions, corresponding to hepatocellular adenomas (HCAs) [1]. FNH and HCAs are the second and third most common benign liver tumours after haemangiomas, respectively [1, 2]. Accurate imaging differentiation of these two types of lesions is essential as the treatment strategies differ considerably. HCAs can present with bleeding or undergo malignant degeneration and often require surgery whereas FNH is a do-not-touch lesion. The recent identification of various molecular pathways altered in these tumours has significantly increased our knowledge of benign hepatocellular tumorigenesis. Moreover, knowledge of the genotype-phenotype correlation in HCA has helped in establishing a new radio-pathological classification. New immunohistochemical and cytogenetic markers have been identified for differentiating various subtypes of HCA. Various studies have identified specific imaging features corresponding to typical and atypical FNH and for differentiating various subtypes of HCA. In this review, we focus on the recent progress in the understanding of the molecular mechanisms and characteristic cross-sectional imaging features with special emphasis on the role of MRI in these two hepatocellular tumours. We also discuss their role in deciding on the different management strategies after diagnosis.

Focal nodular hyperplasia (FNH)

FNH is defined as a nodule composed of benign-appearing hepatocytes occurring in a liver that is otherwise histologically normal or nearly normal. It is the second most common benign liver tumour after haemangioma with a prevalence of 0.9 % and commonly occurs in young females (male:female ratio=1:8) [3]. The majority of FNHs are solitary (80 %), smaller than 5 cm in diameter and occur near the surface of the liver [4]. In contrast to monoclonal HCAs, which frequently bleed, FNHs are polyclonal tumour-like lesions and do not undergo haemorrhage or malignant transformation [5]. Although an association with oral contraceptive use has been speculated, owing to the increased prevalence of these tumours in young women, studies have shown that FNH is not hormonally dependent [6]. Association with vascular diseases such as hereditary haemorrhagic telangiectasia (Rendu-Osler-Weber disease) and congenital absence of the portal vein can be seen [1].

FNH is often an incidental finding at imaging. Distinction between FNH and other hypervascular liver lesions such as HCA, hepatocellular carcinoma (HCC) and hypervascular metastases is critical as the management differs considerably. FNH is asymptomatic in most patients, and in such cases no treatment is necessary. One third of patients may present with abdominal pain or a palpable mass. Typically, FNH follows a benign natural course and remains stable or may even decrease in size at follow-up examination [5].

Molecular cytogenetics and pathogenesis

Genetic analysis of FNH failed to identify somatic gene mutations in the β-catenin gene (*CTNNB1*), *TP53*, *APC* or HNF1α. FNH typically shows dysregulation of the angiopoietin genes, which are responsible for the maturation of blood vessels. An increase in the angiopoietin expression results in uncontrolled maturation and remodelling of vessels, resulting in dystrophic vascular architecture typical of FNH [1, 7]. Wanless et al. postulated that portal tract injury due to either portal tract inflammation or arterial ischaemia is the primary event leading to vascular shunting with hepatocyte hyperplasia and cholestasis [8, 9]. Arterial hyperperfusion and the resultant hyperoxemia lead to increased expression of vascular endothelial and somatic growth factors and activation of hepatic stellate cells leading to the formation of the characteristic central scar [8].

The β-catenin pathway is activated, including the downstream target, glutamine synthetase, which explains the polyclonal over-proliferation of hepatocytes. The molecular mechanisms of this activation are uncertain, but do not involve demonstrable mutations in β-catenin or Axin, unlike HCA [10]. Immunohistochemistry shows a perivenous map-like distribution of glutamine synthetase [11].

Classification

Currently, FNH is divided into two types: classic and non-classic or atypical. [12].

Classic FNH

Classic FNH is characterised by the presence of abnormal nodular architecture, malformed vessels and cholangiolar proliferation. One or more macroscopic central scars are present in most cases that contain fibrous connective tissue, cholangiolar proliferation with surrounding inflammatory infiltrates and malformed vessels. Arterial blood flows centrifugally from the anomalous central arteries. Approximately 50 % of lesions show some degree of fatty infiltration, as opposed to the surrounding liver, which shows signs of steatosis in less than 20 % of lesions. Both the classic and non-classic types contain variable amounts of Kupffer cells [13].

Imaging features

Classic FNH has typical imaging findings enabling accurate diagnosis. FNH is found as an incidental iso- to hypoechoic focal lesion on ultrasound although the isoechoic nature often makes the detection of lesions difficult. A central vascular scar may be seen. Further evaluation with dynamic contrast-enhanced CT or MRI is warranted in most cases for definitive diagnosis. It appears as a lobulated iso- to hypodense lesion on unenhanced CT and shows homogeneous, intense arterial enhancement becoming isoattenuating in the portal and delayed phases with no washout. The central scar showing delayed enhancement because of myxomatous stroma can be seen in 20 % of cases [14].

Magnetic resonance imaging (MRI) has higher sensitivity (70 %) and specificity (98 %) for FNH than US and CT. MRI features include T1 iso- or hypointensity (94–100 %), T2 slight hyper- or isointensity (94–100 %) and a hyperintense central scar (84 %). A scar is usually seen in FNH>3 cm [15]. Lesions show intense homogeneous enhancement in the arterial phase, isointensity during the portal phase and delayed enhancement of the central scar [16] (Fig. 1).

Hepatobiliary-specific contrast agents are being increasingly used in differentiating focal liver lesions. FNH is characterised by an increased density of functioning hepatocytes and hence shows persistent enhancement (iso- or hyperintense) on delayed phase (20 min) gadoxetic acid-enhanced images (Fig. 2). Three patterns of enhancement are described on the 20-min hepatobiliary phase: a homogeneously hyperintense, inhomogeneously hyperintense and peripheral hyperintense rim (hypointense with a ring pattern) (Fig. 3). Approximately 10–12 % of the lesions may not show hyperintensity on the 20-min delayed phase, warranting further evaluation with biopsy or close interval imaging [17]. The presence of abnormal bile ductules that fail to communicate with the normal biliary system possibly results in defective or delayed excretion with persistent contrast agent retention [18, 19]. In contrast, HCA and HCC typically do not show contrast agent retention. A central scar appears hypointense on 10- and 20-min delayed phases because of the predominant fibrous tissue with no well-formed bile ductules [20, 21].

Non-classic FNH

Non-classic FNH lesions always show cholangiolar proliferation like classic FNH but lack either nodular abnormal architecture or malformed vessels. Lack of a central scar, incomplete multinodular organisation and prominent areas of congestion are some of the histopathological features of non-classic or atypical FNH [22, 12].

Imaging features

Typical MRI features of FNH lesions, which include homogeneous iso- to hypointensity on TI-weighted images, homogeneous slight hyper- to isointensity on T2-weighted images and a central hyperintense scar on T2-weighted images, are seen in only 9–50 % of these lesions [23, 24]. Various atypical features described at MRI include [16, 25, 26]:

1. Heterogeneous signal intensity on both T1- and T2 weighted sequences due to sinusoidal dilatation, fatty infiltration and/or small haemorrhagic foci.

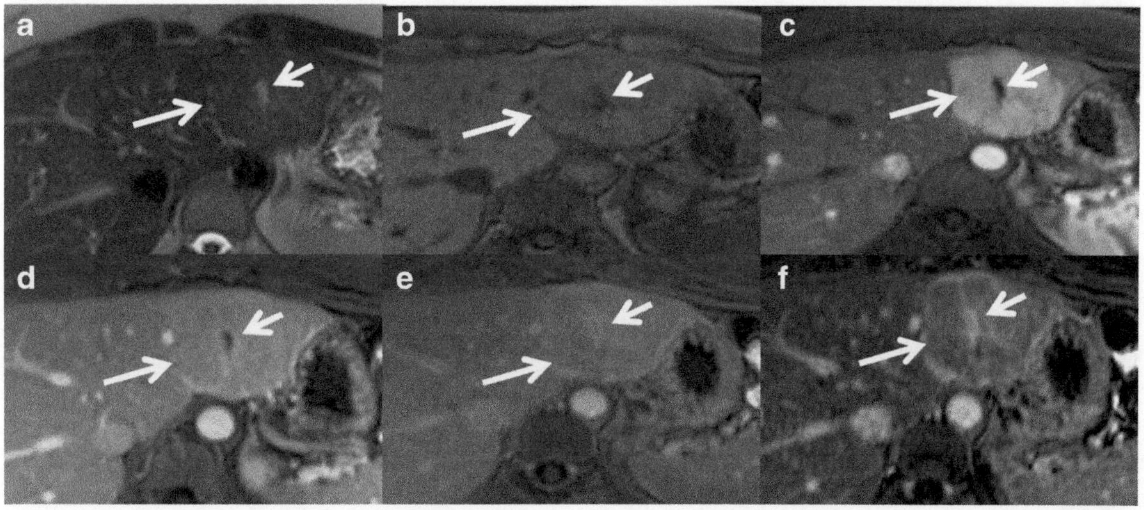

Fig. 1 Classic focal nodular hyperplasia (FNH) in a 40-year-old female incidentally detected on ultrasound (not shown here). (**a**) Axial T2W MRI shows a well-circumscribed T2 isointense lesion (*long arrow*) in the left lobe of the liver with a central T2 hyperintense scar (short arrow). (**b**) Axial T1W MRI shows a well-circumscribed T1 isointense lesion (long arrow) in the left lobe of the liver with a central T2 hypointense scar (*short arrow*). (**c**) Axial post-contrast MRI in the arterial phase reveals intense enhancement of the lesion (*long arrow*) with a non-enhancing central scar (*short arrow*). Axial post-contrast MRI in the venous (**d**) and delayed phases (**e** and **f**) shows the isointense nature of the lesion (*long arrow*) with progressive delayed enhancement of the central scar (*short arrow*)

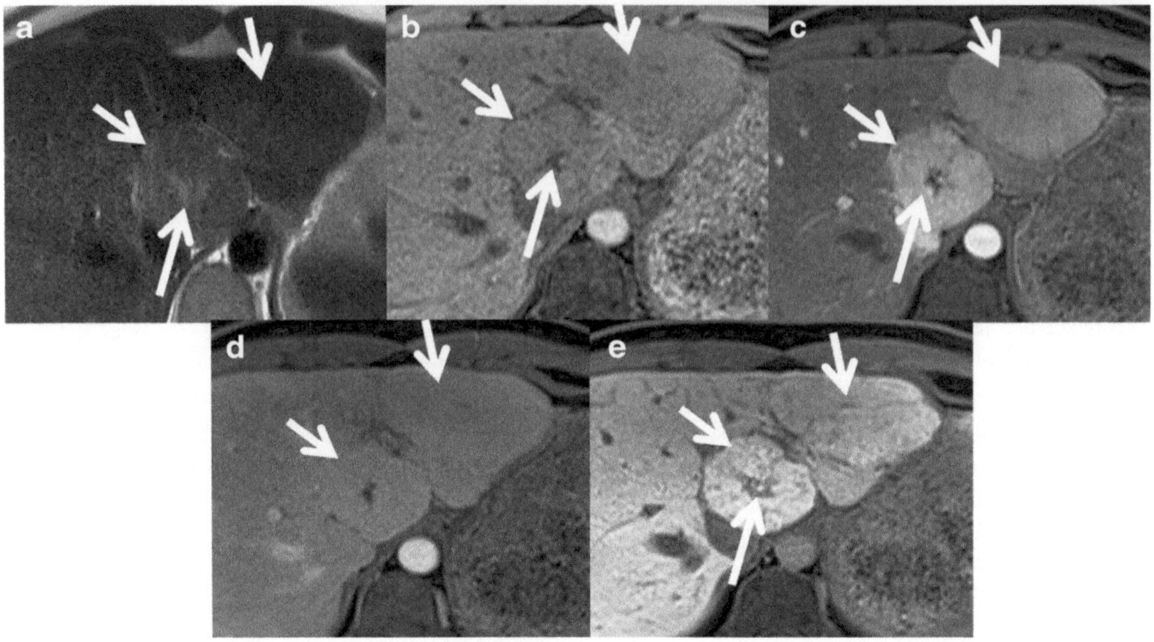

Fig. 2 Classic FNH in a 35-year-old female with hepatobiliary-specific contrast (gadoxetate). (**a**) Axial T2W MRI shows two large isointense lesions in the left lobe of the liver (*short arrows*) with a T2 hyperintense central scar (*long arrow*). (**b**) Axial T1W MRI shows two large isointense lesions in the left lobe of the liver (*short arrows*) with a T1 hypointense central scar (*long arrow*). Axial post-contrast MRI with gadoxetate shows intense enhancement of the lesions (short *arrows*) in the arterial phase (**c**) becoming isointense on the portal venous phase (**d**) and persistent enhancement in the 20-min hepatobiliary phase (**e**). The central scar shows no enhancement (*long arrow*)

2. T1 hyperintensity due to fat, copper accumulation, high protein concentrations, blood degradation products or sinusoidal dilatation.

3. Absense of a central scar, which is typically detectable for lesions greater than 3 cm. The scar can be extremely small or undetectable on CT (16–40 %) and MRI (22 %) [4, 14,

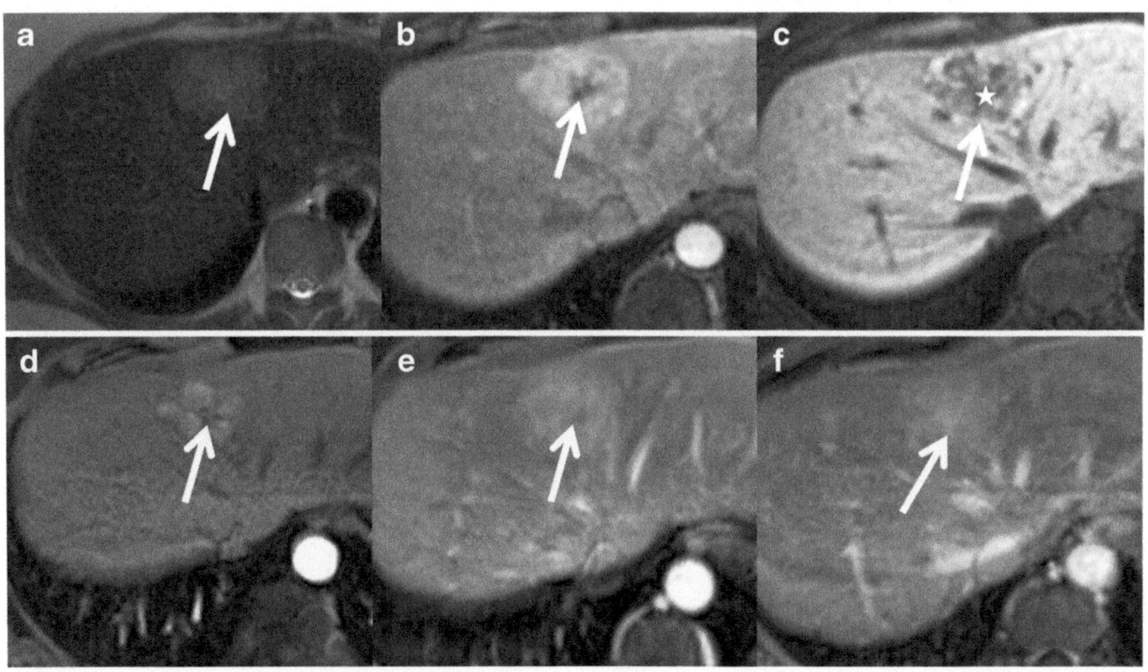

Fig. 3 Appearance of FNH with hepatobiliary-specific contrast (gadoxetate) and a routine extracellular agent (gadolinium). (**a**) Axial T2W MRI shows iso- to mildly hyperintense lesions in segment 4 of the left lobe of the liver (*arrow*). (**b**) Axial post-contrast MRI with gadoxetate shows intense enhancement of the lesions in the arterial phase with a non-enhancing central scar (*arrow*). (**c**) Axial post-contrast MRI in the 20-min hepatobiliary phase shows a peripheral ring of hyperintensity (*arrow*) with central non-enhancement (asterisk). Follow-up MRI with gadolinium after 6 months shows an enhancing lesion with a non-enhancing scar (*arrow*) in the arterial phase (**d**) and persistent enhancement in the portal venous (**e**) and delayed phases (**f**) with delayed enhancement of the central scar (*arrow*)

27]. The central scar can appear hypointense on T2 with no delayed enhancement mimicking the collagenous scar seen in HCA, fibro-lamellar carcinoma, HCC or intrahepatic cholangiocarcinoma likely from obliterative vascular hyperplasia of the central scar [4, 15].

4. A pseudo-capsule due to compressive effects on the adjacent hepatic parenchyma as well as the presence of dilated vessels and sinusoids around the lesion.
5. Interval growth is considered an atypical and worrisome finding in FNH.
6. FNH can rarely show intralesional steatosis, often due to extension from the underlying hepatic steatosis (Fig. 4). Other possible explanations for intralesional steatosis in FNH are hepatic injury associated with steatosis from alcoholic toxicity, obesity, diabetes or malnutrition [28, 29].
7. Telangiectatic FNH is an uncommon entity but the most common among non-classic FNHs. These lesions often show heterogeneity on pre- and post-contrast CT and MRI, and they are strongly hyperintense on T1- and T2-weighted images, often with an absent central scar. Intense arterial enhancement with persistent enhancement during the hepatic venous and equilibrium phases is seen. Recently, a molecular study identified several genetic similarities between telangiectatic FNH and HCA indicating most of these are actually inflammatory hepatic adenomas and have been misclassified as 'telangiectatic FNH' [30].
8. Development of FNH in childhood and presence of symptoms can also be considered as atypical features.
9. Approximately 20 % of patients have multiple FNHs, which are often of a non-classic subtype with atypical imaging features. Multiple FNH syndrome is defined as consisting of two or more FNHs in combination with hepatic liver haemangioma or vascular malformations or intracranial tumours [31, 32] (Fig. 5). Focal disturbance of the hepatic blood supply has been advocated as the most likely causative factor for the concomitant development of these benign hepatic lesions.

Management

FNH with typical imaging features is managed conservatively and does not necessitate surgical intervention. Surgical excision is considered for symptomatic lesions likely from compression of adjacent structures or hepatic capsular stretching. FNH with atypical imaging features needs further evaluation in the form of additional imaging, percutaneous guided biopsy and follow-up. Suspicious lesions could be followed up or surgically excised [33].

Hepatocellular adenoma (HCA)

HCAs are rare benign monoclonal hepatic tumours that commonly occur in females who have been receiving oral contraceptives. The duration of oral contraceptive use and oestrogen content determine the risk of developing HCA. It rarely occurs in children and men (male:female=1:9) [34]. Other risk factors for HCAs include use of anabolic steroids, glycogen storage disease (types Ia, III and VI), haemochromatosis, androgen therapy, and use of barbiturates and clomiphene [35].

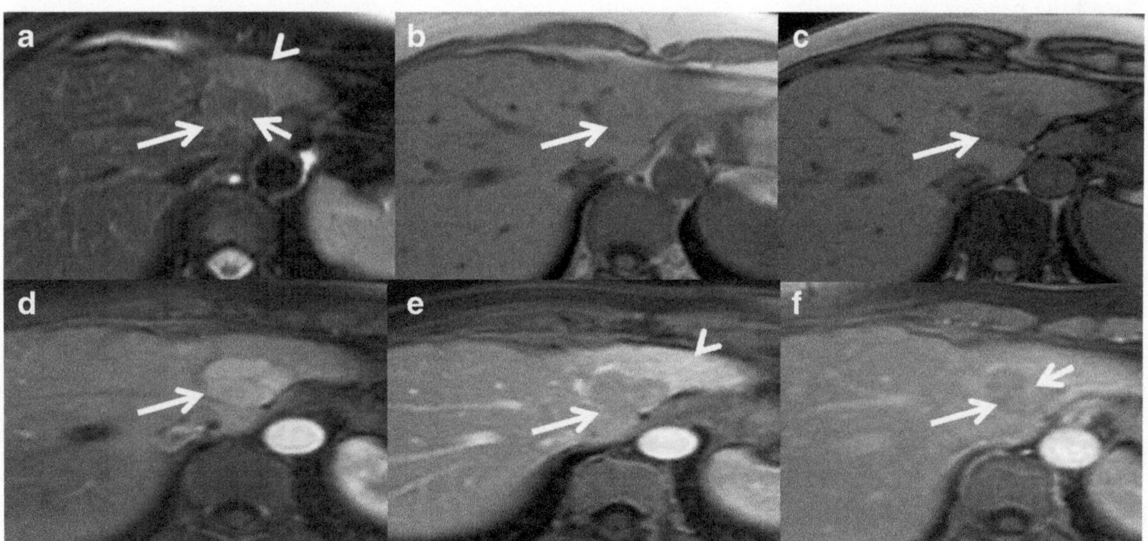

Fig. 4 Biopsy-proven FNH with intralesional steatosis in a 46-year-old female. (**a**) Axial T2W MRI shows an isointense lesion (*long arrow*) in the left lobe of the liver with a faint hyperintense central scar (*short arrow*). Axial T1 in-phase (**b**) and out-of-phase (**c**) MRIs show a drop in signal in the out-of-phase images representing intralesional lipid (arrow). Axial post-contrast MRI shows an enhancing lesion (*arrow*) in the arterial phase (**d**) becoming iso- to mildly hypointense in the portal venous (**e**) and delayed phases (**f**) with delayed enhancement of the central scar (*arrow*). Arrowheads denote transient oedema/enhancement

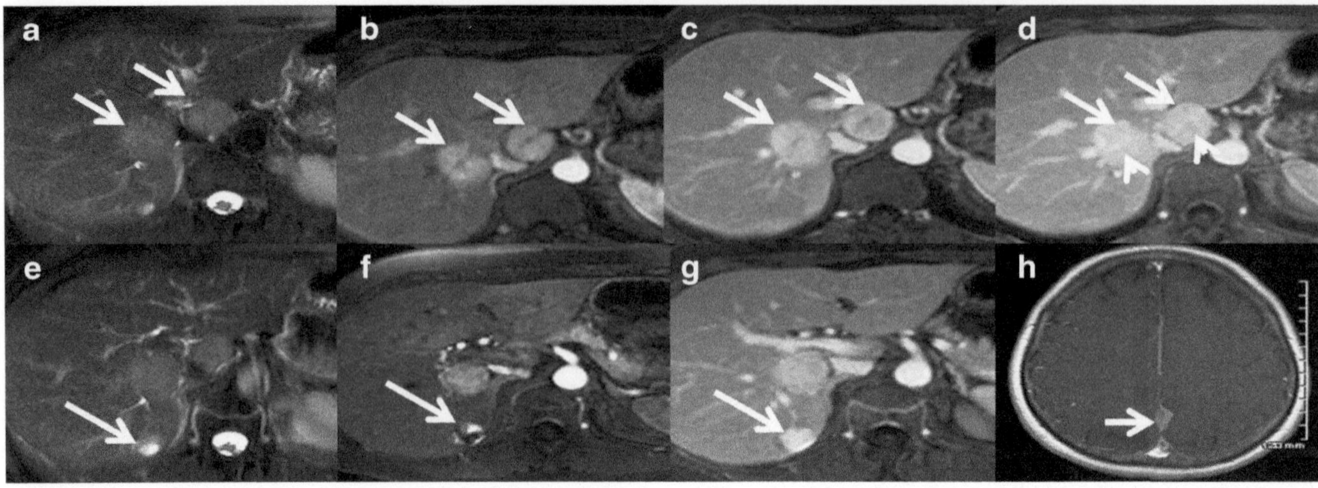

Fig. 5 Multiple FNH syndrome in a 50-year-old female. (**a**) Axial T2W MRI shows two iso- to mildly hyperintense focal lesions (*arrows*) in segments 8 and 4 of the liver. Axial post-contrast MRI shows intense enhancement of the lesions (*arrow*) in the arterial phase (**b**) and persistent enhancement (*arrow*) in the portal venous (**c**) and delayed phases (**d**) with delayed enhancement of the central scar (arrowheads). (**e**) Axial T2W MRI in the same patient shows a small T2 hyperintense lesion in segment 7 (*arrow*). Axial post-contrast MRI shows peripheral nodular enhancement (*arrow*) in the arterial phase (**f**) with progressive centripetal filling (*arrow*) in delayed phase (**g**) in keeping with haemangioma. (**h**) Axial post-contrast MRI brain shows a small enhancing extra-axial lesion in the falx cerebri representing meningioma

Patients may present with right upper quadrant pain or a palpable mass. Up to 50 % of patients are asymptomatic. HCAs can be complicated by life-threatening bleeding or undergo malignant transformation necessitating surgical management [36].

Classification

Initially three MRI patterns were identified corresponding to three pathologic forms, namely the steatotic, peliotic and mixed types [37]. Later, the Bordeaux group divided HCAs into four different subgroups based on molecular genetics, histopathology and clinical features. Various studies have described characteristic imaging features enabling precise diagnosis in select subtypes. Accordingly, HCAs are currently categorised into four distinct genetic and pathologic subtypes: (1) inflammatory HCAs, (2) hepatocyte nuclear factor 1 alpha (HNF-1α)-mutated HCAs, (3) β-catenin-mutated HCAs and (4) unclassified [38, 39].

Inflammatory HCAs

Inflammatory HCAs are the most common subtype and account for about 40–50 % of all HCAs. Inflammatory HCAs include liver tumours previously referred to as “telangiectatic FNH” or “telangiectatic adenomas”. They occur most frequently in young females with a history of oral contraceptive usage and in obese patients. Patients may present with signs of chronic anaemia and/or systemic inflammatory syndrome characterised by fever, leukocytosis and elevated serum C-reactive protein [40].

Sustained activation of the Janus kinase (JAK)-signal transducer and activator of transcription (STAT) pathway (JAK-STAT pathway), with resultant hepatocellular proliferation, is the proposed pathogenesis in the development of inflammatory HCAs. This can happen via two pathways: (1) somatic gain-of-function mutations involving the IL6ST gene, which encodes the oncogene gp130 in 60 % of cases, and (2) STAT3 activation without mutations in gp130 in 40 % of cases [38]. Often there is activation of acute-phase inflammation proteins, such as serum amyloid A and C-reactive protein [11].

Inflammatory HCAs appear heterogeneous with areas of congestion and frank haemorrhage on gross pathology. Intense polymorph nuclear infiltrates, marked sinusoidal dilatation and thick-walled arteries are seen on histopathology. Immunohistochemistry shows homogeneous glutamine synthetase and β-catenin staining [11].

On imaging, inflammatory HCAs manifest as hypervascular liver masses with persistent enhancement on portal venous and delayed phase images. They show diffuse T2 hyperintensity and iso- to mild T1 hyperintensity. Focal areas of microscopic fat may be seen in a small (11 %) subset of patients. Sensitivity, specificity, positive and negative predictive values of marked T2 hyperintense signal with delayed persistent enhancement are 85.2, 87.5, and 88.5 and 84 %, respectively, for the diagnosis of inflammatory HCAs [41]. The atoll sign, present in approximately 50 % of cases, includes a T2 hyperintense rim in the periphery of the lesion (correlating with dilated sinusoids) with central isointensity resembling a coral reef and lagoon respectively (Figs. 6 and 7). Small intralesional T2-hyperintense nodules can be found in the centre of the lesion (small islands) [42].

HNF-1α-mutated HCAs

HNF-1α-mutated HCAs are the second most common subtype and constitute 30–35 % of all HCAs. These develop exclusively in female patients with a history of oral contraceptive use and the tumours are multiple in about 50 % of patients. Often these are incidentally discovered on CT performed for other reasons and are asymptomatic. An association with *maturity*-onset diabetes of the young (MODY), type 3 and familial hepatic adenomatosis has been reported [36, 43, 44].

Biallelic-inactivating mutation of the *TCF1* gene inactivating hepatocyte nuclear factor 1α (HNF-1 α) is the primary event and could be somatic (90–95 %) or germ line (up to 10 %) in origin. The resultant non-functioning HNF-1α protein promotes lipogenesis and hepatocellular proliferation. Also there is suppression of liver fatty acid-binding protein, resulting in impaired fatty acid transport in hepatocytes, leading to intracellular fat deposition. Oestrogens act as endogenous genotoxic agents and cause hepatocyte proliferation by somatic mutations in the TCF1 gene [2, 36, 38].

Excessive lipid accumulation in the tumour hepatocytes is typical on histopathology. No portal tract elements or cytological abnormalities are seen. Immunohistochemistry shows characteristic absence of liver fatty acid-binding protein [11].

On MRI, these tumours show predominantly hyper- or isointensity on T1 with a diffuse signal drop on chemical shift imaging (CSI) because of intracellular steatosis. T1 hyperintensity could also be due to glycogen and haemorrhage. Iso- to slight hyperintensity is seen on T2. Moderate enhancement in the arterial phase with no persistent enhancement in the portal venous and delayed phases is typical (Fig. 8). Sensitivity, specificity, and positive and negative predictive values of a homogeneous signal drop on CSI for the diagnosis of HNF-1α-mutated HCAs are 86.7, 100, 100 and 94.7 %, respectively [41]. Uncommonly macroscopic fat could be identified on CT in approximately 7 %. MRI is more accurate and shows microscopic fat in 35–77 % of cases [45]. Benign nodular steatosis and fat-containing HCC cannot be completely differentiated from steatotic HCA on imaging alone and may need further evaluation with histopathological and/or immunohistochemical analyses [46]. HNF1α-mutated HCA is the least aggressive subtype and has minimal or no risk of malignant transformation. Tumours <5 cm show minimal risk of bleeding [35].

β-Catenin-mutated HCAs

β-Catenin-mutated HCAs are the third most common subtype and constitute 10–15 % of all HCAs. These occur more

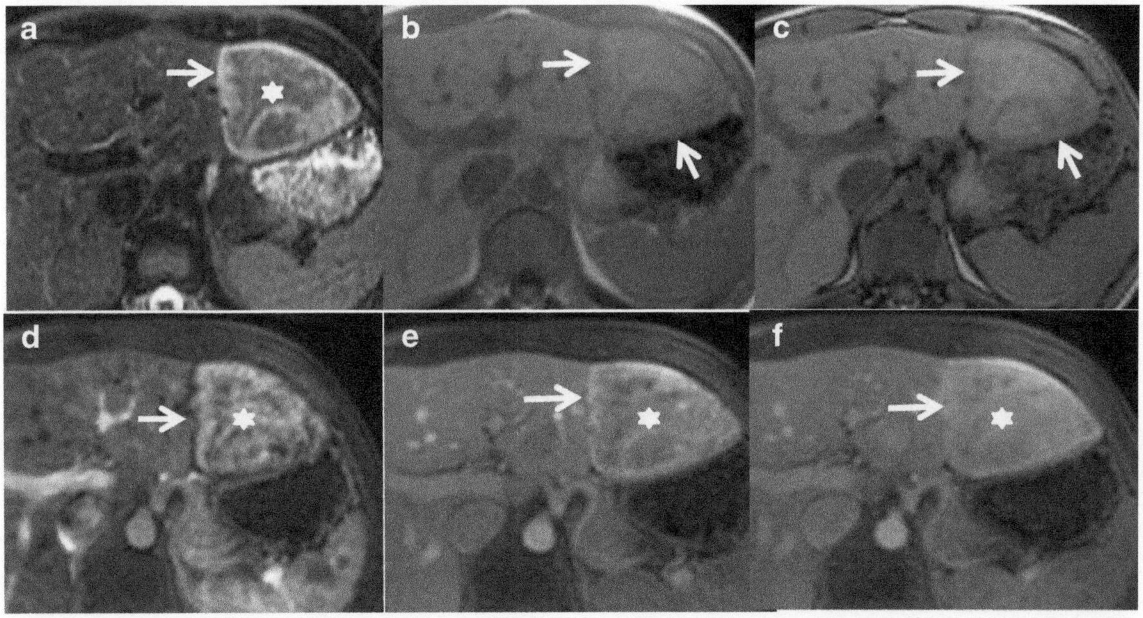

Fig. 6 A 30-year-old female with incidental detection of a hypoechoic nodule on ultrasound. (**a**) Axial fat-saturated T2W MRI shows an iso- to hyperintense lesion (asterisk) in the left lobe of the liver with a peripheral T2 hyperintense rim (*arrow*) representing the atoll sign. Axial T1 in-phase (**b**) and out-of-phase (**c**) MRI shows no drop in signal (*arrows*). (**d**) Axial post-contrast MRI in the arterial phase shows moderate heterogeneous central enhancement (asterisk) and peripheral rim enhancement (*arrow*). Axial post-contrast MRI in the venous phase (**e**) and delayed phases (**f**) shows persistent enhancement (asterisk) with delayed enhancement of the peripheral rim (*arrow*). Surgical resection confirmed the diagnosis of inflammatory hepatocellular adenoma

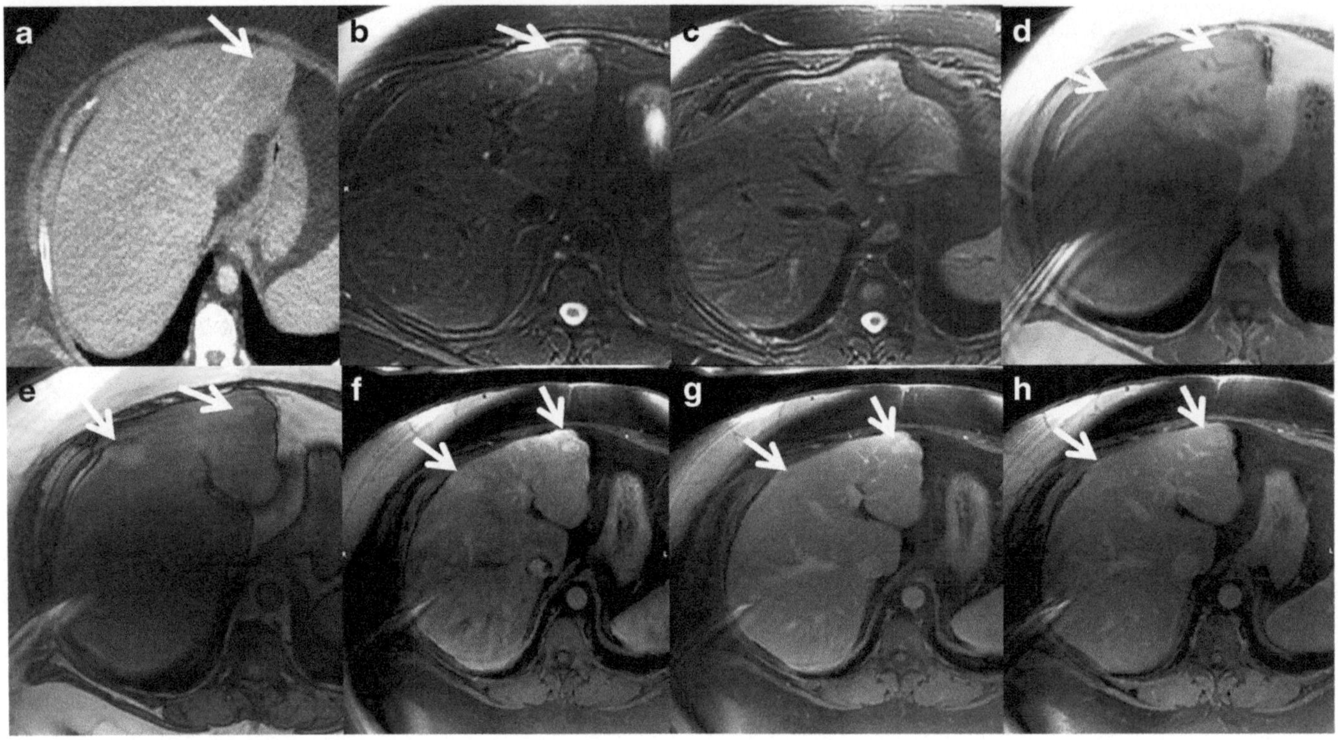

Fig. 7 A 38-year-old female with multiple liver lesions. This morbidly obese patient presented with acute abdominal pain and a solitary liver lesion in the lateral segment (*white arrow*) detected on axial contrast-enhanced CT (**a**). Peri-lesional complex fluid was noted (not shown) and the patient was taken to the operative theatre where a haemorrhagic liver lesion was resected. Four other liver lesions were noted at the time of surgery. The clinical and operative presumptive diagnosis was multiple hepatocellular adenomas, most likely of the inflammatory subtype. The original histopathological analysis described the resected lesion as an atypical focal nodular hyperplasia. Immunohistochemistry was performed several months later. Glutaminesynthetase stains depicted typical perivascular staining consistent with adenoma (not shown). **b** Catenin stains were negative and combined with the history of morbid obesity and metabolic syndrome a diagnosis of inflammatory adenoma was given. Follow-up MR examination was performed 2 years after surgery. Axial fat-suppressed T2W FSE images (**b** and **c**) demonstrate two lesions in the lateral segment (*white arrow*) and in the right anterior lobe (*arrowhead*) with increased T2W signal intensity relative to the liver. There is a faint peripheral rim of increased signal in the lateral segment lesion consistent with an atoll sign. Axial T1W images in (**d**) and opposed (**e**) phase demonstrate moderate diffuse hepatic steatosis and inhomogeneous intralesional steatosis (note the peripheral signal intensity drop) within both lesions (*arrows*). Also note the susceptibility artefact on the in-phase GRE image (**d**) at the lateral margin of the left lobe related to previous resection. Axial fat-suppressed T1W GRE images obtained after injection of extracellular gadolinium during the hepatic arterial (**f**), portal venous (**g**) and 5-min delayed (**h**) phases depict heterogeneous arterial enhancement that persists on delayed phases (*arrows*)

frequently in males and are associated with male hormone administration, glycogen storage disease and familial adenomatosis polyposis [39]. The incidence of HCAs in glycogen storage disease varies from 22–75 and 75 % of these patients older than 30 years harbour HCA. Chronic liver inflammation due to glycogen storage disease leads to the development of HCA and HCC. There is a gain of chromosome 6p and loss of chromosome 6q in these patients, which are also frequently seen in HCC and dysplastic nodules, thereby accounting for the high risk of malignant transformation associated with HCAs in patients with glycogen storage disease [47].

β-Catenin is encoded by the catenin β 1 gene (CTNNB1), located at chromosome 3p21. Mutation results in sustained activation of β-catenin protein, resulting in uncontrolled hepatocyte proliferation. Cytologic abnormalities, such as a high nuclear-cytoplasmic ratio, nuclear atypia and acini formation, are seen on histopathology and mimic well-differentiated hepatocellular carcinoma. Strong and diffuse positivity to glutamine synthase is characteristic of this subtype on immunohistochemical analysis [36].

On MRI, these tumours show heterogeneous T2 signal, which can be iso-, hypo- or hyperintense relative to the liver and shows no intratumoral steatosis. Intense arterial enhancement is seen, which may or may not persist into the delayed phase. Portal venous washout can be seen mimicking HCC [2]. A recent study correlates the presence of a vaguely demarcated scar and poorly delimited high-signal-intensity areas on T2-weighted images to β-catenin positivity [42] (Fig. 9). Tumours occurring in the setting of glycogen storage disease may show diffuse increased attenuation of liver on CT images.

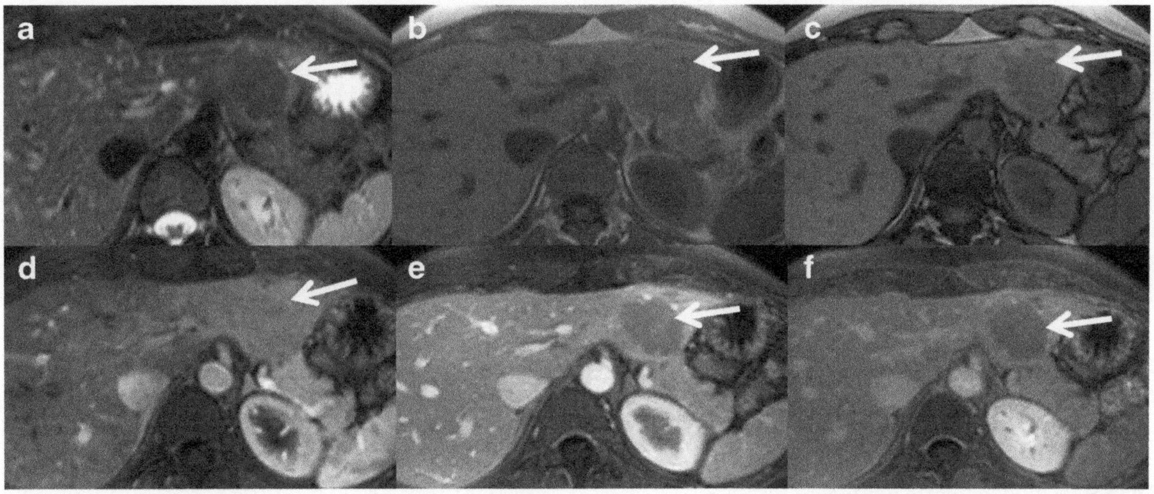

Fig. 8 A 26-year-old female with right upper quadrant pain was found to have an echogenic nodule on ultrasound. (**a**) Axial T2W MRI shows an isointense lesion in the left lobe of the liver (*arrow*). Axial T1 in-phase (**b**) and out-of-phase (**c**) MRIs show a drop in signal in the out-of-phase images representing intralesional lipids (*arrow*). Axial post-contrast MRI in the arterial phase (**d**) shows mild diffuse enhancement of the lesion (*arrow*), not persisting in the portal venous (**e**) and delayed phases (**f**). MRI features are consistent with HNF-1α-mutated hepatocellular adenoma and the patient is on regular follow-up

Unclassified HCAs

This subtype constitutes approximately 10 % and does not show *HNF1* a, *CTNNB1* or *IL6ST* mutations. The predominant molecular pathogenesis and clinical and radiological features of this subset of tumours are poorly understood and further research is warranted [40].

Hepatic adenomatosis

Hepatic adenomatosis has been defined as the presence of multiple adenomas (arbitrarily >10) without any history of steroid therapy or glycogen storage disease [48]. It occurs in females during the 4th and 5th decades of life. Proposed aetiologies include congenital or acquired hepatic vascular

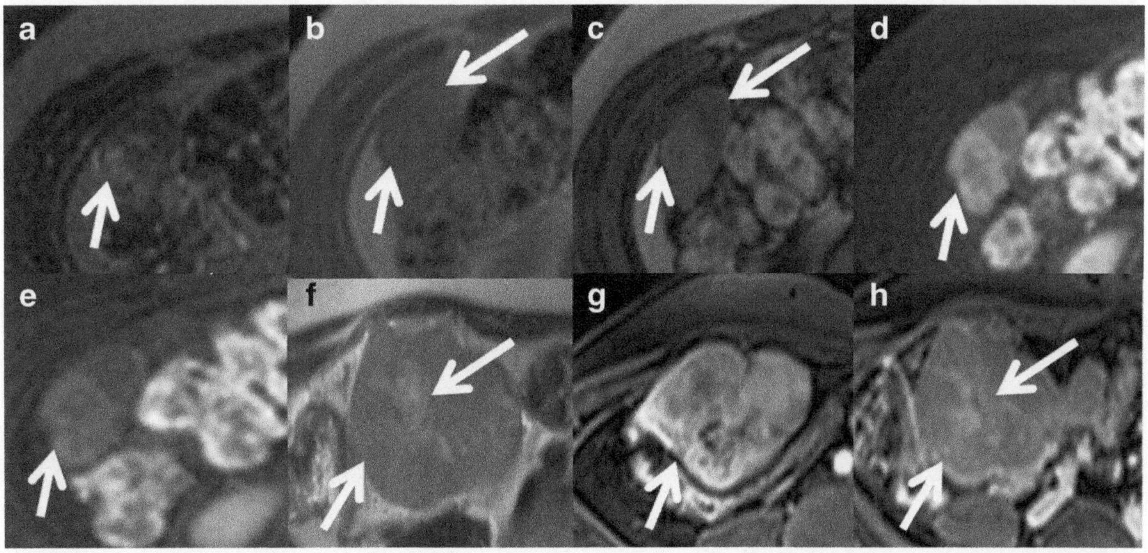

Fig. 9 A 42-year-old female with incidental detection of liver nodule. (**a**) Axial T2W MRI shows a small ill-defined lesion in segment 6 with vague T2 hyperintense areas. Axial T1 in-phase (**b**) and out-of-phase (**c**) MRIs show a drop in signal around the lesion indicating perilesional steatosis. Axial post-contrast MRI shows moderate enhancement (*arrows*) in the arterial phase (**d**) becoming iso- to mildly hypointense on delayed phase (**e**). Ultrasound-guided biopsy revealed hepatocellular adenoma (immunohistochemistry and genetic analysis not performed). Follow-up MRI after 2 years showed significant interval growth (*short arrow*) with vague T2 hyperintense areas (*long arrow*) on axial T2W MRI (**f**). Axial post-contrast MRI shows moderate heterogeneous enhancement (*arrow*) in the arterial phase (**g**) becoming iso- to mildly hypointense on delayed phase (**e**) with mild delayed enhancement of a vague central scar (*long arrow*). Surgical resection showed hepatocellular adenoma with multiple foci of well-differentiated hepatocellular carcinoma and genetic analysis revealed β-catenin mutation

abnormalities, mutations of the *HNF1A* gene and non-alcoholic fatty liver disease. HCAs in patients with hepatic adenomatosis may be of the inflammatory, HNF-1a-mutated or β-catenin-mutated subtypes, and their imaging appearances may vary accordingly [49] (Fig. 10). Contrary to the popular belief of increased complications in hepatic adenomatosis, a recent meta-analysis showed that hepatic adenomatosis per se does not have any increased risk of complications; the tumour size and subtype determine the risks of malignancy and bleeding [50]. Associated MODY should be evaluated in patients with hepatic adenomatosis and liver imaging is recommended in the relatives [51].

Role of hepatobiliary-specific contrast

The appearance of FNH on hepatobiliary contrast has been discussed previously in the article. As FNH is a do-not-touch lesion and HCAs often warrant surgery, differentiating both of them, also from malignant hepatic lesions, is of prime importance. Hepatobiliary contrast is now being increasingly used in atypical cases for differentiation, thereby avoiding invasive biopsies in a good number of cases.

HCAs show mild-to-moderate arterial enhancement in contrast to intense enhancement in FNH. However the inflammatory subtype can show arterial enhancement similar to FNH. The majority of HCAs (93 %) become hypointense on portal venous and delayed hepatobiliary phases with gadoxetic acid, unlike FNH (Fig. 11). The absence of biliary ducts in adenomas, and therefore reduced biliary excretion mechanisms, is believed to be one of the factors responsible for the decreased uptake. Again the inflammatory subtype can show mild hyperintensity on hepatobiliary phase possibly due to pooling of the contrast agent within the peliotic areas [18, 52]. Perhaps the most important recent discovery regarding inflammatory HCA is that it can mimic FNH on MRI. Thomeer et al. and Agarwal et al. both identified that 25 and 46 % of inflammatory HCAs are iso-hyperintense on the hepatobiliary phase on gadoxetic acid-enhanced MRI [53, 54]. In addition, they often mimicked FNH on other imaging sequences. These two recent publications should caution radiologists when using hepatocyte-specific contrast agents to diagnose FNH; if patients are at high risk for the inflammatory type of HCA (obesity, alcohol use), it may not be appropriate to rely on imaging features alone to make a diagnosis of FNH.

Complications

The two major complications of HCAs are *(a)* intratumoral bleeding with or without associated rupture and haemoperitoneum and *(b)* malignant transformation to

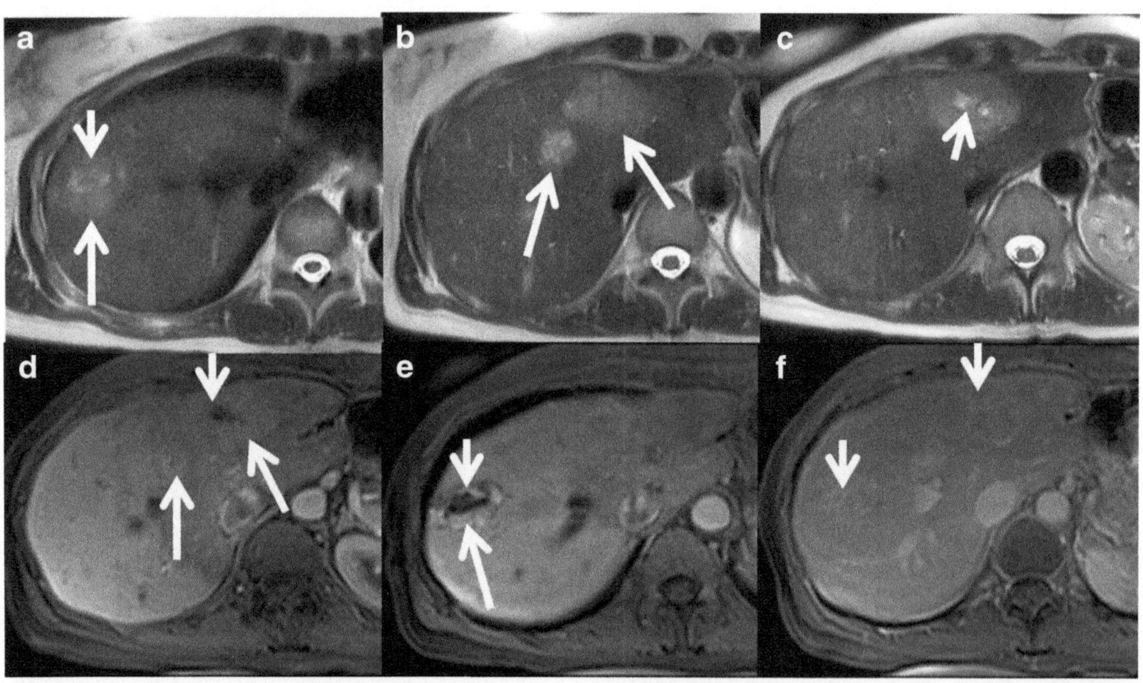

Fig. 10 Hepatic adenomatosis in a 45-year-old male. (**a**), (**b**) and (**c**) Axial T2W MRI at multiple levels shows at least three mildly T2 hyperintense focal lesions (*long arrows*) in the right and left lobes of the liver with vague central T2 hyperintense areas (*short arrows*). (**d**) and (**e**) Axial post-contrast MRI in the arterial phase shows moderate enhancement of the lesions (*long arrows*) with central non-enhancing areas (*short arrows*). (**f**) Axial post-contrast MRI in the delayed phase shows no persistent enhancement with mild delayed enhancement of central areas (*short arrows*). Ultrasound-guided biopsy showed β-catenin-mutated hepatocellular adenoma with no dysplasia. The patient is planned for liver transplantation

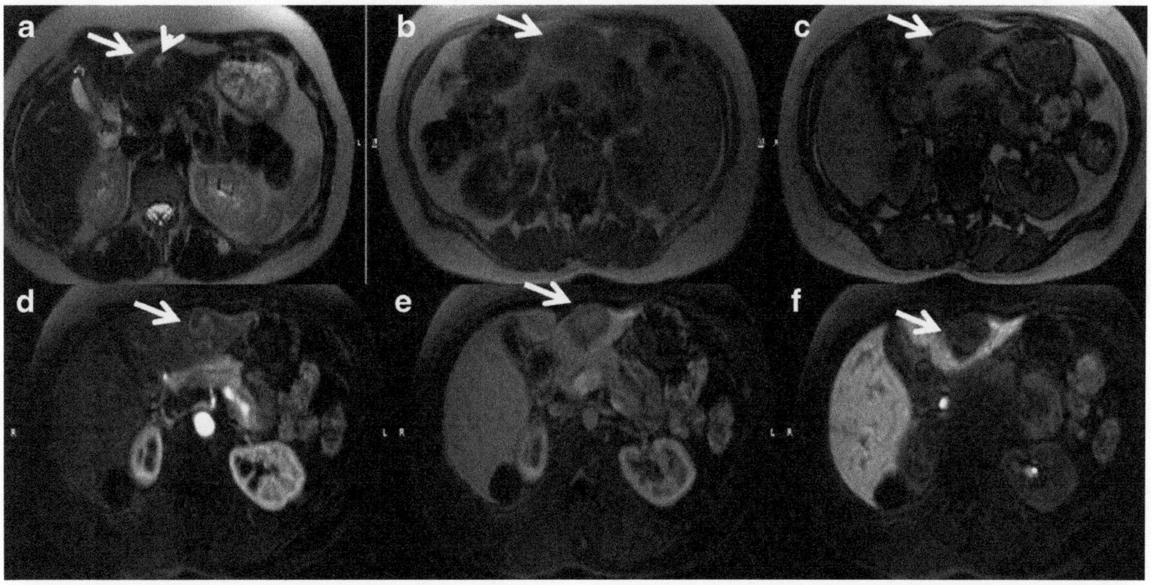

Fig. 11 A 43-year-old female with typical hepatocyte nuclear factor 1alpha (HNF-1alpha)-inactivated hepatocellular adenoma. Axial T2W HASTE image (**a**) demonstrates a well-circumscribed mass in the lateral segment, which is only minimally hyperintense to the adjacent liver parenchyma (*white arrow*). There is a focal region of more increased T2W signal centrally (*arrowhead*). Axial in (**b**) and opposed (**c**) phase T1W dual echo GRE images demonstrate homogeneous loss of signal intensity within the lesion (*white arrows*) but no SI drop in the adjacent liver. Note misregistration between (**b**) and (**c**) as images were acquired in separate breath-holds. Axial fat-suppressed T1W GRE images after the injection of gadoxetic acid during the early arterial (**d**), portal venous (**e**) and 20-min hepatobiliary (**f**) phases demonstrate heterogeneous arterial enhancement with lack of persistent enhancement on portal venous phase and no uptake of gadoxetic acid during the hepatobiliary phase (*arrows*)

HCC. Different subtypes of HCA show variable complication rates.

Haemorrhage can occur in 15–20 % of HCAs [55]. Bleeding can be intratumoral, intrahepatic or extrahepatic (Fig. 12).

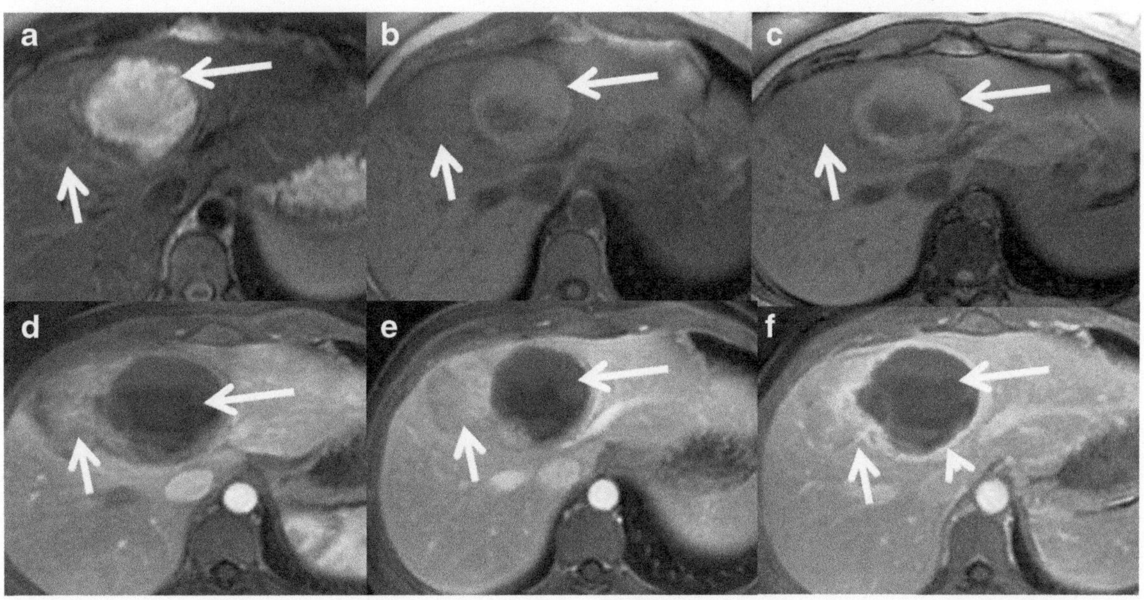

Fig. 12 Hepatocellular adenoma with haemorrhage in a 40-year-old female on oral contraceptive pills. (**a**) Large heterogeneous lesion involving segment 8 and 4 of the liver showing a well-defined T2 hyperintense area along its medial aspect (*long arrow*) and T2 isointense area along its lateral aspect (*short arrow*). Axial T1 in-phase (**b**) and out-of-phase (**c**) MRI shows heterogeneous T1 hyperintensity in the medial portion (*long arrow*) without signal drop representing subacute haemorrhage. Axial post-contrast MRI shows heterogeneous mild-to-moderate enhancement of the lateral part of the lesion (*short arrow*) in the arterial phase (**d**) becoming isointense on venous (**e**) and delayed phases (**f**). The haemorrhagic component in the medial part of the lesion (*long arrow*) shows only peripheral capsular enhancement (*arrowhead*)

Risk factors for bleeding of HCA include a diameter of 35 mm or more, visualisation of central and peripheral intralesional arteries, location in the left lateral liver and exophytic growth [56]. Although peliosis is much more common in the inflammatory subtype compared to the HNF 1-alpha subtypes (52 % vs. 4 %), there is no notable difference in the risk of clinically manifest bleeding between these two subtypes (16 % vs. 9 %) [33]. Bleeding is very rare in the β-catenin subtype although the exact incidence is unknown.

Malignant transformation of hepatic adenoma to hepatocellular carcinoma has been variably reported to occur in 5–10 %, and a recent meta-analysis showed the risk of malignant transformation to be 4% in females and 47 % in males [57, 58]. The important risk factors for malignant transformation of HCAs are male sex, obesity, concomitant glycogen storage disease, anabolic steroid usage, β-catenin–mutated subtype and tumours larger than 5 cm in maximum dimension. β-Catenin-mutated HCAs show the highest risk of malignancy among all the subtypes. Two-thirds of HCAs with malignant transformation show β-catenin mutation and one-third display cell atypias. Also metabolic syndrome is an emerging condition and has been associated with malignant transformation of HCA in males [57]. Hepatocellular carcinomas may develop either as a macroscopic nodule larger than 1 cm in maximum dimension or as multiple microscopic foci. Approximately 10 % of the inflammatory subtype can show additional β-catenin activation and may progress to HCC [36].

Management

Recent classification of HCAs into different subtypes has allowed better understanding of the natural history and biological behaviour of these relatively rare tumours. This has great implications for the imaging and management of these tumours. Many of the previously followed treatment strategies such as surgical resection for all hepatic adenomas and liver transplantation for multiple adenomas are now changing as we have better insight into these tumours because of recent advances in molecular genetics and imaging [35]. Early recommendations on management were made by Bioulac-Sage et al. based on the clinical features, gender, molecular subtype and imaging features [39].

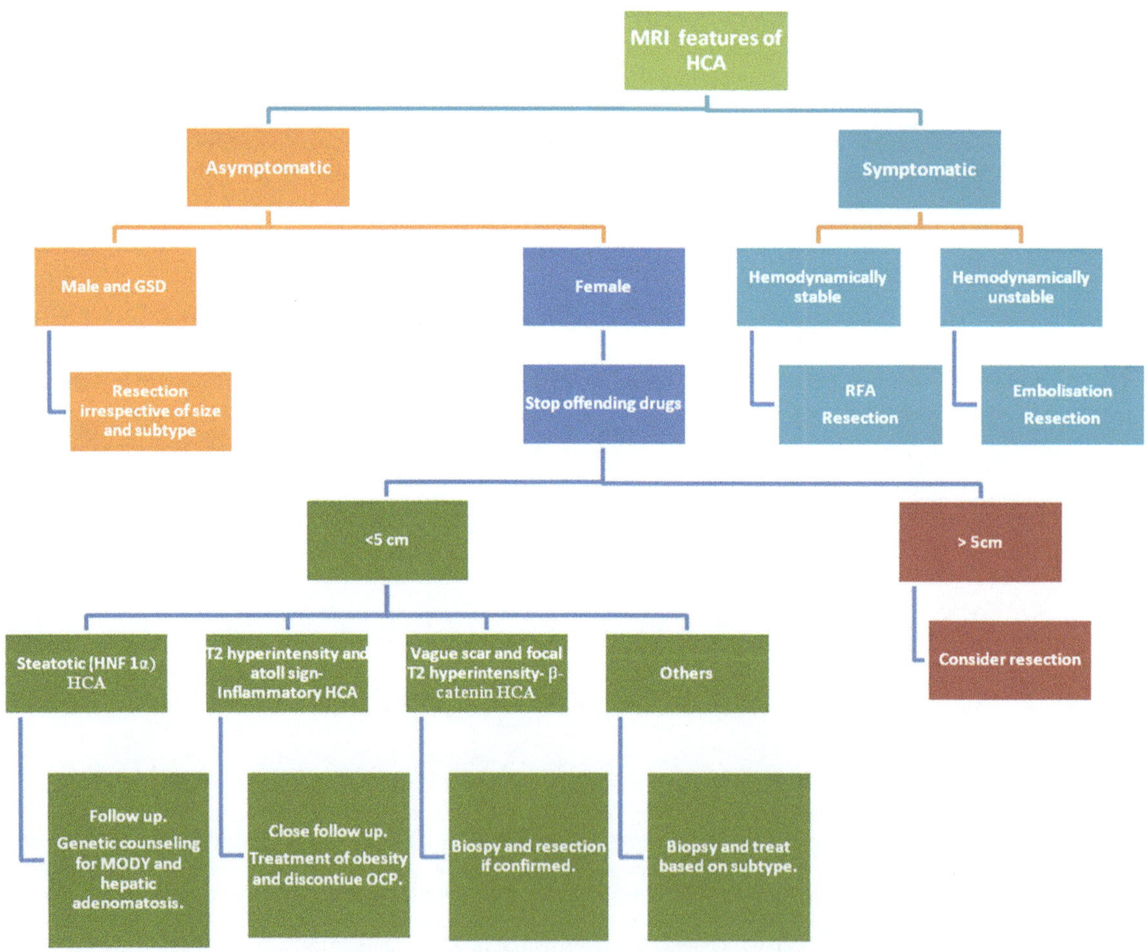

Fig. 13 The algorithmic approach to the management of hepatocellular adenoma (HCA) based on clinical features, gender, imaging and histology

Table 1 Summary of clinical features, demographics, histopathology, immunohistochemistry and molecular genetics of major subtypes of hepatocellular adenoma (HCA) and focal nodular hyperplasia (FNH)

	Subtype	Frequency	Gender	Genetic mutation	Immunohistochemical marker	Histological phenotype	Clinical association	Complications
Focal nodular hyperplasia	Classic	80 %	F>>M	Angiopoietin 1 and 2. β-Catenin activation without mutation	Glutamine synthetase (perivenous)	Abnormal nodular architecture, malformed vessels and cholangiolar proliferation	Hereditary haemorrhagic telangiectasia, congenital absence of portal vein, haemangiomas	Very low risk of haemorrhage. No risk of malignant transformation
	Non-classic	20 %	F>>M	Angiopoietin 1 and 2. β-Catenin activation without mutation	Glutamine synthetase (perivenous)	Cholangiolar proliferation with either abnormal nodular architecture or malformed vessels	Multiple FNH syndrome associated with haemangiomas, cyst and adenoma	Slightly increased risk of bleeding in telangiectatic subtype. False risk of malignancy in inflammatory hepatic adenomas misclassified as 'telangiectatic FNH'
Hepatocellular adenoma	Inflammatory HCA	40–55 %	F>>M	IL6ST (60 %), STAT3 (40 %)	Serum amyloid A (SAA) and C-reactive protein (CRP)	Intense polymorp infiltrates, marked sinusoidal dilatation and thick-walled arteries	Obesity. hepatic steatosis, high alcohol intake and inflammatory syndrome	Increased tendency to bleed. 10 % express β-catenin and are at risk of malignant transformation
	HNF1α-mutated HCA	30–35 %	Exclusively F	TCF1	Lack of LFABP1 expression	Intracellular lipid	Adenomatosis and MODY 3 diabetes	Lower tendency to bleed and very low risk of malignancy. Best prognosis.
	β-Catenin-mutated HCA	10–15 %	F>M	CTNNB1	Glutamine synthase (diffusely positive) and β-catenin	High nuclear-cytoplasmic ratio, nuclear atypia and acini formation	Male hormone and glycogen storage disease	Increased risk of malignant transformation
	Unclassified	10 %	–	–	–	–		

The management strategy is broadly based on the presence or absence of symptoms (Fig. 13). Incidental depiction of hepatic adenoma in an asymptomatic patient needs subtype classification based on MRI as steatotic (corresponding to HNF 1-alpha) and heterogeneous non-steatotic (inflammatory, β-catenin and unclassifiied) hepatic adenomas. Steatotic HCAs have no significant malignant risk; the risk of bleeding is low and hence can be managed by clinical and imaging follow-up without resection or need of biopsy. Heterogeneous non-steatotic HCAs larger than 5 cm, HCAs that continue to grow after stopping use of the offending drugs, HCAs with β-catenin activation, HCAs with malignant changes and all HCAs in males need surgical resection. Resection is effective, with low rates of recurrence [36, 39]. Biopsy is recommended for non-steatotic HCAs less than 5 cm to look for β-catenin mutation, which has a high risk of malignant transformation and needs resection.

In symptomatic HCAs treatment depends on the duration and type of symptoms. Patients who are haemodynamically unstable because of intra- or extrahepatic bleeding require immediate treatment with either hepatic artery embolisation or surgery [59]. Conservative treatment may be considered in haemodynamically stable patients followed by elective definite management, which can be surgery, chemoembolisation or RFA. Transarterial chemoembolisation reduces the risk of bleeding during elective surgery and may avoid surgical resection. Radiofrequency ablation is an effective, less invasive approach for (1) tumours smaller than 4 cm in maximum dimension, (2) patients who are not surgical candidates and (3) those who prefer to avoid surgery after discussion and full understanding of the available treatment options. Radiofrequency ablation has been found to be the most cost-effective approach in the management of small HCAs as compared with surgery, transarterial embolisation and watchful waiting [60].

There are no established guidelines on the optimal interval and duration of follow-up. Yearly imaging surveillance of HCAs is recommended for both solitary HCA and hepatic adenomatosis, and some authors recommend periodic surveillance until menopause [40].

Management of hepatic adenomatosis should depend on the underlying histological subtype and size of the lesions rather than on their number. Symptomatic lesions and asymptomatic lesions larger than 5 cm require surgical resection. Liver transplantation is recommended if there is progressive liver failure or malignant transformation and is no longer advised for patients with asymptomatic familial adenomatosis [61]. Genetic counselling for MODY3 is recommended. Management of HCAs in patients of child-bearing age is complicated because of the possible increased risk of bleeding and growth during pregnancy. Overall treatment strategies are similar to those in non-pregnant females; however close clinical and imaging monitoring is recommended for early detection of complications that may need aggressive management because of increased foeto-maternal morbidity [62].

Conclusion

Recent advances in the molecular genetics and genotype-phenotype correlations in benign hepatocellular tumours have greatly improved our understanding leading to subtype

Table 2 Summary of MRI features of major subtypes of hepatocellular adenoma (HCA) and focal nodular hyperplasia (FNH)

	Subtype	T1W	T2W	In and out of phase	Arterial	Portal venous/delayed	Remarks
Focal nodular hyperplasia	Classic	Iso- to mildly hypointense	Iso- to mildly hyperintense	No signal drop	Intense enhancement	Persistent enhancement	T2 hyperintense scar showing delayed enhancement
	Non-classic	Heterogeneous hypo- or iso- or hyperintense	Heterogeneous iso- or hyperintense	Focal signal drop rarely	Intense heterogeneous enhancement	Heterogeneous persistent enhancement with pseudocapsule	Absent or atypical scar
Hepatocellular adenoma	Inflammatory HCA	Iso- to mildly hyperintense	Diffusely hyperintense	No diffuse signal drop	Intense enhancement	Persistent enhancement	Atoll sign-T2 hyperintense rim. 10 % can have focal intratumoral fat
	HNF1a-mutated HCA	Iso- to hyperintense	Iso- to mildly hyperintense	Diffuse signal drop	Moderate enhancement	No persistent enhancement	
	ß-catenin-mutated HCA	Isointense	Iso-, hypo- or hyperintense	No diffuse signal drop	Intense	Variable. May show portal venous washout	Faint scar and ill-defined T2 hyperintense foci
	Unclassified	–	–	–	–	–	

recognition and better differentiation from other hypervascular lesions. Each of these tumour subtypes has distinct genetic mutations, molecular abnormalities, histopathological features, imaging findings, biological behaviour and prognosis. FNH typically does not bleed or undergo malignant change. HCAs with β-catenin mutations frequently undergo malignant change, inflammatory HCAs commonly bleed, and HNF-1α HCAs typically show a favourable prognosis. Many of these have reasonably specific imaging features permitting accurate diagnosis, which has significant implications for their management (Tables 1 and 2).

References

1. Rebouissou S, Bioulac-Sage P, Zucman-Rossi J (2008) Molecular pathogenesis of focal nodular hyperplasia and hepatocellular adenoma. J Hepatol 48(1):163–170
2. Shanbhogue A, Shah SN, Zaheer A, Prasad SR, Takahashi N, Vikram R (2011) Hepatocellular adenomas: current update on genetics, taxonomy, and management. J Comput Assist Tomogr 35(2):159–166
3. Vilgrain V (2006) Focal nodular hyperplasia. Eur J Radiol 58(2): 236–245
4. Mathieu D, Vilgrain V, Mahfouz AE, Anglade MC, Vullierme MP, Denys A (1997) Benign liver tumors. Magn Reson Imaging Clin N Am 5(2):255–288
5. Cherqui D, Rahmouni A, Charlotte F et al (1995) Management of focal nodular hyperplasia and hepatocellular adenoma in young women: a series of 41 patients with clinical, radiological, and pathological correlations. Hepatology 22(6):1674–1681
6. Mathieu D, Kobeiter H, Maison P et al (2000) Oral contraceptive use and focal nodular hyperplasia of the liver. Gastroenterology 118(3): 560–564
7. Maisonpierre PC, Suri C, Jones PF et al (1997) Angiopoietin-2, a natural antagonist for Tie2 that disrupts in vivo angiogenesis. Science 277(5322):55–60
8. Shimamatsu K, Wanless IR (1997) Role of ischemia in causing apoptosis, atrophy, and nodular hyperplasia in human liver. Hepatology 26(2):343–350
9. Wanless IR (2002) Benign liver tumors. Clin Liver Dis 6(2):513–526
10. Rebouissou S, Couchy G, Libbrecht L et al (2008) The beta-catenin pathway is activated in focal nodular hyperplasia but not in cirrhotic FNH-like nodules. J Hepatol 49(1):61–71
11. Bioulac-Sage P, Cubel G, Taouji S et al (2012) Immunohistochemical markers on needle biopsies are helpful for the diagnosis of focal nodular hyperplasia and hepatocellular adenoma subtypes. Am J Surg Pathol 36(11):1691–1699
12. Nguyen BN, Flejou JF, Terris B, Belghiti J, Degott C (1999) Focal nodular hyperplasia of the liver: a comprehensive pathologic study of 305 lesions and recognition of new histologic forms. Am J Surg Pathol 23(12):1441–1454
13. Hussain SM, van den Bos IC, Dwarkasing RS, Kuiper JW, den Hollander J (2006) Hepatocellular adenoma: findings at state-of-the-art magnetic resonance imaging, ultrasound, computed tomography and pathologic analysis. Eur Radiol 16(9):1873–1886
14. Shirkhoda A, Farah MC, Bernacki E, Madrazo B, Roberts J (1994) Hepatic focal nodular hyperplasia: CT and sonographic spectrum. Abdom Imaging 19(1):34–38
15. Mortele KJ, Praet M, Van Vlierberghe H, Kunnen M, Ros PR (2000) CT and MR imaging findings in focal nodular hyperplasia of the liver: radiologic-pathologic correlation. AJR Am J Roentgenol 175(3):687–692
16. Marin D, Brancatelli G, Federle MP et al (2008) Focal nodular hyperplasia: typical and atypical MRI findings with emphasis on the use of contrast media. Clin Radiol 63(5):577–585
17. Zech CJ, Grazioli L, Breuer J, Reiser MF, Schoenberg SO (2008) Diagnostic performance and description of morphological features of focal nodular hyperplasia in Gd-EOB-DTPA-enhanced liver magnetic resonance imaging: results of a multicenter trial. Invest Radiol 43(7):504–511
18. Bieze M, van den Esschert JW, Nio CY et al (2012) Diagnostic accuracy of MRI in differentiating hepatocellular adenoma from focal nodular hyperplasia: prospective study of the additional value of gadoxetate disodium. AJR Am J Roentgenol 199(1):26–34
19. Campos JT, Sirlin CB, Choi JY (2012) Focal hepatic lesions in Gd-EOB-DTPA enhanced MRI: the atlas. Insights Imaging 3(5):451–474
20. Seale MK, Catalano OA, Saini S, Hahn PF, Sahani DV (2009) Hepatobiliary-specific MR contrast agents: role in imaging the liver and biliary tree. Radiographics 29(6):1725–1748
21. van Kessel CS, de Boer E, ten Kate FJ, Brosens LA, Veldhuis WB, van Leeuwen MS (2013) Focal nodular hyperplasia: hepatobiliary enhancement patterns on gadoxetic-acid contrast-enhanced MRI. Abdom Imaging 38(3):490–501
22. Balabaud C, Al-Rabih WR, Chen PJ et al (2013) Focal nodular hyperplasia and hepatocellular adenoma around the world viewed through the scope of the immunopathological classification. Int J Hepatol 268625(10):14
23. Mattison GR, Glazer GM, Quint LE, Francis IR, Bree RL, Ensminger WD (1987) MR imaging of hepatic focal nodular hyperplasia: characterization and distinction from primary malignant hepatic tumors. AJR Am J Roentgenol 148(4):711–715
24. Lee MJ, Saini S, Hamm B et al (1991) Focal nodular hyperplasia of the liver: MR findings in 35 proved cases. AJR Am J Roentgenol 156(2):317–320
25. Ba-Ssalamah A, Schima W, Schmook MT et al (2002) Atypical focal nodular hyperplasia of the liver: imaging features of nonspecific and liver-specific MR contrast agents. AJR Am J Roentgenol 179(6): 1447–1456
26. Ferlicot S, Kobeiter H, Tran Van Nhieu J et al (2004) MRI of atypical focal nodular hyperplasia of the liver: radiology-pathology correlation. AJR Am J Roentgenol 182(5):1227–1231
27. Shamsi K, De Schepper A, Degryse H, Deckers F (1993) Focal nodular hyperplasia of the liver: radiologic findings. Abdom Imaging 18(1):32–38
28. Stanley G, Jeffrey RB Jr, Feliz B (2002) CT findings and mistopathology of intratumoral steatosis in focal nodular hyperplasia: case report and review of the literature. J Comput Assist Tomogr 26(5):815–817
29. Mortele KJ, Stubbe J, Praet M, Van Langenhove P, De Bock G, Kunnen M (2000) Intratumoral steatosis in focal nodular hyperplasia coinciding with diffuse hepatic steatosis: CT and MRI findings with histologic correlation. Abdom Imaging 25(2):179–181
30. Bioulac-Sage P, Rebouissou S, Sa Cunha A et al (2005) Clinical, morphologic, and molecular features defining so-called telangiectatic focal nodular hyperplasias of the liver. Gastroenterology 128(5): 1211–1218
31. Finley AC, Hosey JR, Noone TC, Shackelford DM, Varadarajulu S (2005) Multiple focal nodular hyperplasia syndrome: diagnosis with dynamic, gadolinium-enhanced MRI. Magn Reson Imaging 23(3): 511–513

32. Vilgrain V, Uzan F, Brancatelli G, Federle MP, Zappa M, Menu Y (2003) Prevalence of hepatic hemangioma in patients with focal nodular hyperplasia: MR imaging analysis. Radiology 229(1):75–79
33. Shanbhogue AK, Prasad SR, Takahashi N, Vikram R, Sahani DV (2011) Recent advances in cytogenetics and molecular biology of adult hepatocellular tumors: implications for imaging and management. Radiology 258(3):673–693
34. Gonzalez A, Canga F, Cardenas F et al (1994) An unusual case of hepatic adenoma in a male. J Clin Gastroenterol 19(2):179–181
35. Dokmak S, Paradis V, Vilgrain V et al (2009) A single-center surgical experience of 122 patients with single and multiple hepatocellular adenomas. Gastroenterology 137(5):1698–1705
36. Zucman-Rossi J (2004) Genetic alterations in hepatocellular adenomas: recent findings and new challenges. J Hepatol 40(6):1036–1039
37. Lewin M, Handra-Luca A, Arrive L et al (2006) Liver adenomatosis: classification of MR imaging features and comparison with pathologic findings. Radiology 241(2):433–440
38. Bioulac-Sage P, Rebouissou S, Thomas C et al (2007) Hepatocellular adenoma subtype classification using molecular markers and immunohistochemistry. Hepatology 46(3):740–748
39. Bioulac-Sage P, Laumonier H, Couchy G et al (2009) Hepatocellular adenoma management and phenotypic classification: the Bordeaux experience. Hepatology 50(2):481–489
40. Katabathina VS, Menias CO, Shanbhogue AK, Jagirdar J, Paspulati RM, Prasad SR (2011) Genetics and imaging of hepatocellular adenomas: 2011 update. Radiographics 31(6):1529–1543
41. Laumonier H, Bioulac-Sage P, Laurent C, Zucman-Rossi J, Balabaud C, Trillaud H (2008) Hepatocellular adenomas: magnetic resonance imaging features as a function of molecular pathological classification. Hepatology 48(3):808–818
42. van Aalten SM, Thomeer MG, Terkivatan T et al (2011) Hepatocellular adenomas: correlation of MR imaging findings with pathologic subtype classification. Radiology 261(1):172–181
43. Bioulac-Sage P, Blanc JF, Rebouissou S, Balabaud C, Zucman-Rossi J (2007) Genotype phenotype classification of hepatocellular adenoma. World J Gastroenterol 13(19):2649–2654
44. Zucman-Rossi J, Jeannot E, Nhieu JT et al (2006) Genotype-phenotype correlation in hepatocellular adenoma: new classification and relationship with HCC. Hepatology 43(3):515–524
45. Prasad SR, Wang H, Rosas H et al (2005) Fat-containing lesions of the liver: radiologic-pathologic correlation. Radiographics 25(2): 321–331
46. Chen ZM, Crone KG, Watson MA, Pfeifer JD, Wang HL (2005) Identification of a unique gene expression signature that differentiates hepatocellular adenoma from well-differentiated hepatocellular carcinoma. Am J Surg Pathol 29(12):1600–1608
47. Lee PJ (2002) Glycogen storage disease type I: pathophysiology of liver adenomas. Eur J Pediatr 161(1):12
48. Flejou JF, Barge J, Menu Y et al (1985) Liver adenomatosis. An entity distinct from liver adenoma? Gastroenterology 89(5):1132–1138
49. Grazioli L, Federle MP, Ichikawa T, Balzano E, Nalesnik M, Madariaga J (2000) Liver adenomatosis: clinical, histopathologic, and imaging findings in 15 patients. Radiology 216(2):395–402
50. Vetelainen R, Erdogan D, de Graaf W et al (2008) Liver adenomatosis: re-evaluation of aetiology and management. Liver Int 28(4):499–508
51. Bacq Y, Jacquemin E, Balabaud C et al (2003) Familial liver adenomatosis associated with hepatocyte nuclear factor 1alpha inactivation. Gastroenterology 125(5):1470–1475
52. Purysko AS, Remer EM, Coppa CP, Obuchowski NA, Schneider E, Veniero JC (2012) Characteristics and distinguishing features of hepatocellular adenoma and focal nodular hyperplasia on gadoxetate disodium-enhanced MRI. AJR Am J Roentgenol 198(1):115–123
53. Agarwal S, Fuentes-Orrego JM, Arnason T et al (2014) Inflammatory hepatocellular adenomas can mimic focal nodular hyperplasia on gadoxetic acid-enhanced MRI. AJR Am J Roentgenol 203(4):23
54. Thomeer MG, Willemssen FE, Biermann KK et al (2014) MRI features of inflammatory hepatocellular adenomas on hepatocyte phase imaging with liver-specific contrast agents. J Magn Reson Imaging 39(5):1259–1264
55. van Aalten SM, de Man RA, JN IJ, Terkivatan T (2012) Systematic review of haemorrhage and rupture of hepatocellular adenomas. Br J Surg 99(7):911–916
56. Bieze M, Phoa SS, Verheij J, van Lienden KP, van Gulik TM (2014) Risk factors for bleeding in hepatocellular adenoma. Br J Surg 101(7):847–855
57. Farges O, Ferreira N, Dokmak S, Belghiti J, Bedossa P, Paradis V (2011) Changing trends in malignant transformation of hepatocellular adenoma. Gut 60(1):85–89
58. Stoot JH, Coelen RJ, De Jong MC, Dejong CH (2010) Malignant transformation of hepatocellular adenomas into hepatocellular carcinomas: a systematic review including more than 1600 adenoma cases. HPB 12(8):509–522
59. Terkivatan T, de Wilt JH, de Man RA, van Rijn RR, Tilanus HW JNIJ (2001) Treatment of ruptured hepatocellular adenoma. Br J Surg 88(2):207–209
60. van der Sluis FJ, Bosch JL, Terkivatan T, de Man RA, Ijzermans JN, Hunink MG (2009) Hepatocellular adenoma: cost-effectiveness of different treatment strategies. Radiology 252(3):737–746
61. Chiche L, Dao T, Salame E et al (2000) Liver adenomatosis: reappraisal, diagnosis, and surgical management: eight new cases and review of the literature. Ann Surg 231(1):74–81
62. Cobey FC, Salem RR (2004) A review of liver masses in pregnancy and a proposed algorithm for their diagnosis and management. Am J Surg 187(2):181–191

Permissions

All chapters in this book were first published in II, by Springer; hereby published with permission under the Creative Commons Attribution License or equivalent. Every chapter published in this book has been scrutinized by our experts. Their significance has been extensively debated. The topics covered herein carry significant findings which will fuel the growth of the discipline. They may even be implemented as practical applications or may be referred to as a beginning point for another development.

The contributors of this book come from diverse backgrounds, making this book a truly international effort. This book will bring forth new frontiers with its revolutionizing research information and detailed analysis of the nascent developments around the world.

We would like to thank all the contributing authors for lending their expertise to make the book truly unique. They have played a crucial role in the development of this book. Without their invaluable contributions this book wouldn't have been possible. They have made vital efforts to compile up to date information on the varied aspects of this subject to make this book a valuable addition to the collection of many professionals and students.

This book was conceptualized with the vision of imparting up-to-date information and advanced data in this field. To ensure the same, a matchless editorial board was set up. Every individual on the board went through rigorous rounds of assessment to prove their worth. After which they invested a large part of their time researching and compiling the most relevant data for our readers.

The editorial board has been involved in producing this book since its inception. They have spent rigorous hours researching and exploring the diverse topics which have resulted in the successful publishing of this book. They have passed on their knowledge of decades through this book. To expedite this challenging task, the publisher supported the team at every step. A small team of assistant editors was also appointed to further simplify the editing procedure and attain best results for the readers.

Apart from the editorial board, the designing team has also invested a significant amount of their time in understanding the subject and creating the most relevant covers. They scrutinized every image to scout for the most suitable representation of the subject and create an appropriate cover for the book.

The publishing team has been an ardent support to the editorial, designing and production team. Their endless efforts to recruit the best for this project, has resulted in the accomplishment of this book. They are a veteran in the field of academics and their pool of knowledge is as vast as their experience in printing. Their expertise and guidance has proved useful at every step. Their uncompromising quality standards have made this book an exceptional effort. Their encouragement from time to time has been an inspiration for everyone.

The publisher and the editorial board hope that this book will prove to be a valuable piece of knowledge for researchers, students, practitioners and scholars across the globe.

List of Contributors

Rosario J. Perea, Teresa M. de Caralt and Marcelo Sanchez
Radiology Department. Hospital Clinic, University of Barcelona, Barcelona, Spain

Jose T. Ortiz-Perez, Susanna Prat-Gonzalez, Xavier Bosch and Antonio Berruezo
Cardiology Department. Hospital Clinic, University of Barcelona, Barcelona, Spain

Manel Sole
Pathology Department. Hospital Clinic, University of Barcelona, Barcelona, Spain

M. Teresa Cibeira and Joan Blade
Haematology Department. Hospital Clinic, University of Barcelona, Barcelona, Spain

Francis Zarb
Department of Radiography, Faculty of Health Sciences, University of Malta, Msida, Malta

Mark F. McEntee
Discipline of Medical Radiation Sciences and Brain and Mind Research Institute, Faculty of Health Sciences, The University of Sydney, Sydney, Australia

Louise Rainford
School of Medicine & Medical Science, Health Science Centre, University College Dublin, Belfield, Dublin 4, Ireland

Massimo Tonolini, Alessandra Pagani and Roberto Bianco
Department of Radiology, "Luigi Sacco" University Hospital, Via G.B. Grassi 74, 20157 Milan, Italy

Giovanni Mauri
Servizio di Radiologia, IRCCS Policlinico San Donato, San Donato Milanese, Milano, Italy
Dipartimento Aziendale di Oncologia, Struttura Complessa di Radiologia Oncologica Interventistica, Azienda Ospedaliera Ospedale di Circolo di Busto Arsizio, Varese, Italy
Servizio di Radiologia, IRCCS Policlinico San Donato, Piazza Malan 2, 20097 San Donato Milanese, Milano, Italy

Luca Maria Sconfienza
Servizio di Radiologia, IRCCS Policlinico San Donato, San Donato Milanese, Milano, Italy
Dipartimento di Scienze Biomediche per la Salute, Università degli Studi di Milano, San Donato Milanese, Milano, Italy

Chiara Mattiuz
Facoltà di Medicina e Chirurgia, Scuola di Specializzazione in Radiodiagnostica, Università degli Studi di Milano, Milano, Italy

Vittorio Pedicini, Dario Poretti and Fabio Romano Lutman
Dipartimento di Diagnostica per Immagini, IRCCS Istituto Clinico Humanitas, Rozzano, Italy

Fabio Melchiorre
Dipartimento di Diagnostica per Immagini, Azienda Ospedaliera San Paolo, Milano, Italy

Umberto Rossi
Dipartimento di Scienze Diagnostiche, Azienda Ospedaliera San Carlo Borromeo, Milano, Italy

Marco Montorsi
Dipartimento di Chirurgia, Azienda Ospedaliera Humanitas (Humanitas Research Hospital), Rozzano, Italy

Pieter Van Dyck, Floris Vanhevel, Jan L. Gielen and Paul M. Parizel
Department of Radiology, Antwerp University Hospital and University of Antwerp, Wilrijkstraat 10, 2650 Antwerp (Edegem), Belgium

Filip M. Vanhoenacker
Department of Radiology, Antwerp University Hospital and University of Antwerp, Wilrijkstraat 10, 2650 Antwerp (Edegem), Belgium
Department of Radiology, Ghent University Hospital and University of Ghent, De Pintelaan 185, 9000 Ghent, Belgium
Department of Radiology, AZ St-Maarten, Rooienberg 25, 2570 Antwerp (Duffel), Belgium

Kristien Wouters
Department of Biostatistics, Antwerp University Hospital and University of Antwerp, Wilrijkstraat 10, 2650 Antwerp (Edegem), Belgium

David M. Grodzki
Siemens Healthcare, Allee am Röthelheimpark 2, 91052 Erlangen, Germany

Rachel Shields, Rajiv Mangla, Jeevak Almast and Steven Meyers
Department of Imaging Sciences, University of Rochester Medical Center, 601 Elmwood Ave., Rochester, NY 14642-0001, USA

Carlos Nicolau
Radiology Department, Hospital Clinic, Villarroel 170, 08036 Barcelona, Spain

Michel Claudon
Children Hospital, University Hospital-Nancy Brabois, Rue du Morvan, 54511 Vandoeuvre Les Nancy Cedex, France

Lorenzo E. Derchi
Emergency Radiology, DISSAL-Radiology, University of Genoa, Genoa, Italy

E. Jane Adam
St George's Hospital, Blackshaw Road, SW17 0QT London, UK

Michael Bachmann Nielsen
Rigshospitalet-Diagnostisk Center, Blegdamsvej 9, 2100 Copenhagen, Denmark

Gerhard Mostbeck
Department of Radiology, Wilhelminenspital, Montleartstr. 37, 1160 Vienna, Austria

Catherine M. Owens
Department of Radiology, Great Ormond Street, WC1N 3JH London, UK

Christiane Nyhsen
City Hospitals Sunderland FT, Kayll Road, Sunderland SR4 7TP,UK

Spyros Yarmenitis
Department of Radiology, Hygeia Hospital, 4, Erythrou Stavrou St, 15123 Maroussi, Greece
European Society of Radiology (ESR)
Neutorgasse 9/2, 1010 Vienna, Austria

Lil-Sofie Ording Muller
Department for Radiology and Intervention, Oslo University Hospital, Oslo, Norway

Paul Humphries
Institute of Child Health, UCL, University College London Hospital NHS Trust and Great Ormond Street Hospital for Children, London, UK

Karen Rosendahl
Department of Radiology, Haukeland University Hospital, Bergen, Norway

V. J. L. Kuijs
Department of Radiology and Nuclear Medicine, Maastricht University Medical Center+, PO Box 5800, 6202 AZ Maastricht, The Netherlands
Department of Surgery, Maastricht University Medical Center+, PO Box 5800, 6202 AZ Maastricht, The Netherlands

M. Moossdorff
Department of Surgery, Maastricht University Medical Center+, PO Box 5800, 6202 AZ Maastricht, The Netherlands
GROW- School for Oncology and Developmental Biology, PO Box 616, 6200 MD Maastricht, The Netherlands

R. J. Schipper
Department of Radiology and Nuclear Medicine, Maastricht University Medical Center+, PO Box 5800, 6202 AZ Maastricht, The Netherlands
Department of Surgery, Maastricht University Medical Center+, PO Box 5800, 6202 AZ Maastricht, The Netherlands
GROW- School for Oncology and Developmental Biology, PO Box 616, 6200 MD Maastricht, The Netherlands

R. G. H. Beets-Tan
Department of Radiology and Nuclear Medicine, Maastricht University Medical Center+, PO Box 5800, 6202 AZ Maastricht, The Netherlands
GROW- School for Oncology and Developmental Biology, PO Box 616, 6200 MD Maastricht, The Netherlands

E. M. Heuts
Department of Surgery, Maastricht University Medical Center+, PO Box 5800, 6202 AZ Maastricht, The Netherlands

K. B. M. I. Keymeulen
Department of Surgery, Maastricht University Medical Center+, PO Box 5800, 6202 AZ Maastricht, The Netherlands

M. L. Smidt
Department of Surgery, Maastricht University Medical Center+, PO Box 5800, 6202 AZ Maastricht, The Netherlands
GROW- School for Oncology and Developmental Biology, PO Box 616, 6200 MD Maastricht, The Netherlands

M. B. I. Lobbes
Department of Radiology and Nuclear Medicine, Maastricht University Medical Center+, PO Box 5800, 6202 AZ Maastricht, The Netherlands
GROW- School for Oncology and Developmental Biology, PO Box 616, 6200 MD Maastricht, The Netherlands

M. Bonatti, N. Vezzali, F. Ferro, P. Pernter and G. Bonatti
Department of Radiology, Bolzano Central Hospital, 5 Boehler St., 39100 Bolzano, Italy

F. Lombardo and G. Zamboni
Department of Radiology, University of Verona, Piazzale L.A. Scuro 10, 37134 Verona, Italy

A. Pycha
Department of Urology, Bolzano Central Hospital, 5 Boehler St., 39100 Bolzano, Italy

Jeffrey S. Quon, Bardia Moosavi, Christopher S. Lim and Nicola Schieda
Department of Medical Imaging, The Ottawa Hospital, The University of Ottawa, 1053 Carling Avenue, Ottawa, ON, Canada K1Y 4E9

Maneesh Khanna
Department of Radiology, Hamad General Hospital, Doha, Qatar

Trevor A. Flood
Department of Pathology, The Ottawa Hospital, The University of Ottawa, 501 Smyth Road, Ottawa, ON, Canada K1H 8 L6

Massimo Tonolini, Marina Petullà and Roberto Bianco
Department of Radiology, "Luigi Sacco" University Hospital, Via G.B. Grassi 74, 20157 Milan, Italy

Anna Maria Ierardi
Interventional Radiology, Department of Radiology, University of Insubria, Viale Borri 57, 21100 Varese, Italy

Virginia Varca and Giacomo Piero Incarbone
Department of Urology, "Luigi Sacco" University Hospital, Via G.B. Grassi 74, 20157 Milan, Italy

European Society of Radiology (ESR)
Neutorgasse 9/2, 1010 Vienna, Austria

V. Dialani and P. J. Slanetz
Department of Radiology, Beth Israel Deaconess Medical Center, 330 Brookline Avenue, Boston, MA 02215, USA

D. F. James
Jefferson Radiology, 85 Seymour Street, Suite 200, Hartford, CT 06106, USA

L. Varennes
Department of Neuroradiology and MRI, University Hospital of Grenoble, CS 10217-38043, Grenoble Cedex 09, France
Department of Radiology, University Hospital of Grenoble, CS 10217-38043, Grenoble Cedex 09, France

F. Tahon
Department of Neuroradiology and MRI, University Hospital of Grenoble, CS 10217-38043, Grenoble Cedex 09, France

A. Kastler, S. Grand and A. Krainik
Department of Neuroradiology and MRI, University Hospital of Grenoble, CS 10217-38043, Grenoble Cedex 09, France

F. Thony
Department of Radiology, University Hospital of Grenoble, CS 10217-38043, Grenoble Cedex 09, France

J. P. Baguet
Department of Cardiology, Mutualist Hospital Group of Grenoble, 38028 Grenoble cedex 1, France

O. Detante
Department of Neurology, University Hospital of Grenoble, CS 10217-38043, Grenoble Cedex 09, France

E. Touzé
Department of Neurology, University Caen Basse Normandie, Inserm U919, CHU Côte de Nacre, Caen, France

Michael R. Torkzad
Department of Radiology, Oncology, Radiation Sciences, Uppsala University, Uppsala, Sweden

Gabriele Masselli
Umberto I Hospital, Radiology Department, Sapienza University, Rome, Italy

Steve Halligan
Center for Medical Imaging, University College London, London, UK

Aytek Oto
Department of Radiology, University of Chicago, Chicago, IL, USA

Henning Neubauer
Department of Paediatric Radiology, University Hospital Wuerzburg, Wuerzburg, Germany

Stuart Taylor
Center for Medical Imaging, University College London, London, UK

Arun Gupta
Intestinal Imaging, St Mark's Hospital, Harrow, UK

Jens Brøndum Frøkjær
Department of Radiology, Aalborg University Hospital, Aalborg, Denmark

Ian C. Lawrance
School of Medicine and Pharmacology, University of Western Australia and Centre for Inflammatory Bowel Disease, Fremantle Hospital, Fremantle, Australia

Christopher J. Welman
Department of Radiology, Fremantle Hospital, Fremantle, Australia

Anne Negård
Abdominal and Children's Radiology, Department of Radiology, Akershus University Hospital, Lørenskog, Norway

Olle Ekberg
Department of Clinical Sciences/Medical Radiology, Lund University; Diagnostic Centre of Imaging and Functional Medicine Lund University Skåne University Hospital, Malmö, Sweden

Michael Patak
Klinik Hirslanden, Witellikerstrasse 40, Zürich, Austria

Thomas Lauenstein
Department of Diagnostic and Interventional Radiology and Neuroradiology, University Hospital Essen, Essen, Germany

European Society of Radiology (ESR)
Neutorgasse 9/2, 1010 Vienna, Austria

Ferruccio Degrassi, Emilio Quaia, Paola Martingano, Marco Cavallaro and Maria Assunta Cova
Department of Radiology, Cattinara Hospital, University of Trieste, Strada di Fiume 447, 34149 Trieste, Italy

Frederik Vandenbroucke, Steven Van Hedent, Gert Van Gompel, Nico Buls, Gordon Craggs and Johan de Mey
Department of Radiology, UZ Brussel (VUB), Laarbeeklaan 101, Brussels, Belgium

Jef Vandemeulebroucke
Department of Electronics and Informatics, Vrije Universiteit Brussel, Brussels, Belgium
Department of Medical IT, iMinds, Ghent, Belgium

Pablo R. Ros
Department of Radiology, University Hospitals Case Medical Center/Case Western Reserve University, Cleveland, OH, USA

Abhishek R. Keraliya, Sree Harsha Tirumani, Atul B. Shinagare and Nikhil H. Ramaiya
Department of Radiology, Harvard Medical School, Brigham and Women's Hospital, 75 Francis Street, Boston, MA 02115, USA
Department of Imaging, Harvard Medical School, Dana Farber Cancer Institute, 450 Brookline Avenue, Boston, MA 02215, USA

Maneesh Khanna
Department of Diagnostic Imaging, The Ottawa Hospital, University of Ottawa, Ontario, Canada
Department of Radiology, Hamad General Hospital, Hamad Medical Corporation, Doha, Qatar

Subramaniyan Ramanathan
Department of Diagnostic Imaging, The Ottawa Hospital, University of Ottawa, Ontario, Canada
Department of Radiology, Al-Wakra Hospital, Hamad Medical Corporation, Doha, Qatar
Al-Wakra Hospital, Hamad Medical Corporation, PO Box 82228, Doha, Qatar

Najla Fasih
Department of Diagnostic Imaging, The Ottawa Hospital, University of Ottawa, Ontario, Canada

Nicola Schieda
Department of Diagnostic Imaging, The Ottawa Hospital, University of Ottawa, Ontario, Canada

Vivek Virmani
Department of Diagnostic Imaging, The Ottawa Hospital, University of Ottawa, Ontario, Canada

Matthew D. F. McInnes
Department of Diagnostic Imaging, The Ottawa Hospital, University of Ottawa, Ontario, Canada